Philip J. Flores, PhD

Group Psychotherapy with Addicted Populations: An Integration of Twelve-Step and Psychodynamic Theory

Second Edition

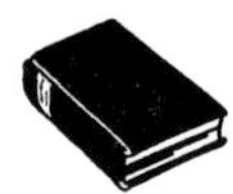

Noteworthy REVIEWS OF THE FIRST EDITION . . .

"The main strength of this book is the way it joins professional and self-help approaches. The author treats the reader to an excellent review of contemporary psychodynamic theory, providing the conceptual underpinning and understanding of substance abusers' needs and how they are addressed in the context of group psychotherapy. He also delves into the spiritual and philosophic traditions behind AA's pragmatic appreciation of the existential plight of alcoholics and addicts, and how AA succeeds by providing individuals with a new and corrective life plan.

This book is important because the author clearly articulates how group therapy for addicted populations is, or should be, different from group treatment for nonaddicts. From the outset, the author builds a strong, and I believe necessary, case that experienced group therapists need to know about addicts, and knowledgeable addictionologists need training in, and understanding of, group psychotherapy. For the novice in either area, there is much to be learned here. For the clinician experienced in the group treatment of addicts, there is a reassuring sense of validation."

The Journal of Studies on Alcohol

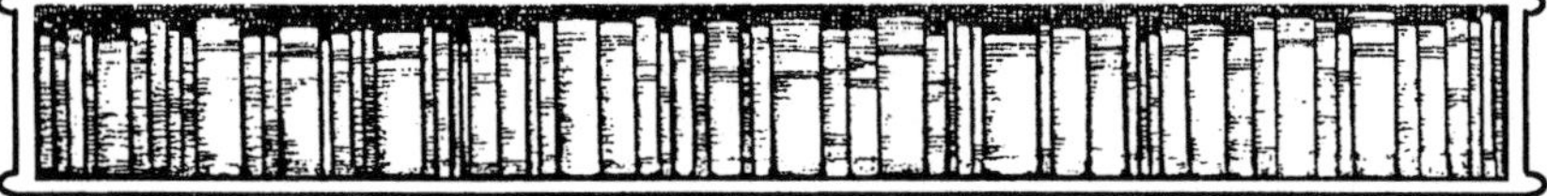

More Noteworthy
REVIEWS OF THE FIRST EDITION . . .

"In the treatment of the addictions, abstinence is a difficult goal to reach and relapse is dispiritingly common. This may lead to the view that treating this group of patients is not worthwhile or, at best, likely to be ineffective. Such gloomy attitudes are not held by Philip Flores, who throughout this book makes a plea for therapeutic optimism tempered with the reminder that however severe the dependence or deprived the circumstances, people retain the capacity to change.

While it is essentially a humanistic message to argue that individuals have worth and that addicted individuals need not remain in that state, the question then arises: how is change to be achieved? The author has long experience as a group therapist, and the best parts of this book form a practical guide to this approach. The difficulties of patient selection and retention, of effecting change, and of leading groups are clearly described, with many suggestions as to their resolution. Underlying theories are derived from the American group-analytic tradition, and especially from the work of Yalom.

This book will be of interest to those applying group therapies to drug and alcohol users."

The British Journal of Psychiatry

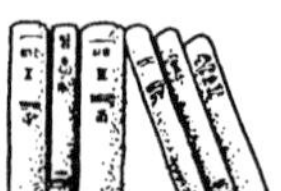

"Although this book stresses group treatment of addictive patients, it should be of interest to all who deal with this population in clinical practice. After describing various group designs, Flores argues for Yalom's interactional model, with variations designed to accommodate the particular defensive styles of addicts. Stressing the need to move slowly as the addict moves along the time line of recovery, the author cites material from such authorities as Mahler, Kohut, Kernberg, and Sullivan. A particularly interesting chapter traces the intellectual origins of AA and presents a well-reasoned analysis of the distinctions and potential complementarity among AA and psychotherapy groups. There is no trace of the dogmatism that often clouds discussions of this important and difficult subject. The literature reviews and bibliographies are excellent, notable for their breadth and scope. Overall, the book is a significant contribution to the existing literature."

Readings: A Journal of Reviews and Commentary in Mental Health

More Noteworthy
REVIEWS OF THE FIRST EDITION . . .

"The subjects of group therapy and addicted populations are integrated in this comprehensive and practical text. The book can be used equally well as college text or treatment handbook, and will surely become a classic in the field.

The 14 chapters deal with such key areas as alcoholism, addiction, and psychodynamic theories of addiction; use of confrontational techniques in the group; inpatient group psychotherapy; characteristics of the leader; transference in the group; resistance in groups; preparing the chemically dependent person for group; and the curative process in group therapy. Ample references at the end of each chapter may steer the reader to further review and study.

Flores discusses theoretical models of groups, contrasts self-help with professional groups, and compares client and therapist variables in the group situation. He presents the benefits of group therapies and some proven strategies and techniques used to help chemically dependent persons to identify and share with others in the safe environment and healing process of the group.

The book presents convincing evidence why group therapy works better than individual therapy for addicted populations."

Guidepost

"A comprehensive and complete dissertation on group therapy in the treatment of addiction. It clearly and succinctly covers the field of alcoholism treatment . . . This book is a must for all therapists who treat addiction and in particular those who utilize group therapy."

Conway Hunter, Jr., MD
St. Simons Island, Georgia

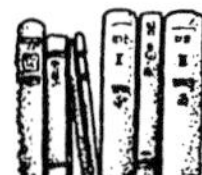

"Philip Flores has written a book that will surely come to be regarded as a classic in the field of group psychotherapy for alcoholics. It belongs on the shelf of every counselor or psychotherapist who sees alcoholics in groups."

John Wallace, PhD
Director of Treatment,
Vice President for Clinical Programs,
Edgehill Newport,
Newport, RI

NOTES FOR PROFESSIONAL LIBRARIANS AND LIBRARY USERS

This is an original book title published by The Haworth Press, Inc. Unless otherwise noted in specific chapters with attribution, materials in this book have not been previously published elsewhere in any format or language.

CONSERVATION AND PRESERVATION NOTES

All books published by The Haworth Press, Inc. and its imprints are printed on certified ph neutral, acid free book grade paper. This paper meets the minimum requirements of American National Standard for Information Sciences–Permanence of Paper for Printed Material, ANSI Z39.48-1984.

Group Psychotherapy with Addicted Populations

An Integration of Twelve-Step and Psychodynamic Theory

Second Edition

HAWORTH Addictions Treatment
F. Bruce Carruth, PhD
Senior Editor

New, Recent, and Forthcoming Titles:

Shame, Guilt and Alcoholism: Treatment Issues in Clinical Practice by Ronald T. Potter-Efron

Neuro-Linguistic Programming in Alcoholism Treatment edited by Chelly M. Sterman

Cocaine Solutions: Help for Cocaine Abusers and Their Families by Jennifer Rice-Licare and Katherine Delaney-McLoughlin

Preschoolers and Substance Abuse: Strategies for Prevention and Intervention by Pedro J. Lecca and Thomas D. Watts

Chemical Dependency and Antisocial Personality Disorder: Psychotherapy and Assessment Strategies by Gary G. Forrest

Substance Abuse and Physical Disability edited by Allen W. Heinemann

Addiction in Human Development: Developmental Perspectives on Addiction and Recovery by Jacqueline Wallen

Addictions Treatment for Older Adults: Evaluation of an Innovative Client-Centered Approach by Kathryn Graham, Sarah J. Saunders, Margaret C. Flower, Carol Birchmore Timney, Marilyn White-Campbell, and Anne Zeidman Pietropaolo

Group Psychotherapy with Addicted Populations: An Integration of Twelve-Step and Psychodynamic Theory, Second Edition by Philip J. Flores

Group Psychotherapy with Addicted Populations

An Integration of Twelve-Step and Psychodynamic Theory

Second Edition

Philip J. Flores, PhD

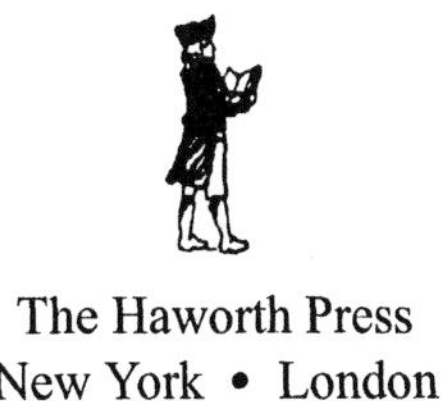

The Haworth Press
New York • London

The Haworth Press, Inc., 10 Alice Street, Binghamton, NY 13904-1580

Cover designed by Marylouise E. Doyle.

Library of Congress Cataloging-in-Publication Data

Flores, Philip J.
Group psychotherapy with addicted populations: an integration of twelve-step and psychodynamic theory / Philip J. Flores–2nd ed.
p. cm.
Includes bibliographical references and index.
ISBN 0-7890-6001-9 (pbk: alk. paper)
1. Alcoholism–Treatment. 2. Group psychotherapy. 3. Substance abuse–Treatment. I. Title.
RC565.F568 1996
616.86'0651–dc20 96-358
CIP

To
Lisa Mahon,

my friend, mentor, teacher, and wife. Without her support, encouragement, advice, patience, and help, this book would not have been possible.

ABOUT THE AUTHOR

Philip J. Flores, PhD, is a clinical psychologist who, for the past twenty years, has worked extensively in the area of addictive diseases and group psychotherapy. He is a Fellow in the American Group Psychotherapy Association and past president of the Georgia Association of Specialists in Group Work. During the last ten years he has served as either treasurer or chair of education and training with the Atlanta Group Psychotherapy Society. He has taught Advanced Group Psychotherapy for a number of universities and private hospitals and was a former member of the Arizona Group Psychotherapy Society before moving to Atlanta, Georgia in 1982. Dr. Flores is currently Adjunct Faculty at Georgia State University and the Georgia School of Professional Psychology where he teaches courses on group psychotherapy and addictions and provides supervision for group psychotherapy. He is also a supervisor of group psychotherapy for Emory University in Atlanta, Georgia. Prior to receiving his PhD in clinical psychology, he worked for a number of years as a certified alcoholism counselor, treating addicted patients in both an inpatient and outpatient setting. Before starting his private practice, he was Director of the Family Outpatient Counseling and Addictive Services (FOCAS), a program that specialized in the outpatient treatment of addictions.

In addition to this book, Dr. Flores has published numerous articles and chapters on addiction and group psychotherapy. He has frequently presented workshops on these two topics throughout the United States while continuing to manage a private practice that specializes in addiction, codependency, ACOA, and other interpersonal related issues. Dr. Flores and his wife, Lisa Mahon, PhD, continue to lead several outpatient psychotherapy groups that meet on a weekly basis.

CONTENTS

Preface

This is a book about addiction and its treatment. However, were that to be the total extent of its author's aim, it would not generate the excitement I think it will stimulate in those who read it carefully. More specifically, this is a book that not only addresses the important topic of addiction, it also outlines sound recommendations for the treatment of addiction within a group therapy setting. In fact, the book presents convincing evidence why group therapy should be the treatment of choice for addiction. It then succinctly outlines how this can be best accomplished within a group therapy setting. And, since group therapy and alcoholism are subjects very dear to me for very different reasons, I am excited to see a book that blends these topics into a smoothly convergent theme.

Alcoholism, the addiction of which I am most familiar, is often called a disease of denial, not only for the alcoholic, but for those who come in contact, professionally and personally, with the alcoholic. If someone is suffering from alcoholism, it is highly unlikely that the person's alcoholism will be diagnosed by a physician, psychologist, or other helping professional. If their alcoholism is diagnosed, the chances unfortunately are poor that the alcoholic will receive an appropriate referral for treatment. Too often, the alcoholic is only admonished to cut down on his drinking and told to straighten himself up and get his life together. If he even is referred to a psychotherapist, the focus of therapy often will be directed towards determining the nature of his "real problem." The message is clearly given that if he were to get at the core of his psychological conflict he could be "cured" and taught to drink normally once again.

To try and cure an alcoholic so they can drink socially and normally is a grave mistake. I know that Eric Berne and Claude Stiener, two very respected associates of mine, believed that an alcoholic could be cured, but I disagree with both of them. I do agree, however, that an alcoholic's life scripts and the games they play, as defined in Transactional Analysis theory, are often important parts in the alcoholic's personality and contribute to the progression of the disease. However, alcoholism is the disease in which chemical dependency and physical addiction result in a condition that leaves the alcoholic with an inability to drink normally. The alcoholic's denial must be broken through first and they must come to learn and accept the undeniable fact that they cannot drink normally because they suffer from a disease called alcoholism.

My writing about alcoholism as a condition in which the person "can't" drink normally may seem surprising to those readers who are familiar with my work, my books, and my theoretical development of Redecision Therapy. Those of you who have participated in workshops at Mount Madonna with Mary and I or have attended any of the many seminars and workshops we regularly give throughout the world, know that I am a person who staunchly believes that the "power is in the patient." There are not many "can'ts" that I acknowledge or recognize as legitimate. For I believe that we too often give up our freedom and responsibility to others too quickly because of early messages we have been given and early decisions we have made as children. The result is that we end up relinquishing the power and excitement in our lives for the safety and security of the past. "Can'ts" for me are usually "won'ts." People who overly utilize words like "can't," "need," and "try," lead me to be very cautious of their motivation in therapy. I consequently watch for how they might try to manipulate and con me. I tell them to turn their can'ts into won'ts, their needs into wants, and get them to realize their "try's" are a relinquishing of their potency and power as an exciting, responsible individual. However, I believe alcoholics "can't" drink and this is one very important exception to the verbal games that most people play in therapy. The realization that "I can't drink," and the alcoholic's denial, must be dealt with directly if they are to progress in treatment.

The recognition of "can't" for an alcoholic is essential to their recovery because the alcoholic suffers from a biological abnormality that prevents them from drinking in a socially appropriate manner. Countless studies have clearly demonstrated that genetics play a crucial factor in the onset of the illness since it has been found that alcoholism definitely runs in families. Children born of alcoholic parents, and then separated from them after their birth and raised in totally different environments, have a much higher chance of developing alcoholism than children born of nonalcoholic parents. Recent biological research is uncovering numerous possibilities that exist between genetics, biochemical abnormalities, and alcoholism.

The personality of the addicted individual, their genetic makeup, constitutional resistances to the illness, and many environmental variables (along with untold numerous other influences) can cause the illness to appear in an unending variety of forms. Because of the great variability of the illness and the frequent uninformed, naive status of the observer, addiction is frequently unrecognized for what it is and misdiagnosed and left untreated. The course of the addiction is usually a very gradual and progressive one in which undetectable changes in personality are easily attributed to other causes and influences besides the use of a chemical substance. The changes usually result in inexplicable deviations of long-established values and social behavior. The individual's ability to achieve in his or her personal life or occupational pursuit is frequently impaired, resulting in frustration, anger, and irritation. Unfortunately, the effects of addiction are often only detectable at autopsy when multiple effects to the heart, brain, and liver are finally diagnosed.

Because of the progressive and insidious nature of alcoholism, the recognition of the disease and the breakdown of denial is essential, as Alcoholics Anonymous readily recognizes. The first three steps of the AA program readily address this issue: (1) We admitted we were powerless over alcohol–that our life had become unmanageable; (2) We came to believe that a Power greater than ourselves could restore us to sanity; (3) We made a decision to turn our will and our lives over to the care of God as we understood Him. And, as I have stated elsewhere, I believe the second and third steps are really Redecisions (as defined by Redecision Therapy) because they require an act of faith from the alcoholic's Free Child. Promoting and encouraging the alcoholic's Redecision not to drink ("I can't drink") is the most important therapeutic event that can be achieved in treatment. The power of the group to confront the alcoholic's denial and to reinforce their Redecision not to drink is why group therapy is such an important component to the recovery process.

This book addresses both of these very critical therapeutic issues in the treatment of addiction. First, it places alcoholism within the realm of a disease paradigm and defines the importance of requiring the alcoholic to maintain his sobriety if he is to obtain any change in his destructive life script. Secondly, its author outlines how the attainment of sobriety and the maintenance of the Redecision that "I can't drink" is to be achieved within a group therapy setting. The Redecision to not drink, ("I can't drink because I am an alcoholic") is one that requires careful monitoring because the pull of the alcoholic's physical and psychological dependency is so strong and pervasive.

Group therapy can be an exciting adventure and I believe, as AA does, that people have the capacity to change. People (not only alcoholics) can change if they are helped by the therapist to cure themselves. Mary and I strive to teach our patients how they have deadened themselves–made themselves depressed, phobic, or anxious–while giving them the encouragement and permission to enjoy life instead. For the drinking alcoholic, this is impossible to obtain unless they first stop drinking and remain free of chemical use.

The alcoholic's Redecision to not drink is a new journey, which is both exciting and frightening. This movement can be sustained and encouraged through the feelings of identification, support, and belonging, which are generated in the therapy group and AA. Because alcoholics early in their recovery need support, group therapy and AA can meet their dependency needs while allowing them to regulate and set their own pace and involvement in their recovery. During the early stages of recovery, alcoholics usually find it easier to place themselves in a dependent position among others with whom they can identify and feel comfortable. Ultimately, alcoholics must come to assume responsibility for their own sobriety without dependency on others; but the group can provide the structure for this until they decide they are ready to move through this transitional period. A point this book makes repeatedly is that recovery is a time-dependent process in which the initial stages of treatment are different from the later stages of treatment. After the breakdown of denial and abstinence is obtained, a therapy group can be used to deal with the array of emotions that usually accompany the first few months of abstinence.

The author outlines how the group can be utilized in the later stages of the recovery process to examine the ways that life scripts and games help maintain the alcoholic's psychological dependence on alcohol. This book correctly examines the many ways that unaltered, untreated, and unexamined psychological factors can lead to a relapse. The alcoholic's life script may not be a factor in all cases, but its associated games, cons, and repetitive patterns can lead to a reemergence of denial and return to the addictive use of chemicals.

Unfortunately, many therapists hold the erroneous assumption that if alcoholics only knew how to express their feelings better, they could be cured. I have said before that I have yet to see a cure coming from just the facilitation of the expression of feelings. Those familiar with my work with Gestalt Therapy and my association with Fritz Perls and Jim Simkin, know that I am not one to shy away from the expression of feelings. However, the cessation of alcohol intake must be obtained first. Then the alcoholic must come to acknowledge the severity of his problems (which requires a Free Child Redecision). Finally, a sound group therapeutic format must be established which allows the alteration of disruptive life scripts, the confrontation of gains, and the strokes for positive change.

All of these sound principles of treatment have been carefully outlined in this book. I hope all of you who read it find it helpful in your understanding of addiction and useful in your treatment of the chemically dependent patient. Because this book outlines how addiction can be treated within a group therapy session, it will be invaluable for those who are either knowledgeable about addiction or uninformed about group therapy. Both of these important subjects are brought together in a complementary and concise fashion.

Robert Goulding, MD
Distinguished Fellow
American Group Psychotherapy Association;
Co-Director of Western Institute
of Group and Family Therapy;
Past President
American Academy of Psychotherapists

Introduction

This is a book that does a notable job of integrating two widely disparate variables: alcoholism and group treatment. Dr. Flores has done a painstaking objective blending of the shared setting with probably the most endemic pathology of our time. To practitioners familiar with the group approach and the remarkable work of Alcoholics Anonymous (AA), it is a puzzlement that group therapy is not the treatment of choice for all oral addictive pathology. Group therapy is now becoming recognized by more and more of the leading group theorists and practitioners as the treatment of choice for both addiction and its associated character pathology.

Because the group method was solidly grounded on individual treatment for so many years, it was assumed that there was basically little difference in the effect of individual treatment and group treatment. The only reason group was recommended was that it was a low-cost modality and many patients could be approached at the same time, but it was generally considered a social adjunct rather than a viable therapeutic instrument in its own right. What we have discovered in the last twenty years with new developments in group treatment is that this is patently not so. In fact, a well-conducted group in conjunction with AA has a substantial impact on the treatment effectiveness with this population. Dr. Flores devotes a great deal of time and effort to describing how these divergent approaches can be smoothly integrated into one complementary treatment effort.

Dr. Flores makes the point that the disease model and the mental health model are not as dissimilar as many see them. They are in most ways closely related. And to take a position on either side is an awkward effort to separate two approaches that have much to contribute to a totalistic one. One important accomplishment of this book is that it demonstrates how these different ways of defining and treating addiction can be applied effectively within the group therapy format.

Dr. Flores expands the work of one of the most popular writers in group therapy today–Dr. Irvin Yalom. New additions to Dr. Yalom's findings have made his original contribution dramatically more effective. Throughout his book, Dr. Flores draws on some of these findings to help explain and expand Yalom's model. He shows how the model can be adapted and applied more effectively with this population. Dr. Flores suggests specific alterations and special considerations in technique to fit the unique problems of the addicted. He pays special attention to the opening stages of treating the addicted personality and describes the techniques needed. After initial resistances are resolved, the practitioner can readily apply the more recent advances in group treatment.

Dr. Flores presents convincing evidence that it is the alcoholics' and addicts' inability to establish and maintain healthy interpersonal relationships that contributes not only to their addiction, but also to their difficulty maintaining sobriety and abstinence. It is in the later stage of addiction treatment that Dr. Flores believes that modern views and recommendations for group therapy would be especially helpful. It would be helpful to review some of the developments that have occurred since Dr. Yalom's original book was published in 1975.

Adaptation of Modern Approaches

To begin to understand how modern group approach can be helpful in treating this population, it is important to note that all modern group therapy is aimed at resolving impediments of its members to saying new things and establishing new relationships. A number of techniques have been introduced that have increased the efficacy of the modality. These are bridging, focusing on immediacy, establishing the observing ego, developing the insulation barrier, and accentuating emotional communication. A word about each.

Bridging

Skilled leaders use bridging with addicted personalities to melt barriers of isolation. Instead of they themselves approaching the withdrawn person, they use an oblique approach linking other members with the patient who is out of reach. Such patients are more apt to respond to peer influence rather than to authoritative influence. There are many types of bridging. In similarity bridging, group leaders seek a member who shares some aspect, behavioral or otherwise, of the member they want to bring into the group flow, and the leaders connect the two members. In reactive bridging, group leaders ask a person on the sidelines how the speaker comes across and so forth.

Focusing on Immediacy

Dr. Flores touches on the concept of immediacy, which Dr. Yalom calls the here and now. Therapists have found that there are all types of resistances to immediacy and have delineated them. These resistances are caused by the anxiety signals a person experiences in the present brought on by the danger of closeness, the danger of being swallowed, the danger of being rejected, the danger of experiencing aggression, and other forms of unacceptable responses and feelings. Many people avoid the immediate by bringing in problems. They do not have to relate to the people in front of them in a give-and-take way. They simply present their problems to the group and await magical answers.

Another device people use to avoid immediacy is flight into time. This includes the immediate past, the recent past, and the remote past. It also includes flight into the future–into fantasy, into promises, into a description of fears. A group in which resistances to immediacy are resolved is a group that brims with life.

Establishing the Observing Ego

It has been recently noted that all members of a group, no matter how narrow or small, have a conflict-free part of their perceptual apparatus that sees things as they really are–uncluttered by distortion. There are always people in the group who have a conflict-free perception about what is going on. Therapists have learned to utilize these people to describe to the members caught in the tangled web of their history what they are doing and how they are creating their present world. The members with conflict-free perceptions serve as transitional observing egos. What these members see clearly now will help group members learn how to see themselves clearly later. The more members of a group can witness how they function without seeking to change it, the greater the freedom part of their personality has to master it at its own pace.

Developing the Insulation Barrier

One characteristic of people suffering with oral addictive personalities is their fragile and easily penetrable psychic skein. Stimuli that impinges upon these people, which may be toxic and rejected by those with a tough psychic skein, find an easy access to a member's ego and inflicts damaging wounds. These people cannot resist temptation, cannot subdue their own appetites, and cannot differentiate what is good from what is bad for them. They are always vulnerable. Through the group experience, therapists have learned how to strengthen and thicken these insulation barriers so that these people can more successfully wall off what is noxious to their function and sense of self.

Accentuating Emotional Communication

One of the most important technical operations in which the leader in modern groups can engage is to keep the group on an emotional level. Melanie Klein, Hyman Spotniz, and others have pointed out that characteristics form during the pre-oedipal period, that is, the period between birth and three-and-a-half to four years of age. Most character structure is established during these early years when audiations, thoughts, and cognitive verbal communications have little reality. What does influence and shape the way people's characters are formed are impulses and feelings. Impulses are primitive forms of communication. Emotions are refined impulses. Both impulses and emotions dominate the child before he or she is able to speak. Therefore, all addiction problems have a base in the earliest periods of development when emotions are the dominant focus of communication. In group, if we work strictly on an emotional level, we are awakening that formative period in life. It is here in this cauldron that character and personality changes that affect addictions will take place.

These are only a few of the technical innovations that are becoming popular in the therapeutic armentarium of the modern group therapist. There are also environmental arrangements that have been singularly effective, such as combining group treatment with AA. Another intervention, combining group treatment with individual treatment, is an arrangement known as conjoint therapy; that is, every person with an addictive problem should be in group once a week and in individual therapy once a week (with different therapists). In this way, one therapist may pick up what the other may overlook. The group serves as a chorus, a leverage factor, and a multidimensional holding environment.

What Dr. Flores has achieved here is a synthesis of many divergent innovations in the treatment of one of the most important segments of our society. The way Dr. Flores adroitly utilizes these concepts separates this work from the voluminous literature in the field. He knows what he is doing and can delineate it. Those people who do work in this field are obviously making one of the most important contributions to our culture. Any tool that can be placed in their hands that will aid them in their task must be welcomed and cherished.

Louis R. Ormont, PhD

Chapter 1

An Introduction to Group Psychotherapy and Addiction

Within the last thirty years, there have been significant and dramatic changes in the understanding of addiction and its treatment. Foremost among these changes is the utilization of group psychotherapy as an important, if not the most crucial, component of an alcoholic's or substance abuser's treatment regimen. However, as important a development as this has been, the recognition and acceptance of addiction as a disease and a primary disorder that must first be addressed has had more of an impact on the way that addiction is treated. Addiction to chemicals, whether it be to alcohol or drugs, is no longer viewed as a symptom of a more serious core issue. Rather, it is seen as a primary condition that must first be arrested if any progress in treatment is to be achieved and abstinence from all chemicals must be the first goal of recovery. Put another way, substance abusers and alcoholics cannot benefit from psychotherapy as long as they continue to use chemicals. Not only has this stance legitimized the treatment of addiction and created a philosophy of treatment completely independent of the more classical and traditional approaches to psychological difficulties, but it also raises the question of whether addiction is purely a psychological phenomenon. The disease concept has also lent support to Alcoholics Anonymous's (AA) lifelong contention that addiction is a disease and total abstinence (AA's first step of its twelve-step program) is a necessity if addiction is to be treated successfully.

Prior to this shift in treatment philosophy, intra-psychic conflicts and intra-personal dynamics were usually viewed as the cause of addiction. However, the disease concept stands that view completely on its head. Depression, anxiety, and character pathology are now viewed as symptoms–the result, not the cause–of addiction. Addiction specialists discovered that once they persuaded the alcoholic and substance abuser to abstain from the use of chemicals, these symptoms either completely subsided or at least greatly diminished in many cases. In their classic longitudinal study, Vaillant and Milofsky put a final nail into the controlled drinking versus the disease concept controversy of the late 1970s when they concluded, "Thus, the etiological hypothesis that viewed alcoholism primarily as a symptom of psychological instability may be an illusion based on retrospective study" (1982, p. 494). Consequently, Vaillant and Milofsky verified what everyone within the AA community and the addiction treatment field has know for years. Vaillant put it best when he later wrote "Prospective studies are gradually teaching psychiatrists the astonishing fact that most of psychopathology seen in the alcoholic is the result, not the cause of alcohol abuse. Put differently, alcoholism is the horse, not the cart of mental illness" (1983, p. 317).

Not only has the treatment of addiction been legitimized, addiction has become recognized as one of the most significant and major health problems in this country. Previously, treatment for addiction was available only through AA, other twelve-step programs (e.g., Cocaine Anonymous, Narcotics Anonymous, etc.), or an occasional obscure hospital or treatment program in some distant part of the country. Now it is rare to find any major metropolitan area that does not have at least one hospital or outpatient treatment program that specializes in addiction treatment. The increase in the need for more treatment facilities is a direct result of the increased use of alcohol and substances in our present-day culture. The most crucial precipitating factor in addiction is the degree of availability and access to a particular drug. Thus, no matter how tolerant an attitude for addictive practice society has, or how strong individual personalities or genetic predispositions are, no one can become addicted unless they have ready access to the drug. Thirty years ago, addiction treatment was less complicated. The addicted person was instructed to stop drinking, then was detoxed if necessary, and was told to start going to AA meetings. Now, it is rare to find an alcoholic, especially one under thirty years of age, who is not also using and abusing numerous other drugs. The concept of cross-addiction, namely, stopping the use of one drug only to become addicted to another, is common practice for most substance abusers and alcoholics. The term "poly-drug abuser" is becoming more of a common diagnosis. It is now necessary to inquire what is the substance abuser's "drug of choice." Certainly, the onset of increased drug use in our culture has complicated the diagnostic and treatment picture.

Increased drug use has also resulted in increased demands for effective treatment for chemical dependency. Consequently, group therapy has also increased in popularity and has become the treatment of choice for all chemical dependencies and substance abuse disorders. Initially, the increased utilization of group psychotherapy may have been due in part to the cost effectiveness of group treatment and the influence of the popular support group format of Alcoholics Anonymous (AA) and its twelve-step program. Nevertheless, most professionals who work with substance abusers on a sustained and prolonged basis (Khantzian, Halliday, and McAuliffe, 1990; Flores, 1993; Flores and Mahon, 1993; Vannicelli, 1992; and S. Brown, 1985; Brown and Yalom, 1977; Washton, 1992; Matano and Yalom, 1991) now agree that there are far more important reasons why group therapy is an essential and crucial ingredient in the treatment of addiction. These reasons have to do with a number of important factors, including–but not limited to–the nature of the addiction process itself, which either produces or exacerbates depression, anxiety, isolation, denial, shame, transient cognitive impairment, and character pathology. It is now recognized that many of these issues, whether the person is addicted or not, respond better to group treatment than to individual therapy. There is also an emerging appreciation for the special advantages of group therapy, and it is no longer viewed as a secondary or inferior form of treatment. It is now seen as the source of powerful curative forces that are not typically available for the patient being treated in individual therapy. In the hands of a skilled and well-trained group leader, these forces can be harnessed and utilized in a way that provides a vital and unique therapeutic experience for an individual that would not be possible in individual treatment.

The increased recognition and acceptance of group therapy as a legitimate form of treatment in its own right coupled with the alarming increase of substance abuse in our culture has resulted in an increased demand upon degreed and non-degreed professionals to lead groups with these patients. This demand has often been made of group leaders who have not been adequately trained in group psychotherapy and who therefore are forced to apply models of group treatment that are poorly suited to the addicted patient. Since group therapy is an intricate component if not the most crucial element for both inpatient and outpatient treatment programs as well as after care and relapse prevention, it is crucial that a practical and effective model of group therapy be outlined and established if treatment is to reach its full potential.

SPECIFIC IMPLICATIONS OF GROUP THERAPY WITH CHEMICAL DEPENDENCY

Consequently, the answer to the intricate question regarding the effectiveness of group psychotherapy for addicts and alcoholics must be asked and answered more precisely. Why indeed is group psychotherapy such an effective mode of treatment for alcoholics and addicts? Part of the answer lies within the typical defensive style of the addicted individual. This is a characterological style that involves the defensive posture commonly referred to as denial. Addiction is, in fact, frequently cited as a disease of denial. However, the chemically dependent individual usually presents with a much more complex set of defenses and character pathology, and the group leader must have a clear understanding of each group member's defensive process and character dynamics if he or she intends to help each of them benefit from treatment. Nearly twenty years ago, John Wallace (1977a) addressed this important issue in an informative essay on the alcoholic's defensive style and referred to these characterological defensive features as the alcoholic's preferred defense system. Khantzian, Halliday, and McAuliffe (1990), Krystal and Raskin (1993), and Flores and Mahon (1993) have since expanded on Kohut's (1977a) earlier hypothesis that addiction is a disorder of the self. Evidence will be presented in the following chapters outlining the way group treatment helps break through the substance abuser's preferred defense system and wall of denial while dealing with his or her disorder of the self. The characteristics of the typical addicted patient from an object relations and self-psychology perspective will be dealt with in more detail in Chapter 6. For now, it is important to note that the advantages group psychotherapy provides by confronting and altering the addict's and alcoholic's defensive style is a theme that will be addressed throughout this book.

Despite the special issues that must be considered when treating the addicted patient, there are important advantages to group psychotherapy that are not limited exclusively to the addicted population. Within group psychotherapy there is a phenomenon surrounding its curative process that cannot be explained completely from a psychological perspective or put in an exclusively psychological framework. Chapter 7 will give an alternative view of these forces from a phenomenological, existential, and anthropological perspective, especially as these forces apply to addiction and Alcoholics Anonymous. Chapter 15 will deal primarily with the psychological aspects of the curative process in group and will examine the ways group plays an intricate part in the healing, treatment, and arrestment of addiction. But there are other important reasons why groups are so effective in producing change in an individual's life, and one way of understanding the significance of this impact is to view group psychotherapy from an anthropological perspective. Jerome Frank, for instance, has written an excellent book (1961) in which he creatively draws parallels between healing rituals in primitive cultures and similar rituals in modern

Western medicine that play an equally intricate part in the principles of cure and healing existing in our present day society. Exploring the ramifications of healing from a cultural perspective, Frank convincingly argues that the group provides a much more powerful curative force than individual therapy because it alleviates the isolation and the demoralization that, for Frank, is the central issue for individuals seeking psychiatric help in our society. Speaking from an anthropological perspective, Frank sees many advantages and benefits of group psychotherapy over individual therapy. The roles that culture and society play in addiction and its subsequent treatment is a topic beyond the scope of this book. However, it is important to note at this point that the chemically dependent individual responds more favorably to group because the cultural and societal forces that contribute to addiction can be used in turn by the group to heal and treat the very deficit they have created. These are the sentiments expressed by Ettin (1988) when he wrote, "By the crowd, they have been broken, by the crowd they shall be healed."

Consequently, as Frank succinctly outlines, the group offers its members many advantages over individual treatment. The empirical research on the advantages of group treatment is abundant. In a review article on the effectiveness of group psychotherapy, Allen (1990) cited countless outcome studies that led him to conclude that "the effectiveness of group cannot be disputed." In another extensive review on the efficacy of group treatments, Dies (1992b) stated that after four decades of empirical investigation "there is relatively little differential outcome of individual and group treatments." He concluded that in the face of mounting pressure to justify the expense of psychotherapy, group therapy will become the treatment of choice in the future.

Specific empirical research into the effectiveness of group psychotherapy with chemical dependency has until recently been either limited, anecdotal, or equivocal. A review of the current research with addictions will be presented more thoroughly in Chapter 12. For now, it will suffice to report that within the last ten years there have been a number of major books and articles on the subject and a surprising consensus has been reached independently by a number of researchers and practitioners who regularly work with addicted patients in a group therapy format (Khantzian, Halliday, and McAuliffe, 1990; Vannicelli, 1992; Flores and Mahon, 1993; Matano and Yalom, 1991). Their recommendations will be thoroughly examined and presented in Chapters 3, 4, and 5. Previous to these publications, the use of group therapy had been enthusiastically recommended, supported, and applied, although a systematic, well-organized, or clearly defined rationale for its application had not existed.

The trend toward the use of group psychotherapy had been hindered previously by the popular misconception that group psychotherapy with addicted patients did not require specially qualified leaders because groups could take care of themselves. However, this is not the case. In order for group treatment to fulfill its potential, it requires a special understanding of group process, group dynamics, stages of group development, and countless other issues that only come with extended training and experience in leading groups. Too often, therapists trained only in individual therapy or experienced with nonaddicted patients were thrust into group psychotherapy leadership roles. Similarly, many alcohol counselors knowledgeable about addiction and the disease process because of their own addiction were often placed in the role of group leader without the benefit of formal training in group psychotherapy. Because group psychotherapy, as it should be applied, is difficult, and because addicted patients pose special and unique problems for the group leader, group psychotherapy with this population requires a number of specifically trained skills. Many groups led by untrained or poorly trained leaders did not fulfill their potential or may even have had negative effects on a patient's recovery.

Clearly, a need exists for training and educating potential group therapists who are or will be leading groups composed primarily of chemically dependent individuals. This is necessary because working with chemically dependent individuals within a group setting poses numerous difficulties for most group psychotherapists. It matters little whether the group therapists are recovering addicts or alcoholics themselves, or if they have followed the more traditional course of academically based training. In either case, the problem is usually related to two contributing factors. Either there has been a lack of effective group psychotherapy training opportunities for these group therapists, or they have been taught a model of group psychotherapy that is inadequate for patients who are chemically dependent.

Unfortunately, most contemporary approaches to group psychotherapy have not taken into consideration the special characteristics of chemically dependent patients and the special problems these patients pose for the group leader. Consequently, group leaders have often desired more direction, better training, and more practical suggestions for effectively leading groups composed of addicted patients. Compounding this difficulty is the well-known fact that group therapy is usually a very integral part of an alcoholic's and addict's treatment in both inpatient and outpatient settings. Subsequently, group leaders have frequently found themselves thrown into a "sink or swim" situation. Most have been able to respond creatively by adapting skills they have acquired for individual psychotherapy. However, what often gets passed off as group psychotherapy is usually little more than individual therapy within a group setting. Individual therapy, whether done in a diad or in a group, is not group psychotherapy. Therapists will also find that principles which work well for individuals are totally inappropriate for group psychotherapy. Beyond this, the rich potential for self-understanding, psychological growth, emotional healing, and true intimacy that exists only in a group setting is left unfulfilled. Group leaders must be familiar with and sensitive to the basic issues that manifest in group psychotherapy or else they will find themselves in waters filled with treacherous undercurrents.

Many group therapists have responded to this situation by utilizing procedures they have intuitively adopted from Alcoholics Anonymous and other twelve-step programs. This is not to say that the principles of Alcoholics Anonymous are inadequate. To the contrary, recovery from addiction for most individuals is often impossible without the utilization of the principles of the AA program. This is why most successful treatment programs in this country require that attendance in AA and other twelve-step meetings be a mandatory part of the treatment process. However, AA and other twelve-step programs are not group psychotherapy, and the two different treatment modalities should not be confused. On the other hand, group psychotherapy is not Alcoholics Anonymous and group psychotherapy should never be intended to be a substitute for AA or its other affiliated twelve-step programs. Twelve-step programs and group psychotherapy provide important complementary components to the recovery process and in the hands of a skilled clinician, group psychotherapy can be a very important tool in the treatment process. Twelve-step programs such as AA can keep chemically dependent individuals sober or clean while the group can speed along the recovery process by giving them an opportunity to understand and explore the emotional and interpersonal conflicts that are secondary or contributing to their addiction.

Even though group psychotherapy is an important therapeutic modality in most contemporary inpatient and outpatient addictive treatment programs, the model upon which it is based has been, for the most part, derived from the practice of outpatient psychotherapy with nonaddicted patients. However, the theoretical and practical considerations underlying outpatient group psychotherapy with a nonaddictive population is not always applicable to individuals suffering from chemical dependency. Even Yalom (1975) suggested that alcoholics and persons with character disorders be omitted from group psychotherapy because they are inappropriate candidates for this mode of treatment. Consequently, currently accepted principles of group psychotherapy need to be altered in order to meet the realities and necessities of treating the addicted patient. This problem is further complicated by the fact that most addicted patients, as well as staff members, often become confused about the different types of group treatment modalities. For instance, AA, NA, and CA groups, "step-work" groups, discussion groups, educational groups, aftercare groups, and support groups are just a few of the variety of group treatment modalities that many patients are exposed to during their treatment process. It is not surprising that patients often become confused about the principles of group psychotherapy and that the staff fails to appreciate the significance of the impact that group psychotherapy can make on an individual's recovery. It is also important to take into consideration the time factor involved in an individual's recovery. What a group leader does in group psychotherapy with patients in an inpatient setting in a hospital during the first few days of recovery will be dramatically different from what that same group therapist would do with the same recovering person who has six months of sobriety in an aftercare group.

Therefore, the purpose of this book is to examine and present a systematic model of group psychotherapy as described and practiced by the leading theorists in the field of group psychotherapy and addiction (Yalom, 1975; Brown and Yalom, 1977; Wallace, 1978; Vanicelli, 1992; Khantzian, Halliday, and McAuliffe, 1990; Washton, 1992; Vannecelli, 1988; Flores and Mahon, 1993). This book is an attempt to define proven strategies and articulate suggestions for improving the treatment of the chemically dependent patient by providing a cognitive understanding of the special problems that chemically dependent individuals bring to group psychotherapy. Although group psychotherapy has long been an essential component of treatment programs, group orientations vary enormously from one setting to another. Nevertheless, most professionals who work with alcoholics and addicts on a sustained basis agree that abstinence is a necessary first step in treatment. Once that is obtained, the consensus is that the therapy group offers chemically dependent individuals unique opportunities to learn about themselves and their addiction.

Washton (1992) summarizes some of the advantages of group therapy in the following manner:

1. mutual identification with and acceptance from others going through similar problems,
2. positive role modeling for abstinence and reality testing about chemical use is enhanced because the addicted person has the opportunity to better understand their own attitudes about addictions and their defenses against giving up chemicals by confronting similar attitudes and defenses in others,

3. confrontation, immediate feedback and positive peer pressure for abstinence,
4. affiliation, cohesiveness, social support while learning to identify and communicate feelings more directly,
5. structures, discipline and limit setting while permitting experiential learning and exchange of factual information about recovery and drug use,
6. installation of hope, inspiration for the future and the pursuit of shared goals and ideas.

As a group psychotherapist, consultant, and trainer for nearly twenty years, I have had the opportunity to work with and supervise numerous therapy groups in both inpatient and outpatient settings in both the public and private sector. I am currently involved in an ongoing project aimed at adapting the principles of group psychotherapy to addictive populations. The importance of such an endeavor can hardly be overestimated in view of two simultaneously occurring, although not necessarily related, trends in modern addiction treatment. The first is the greater utilization of recovering people themselves as a source of professional treatment personnel. The second is a trend for most treatment programs to include group psychotherapy as an essential component of the treatment effort. Unfortunately, most professionals have not received adequate training in either group therapy or addiction during their academic careers. Certainly, most of them have not been exposed to the principles of group psychotherapy with an addictive population. It therefore becomes necessary to define a set of theories and practices that are specialized to meet the needs of the addicted patient in group psychotherapy.

THE DISEASE CONCEPT AND GROUP PSYCHOTHERAPY

As a group therapist, if you believe that addiction is a disease, it will affect the way you approach treatment and conduct your psychotherapy groups with addicted patients. The disease model requires that you view addiction as primary illness that cannot be cured, only arrested. Furthermore, the disease model requires viewing addiction to alcohol and drugs much like one views many chronic illnesses, such as heart disease or diabetes. Since chronic diseases are those prone to relapse, constant monitoring of the afflicted individual's lifestyle and alteration of his or her behavioral habits is necessary in order to reduce the risk of relapse. Accepting addiction as a disease means viewing this condition as a physiological illness with emotional, behavioral, and conditioned response components, not as a secondary sign or symptom of some underlying mental or emotional disorder. Group psychotherapy from this perspective, especially at the beginning of treatment, is aimed not at uncovering psychological pathology, but at identifying the defenses and characterological deficits that prevent compliance with abstinence and recovery. The ability to deal with uncomfortable feelings triggered by interpersonal conflict is an equally important component of the recovery process. Group psychotherapy should be used to enhance adherence to the principles of Alcoholics Anonymous and other twelve-step programs, while allowing a closer examination of the difficulties recovering people have with their interpersonal relationships. It is rare to find a chemically dependent individual who hasn't relapsed because of the strong affect that has been stirred up as a result of interpersonal conflict.

Furthermore, the disease model requires accepting the chemically dependent individual's metabolic and physiological response to ethyl alcohol and other chemicals as entirely different from that of the non-chemically dependent individual. A vast amount of evidence involving the brain and liver, endorphin and receptor sites, permeability of nerve cell membranes, specific hereditary electroencephalograph patterns, and metabolic differences, as well as a number of hereditary studies that control for parental alcoholic environment in several ways, substantiate the scientific basis for accepting addiction as a disease. Thus, there is little question that the history, symptoms, and signs of addiction form a recognizable pattern. Individuals who become dependent on alcohol and drugs will deteriorate in all areas of life–physical, mental, emotional, moral, and spiritual. The well-known, total destructiveness of addiction need not be repeated. Attitudes, individual responsibility, and public recognition are crucial factors that must be recognized before addiction can be treated effectively. The reason that it is important to recognize addiction as a disease is to remove the stigma that often accompanies it and legitimize its treatment. Finally, the disease concept establishes addiction as the primary illness and not some underlying symptom that will be alleviated once the real problem is solved.

The debate on whether chemical dependency is truly a disease is a common one. Opponents of the disease concept argue that addiction does not truly fit the criteria of a disease because, substance abusers make an active choice (i.e., to use chemicals or not to use chemicals) to inflict the disease upon themselves while diabetics, for instance, do not. Nor do diabetics derive pleasure from that choice. Furthermore, opponents would argue, addicts and alcoholics choose to pursue their drug use because they derive pleasure and satisfaction from it, and it is their pursuit of pleasure that leads them to become "sick." However, as Donald Goodwin cogently argues (1979), few opponents of the disease concept have difficulty accepting syphilis and gonorrhea as diseases, and these maladies parallel addiction in their etiology. All are derived from a choice to pursue a pleasurable activity that results in individuals suffering an infliction primarily because of their exposure to an external foreign agent or dangerous substance that would have not entered their physiological system had they not chosen to pursue that activity.

In fact, afflictions associated with improper habits and lifestyles that are incongruent with good long-range health contribute more to all diseases than is usually acknowledged. The crucial connection between lifestyle and disease has emerged largely because of a revolution in the healthcare requirements of the American people within the last seventy-five years. This revolution is one that Western industrial societies are just beginning to recognize and that the medical profession itself is just coming to grips with. The revolution in question is that the morbidity and mortality rates of Americans are no longer related to the infectious diseases prevalent at the turn of the century. Instead, the diseases that are most prevalent today are those related to chronic disorders associated with our lifestyles. Influenza, pneumonia, tuberculosis, gastroenteritis, and diphtheria have been replaced by heart disease, cerebrovascular disease, respiratory disease, various cancers, and alcoholism–all of which are in part a product of how we live and behave. How much we drink and eat, whether or not we smoke, how we deal with daily stress, and how much we exercise are the most important contributing factors to our health and our susceptibility to disease. In one sense, the most serious medical problems that plague the majority of individuals today are not ultimately medical problems at all; they are behavioral problems requiring the alteration of characteristic response patterns and thus, are directly related to lifestyle and attitudes toward lifestyle (Stachnik, 1980).

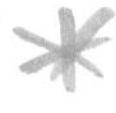

As modern medicine has begun to recognize that attitudes, lifestyles, and behavior play an important part in what is commonly called a disease, there has also been a growing awareness of the need for a "new medical paradigm" to help explain this phenomenon. The old medical formulation for identifying diseases has been criticized by many as relying too heavily on the mind-body split imposed on Western medical practices by René Descartes' sixteenth-century philosophical dualism. Thomas Kuhn (1962) pointed out years ago in his book, *The Structure of Scientific Revolutions*, that paradigm shifts only occur in science when enough anomalies begin to turn up, thus forcing a paradigm crisis. As he observed, scientific discovery, contrary to some popular misconceptions, is never achieved in a nice, orderly fashion as the result of the steady accumulation of more and more information. As more researchers and scientists explore the relationship between healing and physical illness, they are becoming aware that the relationship of the mind to both disease and recovery is an intricate one that challenges many of the conventional attitudes toward sickness and health.

Correspondingly, as addiction has moved from the fringes of our society into the mainstream of our everyday lives within the last three decades, it has had a profound impact on the way that our culture defines addiction and the way it treats it as a disease. Previously, addiction was almost exclusively limited to alcohol and drugs, but now it is not uncommon to hear people speaking of themselves as "excitement junkies," or "hooked" on tennis, running, racquetball, or other forms of exercise.

As the abstinence model of Alcoholics Anonymous gained popularity in the treatment of addiction, it legitimized the disease concept. In the 1970s, treatment centers began treating substance abusers in their alcohol recovery programs. While the treatment results of the integration of these two different addictions hasn't been as promising as first anticipated (because of reasons that will be outlined in Chapter 8), treatment personnel found there were many similarities and that the disease concept model worked better than anything else that was available at the time. It was discovered that although the behavior of the alcoholic patient differed from that of the addict, the recovery process was remarkably similar (Early, 1994). Gradually, treatment centers and addiction specialists began to recognize that there were many other obsessive-compulsive disorders and behaviors (e.g., gambling, food, sex, work, and even relationships) that were very similar in nature to the qualities that the alcoholic or addict shared in their addiction. More important, they were having similar success in their results when they addressed these disorders with the twelve-step model. At the same time, as counselors, psychiatrists, and other medical personnel continued to work with these patients on a sustained basis, they began to recognize that if an individual had one disorder, there was a very strong possibility that they would have another related disorder. It also became evident that for a vast number of these patients, eliminating one disorder (e.g., cocaine dependence) was likely to result in an increase in another disorder (e.g., sexual addiction).

The identification of co-dependency and Adult Children of Alcoholics (ACOAs) as other variations of this addictive process began to teach addiction specialists that addictions were related not by the substance used, but by the behavior and attitudes that typified all addictive diseases.

For instance, treating patients with eating disorders by the addictive model taught addiction specialists that the treatment efforts for all addictions should be focused inward, away from the substances and toward the thoughts, feelings, and actions that preceded or followed the compulsive consumption of substances or food. Approaching co-dependency and ACOA issues with similar strategies revealed that the addictive drive is an internal compulsion that need not be attached to a substance; it can manifest itself with an activity, a ritual, or even another person.

Addiction is now recognized as a disorder that can take many forms and manifest itself across a myriad of patterns. Schaffer (1995) for one has acknowledged that he has gradually come to hold the position that addiction is best understood as an altered state of consciousness that involves components of biochemical and physiological alterations of brain operations that are tied into adaptation in brain reward circuitry which results in long-term changes in brain functioning. It is these physiological adaptations of brain functioning that underlie compulsive behavior in response to conditioned cues. Consequently, addiction has more to do with learned behavior (conditioned responses due to powerful, emotional reward experiences) and deficits in cognitive and emotional functioning than it has to do with dependence on a drug or withdrawal symptoms related to abstinence. Once an addictive style or obsessive-compulsive pattern of responding and thinking is established in the brain because of a substance's biochemical impact, the person is conditioned or prone to substitute one manifestation, compulsion, or object of addictive preoccupation for another. The general consensus in the neurosciences about addiction is voiced by Steve Heyman (1995) who is of the opinion that addiction is best defined as a "brain disease." Based on years of accumulated data derived from the neurosciences, he views addiction as a disease uniquely tied into neural underpinnings of motivation and emotion; the pathophysiology of which involves drug-induced, long-lived molecular changes in the brains of vulnerable individuals. This results in a perversion of the normal volitional control of behavior. Heyman believes this ingrained behavioral pattern cannot be altered as long as chemicals are being used and "like all patients with a serious chronic disease, the addicted individual can be asked to comply with treatment and to avoid behavior that put himself at high risk of relapse."

ADDICTION, ABSTINENCE, AND THE DISEASE CONCEPT

Accepting addiction as a disease has other important implications because the disease concept always requires that abstinence be the necessary first step in treatment. For a number of years there has been a hotly debated controversy surrounding the issue of whether abstinence is always a necessary requirement in the treatment of alcoholism. Behaviorally and cognitively oriented researchers have advocated offering controlled drinking as a treatment alternative (Martlatt, 1983; Sobell and Sobell, 1973a; Pendery, Maltzman, and West, 1982). During the early 1980s, this controversy was somewhat resolved in favor of the abstinence position, after numerous follow-up studies on controlled drinking found that claims that alcoholics were able to maintain self-control while drinking were either greatly exaggerated or misleading. Vaillant (1995) demonstrated in a very well-controlled, long-term, follow-up study that 80 to 90 percent of previously identified successful controlled drinkers had relapsed. Even the media and the popular press got caught up in the debate when a popular television news program (*60 Minutes*) conducted its own follow-up on a study that claimed to have successfully treated alcoholics with controlled drinking. To the researchers' embarrassment, *60 Minutes* discovered that their findings were grossly misleading. Of the twenty successfully treated alcoholics, it was discovered that nineteen had either relapsed or died drinking.

In the last few years, this debate has once again reared its controversial head in the form of the Natural Recovery research of Sobell (1995) and the Moderation Management (MM) program advocated by Alan Marlatt and others. In both instances, the emphasis is on identifying those individuals who can either drink moderately, cut down on their consumption of alcohol, obtain "nonabstinent recovery," or stop drinking on their own without treatment or AA.

Certainly, the AA approach to the treatment of addiction is not for everyone and there are individuals who may respond better to other avenues of treatment. Researchers such as Marlatt (1983) and Sobell (1995) should be applauded for their attempt to identify and explore alternative treatment options for those who fail to respond to AA and other twelve-step approaches. The problem arises when there is inconsistency in the diagnostic criteria for determining who is or who is not an alcoholic or addict. The implication of this confusion in criteria can have far-reaching effects. Certainly, there are many individuals who experience dependency and physical or psychological withdrawal symptoms who are not necessarily addicted based on the criteria that AA and other twelve-step programs use in their definition of addiction. Drug abusers and sporadic heavy binge drinkers may not necessarily be identified as addicted by AA standards and would be by Sobell's or Marlatt's criteria.

The Natural Recovery research by Sobell (1995) attempts to demonstrate that some individuals can either reduce or stop drinking on their own without AA or any formal treatment. Sobell is attempting to identify the characteristics of those individuals who resolve their difficulties without treatment or self-help groups. She is also attempting to identify the percentage of recoveries that are "non-abstinent drinking recoveries." Similarly, Marlatt's Moderation Management approach maintains that some drinkers can learn to manage their drinking without eliminating it entirely. There are two important aspects of these research efforts that need to be questioned. Aren't the substitutions of new terminology such as Natural Recovery and Moderation Management really just variations of the old controlled drinking controversy dressed up in new clothes? Most good follow-up studies essentially demonstrated that any reports of successful controlled drinking diminished with the passage of time. Most alcoholics can control their drinking or abstain from drinking for short periods of time. AA has always known this. Those who can stop on their own or can drink moderately are not alcoholic according to AA. Abstinence and AA are only for alcoholics who want to stop drinking and want help in doing so.

Second, Marlatt's and Sobell's research is showing that those individuals with less severe symptoms and shorter periods of problem drinking do not have to abstain in order to experience recovery. AA would simply counter by saying those people are not and never were alcoholics. Alcoholics, by definition, cannot control or manage their drinking successfully over an extended period of time. Neuropsychological and neurophysical research findings support the reported individual experience of every alcoholic and addict who is in a twelve-step recovery program. Abstinence is the necessary first step if long-term recovery is to be obtained and then maintained. From this standpoint, AA and other twelve-step programs depart widely from the more behaviorally oriented treatment philosophies, which are more likely to look at alcohol consumption and its control as an end result of their efforts. For AA, abstinence—or more correctly, sobriety—is the beginning of treatment, not the end. As one recovery addict said recently in an AA meeting: "AA didn't give me back my life, it gave me my life for the first time."

Marlatt's and Sobell's research is demonstrating the importance of establishing a consistent diagnostic criteria if useful research is to be conducted. Twelve-step programs and behaviorally oriented researchers just do not look at, define, and understand addiction in the same way. For recovering alcoholics and addicts, addiction is much more than a bad habit that needs to be changed. It involves an attitude, a belief system, and the values that one holds which dictate the way a person will live his or her life. While the intensity of this debate is fueled by strong personal beliefs and passionate professional territoriality, it has relatively little clinical effect outside the arena of academia and those few treatment programs that utilize aversion and behavioral therapy. The majority of clinicians and treatment program counselors in this country know by their experience what recovering addicts and alcoholics and AA, NA, and CA have always known: abstinence is the only treatment alternative for the addict and alcoholic. Yet the controversy has far greater implications than merely academic ones. As every person who is either addicted or who has worked with chemically dependent individuals on a sustained basis knows, there is nothing that alcoholics or addicts want to hear and believe more than the statement that they can learn to control their alcohol and drug use in a socially accepted manner. Put ten alcoholics in a room and tell them that research shows that one out of ten can return to normal drinking and each one will believe that they are the one special case. As Wallace (1984) demonstrated in an informal survey of 160 alcoholics currently in treatment, all 160 had in the past tried controlled drinking and failed. Considering that these 160 failures may not be as unfortunate as the ones who fatally succumbed to their disease, the controversy takes on an added sense of urgency. This is especially true in light of the evidence which suggests that abstinence has few, if any, detrimental effects for a person, even if that person is "only" an abuser and not "really addicted." To the contrary, abstinence usually leads to increased health and satisfaction with one's life. Therefore, the risks of abstaining from drugs and alcohol must be carefully weighed against the probable cost to the person who tries controlled use and fails. In many cases, this can be a fatal mistake.

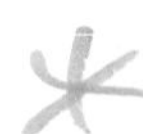

As implied earlier, the controversy surrounding controlled drinking, Natural Recovery, and Moderation Management is also complicated by the differences in diagnostic criteria that many professionals use when they are conducting controlled drinking research. An individual diagnosed as an alcoholic in one study might not fit the criteria for an alcoholic in another study. Certainly, many individuals defined as alcoholic by Alcoholics Anonymous would fail to be diagnosed as such by someone using the *DSM-IV* criteria (American Psychiatric Association, 1994). What many professionals fail to appreciate is that the *DSM-IV* criteria for alcoholism is not better than AA's, it is just different.

Curtis Barrett summed up this controversy nicely when he wrote:

> To illustrate how very diverse diagnostic or intake criteria might be these days, it is instructive to contrast those used by the DSM-III criteria (American Psychiatric Association, 1980), with those used by the venerable self-help group, Alcoholics Anonymous. In DSM-III one

> is first struck by the fact that "alcoholism" is not listed as a mental disorder. However, careful reading reveals the statement that "Alcohol Dependence has been called alcoholism" (American Psychiatric Association, 1980, p. 169). To diagnose Alcohol Dependence the following are required: (a) either a pattern of pathological alcohol use or impairment in social or occupational functioning due to alcohol use, and (b) either tolerance or withdrawal. The distinction between alcoholism and alcohol abuse boils down to whether one finds tolerance or withdrawal. Thus, a person with a history of blackouts, binges, failure to control excessive drinking, loss of job and legal difficulties (e.g., driving while intoxicated), may not be diagnosed as being alcoholic/alcohol dependent if one uses DSM-III criteria. (1985, p. 19)

AA, as always, avoids such controversy and, true to its tradition, "keeps it simple." AA members are told to diagnose themselves. Another's diagnosis of someone else's alcoholism is held secondary to that individual's diagnosis of him or herself. AA members are alcoholic if they say they are alcoholic. AA does provide the literature and the information necessary if the person so desires it. But characterization of oneself as alcoholic is the cornerstone of the AA program.

Barrett (1985) adds,

> In a chapter in "How it works" (AA World Service, 1939, p. 58) one reads that a person who wants what AA has should consider taking certain steps that are "suggested as a program of recovery." The first of these is: "We admitted we were powerless over alcohol–that our lives have become unmanageable." If the person wants further help in self-diagnosis there is material that will permit a sort of matching operation that is not too different from that followed in the DSM-III. (1985, p. 19)

Sobriety is clearly the goal of AA. However, AA is a program of recovery which addresses the difficult adjustments that are necessary if one is to remain alcohol- and drug-free. "AA does not teach us how to handle our drinking . . . It teaches us how to handle our sobriety" (Alcoholics Anonymous, 1939, p. 554). AA does not rule out the possibility that the alcoholic may return to controlled drinking, but that it is a goal that cannot be achieved if a person is a true alcoholic. Thus, AA recognizes that those alcoholics who return to controlled drinking were misdiagnosed.

Considering these criteria problems, it is conceivable that a competent researcher utilizing the *DSM-III* or *DSM-IV* criteria for alcohol dependence would fail to define as alcoholic an individual whom AA sees as alcoholic, even if this person so defined themselves. Such difficulties help explain why the controlled drinking, Natural Recovery, and Moderation Management studies have resulted in such controversial and contradictory conclusions.

Those whose interest in addiction is only passing or purely academic fail to understand the significance of this criteria problem. For alcoholics and substance abusers struggling with their disease, it is literally a matter of life and death. For instance, Wallace (1984b) sees the ideological base of AA providing a crucial component in the alcoholic's and addict's recovery process. In fact, he contends that the alcoholic and addict need AA's somewhat biased view of reality. "The alcoholic can ill afford the dispassionate, disinterested, and indeed, almost casual play upon words and ideas of the inquiring academic intellectual" (1975, p. 7).

Wallace strongly feels that the chemically dependent individual recognizes intuitively the need for a stable and enduring belief system if he or she is to stay sober and clean. Wallace has more difficulty in comprehending and discerning the equally biased view of reality of the academician. His contention is that:

> Hidden neatly beneath the rhetoric of science and scientism are the actualities of dreadfully inadequate personality measuring instruments, inappropriate sampling procedures, inadequate measuring operations, improper choice of variables for study, grossly violated statistical assumptions, data gathering, recording and analyzing errors, and so on and so forth. Is it any wonder then that the most outstanding quality of most academic research is now you see it, now you don't? Are we really amazed to find sober alcoholics clinging to their belief systems like drowning poets to their metaphors in a sea of confusion? (1975, p. 7)

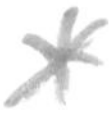

Wallace also recognizes the importance of helping individuals achieve a self-attribution of alcoholic and, hence, an explanatory system for their behavior. Treatment from this standpoint is very much the teaching of an "exotic belief" whose true value of actually describing what has occurred to individuals because of their addiction is held as irrelevant. Its true value is determined by the fact that it (1) helps explain the past in a way that gives hope for the future; (2) allows alcoholics and addicts to cope with their guilt, anxiety, remorse, and confusion; and (3) provides them with a specific behavior–staying sober or clean and working the twelve steps of the program–that will change their lives in a desired direction. As Wallace says, alcoholics or addicts have a lifetime of sobriety in which to recognize the fact that not all of their personal and social difficulties are the result of their addiction. But they can come to this realization after they have gotten the alcohol and drugs out of their system and have steered their lives in the desired direction. As Martin Buber (1964) recognizes, persons in crisis need direction; it is only after sobriety has been maintained that they can start to investigate some of the deeper psychological issues in their lives.

Recent neuropsychological research has shed some light on the importance of providing alcoholics and addicts with a clear, structured program that they must follow during their first months of abstinence. New members of twelve-step programs are told not to make any major decisions during the first year of recovery. They are instructed not to analyze the program. They are told, "The program works because it works! Go to ninety meetings in ninety days! Take the body and the mind will follow!" Each of these suggestions is based on AA's and other twelve-step programs' intuitive understanding that alcoholics and addicts, during the early stages of abstinence, are incapable of thinking clearly and do not possess the intellectual capabilities necessary for rational, intelligent decisions. The program provides them with twelve clear steps that they must follow. New members are told to "keep it simple." After they finish the first step, they are told to complete the second step and then proceed on to the third step, and so on.

On neuropsychological tests sensitive to abstract reasoning, flexible thinking, fluid intelligence, and new learning, alcoholics and addicts consistently score in the brain-impaired range (see Chapter 8). Yet their verbal intelligence and old learning remains pretty much intact. Consequently, they will often appear unimpaired to the unsuspecting observer. Their level of impairment is usually not permanent and does not involve cortical structural damage. Rather, their brain dysfunction is of a diffuse nature, usually the result of an alcohol-induced encephalopathy exacerbated by nutritional and vitamin deficiencies. Most alcoholics and addicts experience "spontaneous recovery" from the loss of cortical functioning if they remain alcohol- and drug-free and improve their vitamin and nutritional intake. This recovery of cognitive functioning is gradual and steady. The greatest improvement is usually experienced in the first months with total recovery achieved after one to two years of abstinence.

Considering the implications of this research, the structure and direction that AA and other twelve-step programs provide at the beginning of the alcoholic's and addict's recovery are vital. However, there is another important aspect of twelve-step programs that many professionals fail to appreciate. The twelve-step program provides the newly recovering addict and alcoholic with hope and inspiration. Jerome Frank would say AA and other twelve-step programs help combat the alcoholic's and addict's demoralization. Yalom would speak of the instillation of hope and the Buddhist teachings emphasizing the necessity of "vital lies" in our life. This is very close to what Wallace prescribes when he suggests teaching the alcoholic and addict an "exotic belief." Twelve-step programs work because they do not overlook the significance of belief and inspiration in an individual's life.

The differences between the way that the AA community and the academically oriented professional view and understand addiction can best be captured by referring to how Sogyal Rinpoche, a Tibetan monk and the author of *The Tibetan Way of Living and Dying* (1992), described his experience when he left his native country of Tibet and began to lecture on the Buddhist teaching here in the United States. To his surprise, he discovered that individuals who belonged to Western cultures responded in a dramatically different way than did individuals of Eastern cultures or his own country of Tibet. Those in the West would find the teaching "interesting," while those in the East would find the Buddhist teaching "inspiring." He discovered a totally different expectation and response from those with different cultural experiences and values. Rinpoche was acutely aware that we are a product of our Western heritage and that our culture has a tendency to value the intellect over the emotions, the rational over the spiritual, and the mind over the heart. Our experience dictates what it is that we will see, know, and ultimately respond to.

This point was dramatically brought home to me in a very personal way early in my professional career many years ago when I was recruited to join a private practice psychiatric group in Atlanta that specialized in addictive medicine. There were a number of physicians in this practice who were recovering from their own addiction to chemicals and alcohol. All of them had become clean and sober either through AA or treatment programs that emphasized the disease concept and the twelve-step approach to recovery. All of them, even though they had been clean and sober for years, were still very active in the program. Consequently, the twelve-step approach to treatment was heavily reflected in their own approach and treatment with their addicted patients. After I had been working with this practice a number of months, one of the psychiatrists (I'll call him Sam) who had been sober and active in AA for nearly twenty years stepped out of his office, which was next to mine, and asked how I was doing and adjusting to a practice that specialized in addiction. Part of the reason for his inquiry had to do with his curiosity about my recent attendance at the SECAD (Southeast Conference on Addictive Diseases) conference that was held each year in Atlanta. For those readers who have never attended or are unfamiliar with the conference, it is a six-day event that is focused exclusively on the twelve-step and disease concept approach to treatment. It is heavily attended by health service professionals who are in their own recovery from addiction. Sam was interested in my reaction to the conference since he knew this was the first time I had attended SECAD. But he was also a little suspicious of my attitude toward addiction and the AA program since he viewed me as someone fresh out of academia and "outside of the program." I suspect that he wasn't sure if I was one of those "ignorant professionals" that he and other members of the program had learned to be distrustful of because of the poor treatment, poor management, and misdiagnosis they had experienced during their own addictions. In response to his questions of what I thought of the conference, I answered in all honesty that I wasn't much impressed with it. When he asked why, I told him that I didn't hear or find a lot of useful or new information about treatment and addiction. He laughed good-naturedly, shook his head, and said, "Phil, you missed the whole point, people don't go to SECAD to get information, they go to get inspired."

In the same way, the recovering addict or alcoholic doesn't go to AA for information; they go for inspiration. Much like Rinpoche has written in his book on Buddhism, inspiration is a very crucial part of treatment and that is why the program works and why many academicians will never understand it. They forget or are not in touch with the psychic pain, emptiness, and desperate feeling of demoralization that alcoholics or addicts are struggling with. Addicts and alcoholics need more than information; they need to be inspired and touched emotionally by someone. Their addiction has isolated them and shut them off from genuine authentic human contact. Much in the way that Yalom (1995) writes about the importance of identification, altruism, and instillation of hope as powerful curative factors in group, so are these forces working in a twelve-step meeting. One must never forget that behind the label of alcoholic or substance abuser is a lving, breathing, human being who is suffering, confused, isolated, and desperately in need of a belief and a direction in the midst of his or her crisis.

An illustration from the Buddhist religious tradition might help clarify the importance of vital lies, instillation of hope, exotic beliefs, and inspiration in the treatment of addiction. The concept of "useful illusions" is a central one in the Buddhist religion. The Buddhist monk and religious teacher realized the importance of mobilizing an individual's faith and hope during the early stages of doubt and confusion in his or her life. It is "useful" to create an "illusion" which may allow individual disciples to grasp an important principle of life that they might not otherwise be ready to accept in the early stage of their journey to self-understanding.

Hutchinson (1969) sums up the Buddhist position when he describes the aim of the Noble Eightfold Path:

> What was the content of this experience? Buddha's answer resembled a physician's terse diagnosis and prescription of therapy for a disease, Buddhist tradition has communicated Buddha's truth in the form of the Four Noble Truths and the Noble Eightfold Path. The first two of the Four Truths may be termed diagnosis and the third and fourth, therapy. The first asserts that all existence is misery, or *dukkha*, and the second that misery is rooted in ignorant craving, or *trishna*. The third truth asserts that misery may be abolished by abolishing ignorant craving, and the fourth truth asserts that this can be done by the Noble Eightfold Path. Thus as one Buddhist writer puts it, Buddha "had found the sovereign remedy for all the major ills of mankind." (p. 111)

Central to Buddhist teaching is the "blowing out" of the flame of passion. Often confused with annihilation or death, the aim of the Buddha was to get the disciple to extinguish the "ignorant cravings" that produced misery. Much like the Buddhist disciple in the excerpt above, alcoholics must "surrender" what they think will make them happy (drinking) and come to recognize that it is their misconception of happiness (ignorant craving) that causes their suffering. The breaking of this cycle is enhanced by useful illusions.

The Buddhist disciple would approach the Buddhist monk with the question of the meaning of life and the desire to experience Nirvana. The disciple was told to meditate and practice the eightfold path to enlightenment, which included right action and right thinking. After six months of meditation, the disciple again visited the teacher for instructions, as he had not yet reached enlightenment. Two years later, the disciple again asked for a meeting with his teacher, complaining that he had done all that he had been instructed to do and had not yet reached Nirvana. The student tried to remain accepting as he was told that he must be patient and continue to practice the eightfold path to enlightenment. Finally, after five years of dutiful meditation and practice, the student could no longer contain his frustration and finally confronted the Buddhist monk with his anger, saying, "I have done all that you have told me! I practiced the eightfold path to enlightenment! I have meditated daily and practiced the principles of right thinking and right action! I have done all these things, and I have not reached Nirvana!" To this, the Buddhist monk answered with love and understanding, "My son, there is no Nirvana, but because of your meditation and practice of the eightfold path, you are better off, aren't you?"

Much like the Buddhist disciple, recovering alcoholics who have worked the twelve-step program of recovery are better off. Their lives, which were in a shambles, have some direction and are now in order. Their health, both psychological and physical, is usually restored. Now, after five years of sobriety, they can realize that all of their problems were not really caused by their alcoholism. They have not reached enlightenment, but they are better off than they were when they were drinking or using drugs.

This is the significant issue that the controlled drinking, Natural Recovery, and MM advocates clearly miss. Why even bother to teach an alcoholic or addict to drink moderately or use drugs recreationally? Alcoholics Anonymous, as advocated by its founder Bill Wilson, was far more interested in alcoholics' or addicts' lifestyles and their distorted, bankrupt philosophy of life. While facing the issues of drinking, drug use, and abstinence is of crucial importance to the program, it is only the first step in the twelve-steps of recovery. An often unnoticed fact is that the first step of the AA and other twelve-step programs is the only step that explicitly mentions drinking or drug use. The other eleven steps are there for alcoholics and addicts to use as a guide to change their lifestyles and the bankruptcy of their values. Such a viewpoint leads one to wonder why training substance abusers to moderately use chemicals is so attractive. It is such a paltry goal and misses the boat completely. As McCrady (1985) writes,

> People who earn an alcoholism diagnosis have worked hard for it–they have consumed enormous quantities of ethanol and have created terrible personal pain in their lives because of their alcohol consumption. Why, then, continue to attempt to drink and risk the pain over and over? Instead of trying to help alcoholics drink, therapists might better view such a desire to drink as an "irrational belief." Psychologists' burgeoning knowledge of cognitive behavior modification could then be used to help alcoholics challenge the irrational belief that C_2H_5OH is so important that it cannot be totally eliminated from their lives. (p. 370)

Furthermore, if the Natural Recovery and Moderation Management advocates wanted to demonstrate that alcoholics can drink with control for a time, then it would only confirm what most people familiar with Alcoholics Anonymous have known for a long time. Alcoholics often drink with control for years before they either quit or die. They also have usually been able to control their consumption for weeks at a time, even months. Yet, it is the emotional suffering and the bankruptcy of their lives that need to be changed and treated. Most alcoholics would admit that control only spoils their drinking. Many ask, Why would I want to have only one beer? Within this viewpoint, control is not a desirable goal for those addicted because control actually inhibits the freedom that alcoholics most strongly want to pursue. Control is a problem for every addicted individual, not the solution. As Stewart (1985) writes,

> Alcoholics in trouble suffer more from the use of control than its loss. A truly free alcoholic is not concerned with maintaining control. He or she is much more interested in ongoing freedom. The alcoholic in control, fearing its loss, is not a good example of enjoyable sobriety . . . Abstinence is one condition of enduring freedom for the alcoholic. Most alcoholics who have been sober for years would support that belief, but one is not sober on abstinence alone. There is a creative discipline in sobriety that is not present in mere abstinence for its own sake. Abstinence for itself, by willpower, is a control, but abstinence and devotion to sobriety is a disciplined act of love. (pp. 373-374)

What appears reasonable as a possible solution to this controversy is to ask that the patients themselves weigh the risks and benefits of abstinence-oriented vs. Moderation Management treatments. However, since addicts or alcoholics in the throes of their addiction are usually incapable of making such an important and rational decision, the risks associated with abstinence-oriented therapy do not seem great since many persons choose to be abstinent and do not appear to be harmed by their abstinence. Why not develop a partnership between Alcoholics Anonymous and professionally oriented treatment approaches and combine the two different sets of knowledge and expertise? By doing so, the chances are greater of developing an innovative treatment model that may actually help more alcoholics and addicts, rather than continuing the destructive territorial fighting that is presently occurring. This is precisely the aim of this book and will be a constant theme that runs throughout its presented alternatives to the successful treatment of the chemically dependent individual.

Those professionals who are suspicious or antagonistic toward twelve-step programs might have something valuable to learn if they were instead to direct some of their energy toward understanding what the programs are about and how they work. More than anything else, AA is a pragmatic program that is less concerned with whys than it is with how. Instead of trying to discredit it or tear it apart, both the professional and the addicted patient would be better served if AA were understood for its results. As new members of the program are often told, "If it's not broke, why fix it?" Those critical of the program only see its spiritual roots and judge it to be a religious organization with an ideology that fosters debasement, compliance, mind control, and dependence. Many critics, whose own ideological beliefs are deeply rooted in Western rational philosophy and the science of psychology, might be more understanding and accepting of AA if they were to recognize that many of the program's historical roots can be traced back to William James, one of the early pioneers of the science of psychology and the philosophy of Pragmatism. James's writings and his classic text, *The Varieties of Religious Experience* (1902), had a profound effect on Bill Wilson, the chief architect of AA, the Big Book, and its twelve-steps and twelve principles. One main tenet for James, as it was for all Pragmatists, was that the process of determining the value and truth of something was closely related to its utility and practical usefulness. If something worked, it was judged to be true. The Pragmatists were far less interested in grand, abstract, and obtuse theories, or what John Dewey came to call "spectator knowledge," than they were in the nitty-gritty practical aspects of knowledge that came from the experience of something working after it had been tried and tested.

AA members are told "Utilize! Don't analyze; go to ninety meetings in ninety days!" Following James's recommendation that if you want to change the way you are thinking or feeling, first change the way you are behaving, AA members are told "Take your body to a meeting and your mind will follow." Nowhere is this pragmatic influence more clearly demonstrated than with Father Martin, a Catholic priest and early AA enthusiast who is the living embodiment of AA and its philosophy. Once, when asked why AA works, Father Martin responded in his own unique style by saying, "AA works because it works!" The utility of teaching the addict or alcoholic to behave according to the principles of the twelve-step program determines its usefulness and its truth.

Since the publication of the first edition of this book (1988), there has been a growing number of professionals who have been much more accepting and knowledgeable about AA and its twelve-step philosophy. They see the disadvantages of working against AA and have sought ways of bringing AA and professional treatment programs together. Minkoff (1995) for one has suggested the value of a complementary integration of twelve-step and mental health treatment philosophies. He believes there is a need for a "unified conceptual model" of treatment that considers both the disease model of addiction and a disease model of mental illness. While Minkoff is specifically focusing on the dual diagnosis patient who may be psychotic as well as addicted, his attempt to view addiction as a disease that involves two independent and primary but interactive illnesses has merit because he recognizes that the split between the mental health model and the disease model is an unnecessary one. He recognizes that the historical roots of the split originated in the medical establishment's failure to adequately treat or understand alcoholics. Essentially, modern medicine had turned its back on the alcoholic's plight, and it was this failure of the medical establishment in the 1930s that forced Bill Wilson and other suffering alcoholics to create their own treatment method. They were more concerned with one that worked and were less concerned with the prevailing beliefs and philosophies of the day that dictated what was properly an illness and what properly constituted treatment.

Minkoff challenges the typical hierarchical medical approach to treatment and its tendency to foster this separation between the mental health model and the disease model. He asks us to consider how ridiculous this situation would be if we were to practice it with other aspects of psychiatric care. Imagine if someone with anxiety could only be treated by an anxiety disorder specialist and if there were any signs of depression, a depression specialist would have to be called in.

Fortunately, there are a growing number of professionals and researchers who are starting to appreciate the advantages of AA and other twelve-step programs. They are discovering that the integration of the two can be quite complementary. For instance, Dodes (1988) commented that based on his experience with more than 500 patients treated with a combination of psychoanalytic psychotherapy and twelve-step programs, he found that "patients appear able to implicitly grasp a dual level of functioning within themselves and therefore to accept the dual level of therapeutics approach" (p. 288). In a similar fashion, Brown reported comparable results in her excellent book, *Treating the Alcoholic: A Developmental Model of Recovery* (1985), based on a ten-year study that she conducted on recovering alcoholics who had successfully stopped drinking. While she was primarily interested in identifying what worked for these AA members and why, her other main impetus for the book was an attempt to form a "synergistic partnership between the domains of AA and professional helpers," because she was acutely aware of the mistrust and competitive animosity between the two. While she states that she is clearly on the side of the alcoholic and that her "book is a challenge to professional helpers and nonalcoholics from all disciplines to reexamine their own beliefs, values and theories about alcohol and alcoholism," she believes strongly that "the alcoholic badly needs the professional." Her book is one example of a growing number of appeals for a "synergistic working relationship" that is starting to come from the professional community.

Aware of the reasons for the split, Brown cautions the alcoholic about the dangers that are still inherent in the professional community when she writes:

> If you are suffering from alcoholism, it is likely that your alcoholism will not be diagnosed by physicians, psychologists, or other helping professionals. If your alcoholism is diagnosed, the chances are good that you will receive an inappropriate referral for treatment. You may be told to "cut down" on your drinking, or you may be sent to a psychiatrist to determine what the real problem is. If you are abstinent and recovering from alcoholism and need professional help for other life problems, the chances are good that you will be too afraid of the professionals to seek the treatment you require. Of course there are many exceptions, but it is a bleak picture. (p. ix)

Brown's conclusions help explain why recovering addicts or alcoholics may be distrustful of professionals. Certainly many members of twelve-step programs have earned the right to be suspicious of "ignorant professionals" who have often misdiagnosed them and offered little help in their struggles with their individual addictions. For example, alcoholics frequently report a personal downward spiral when they were advised "to cut down on their drinking" while the professional sought to get at the "real core" of their problem. One need only attend a few AA meetings to hear the horror stories told by many members. In fact, AA would have never come into existence if it had not been for the kind of help alcoholics desperately needed. AA, as a social phenomenon, is an example of how a certain portion of an inflicted population banded together in a community of help because society's sanctioned mode of treatment was inadequate. Yet the founder of AA himself–Bill Wilson–had no doubts about the mutual cooperation of AA and professional help in his own treatment and recovery from alcoholism. He twice returned to long-term individual psychotherapy with his friend and advocate, psychiatrist Harry Tiebout. Research conducted by AA reveals that 60 percent of AA membership has sought some form of psychological treatment in the past and this percentage is increasing each year (Alcoholics Anonymous, 1990).

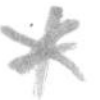

Most of the criticism of Alcoholics Anonymous in the past has focused on its ideological and religious overtones, with the implication that AA puts pressure on its members to accept the AA belief system and that this pressure harms them in some way. For instance, Tournier (1979) criticized AA's effectiveness because he felt that it was a treatment method that had never been scientifically established and that the fellowship's ideology dominated the treatment field, which resulted in a situation that limited new ideas. Jones (1970) also criticized the AA program as an "acceptance of totalitarian ideology" (p. 195). Unfortunately, these types of attacks are short-sighted and reflect ill-informed beliefs about the treatment philosophy of Alcoholics Anonymous. Chemically dependent individuals would be better served if critics of AA would direct their energies toward understanding the ideological differences that exist between themselves and the AA program. If they would gain a more accurate understanding of AA, they would find that the disparity between their position and AA's is actually not that great. Professionals may actually learn a great deal more about psychotherapy and treatment, not only for the addicted individual, but for the person who does not suffer from an addiction problem. It is within the realm of group psychotherapy that these two opposing views can best be merged into a supportive approach to therapy. The marriage of the principles of Alcoholics Anonymous and group psychotherapy could result in an exciting and extremely complementary enterprise.

Chapter 2

Different Models of Group Psychotherapy

Abraham Maslow is attributed as once saying, "If the only tool you have is a hammer, every problem you see will look like a nail." Maslow's satirical but cogent statement summarizes precisely the potential dilemma of adapting wholeheartedly and unquestioningly any one single theory of treatment and "cure" for addiction. Despite this book's blatant bias for utilizing the disease concept, looking at addiction only from the disease perspective can lead an unsuspecting observer to see only the nail (i.e., the disease of addiction) which has to be pounded into place by the only tool available (i.e., Alcoholics Anonymous, for instance). However, AA is not the only organization that has certain members who are myopically limited because of their tunnel vision. Group psychotherapy, as well as most formal schools (i.e., the psychodynamic, Rogerian, Gestalt, etc.) of psychotherapy have more than their share of adherents who believe their way is the only right way to treat patients who suffer from addiction. Unfortunately, such factionalism is short-sighted and limits the number of options available for utilizing different tools in the treatment of addiction.

This chapter will focus not so much on the necessity of twelve-step programs and professionals banding together in a spirit of mutual cooperation, as it will be directed toward providing a systematic model for treating the chemically dependent individual within a group setting. Group psychotherapy, as it is taught and practiced today, suffers from its own form of factionalism. Adherents of different group psychotherapy models frequently attest to the superiority of their particular approach to group treatment. Each model of group psychotherapy has something unique to offer to a certain population and in the hands of skilled clinicians, these different models can provide powerful therapeutic experiences for its group members. However, a model has to be matched with the needs of the particular population being treated, and the goals of treatment also have an important influence on the model that is chosen. If group psychotherapy is to be a powerful adjunct in the treatment of addiction, a number of important questions must be asked and ultimately answered. For example, at what particular stage of recovery is the addicted individual? A group made up of individuals with two to three days of sobriety is far different from a group of individuals with one to two years of sobriety. Second, what is the aim of the group? More specifically, is abstinence from alcohol and drugs the goal of treatment, and how can this be enhanced in a group psychotherapy setting? The aim of this chapter is not to advocate one approach to group psychotherapy over another as much as it is to discern which model best meets the needs of the chemically dependent individual at that individual's stage of recovery. Each particular model of group psychotherapy to be presented here requires that the group leader analyze certain aspects of the group or group members' behavior differently.

Different ways of analyzing groups have a tremendous impact on what the leader observes and ultimately responds to in a group. This, in turn, is influenced by the basic task that the group hopes to accomplish and subsequently affects the different levels of intervention that a group leader chooses to make. These are decisions a group leader and a treating institution have to make before members are placed in a group setting. These crucial aspects of group psychotherapy will be discussed in relation to the most common and popular approaches to group psychotherapy. Each particular model available to the potential leader will be critiqued in relation to the special difficulties it poses for the group leader of a group whose members are suffering from an addiction problem.

SOME MODELS OF GROUP PSYCHOTHERAPY

Successful group psychotherapy, whether it be with chemically dependent members or non-addicted members, requires that two conditions be adhered to and maintained. First, the group task and structure should fit and be matched with the members' needs. If the leader and the treating institution adhere to the disease model, abstinence must be the goal and the group task should be structured to accomplish this end. Second, the leader's decision and technique should be adapted so that there is a match to the overall task or purpose of the group. Unfortunately, group goals are often vague or confusing, with not enough emphasis on a systematic plan for accomplishing these goals. Leaders and members often tend to view groups in terms of techniques (i.e., communication exercises, hot seat, etc.) or theoretical orientation (psychodynamic, Gestalt, etc.) rather than in terms of a goal or a task to be accomplished. Techniques and theories can become sacred rituals rather than tools for the accomplishment of the tasks that are the specified purpose of the group. In the same vein, a variety of group approaches that emerge to serve special purposes, as in twelve-step programs and group psychotherapy, are often seen as competing enterprises rather than different modes for achieving similar ends.

Singer et al. (1975) have outlined a heuristic "cognitive map" of the group psychotherapy field that categorizes the group event in terms of two basic parameters: (1) the task system of the group event; and (2) psychological levels of the systems involved in that task. This cognitive map will be presented here in an adapted form in order to give potential group leaders a better understanding of the alternatives available in their approach to conducting a group with chemically dependent individuals. Group events for Singer fit somewhere on a hypothetical continuum that has learning at one end and psychological change at the other. Despite the dangers of oversimplification, group members involved in such a presentation can be thought of as being placed in small group for two primary reasons. They are gathered together either to learn some new information or to change some aspect of their behavior.

Within Singer's context, learning is defined as that which occurs within an individual's experience that results in a cognitive or perceptual change. Anyone reading this chapter is hopefully attaining a cognitive change as result of learning new information. Psychological change is defined in the sense of altered coping capacity, personality structure alteration, or response repertoire expansion. Psychological change from this perspective is usually associated with an experiential component of the group event, with less emphasis on the alteration of a member's cognitive set. Every gathering of members within a group is usually geared toward one of these two components. A particular orientation of the group and its leader plays an important determining factor in the amount of emphasis that will be placed on learning or on change in a particular group. Certainly, learning and change are not mutually exclusive and indeed often mediate each other. Yet, in any particular group psychotherapy setting, there should be an implicit, if not explicit, priority that determines which task (i.e., learning or change) will be pursued at the expense of the other. Within a group psychotherapy setting with chemically dependent members, if one considers the possible consequences of continued alcohol consumption for many practicing alcoholics, change must take priority over learning, at least during the early stages of treatment. Therefore, tasks within a group psychotherapy setting can be defined along a three-point continuum: (1) learning; (2) learning and change; and (3) change. (See Figure 2.1.)

FIGURE 2.1

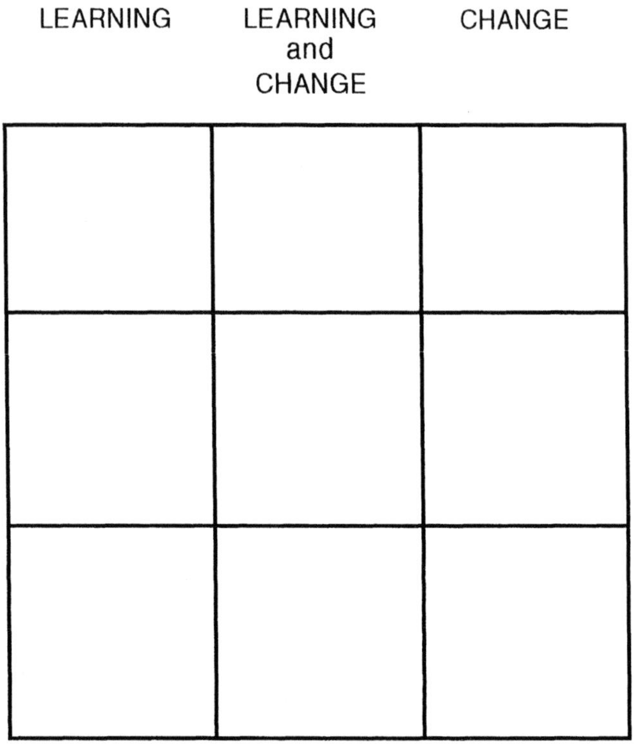

LEARNING	LEARNING and CHANGE	CHANGE

Source: Singer et al. (1975)

PSYCHOLOGICAL LEVELS OF INTERVENTION

A group leader has at his or her disposal a number of viable options for how to analyze and intervene in a group psychotherapy setting. The relevant levels of psychological intervention can generally be placed within three broad, yet distinct, categories. First, the group leader can choose to intervene on a group process level (i.e., What is the particular group event and what are the dynamics that have led to the current set of responses for a particular member or members within the group setting at this particular moment?). Second, the group leader has the choice of focusing on the interpersonal process within the group (i.e., What is the particular interaction occurring between certain members of the group? Why does one member react in a supportive fashion with most of the other group members, only to respond in an attacking manner with another member who presents himself within a similar set of circumstances?). Third, the group leader can decide to focus on the intrapersonal process with each particular member (i.e., How does each member defend, react, and deal with his or her anxiety, anger, and stress?). Each process is a system conceptually different from, but related to, the others. Since behavior is multidetermined, any event occurring within a group can be understood as a product of processes occurring on all levels simultaneously. Consider the following example of the first session of a group of newly recovering alcoholics:

> Early in the group meeting, Sam, a rather boisterous and provocative individual who has a long and rather complicated drinking history, starts the group by wanting to discuss his anger and difficulty trusting a roommate with whom he shares an apartment. His primary complaint centers around his lack of trust because of his roommate's constant use of drugs. Sam, himself, does not use drugs and is presently struggling to decide whether he should stop drinking or cut down on his consumption of alcohol despite repeated failures at controlled drinking over the last few years. His repeated relapses have resulted in a recent divorce. Group members are divided in their reaction to Sam's presentation; most support him and express concern about his present dilemma. However, Sharon, a quiet and anxious woman struggling with her addiction to prescription tranquilizers, strongly objects to Sam's lack of trust in his roommate and becomes uncharacteristically vehement in her attack upon him.

On the group level, this transaction can be viewed a number of ways. Certainly, the question of trust, which Sam has focused on in his relationship with his roommate, is one issue that the entire group may want to address directly. This is especially true since the group is composed entirely of new members and each person is likely to feel unsure about the level of alliance, support, and safety within the group setting. Picking the issue of trust and treating it as an outside phenomenon may be the group member's way of avoiding the intensity of the issue in the here and now. The group's flight from dealing directly with their feelings surrounding their lack of trust in the group's leader and its members could also be a displacement of the general uneasiness that each member feels because of the new and unfamiliar group setting.

On the interpersonal level, there may be a triggering of old resentments between members, or more correctly, the transference figures certain members represent to each other. Sharon's strong response to Sam actually reflects her own anger at not being trusted by her husband and other important individuals in her life. Her anger is fueled by Sam's lack of understanding for his roommate's drug problem. She strongly identifies with his roommate's dilemma because she feels she has been judged unjustly by others, which is made even more intolerable to her because she trusted and now feels betrayed by the physician who had prescribed the tranquilizers for her.

Sam's provocative style, coupled with his lack of tolerance for another's problems and his own insistent denial that he is an alcoholic, may trigger Sharon's memories and intolerance of her own father's denial about his alcoholism while he continued to criticize her mother for her lack of trust in him.

On an interpersonal level, like all of us, the two members in question have long-standing anxieties, conflicts, fantasies, defenses, and compensations that they brought with them into group. Sam, in particular, may be deflecting the focus from his own difficulty with recovery and abstinence by getting the other members to deal with his roommate's problems, while at the same time giving the appearance of being actively involved with the group on a personal level. At the same time, Sam gets to hook the group into an endless debate about whether his roommate is an addict, a crucial issue that Sam needs to address and answer about himself. Sam's provocative and evasive defensive style needs to be understood, explored, and ultimately confronted in a therapeutic manner. A full understanding of this group session would require data on all three levels. Only then would there be enough information to explain why this behavior became salient to these members in this group at this particular time. However, before these issues are decided, the group leader must return to the first important question: What is the goal of this group? (See Figure 2.2.)

To help answer this question, group leaders now have within their conceptual map a choice of interventions based on the possible tasks and goals available to them.

In relation to a learning task or insight-oriented group, the three levels (i.e., group level, intrapersonal level, and interpersonal level) refer to the process or system that is the object of study. The group leader chooses which of the three will best serve the interests and needs of the group members. Are the group members there primarily to understand themselves better, and how can this best be accomplished? Within the context of change, the concept levels refer to those processes utilized as the vehicle for intervention to produce change. For example, peer group pressure (group level), a therapeutic relationship with the leader and group mem-

FIGURE 2.2

	LEARNING	LEARNING and CHANGE	CHANGE
GROUP PROCESS			
INTERPERSONAL			
INTRAPERSONAL			

Source: Singer et al. (1975)

bers (interpersonal level), and interpretations and confrontations of defensive structures (intrapersonal level) are all possible ways of altering a chemically dependent individual's behavior.

Most models of group psychotherapy can be placed within the following four categories: (1) Focused criteria change groups; (2) Individually oriented growth and personal change groups; (3) Interpersonally oriented groups; and (4) Process-oriented psychodynamic groups. These four types of groups will be described further and will be systematized in Figures 2.3 to 2.7. Although devised on the basis of Singer et al.'s (1975) informal observations of tasks and structure in different possible group events, the "cognitive maps" presented here are simplified, but consonant with the empirical, analytical observations of Lomranz, Lakin, and Schiffman

(1972), upon which Singer and his cohorts built their schema. Of course, there are many group events that defy categorization and do not fit neatly within this typology. Despite the shortcomings of such a typological classification, the presentation and forced fit of the different approaches of group psychotherapy will hopefully provide beginning group leaders with a better understanding of the possible options available to them in their treatment of addiction within a group setting.

Focused Criteria Groups

Focused change groups are specifically designed to change, alter, or eliminate a group member's self-destructive or self-defeating target behavior. Such groups are usually short term and historically have been used with addictive types of behavior (smoking, eating, taking drugs) as well as when the focus is on symptom reduction (shyness, grief, panic disorders, divorce recovery, pain management) or behavioral rehearsal (assertiveness, conflict resolution, etc.). Usually, these groups are either highly confrontive or highly supportive. The leader is often very active and since the focus is on altering and changing behavior, little importance is placed on insight or learning about oneself.

Since the criteria for establishing these groups is a shared emphasis on symptom reduction or behavioral change, they are highly specific and consequently usually very homogeneous in nature. Unlike heterogeneous groups that encourage learning by way of the differences manifested by each individual group member, homogeneous groups look for similarities in group members' lives as a way to mobilize compliance and behavioral change. While a homogeneous focused criteria group can be conducted in an outpatient setting, there is a propensity for these groups to be established in institutional settings that cater to specific populations.

It is important here to examine more clearly what is meant by homogeneous and heterogeneous group composition. Yalom (1975) reviewed extensively the relationship of these factors to group composition and treatment outcome. He concluded that there was "a general clinical sentiment that heterogeneous groups have advantages over homogeneous groups for intensive interactional group therapy" (p. 261). While homogeneous groups are more likely to become cohesive more quickly and provide immediate support (and consequently have fewer dropouts and less conflict), they are also more likely to remain at a superficial level, thus providing less opportunity for altering character structure.

Since altering character structure is such a necessary component of successful, long-term treatment of the chemically dependent individual, the need for heterogeneity will be of greater importance in group therapy the longer the alcoholic or addict is free of chemicals. Utilizing Yalom's recommendations, a focus on the homogeneity of group will be more beneficial early in treatment and attentiveness to the heterogeneous factors will have more significance later in treatment when the chemically dependent individual is in aftercare, relapse prevention, or a long-term outpatient group.

However, as Yalom suggests, there are other factors to consider when determining the appropriate use of homogeneity or heterogeneity. He recommends striving for maximum heterogeneity with group members' patterns of coping and conflict areas, while seeking homogeneity in each member's degree of vulnerability and capacity to tolerate anxiety. As any experienced addiction specialist knows, chemically dependent persons do not handle vulnerability or tolerate anxiety and uncertainty well early in recovery. However, they must develop this capacity later in recovery if they are to remain sober or clean, since they will no longer have the luxury of using chemicals as a way to self-soothe. As Anne Alonso (1985) recommends, the group functions best when the group leader keeps it running at the highest level of *tolerable* anxiety. Early in recovery, addicts and alcoholics cannot tolerate much ambiguity or uncertainty. Later in recovery, it will be crucial that they learn how to deal with such feelings without the use of chemicals. Singer et al. (1975) submitted a very unflattering description of such a group when an addiction treatment group was used as an example of such an approach. (See Figure 2.3.)

> All of the target behavior are addictive in nature; each has become a way of avoiding anxiety, despair, depression, meaninglessness, or powerlessness, and each has been psychologically reinforcing in addition to any physical dependence. The programs in which these events are nearly always embedded (e.g., Phoenix House, Weight Watchers) and their leaders first utilize rituals of entry, such as confession and humiliation, to promote a powerful identification with the program and the group. The substitute dependency makes withdrawal from the target behavior possible. Leaders foster group pressure, supportive sanctions–not interpretations or didactic transferences–to help members stay abstinent after the initial withdrawal. . . . Focused Criteria Group leaders make it appear that intrapersonal and interpersonal process are key vehicles for change. Closer inspection suggests to us that group processes–covertly utilized–are the primary change inducers. (Singer et al., 1975, p. 146)

Historically, what has often been passed off as group psychotherapy with addicts and alcoholics was actually a variation of a homogeneous

FIGURE 2.3

	LEARNING	LEARNING and CHANGE	CHANGE
GROUP PROCESS			
INTERPERSONAL			
INTRAPERSONAL			

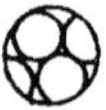

3) Behavior Management, Overeaters Anonymous, Smoking Cessation, etc.

Source: Singer et al. (1975)

focused criteria group. Usually, the leader, who was very active, confrontive, and directive, worked sequentially with each member in group until everyone got his or her time on the "hot seat" within a group setting. The rest of the group essentially served as an audience or auxiliary, either confronting or supporting the patient, depending on the leader's power to influence and direct.

While Singer and his co-authors failed to specifically include twelve-step groups like Alcoholics Anonymous, Narcotics Anonymous, and Cocaine Anonymous within their focused criteria group format, many of the characteristics of this type of group occur within these programs. However, it is fortunate that they excluded AA, NA, and CA from this category because, while their description of a focused criteria group as it applies to addiction is an accurate one, it fails to accurately describe the significance of the twelve steps of AA and other abstinence-oriented programs. The twelve steps form a unique learning component of the group process that is the real secret of the program's success. As any recovering alcoholic or addict would readily acknowledge, just going to meetings will not guarantee them long-lasting sobriety or abstinence. That only comes from working the twelve steps of the program. If twelve-step programs are able to offer more effective help to their chemically dependent members, why do AA, NA, and CA need professionally led groups? They don't need professionally led groups if the only purpose of the group is to provide support and ensure abstinence. Group psychotherapy should never be intended as a substitute for AA, NA, and CA. Group psychotherapy by itself will not keep an alcoholic sober or an addict clean. The programs of AA, NA, and CA can accomplish this task much more effectively. What group psychotherapy has to offer the chemically dependent individual is an understanding of the intrapersonal and interpersonal conflicts that interfere with compliance and acceptance of the program as well as the forces that can lead to a relapse. Group psychotherapy can also speed up the recovery process and reinforce the steps of the twelve-step programs for those individuals who have difficulty understanding, accepting, and working the twelve steps of recovery.

Individually Oriented Change Groups

Groups conducted from an individual change format also have as their primary task the goal of producing change in the individual's behavior, whether it be a reduction in suffering, increased awareness, or an increased capacity for more creative functioning. Consequently, this approach has some similarities to a focused criteria group. However, there is a significant difference in their application of individual treatment within a group setting. While this approach also has a tendency to use the rest of the group as either an auxiliary or an audience while working sequentially with one group member at a time, there is usually a well-developed rationale or theory that guides the techniques and strategies used in its application. Unlike the focused criteria group, where the group leader does individual therapy within the group, some of these approaches (i.e., psychodrama, psychomotor) use the rest of the members of the group in a very structured and directive manner that enhances the experience for the group members in a way that could never happen in individual treatment. (See Figure 2.4.)

While this format reflects a wide range of technical and theoretical approaches to group psychotherapy, including Redecision Psychotherapy (e.g., Goulding and Goulding, 1979), Psychodrama (e.g., Moreno, 1971), Gestalt (e.g., Perls, 1969), Bio-Energetics (e.g., Lowen, 1969), and Psy-

FIGURE 2.4

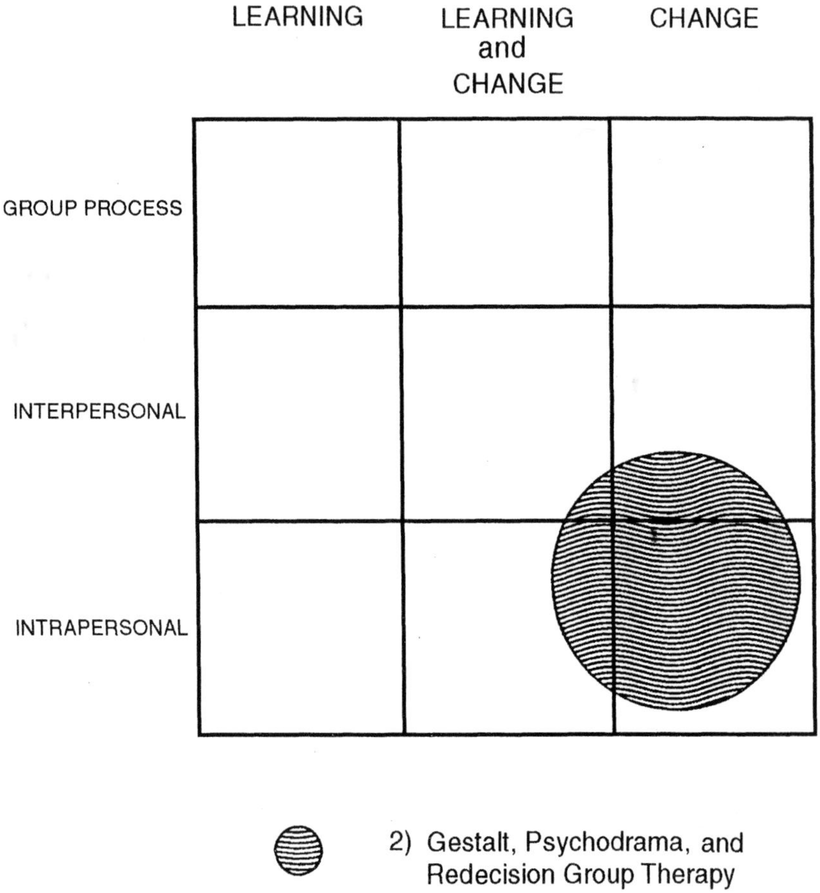

LEARNING
LEARNING and CHANGE
CHANGE

GROUP PROCESS
INTERPERSONAL
INTRAPERSONAL

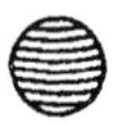

2) Gestalt, Psychodrama, and Redecision Group Therapy

Source: Singer et al. (1975)

chomotor (e.g., Pesso, 1991), a vehicle for change in all of these approaches is an intrapsychic focus coupled with group leader intervention. The group is regarded as an aggregate of individuals and the leader essentially works with one group member at a time while the rest of the group members function vicariously as observers, contributors, alter egos and "significant others." Group processes, with the exception of peer support or the provision of multiple transference figures, are typically viewed as distractions or constraints upon the treatment and are not actively utilized in the work. Emphasis is placed on change, with insight or learning sometimes viewed as a hindrance or obstacle to change. The stereotypic prototype of this model is the Perlsian-lead Gestalt psychotherapy group where members take turns working in the "hot seat" with the group leader. Intellectualization, insight, and learning are viewed, in Perlsian terminology, as "mind fucking" and indications of cognitive defenses. Group members are encouraged instead to focus on their intrapsychic experience and increase their awareness. As Perls frequently admonished, they must "lose their mind and come to their senses." Change is the primary focus of each session and little emphasis is placed on understanding as it applies in the usual sense. Not all Gestalt therapy is Perlsian in nature, however. This overly stereotypic presentation of Gestalt is only used as an illustration and does little justice to other Gestalt therapists like Erv and Miriam Polster who infrequently, if ever, used the classical empty chair technique or "hot seat" in their group or limited their options while doing psychotherapy by following such rigid procedures.

The Polsters and Gouldings represent excellent therapists who utilize this approach to group. Each will be described in some detail to help illustrate the advantages of this model. The Polsters describe Gestalt therapy as phenomenologically rooted existential psychotherapy. It is phenomenological in that it emphasizes the individual's awareness of what he or she is experiencing now. It is existential in that its focus is on responsibility, freedom, and choice. Gestalt therapy started as a revision of classical psychoanalysis (Perls, 1969; Polster, 1975). It quickly became a whole and autonomous system for integrating wisdom from diverse sources into a unified clinical methodology (Perls, Hefferline, and Goodman, 1951). Its popularity had in the past almost singularly been attributed erroneously to Fritz Perls. However, not all Gestalt therapy is Perlsian (Dublin, 1976; Dolliver, 1981). Gestalt therapy has been strongly influenced by others (e.g., Laura Perls [1976], Erv and Miriam Polster [1976], James Simkin [1976], and Joseph Zinker [1977]). It is with these others in mind that a very brief explanation of Gestalt's historical roots and influence will be explored.

Gestalt therapy is tied to the Gestalt psychology at the Berlin School of Wertheimer, Kohler, and Koffka, in that both are forms of phenomenological field theory. The chief characteristic is the total immediate experience, here and now, with introspection usually seen as a source of bias. Experience, in this schema, must be differentiated from assumptions and inferences. Awareness is used to gain basic insight into the basic situation of the field. Intellectualization and rationalization are seen primarily as defenses and resistances that must be observed and explored by the therapist.

Early experimentation in Gestalt psychology indicated that there was an inherent tendency of the organism to organize perceptions in an orderly manner, and a completed organized configuration was labeled a *complete gestalt.* Unfinished business that persisted troublesomely in an individual's memory later came to be designated as *incomplete gestalts.* It was postulated that these incomplete gestalts must be re-experienced and completed lest they remain figure and distort present experiences by interfering with the process of assimilation that is required before a completed experience can become ground.

Change only occurs through heightened experience, and anxiety is frequently seen as a signal of the source of discomfort which must be experienced and completed. Neurosis occurs because of impasses that contribute to fixation and distortion of present experiences. Individuals stuck at an impasse remain unaware and doubt their own ability, which further stops the spontaneous flow of awareness. Interference with awareness results in a constricted I-boundary, which in turn interferes with either a lack of separateness or excessive dependence in the environment. The goal of therapy is frequently to expand I-boundaries and to heighten the fluidity of awareness so that figures succeed one another freely, allowing the individual full contact with the environment. I-boundaries are expanded primarily through contact.

The experiment is the key to Gestalt therapy and the attempt is to "work through" the impasse. Since thinking is viewed as a primary defense against assimilation, Gestalt therapy frequently draws on action methods to heighten awareness and increase contact. Fritz Perls expanded on Wilhelm Reich's theory of body armor and character structure, consequently providing Gestalt theorists with a rationale for bypassing cognitive defenses through an emphasis on somatic defenses and restriction. Moreno's psychodramatic techniques served as a prototype for developing action methods such as two-chair dialogue, enactment, and directed fantasy, which facilitated the increase of awareness necessary for contact, thus expanding I-boundaries and allowing impasses to be worked through more readily. It must be remembered that the premise of Gestalt therapy is that human nature is organized into patterns and wholes. However, as Polster and Polster (1976) and Kelly (1955) have demonstrated, every concept implies an opposite; our minds and senses constantly react to dualities in our environment. Gestalt therapy parallels a Hegelian philosophy of thesis, antithesis, and synthesis in its treatment philosophy.

Thus, in summary, Gestalt therapy, like no other therapy before it, outlines and articulates a theory of optimal human functioning. In one sense, it is a belief system that describes how the individual can live fully and freely from one moment to the next, autonomous and independent.

Gestalt theory and Fritz Perls's influence are also evident in Redecision Therapy. Bob Goulding, half of the team that originated this theoretical approach, spent a great deal of time working with Fritz Perls. The Gouldings have, in fact, incorporated Gestalt theory (or at least Gestalt techniques) in their Redecision Model. The Gouldings also emphasize responsibility, freedom, choice, and the present. Unlike the therapy of the pure Gestaltists, the Gouldings's therapy has a strong cognitive component that was inherited from Bob's relationship with Eric Berne (1961). Berne worked to develop a behavioral theory that would help explain the nature of man. Berne was a scientist and he was interested in understanding, predicting, and controlling both behavior and feelings. His approach was primarily cognitive rather than purely psychoanalytical. However, he too was strongly influenced and trained in Freudian psychology. Some claim that his ego states (Parent, Adult, Child) are just a substitute for Freud's Ego, Id, and Superego. However, Transactional Analysis is far more than ego states. It has developed into a sophisticated theory that focuses far more on decision and change than any other theory before it.

Observers soon learn that the Gouldings are tenacious in their commitment to bringing about change. They insist on working in short, twenty-minute segments and are convinced people can change in one session. They are radical existentialists in the sense that they insist individuals recognize that they are completely responsible for how they think, behave, act, and feel. Consequently, individuals must then learn that they alone have the power to bring about change in their life.

The Gouldings operate out of a simple but effective model that generally follows three principles of intervention: (1) contract work; (2) impasse clarification work; and (3) redecision work. However, there is much more going on in the Gouldings's therapy approach, and the interested reader should examine John McNeel's (1977) excellent analysis of the seven components of Redecision Therapy for a succinct description of a Gouldings' workshop.

When we feel bad, the Gouldings insist, we are frequently doing one of three things; we are either in another place, another time, or somewhere else stuck in a fantasy or in a "game." The game and fantasy for the Gouldings is paramount, for without them it is not possible for "rackets" and bad feelings to persist. These racket feelings can frequently be traced to early decisions made in childhood, and it is here that the Gouldings make their most important and unique theoretical contribution. In Transactional Analysis theory, decisions, even forgotten ones, no matter how strongly encouraged by early parental programming, or how necessary for survival during childhood, are ultimately self-determined and to some extent reversible. Each of us, according to this schema, have made necessary early decisions as children in order to survive in the world as we then experienced it. However, while these early decisions served survival purposes at the time they were made, they now remain out of our awareness at an unconscious level and frequently contribute to the problems we are now experiencing. Hence, erroneous decisions made with inadequate information at a primitive level must be brought into awareness, discarded if necessary, and replaced with *redecisions* based on reality and factual data.

The Gouldings' genius is in the pragmatic effectiveness of their model in bringing about redecision and change. The now classical Libermann, Yalom, and Miles (1973) treatment effectiveness outcome study clearly illustrates that Bob Goulding was the most effective of all the therapists evaluated in the research project. His effectiveness in part was determined by two factors. First, in the language of Lieberman, Yalom, and Miles, he was identified as a moderate affective stimulator, meaning that he provided enough arousal for his group members but did not overwhelm them with his interventions or confrontations. Secondly, through his integrative use of cognition (T.A.) and catharsis (Gestalt), he was able to bring together two crucial components for effective change. Research has demonstrated that insight alone is not enough for behavioral change. Unless there is emotional arousal accompanying this insight, lasting change will not be experienced.

Within the last ten years, this model represented by Perls, Polster, and the Gouldings has been evolving in its development and has also gained some popularity in its use. Although Psychodrama (Moreno, 1971) has been around for almost as long as Freud and is the granddaddy of the individually oriented approach to group treatment, there has been an integration of similar but divergent theories into a generic format commonly referred to as either regressive therapy or Intensive Expressive Psychotherapy (IEP). While there was a renewal of enthusiasm for this approach in the treatment of addiction, some of the excitement about its efficacy has waned because of its tendency to produce causalities (see Chapter 15). However, it is still widely used in various treatment programs and by many therapists throughout the country.

IEP's popularity was renewed after it was applied nationally by different treatment programs as a treatment modality for co-dependency and Adult Children of Alcoholics (ACOAs). However, it gradually evolved into the treatment of choice for addicts and alcoholics who had failed to respond to the more traditional forms of treatment and the twelve-step-oriented alcohol and drug treatment programs. It was hoped that this approach might work for those addicts and alcoholics who were suffering multiple relapses and were unable to maintain sobriety for any length of time even though they were diligently and faithfully working the twelve steps of the program. Eventually, the IEP model was applied with some success to patients suffering from eating disorders, sexual abuse, and many forms of dissociation, especially posttraumatic stress disorders. It was found that in some cases it could also be helpful for the overly controlled and emotionally constricted patient who had failed to respond to either medication or the more traditional form of "talking therapy." Adherents of this approach believed that the only patients who were contraindicated for IEP were those suffering from a thought disorder (schizophrenia) or those who were actively psychotic.

Treatment program personnel were motivated to utilize this model because they were trying to find ways to impact chemically dependent individuals quickly on an emotional level since many of these patients were so out of touch with their feelings and were resistant to less evocative approaches. Certainly, the frustration of dealing with the characterological defenses and features so common with this population prompted a need to find alternative and more effective methods of treating them. Though the frustration of attempting to treat character pathology is not limited to addiction, the two frequently go hand in hand. Practitioners have long sought ways to impact such patients and effectively treat them. Louis Ormont (1992) refers to such individuals as suffering from pre-oedipal conflicts. He contends that they pose special problems because their difficulties arose before they learned to use words effectively. As a result, they are prone to act or emote rather than talk. Usually, they do not respond well to interpretation. Ormont suggests that they must be approached and influenced through feelings and actions. Consequently, some have argued that an IEP approach, with its emphasis on action rather than talking, might have more therapeutic impact than other methods of treatment have for these patients.

A pre-oedipal personality is generally understood to be one whose development was arrested before the child could use words to conceptualize thoughts. Because the personality solidified before the child had achieved sufficient ego strength, the adult who presents in treatment finds it hard or impossible to articulate conflicts, difficulties, and feelings. The early origin of the disturbance implied that the difficulties developed largely or entirely before the child could find even rudimentary language to express him or herself, or to cognitively make sense of his or her experience. Building on this explanation of disturbance, IEP therapists believed it was of little use, when working with such individuals, to use words or interpretations as therapeutic techniques. Insight and learning was impossible or of little consequence. Affect was a necessary first requirement to produce change. It was believed by IEP therapists that one of the most frequently used tools in the treatment of addiction–confrontation–was also of little benefit since these individuals could not usually experience their inner selves. This is why some of the strategies advocated by John Bradshaw (1993) were believed to be so valuable. IEP therapists were trying to reach what Bradshaw and others were referring to as the "child within," whose feelings and emotions were either dissociated or "frozen in time" around the original trauma. IEP utilized those techniques that were believed to help break down or dissolve these dissociative barriers, thus releasing frozen emotions that supposedly help the pre-oedipal patient gain an experience of his or her "true self" or "inner child."

While IEP may have appeared at first as a new technique to the inexperienced group therapist, the principles that guided its application had a long history and tradition. One primary theme of the IEP approach is that it is usually applied in a group setting and is an "action-oriented" psychotherapy. IEP can best be described as a loosely organized body of techniques and applications that is grounded in the theoretical principle that instead of "just" having individuals talk about their feelings, thoughts, or past events, it is much more beneficial to utilize methods that will help them gain an experience of their thoughts and feelings in the "here and now" of the group. Members are guided and encouraged to give their experiences expression behaviorally and emotionally.

A frequent criticism of IEP is that it is an assortment of techniques in search of a theory. While this may be somewhat true, it is not a completely fair assessment of its application. Many of the theoretical principles that guide its application go back to early Freudian psychodynamic theory with its emphasis on catharsis, abreaction, and the corrective emotional experience. IEP is primarily interested in patients' emotions and the expression of these emotions. An IEP therapist would much rather have patients experience their emotions and give them expression either physically or emotionally than hear what they think or have them analyze and intellectualize their feelings. Thinking and insight are not necessarily seen as having no value; rather they are viewed as secondary to the experience of one's feelings and the expression or release of these feelings.

An important part of IEP's legacy is tied to "action-oriented" psychotherapy. Its roots go back to the 1930s when Jacob L. Moreno discovered it was more beneficial to have his patients act out their conflicts and difficulties in Psychodrama than just have them talk about them. Moreno first called this approach the "Theater of Spontaneity." Over the years, his early theories have been expanded by others (i.e., Fritz Perls with Gestalt, Bob and Mary Goulding with Redecision Therapy, Alexander Lowen with Bio-Energetics, Al Pesso with Psychomotor) who see that intellectualization, rationalization, and isolation of affect are often the primary obstacles to overcome in trying to get patients to "work through" their unresolved traumas and impasses.

Over the last decade, these theories have been synthesized and consolidated into a loosely defined body of knowledge that regards the expression of emotions and the release of pent-up or blocked feelings as the primary goal of psychotherapy. Intellectual understanding and insight alone is usually not enough to free a person from his or her crippling anxiety, depression, repetitive self-defeating behavior, and addiction. Specific techniques have been developed to achieve this end, and it is a widely held opinion that this approach works best when applied in a group setting. The group provides the necessary balance between stimulation, support, and identification to help patients work through the feelings of fear, shame, and isolation that always accompany these types of difficulties and the subsequent necessary therapeutic work.

Interpersonal Learning and Change Groups

The interpersonal learning groups have their roots in the now classical sensitivity training or T-groups. Currently, this group approach has been defined and placed under the Singer label of interactional group psychotherapy; an approach most commonly associated with the work of Irvin Yalom (1985). The stated aim of this approach is to help group members understand the effects their behavior has on others and in turn how others' behavior affects them. Feelings and emotional expressions are explored in the belief that they play a substantial part in motives, communication, and behavior. Thus, the primary learning task in the T-groups is the emphasis these groups place on the interpersonal interactions that occur in groups. (See Figure 2.5.)

Yalom, for one, has added variants to this approach by utilizing behavioral unfreezing as another way to foster subsidiary change in a group member's behavior. The leader's task is to be a role model, giving feedback, without making evaluations of the group member's behavior. Expe-

FIGURE 2.5

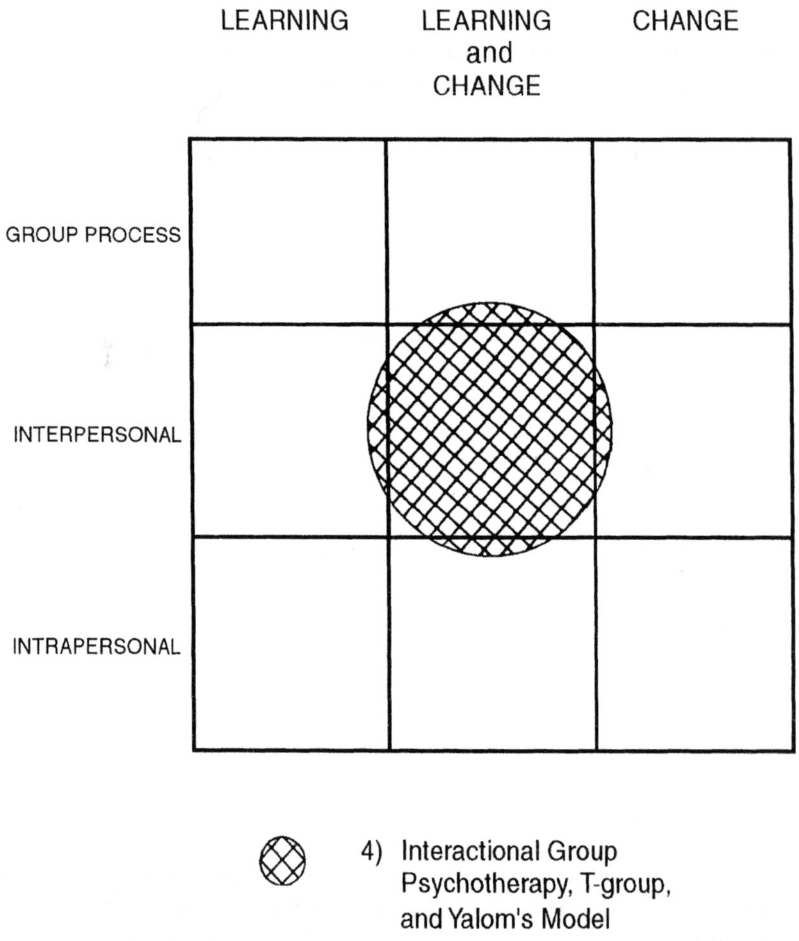

LEARNING

LEARNING and CHANGE

CHANGE

GROUP PROCESS

INTERPERSONAL

INTRAPERSONAL

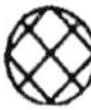

4) Interactional Group Psychotherapy, T-group, and Yalom's Model

Source: Singer et al. (1975)

riences are validated through the group leader's direction, allowing individuals within the group to get a consensus from the other group members, and enabling them to learn how their behavior and actions affect others. Yalom views learning and change as inseparable occurrences, arguing that neither can occur without the other.

Yalom's view on change and learning takes on added significance when dealing with the chemically dependent individual. Any group leader who has had contact with twelve-step groups on a sustained basis knows that chemically dependent people can either drink themselves to death or drug themselves into oblivion while they explore the reasons why they are drinking and doing drugs. An approach that focuses only on insight, self-understanding, and learning will usually have little long-lasting beneficial effect on chemically dependent individuals during the early phase of their treatment and recovery.

Yalom's model and the interpersonal approach will be explored at great length in Chapters 4 and 5. For now, it is important to know that this approach is one in which the interpersonal interactions between the group members are a cornerstone of treatment. Little attention is paid to group-as-a-whole or intrapsychic dynamics. Yalom emphasizes maintaining a balance between the cognitive and the emotional while ensuring that group members have the opportunity both to learn about themselves and change their behavior. With the group serving as a social microcosm, the members get a chance to learn about themselves in relation to each others while having the opportunity to practice the new behavior in their exchanges with each other. If they can do it in group, the new behavior will be more generalizable to the "real" outside world.

Group Process in Psychodynamic Groups

The last model to be presented was chosen in this sequence because it is the approach that is most widely practiced and is more thoroughly grounded in a solid theoretical rationale for its application. Because of the sophistication of its theoretical foundation, it is the approach that most easily allows for the incorporation of the other three models and the integration of affect, change, insight, and learning. As you will soon gather from the summary to be presented, the psychodynamic approach to group therapy has a wide spectrum of influence and many diverse interpretations of what needs to be emphasized in its application.

What is now called psychodynamic group psychotherapy has evolved into a generic model of group treatment which recognizes that there are three primary forces operating at all times in a therapy group: intrapsychic or individual dynamics, the interpersonal dynamics or the system, and group-as-a-whole dynamics). The task of the group leader within this approach is to integrate all of these components into a coherent, fluid, and complimentary flow, remembering at all times that there is a plethora of variables (stage of group development, ego strength of individual group members, target population being treated, individual resistances operating in concert with group resistances, group role inductions, etc.) that influences which type of intervention (group-as-a-whole, individual, or interpersonal) needs to be emphasized at a particular time in group. The experienced psychodynamic group leader also knows that the intervention level he or she chooses at a particular time will have an impact on the other two levels. The group leader is also well aware that an overemphasis on one level of intervention comes at the cost of the other two levels, reducing their impact and relevance to treatment. The level of intervention that takes priority for the psychodynamic-oriented group is in part determined by the therapist's theoretical persuasion, training, experience, and personality. Consequently, it is rare to find two psychodynamically oriented group leaders who write about and conduct group therapy in exactly the same manner.

Within the defined area of psychodynamic process-oriented group psychotherapy, there exists a wide range of diversity. A student of process-oriented group psychotherapy will soon learn that the way Wilfred Bion (1961) teaches group psychotherapy is far different from other recognized authorities such as Alexander Wolfe and Ernest Schwartz (1962). These theorists, in turn, are far different in their approaches to psychodynamic group psychotherapy than the brand of psychodynamic group process that is exemplified by Helen Durkin (1964), Henriette Glatzter (1969), Anne Alonso (1985), Scott Rutan and Walter Stone (1993), and Louis Ormont (1992).

However, before one can understand the subtleties and differences between these different approaches to group psychotherapy, one must be aware that the foundation of each is built upon Freudian psychodynamic theory. Sigmund Freud's (1921) contribution to group psychology cannot be ignored. Every major school of group psychotherapy has been directly or indirectly influenced by Freudian thought. Fritz Perls in Gestalt, Eric Berne in Transactional Analysis, J. L. Moreno in Psychodrama, Harry Stack Sullivan with his interpersonal theory of personality and its subsequent influence on Irvin Yalom, as well as every psychodynamic process-oriented group psychotherapist from Wilfred Bion to Alexander Wolfe have had the foundations of their approaches to group psychotherapy firmly set in Freudian psychology.

Before venturing to describe the similarities and differences between these particular schools of group psychotherapy, a cursory examination of Freud's early writings on group psychotherapy is in order. Freud's notion of regression in groups is paramount to understanding the dynamics that occur within any group setting and reflects his most important contribution to group psychology. Freud held an overwhelming bias that the group or herd instinct is mindless, primitive, and ultimately destructive. Group members will repeatedly, although often unconsciously, try to determine how they are to survive in a newly formed group setting. Therefore, individuals in a strange group setting will be forced to deal with primitive emotions like aggression, fear, anger, and anxiety because they are caught in a regressive response to a basic survival situation. Freud, more than anyone else before him, defended the individual against the compelling forces of the herd instinct and perceived each individual as being at battle with the pressures of society to conform to the norms of the group. The conflict is always between the individual–whom Freud defended–and society or the herd instinct, which Freud abhorred. Freud saw the group as a source of contagious reduction of mentality that resulted in each member denying his or her individuality when placed within a group setting. Group members have a thirst for obedience and a need to conform; they depend upon a strong group leader. Individuals within the group will thus succumb to these unconscious pressures and project their ego ideals onto the group leader. The group ideal is subsequently personified in the group leader and this is, in turn, substituted for the ego ideal of each person in the group. There is a need for the group to make the leader bigger than life. While group members want their leader to be greater than he or she actually is, because this belief ensures them protection, they want simultaneously to dethrone and destroy their leader. The members' ambivalence is related to the more primitive stages of their development and is reflected in Freud's myth of the primal horde (i.e., where the brothers form a blood bond after the killing of the father). Group members will then attempt to create a mythical hero who will hopefully accomplish the task of becoming bigger than life in the belief that this will protect them from the guilt and anxiety that accompany their individuality and is usually associated with the responsibility that follows free choice. All life, for Freud, is a struggle with the ambivalence brought upon by the individual's dualistic view of wanting to fight authority and desiring to succumb to the safety of identifying with the group mind. Each member's denial of his or her individuality leads eventually to personal pathology, and this is seen as a by-product of the collective forces of the herd instinct and society's pressures to conform.

The most important aspect of Freud's contribution to group psychotherapy is the significance he places upon the notion of regression in groups. Regression is a phenomenon that is primary to any group setting. If the group leaders fail to acknowledge the importance of regression and its subsequent relation to safety and trust for individuals who are chemically dependent, there is little chance that the group experience will be helpful in their treatment. The significance of trust, safety, and cohesion in a group setting will be discussed at length in Chapter 15 when Yalom's curative factors are explored in relation to group psychotherapy with addicts and alcoholics. For now, the different theoretical perspectives within psychodynamically oriented groups will be explored.

Group-as-a-whole perspectives are best exemplified by the Tavistock-type small group or study group (Bion, 1961; Rice, 1965). In a strict Tavistock approach to groups, group process learning events have a unitary learning task that focuses on group level performance, particularly those surrounding authority issues and covert processes. Secondly, emphasis, if any at all, is placed on interpersonal phenomenon. (See Figure 2.6.)

Interpretation and intervention are focused on the here and now phenomena occurring within the group as a system, and rigorous observation of time, role, and task boundaries are the prime leader techniques. Emphasis is placed on authority relationships and reactions to leadership by group members. Feelings in group are usually focused first on the group leader and then eventually on the other group members. Such groups are usually difficult to lead and many Tavistock leaders will admit that a strict Tavistock group is not a psychotherapy group and should never be intended as such (Kline, 1983). Tavistock groups will teach members how they respond to authority and react to stressful ambiguous situations. Any recovering alcoholic or addict who is an active member of AA, NA, or CA can answer those questions unequivocally. The chemically dependent person usually has extreme difficulty in both areas of his or her life. Consequently, such a group approach with newly recovering alcoholics and addicts will only add to their problems rather than give them any help in addressing their abstinence.

Wilfred Bion (1961) is the theorist most closely aligned with the Tavistock approach. Bion's model ignores the individual in the group and goes so far as to advocate that if the leader addresses individual problems within the group setting, the leader is colluding with the group members in their attempt to avoid group work by allowing them to shift the focus from the primary group issues. Within Bion's framework, when individuals are brought together in a group setting, they regress into a group mind. Bion prefers to view the group as an aggregate of individuals in a state of regression. The group members will attempt to resist the emergence of psychotic or neurotic residuals by employing three basic assumptions (i.e., fight-flight, dependency, and pairing). These assumptions will be explored

FIGURE 2.6

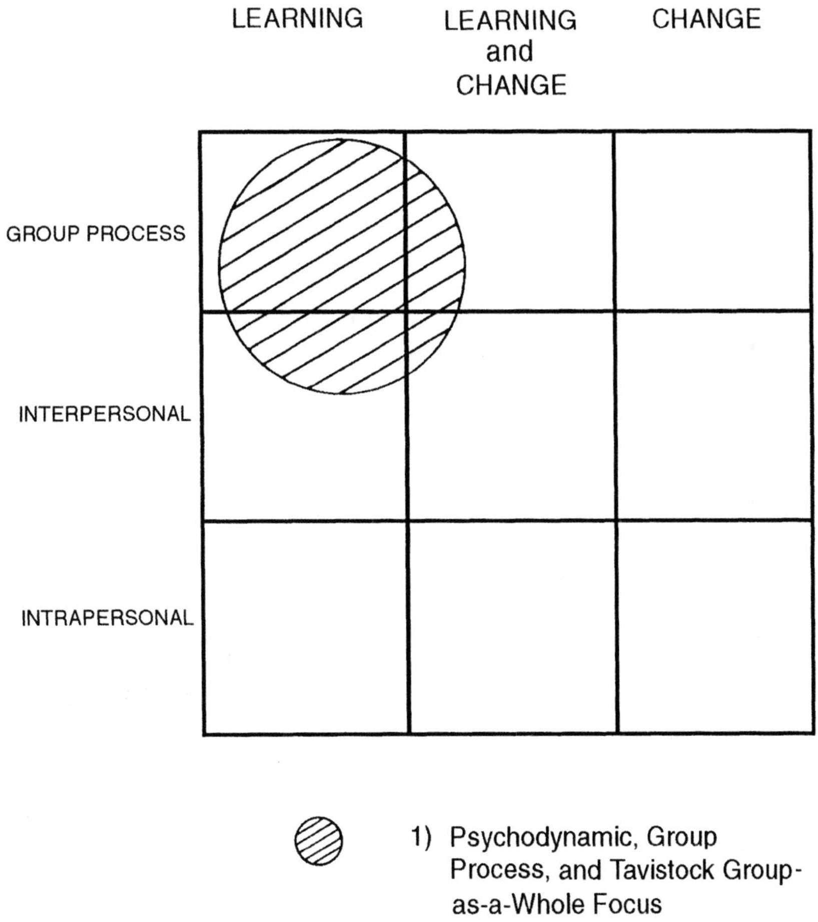

	LEARNING	LEARNING and CHANGE	CHANGE
GROUP PROCESS			
INTERPERSONAL			
INTRAPERSONAL			

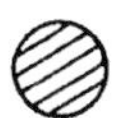

1) Psychodynamic, Group Process, and Tavistock Group-as-a-Whole Focus

Source: Singer et al. (1975)

in more detail in Chapter 14. For now, it is enough to say that Bion views these assumptions as a form of group resistance that needs to be interpreted and ultimately addressed. The individual cannot be treated in group, and the only appropriate target for treatment, from Bion's perspective, is the commonly shared anxiety of the group and the defenses erected against this anxiety.

Within the last few years, Agazarian (1992) has developed a somewhat unique and different application of a group-as-a-whole approach. She has taken many of the principles of General System Theory (GST) and applied them to group treatment. She holds the position, as most GST practitioners do, that all systems possess a fundamentally common structure and because of *isomorphy*, you cannot help but alter one part of a system when intervening on another level of that system. Within Agazarian's perspective there are three systems always operating within a group. There is the group-as-a-whole system, there is a subsystem (two or more group members) within the larger system, and there is the individual, who has his or her own internal system of object and self-object representations. This three-tier system of group operates within the larger context of a fourth system, which can be the institutional setting or the facility where the treatment is being provided. Each part of the system impacts on the other three parts.

Her model is relatively new, and she has been evolving her theory as she gathers more experience and information. At first, she only advocated dealing with the suprasystem (group-as-a-whole) and recommended that the group leader gradually work on down the system. Within the last few years, she has utilized more of the subsystem in her treatment. Like most systems theorists, she believes that an individual in group *never* speaks for themselves and is *always* giving voice to the common group tension. The regressive pull of the suprasystem (group-as-a-whole) would interface with the group members' personal dynamics and they in turn would be induced to play the role they played in their family or in their lives. Consequently, through the regressive pull of the group dynamics, each person's individual dynamics would get repeated in group through the force of the repetition compulsion.

General Systems Theory places a great deal of emphasis on roles that members will take on in a group. From a systems perspective, opposite positions and views have to be articulated in group by at least one member since the theory holds that each action within a system produces a reaction. For instance, if there were a regressive pull for a group consensus that there be no aggression or hostility in the group and if this denial of reality took the form that "this is safest group ever and nobody could ever be harmed in here," a deviant voice must speak to the other end of this continuum by saying, "I don't feel safe here." Having someone speak to all sides or opposite poles of an issue not only places boundaries on the limits on the group experience, it also provides reality testing. Agazarian's use of the subgroup to voice an opposite position is motivated by her awareness that it is often too difficult or threatening for any one person alone to take on a deviant role in group. Often, the person who speaks a truth that a family or a group does not want to hear can become the scapegoat. Agazarian is well aware that there is a regressive pull in group to have group members placed into roles and that the scapegoat and the identified patient are the two most frequently used roles. If the rest of the group can either spend their time attacking one member for containing all the badness (the scapegoat) or helping someone who contains all the sickness (the identified patient), they do not have to deal with themselves.

Agazarian sees psychopathology largely as the result of people wanting to disown or deny negative aspects of self, resulting in a projection of these disowned parts onto another. Jung would describe this as a failure to want to become familiar with or own our dark side. Anything denied will stay hidden, influencing one's actions unconsciously. Closely tied into this defensive process is the tendency for individuals to hold all-or-nothing positions. Addicts and alcoholics are notorious for this, and twelve-step programs refer to it as their tendency to get into "black and white thinking." Such a rigid position is a defense against anxiety. Placing a person or situation into distinct categories like good or bad, reduces the ambiguity and makes the world appear more predictable and safe. Of course, this comes at the cost of denial of reality and the need to have someone contain all the bad or all the good. Agazarian pushes her groups to deal with the ambiguity inherent in life by insisting the members focus on opposites and splits within the groups. She wants each person to live in the ambivalence of their actual existence. She wants it worked through without denial and not acted out through the repetition compulsion.

Her premise is that if the group leader focuses on the larger suprasystem of the group, the evolving dynamics inherent in this or any system will produce anxiety and conflict as individuals within the system are forced to recognize and work through their individual differences. Put another way, each member's individual dynamics will clash with the group dynamics. As these issues are worked through and mastered on a group level, through the process of isomorphy or osmosis, these differences will be contained by the subgroups and eventually integrated and mastered by the individual members within the system. Most individuals are too defended against uncomfortable anxieties or aggression and have different levels of tolerance and awareness for their occurrence. The group provides its members with a holding environment and a composite "group ego" (composed of all the other members' observing egos), which increases the flexibility and resources available because everyone contributes to observations or feelings that would normally be contained or cut off from any individual member alone. Consequently, this increases the observations and awareness of all individuals within the group. The entire system and its subsystems serve as containers for members' feelings and thoughts, providing them with the opportunity to be modulated and integrated. Very similar to a dialectic process of thesis, antithesis, and synthesis, the system approach allows a tolerance for splits and opposites to be experienced. The task for the group leader is to increase communication across the boundaries of these splits. How the group communicates is much more important than what it communicates. These strategies open the boundaries for increased communication and the development of better understanding of walled-off aspects within oneself.

In sharp contrast to Agazarian's and Bion's position, Wolfe and Schwartz (1962) view the group and group process as a metaphor, an illusion that does not exist. Wolfe has satirically commented that the group leader must always remember "that individuals come for treatment, not groups." To this, he adds the penetrating criticism that "group dynamics never cured anybody." For a group leader to address interpretations to the group only adds to and helps create the illusion of group consciousness. Wolfe cautions the group leader against reinforcing such a belief because groups try to make all members alike. Groups coerce each member to regress and behave as the most dominant member within the group does. The group ego is a mystique, an artifact resulting from group conformity, pressures, and identification. This tendency of producing a unified group consciousness, according to Wolfe and Schwartz, must be challenged, as it reinforces an illusion and encourages regression and compliance while minimizing the individuation of group members. Instead, the focus in group should be on the members' separateness, individuality, and transference distortions. Because the group setting allows individual conflicts to manifest in relation to other group members, the group leader has more material to work with than he or she would in an individual psychotherapy setting. Individual therapy within a group setting reduces a transference intensity that exists within an individual setting, allowing the individual to profit more from treatment.

Durkin (1964) and Glatzter (1969), in turn, advocate a combination of the intrapersonal and the group process focus in their orientation toward group psychotherapy. Durkin's and Glatzter's roots are set in the British School of Ego Psychology, and they view the analyzing of ego traits and defenses within a group setting as the primary task of the group leader. Within their schema, they focus on the developmental assessment of the ego in the belief that analysis should be directed toward the maladaptive compromises that the ego has had to make in order to survive in a stressful and dysfunctional situation. Psychopathology is part of an ongoing process of the ego's effort to cope, and it is within the member's transference distortion that these maladaptive efforts most readily appear. The group allows for more sources of transference distortions and the leader has a readily accessible laboratory to see how individual members act out their pathology, rather than just having them talk about it in an abstract manner. The purpose of group, according to Durkin and Glatzter, is to analyze these transference resistances and show members how their past continues to impact on their present functioning.

The group setting allows a group leader to deal more effectively with the defenses that are ego-dystonic. Ego-dystonic defenses differ from ego-systonic defenses in that the latter represent a defensive posture that is more ingrained and characterological in nature. Such a defensive stance usually causes the individual little overt concern. In contrast, individuals with ego-dystonic defenses experience little difficulty within themselves. It is the alcoholic's and addict's defensive style (i.e., narcissistic acting out, addiction, etc.) that causes others more difficulties and frequently leads such individuals to be sent to or brought into treatment by disgruntled bosses, unhappy spouses, and frustrated significant others in their lives. A group setting, through the transference distortions and confrontation of other members, allows ego-systonic defenses to become dystonic, thus prompting the individual to become more motivated for change. Why else would such individuals want to change if they have little discomfort in their behavior and firmly believe it is others who are having the problem because of their difficulty in dealing with them?

The group, within Durkin and Glatzter's model, also allows the leader more opportunities to avoid both negative and positive transference distortions. An overly compliant, passive-aggressive individual who experiences positive transference to his or her therapist during individual therapy is more likely to cover over and hide feelings of anger. Group members are more likely to be accessible targets for such an individual's anger. Group members' needs for support and understanding are also more easily met since other group members are more likely than the group leader to be able to respond spontaneously in a supportive manner in their interactions with each other.

The most current and comprehensive approach to psychodynamic group theory is represented by Rutan and Stone (1993). They have been able to incorporate many aspects of the different theoretical positions described so far while adding important elements from both an object relations and self-psychology perspective. More will be presented on this approach in the following chapters on the psychodynamics of addiction and long-term strategies for addiction treatment.

SPECIFIC APPLICATIONS FOR ADDICTIONS TREATMENT

While this summary of the different levels of intervention available in group was intended to illustrate the advantages and disadvantage of each model, the key question that must be addressed is, Which approach would work best with the chemically dependent individual? Unfortunately, that question cannot be answered categorically because there are so many intervening variables that must be considered in determining the best strategic approach when working with alcohol and substance dependent patients in a group. What works best for the non-addicted patient does not necessarily work with the addicted individual. Treatment as a time-dependent process (what works early in treatment will not necessarily be beneficial later in treatment) must be the guiding principle when working with the addicted patient. Underlying character pathology, ego strength, and even drug of choice are other considerations that must be evaluated carefully if group treatment is to be effectively maximized.

It is important to remember the balance that must be maintained between affect and cognition, learning and change, structure and ambiguity, and the individual and the group when working with this population. The group leader must constantly keep in mind that each intervention must be carefully weighed against the need for maintaining abstinence while promoting the exploration of self, the uncovering of characterological patterns, the easing of defenses, and the releasing of repressed emotions. Too much of one or too little of another will increase the likelihood of a return to using alcohol or substances. If this happens, treatment is essentially ineffective and abruptly halted.

The interpersonal approach, exemplified most cogently and completely by Yalom's interactional model, is the group treatment method that is most likely to capture all of the diverse considerations necessary to treat the chemically dependent individual most effectively. Yalom's recommendations provide the most easily adaptable approach to group treatment so that modifications can be easily applied across the continuum of the alcoholic's or addict's recovery needs. His model can be tightened up (more structure added as he outlines in his inpatient recommendations) early in treatment and then can be loosened up (less structure utilized as it incorporates some of the more sophisticated theoretical considerations of self-psychology and modern analytic approaches) later, once abstinence has been solidified and there is less danger of relapse.

To help illustrate some of the common difficulties that the chemically dependent person poses for the group leader, a number of vignettes will be presented. The first has to do with the common mistake of failing to make abstinence a priority in treatment and holding on to a theoretical position that insight or learning alone will supply all of the necessary components for successful treatment.

> Bob was referred for an evaluation following a DUI (Driving Under Influence) arrest. A financially successful and prominent real estate broker, he had gained some recognition in the community for his philanthropy and willingness to donate much time and effort to community causes. He was also a gifted tennis player ranked locally on an amateur level. During the interview, he was very articulate, open, and honest, demonstrating that six years of psychoanalysis and two years in a weekly outpatient psychotherapy group had helped give him an impressive insight into himself and his relations to others. He confided that his drinking has concerned him for years, but that whenever he voiced this concern in his previous treatment, little regard was paid to it. He had twice previously stopped drinking on his own to "see if I could do it." One period of abstinence had lasted six months, following a black-out when "I had made a total ass of myself at a social event." His ability to stop on his own and the opinions of doctors, therapists, and even his wife that he could not possibly be "one of them" repeatedly convinced him that his expressed concerns were of no consequence. Prior to the end of the interview, the therapist summarized evidence (repeated black-outs, DUI arrest, periodic attempts at control, familial history of alcoholism, repeated shameful experiences when drinking, loss of control indicating he could not be sure when he started to drink whether he would get intoxicated, even though that was not his original intent) that suggested he could very well be an alcoholic. Bob looked immediately relieved at this information and said he had spent years trying to get someone to understand his experience. Informed by the therapist that a self-diagnosis was the only diagnosis of alcoholism that really mattered, he was encouraged to go to a number of AA meetings next week, return for another appointment, then determine what he thought and felt about his possible alcoholism. He returned to the next session, practically beaming, and presented his white chip to the therapist, and said, "I feel like I found a home. These people relate to me and I feel I can relate to them."

This vignette illustrates that at times, no amount of learning and insight alone can alter the progression of addiction. Not all addicted individuals need to be confronted and have their wall of denial stripped aggressively away. As this case illustrates, sometimes the addicted individual just needs to be carefully listened to and to have his or her experience either confirmed or clearly validated. The pitfalls of a total learning approach to treatment can be demonstrated by another example.

> Donna, a forty-one-year-old divorcée, has been married to two alcoholics and is herself addicted to benzodiazepines "to help settle my nerves." In and out of psychotherapy for the last fifteen years, she has never remained in therapy longer than a year and a half (three different times) and has never been out of therapy longer than nine months. She usually picks psychotherapists who place an inordinate amount of emphasis on understanding and insight, usually terminating treatment when she is challenged to give up her medication and change her behavior. At cocktail parties, she can readily and accurately tell her acquaintances the reason she has difficulties in relationships with men and why her failure with her own children is similar to her parents' failure with her. Yet, she does not change. She continues to repeat the perpetual self-destructive and self-defeating interpersonal style that has plagued her since childhood while remaining capable of explaining and understanding the reasons that compel her to act as she does. Since her defense system is composed primarily of the defenses of intellectualization, rationalization, and isolation of affect, her continual involvement with psychotherapists who only feed her defensive style helps her not to change and prevents her from looking at the feelings associated with her difficulties. Her addiction has never been addressed and it prevents an altering of her characterological style. The rationale for her continual prescription to benzodiazepines is difficult to justify. Attempts to stop the use of benzodiazepines has resulted in her substituting alcohol to "help calm her nerves." She justifies her use of medication because it was prescribed by a family physician who was concerned about her drinking and suggested she take Valium instead. This lends support to Joe Pursh's keen insight that "physicians have been treating alcoholics for years as if they were suffering from a Valium deficiency."

Of course, a group leader operating at the other extreme of the spectrum can also suffer limiting effects of a treatment approach that stresses only change and the expressing of feelings and discourages insight. Group "groupies" who are "into discovering themselves" are often prone to manipulating the group therapy situation to their advantage. Mary Goulding, herself a gifted group psychotherapist, is well aware of the "games" that many group members can be involved in and warns unsuspecting group leaders to be cautious in their application of an intervention that is only experiential. Mary Goulding tells a story of one such woman who had participated in one of her groups (1980).

> A woman entering a weekend marathon group started the group talking about her grief in relation to her deceased mother. The woman quickly plunged into an empty chair dialogue with her departed mother, crying and eventually expressing an abrupt explosion of anger at her mother for dying and leaving her alone. By this time, most of the members in the group were in tears themselves or at least very strongly affected by the woman's emotional outpouring. As she was encouraged by the group leader to complete her "work" with the deceased mother, the woman tearfully said, "And this is the last time I will say good-bye to you, mother." To this, the group leader quickly asked, "The last time?" "Oh yes!" the woman exclaimed, "I said good-bye to my dead mother in California with Fritz Perls in 1960, in 1972 with Erv and Miriam Polster while they were both in Cleveland, and with another therapist in New York!"

This vignette illustrates one of the dangers that may befall an unsuspecting group leader who is too readily taken in by a group member who is all too willing to express affect that is dramatic and easily accessible. However, a more prevalent danger in working with chemically dependent individuals in a group setting is the possibility of the group member being overstimulated and flooded emotionally by a group leader who employs a format that only encourages the expression of affect. This has certainly been the case on a number of occasions when I have had the opportunity to direct and participate in a psychodrama group at a Veterans Administration Hospital inpatient unit for chemically dependent veterans.

> Mike, a thirty-two-year-old, single, Caucasian male had "volunteered" to be a protagonist in a psychodrama group that met once each week during the patient's stay on the inpatient drug dependence unit. Mike, a quiet and somewhat shy man, began talking about his girlfriend who had died in an automobile accident that had resulted from Mike's inability to negotiate a turn in the road while he was driving her car. His difficulty in controlling the automobile was due to the fact that he was heavily intoxicated at the time he was driving. A powerful and explosive psychodrama scene was enacted with auxiliary alter egos played by supporting members in the group. In the final scene, Mike tearfully and painfully enacted pulling his dead

> girlfriend from the automobile, desperately trying to evoke some response from her lifeless body by shouting and begging for her forgiveness. At the close of the group session, the two co-therapists and many of the group members congratulated the director of the psychodrama for the powerful and masterful direction he had given Mike during this very dramatic encounter. Unfortunately, upon arriving on the unit the next morning, it was learned that Mike had left the hospital AMA (against medical advice) during the previous evening.

Undoubtedly, the stirring and flooding of intense feelings associated with this long-repressed experience had proved too threatening and overwhelming for Mike. This scenario was repeated too often on this unit. The consequences were not the same every time, but occurred with enough consistency to warrant the judgment that the risk of overstimulating a patient was not worth the infrequent benefits of such an approach to group psychotherapy with a chemically dependent population.

A more recent experience with a similar situation in a different group format produced far better results.

> Martha, a thirty-one-year-old recovering alcoholic with three years of sobriety, had entered an outpatient psychotherapy group because of her difficulty dealing with a recent loss (divorce from her husband) in her life. Early in the third session of the group, Martha spoke briefly about her present feelings surrounding her divorce and how they were quite similar to her feelings regarding the loss of a friend who had died in an automobile accident that occurred while Martha was driving intoxicated. The therapist's decision at this time was to focus on the feelings stirred up by the divorce and not to pursue the feelings surrounding the death of her friend. This decision was made because the group leader was not sure of the support Martha might receive from the other group members as well as the amount of ego strength she now possessed because of the acute state of her present stressful marital situation. The group leader also wanted more time to carefully assess the extent of her capacity to deal effectively with such a traumatic experience, as well as give her time to gain more trust and cohesion with the other group members. Approximately six months later, she once again mentioned the incident in passing. The group leader, at this time, decided to pursue it in more detail. As Martha told her story of guilt and eventual suicidal contemplation because of her friend's death, the other group members were encouraged to respond to her sharing of her story. Since the group had been conducted within an interactional format, her

> fears of condemnation from the other group members were explored and eventually discovered to be unfounded. The other members' support and sharing of their acceptance of her, despite what she had felt was an unforgivable incident in her life, was very cleansing and releasing for Martha. She returned to the group the next week with a noted improvement in affect, speaking of the dramatic change in herself, adding that she felt "as if a weight has been lifted off my chest."

The difference in the therapeutic outcome between Mike's and Martha's experiences illustrates an important decision that a group leader must make when choosing which group format to apply in addiction treatment. While one approach may be better suited for other populations, it is suggested here that a method which takes into careful consideration the special circumstances of the addicted patient be applied in a way that produces change and learning in a steady, controlled, and effective fashion. This is the primary reason why the rest of this book will be addressed toward outlining and articulating the interactional group model as the preferred mode of treatment for the chemically dependent individual. Yalom's particular brand of interactional group psychotherapy is the model that best serves the tasks and goals that must be established if group psychotherapy is to be an effective tool in the treatment of addictions. While there are modifications that must be made in Yalom's model, it is important to understand the basics of this approach before any alterations of the model are implemented by the group leader. Chapter 4 will be directed toward describing Yalom's approach to group psychotherapy. Before completing this chapter, a final conceptual map (see Figure 2.7) will be presented to permit potential group leaders to see that all of the options they have before them are dependent upon the tasks, goals and focus of interventions they wish to make in order to ensure that their particular group members' needs are met in the most beneficial and productive manner.

FIGURE 2.7

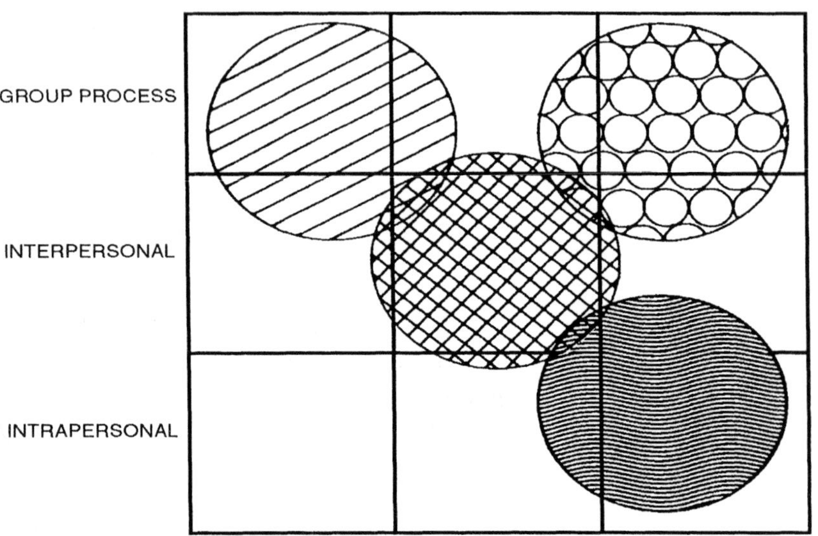

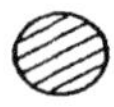 1) Psychodynamic Group Process and Tavistock Group-as-a-Whole Focus

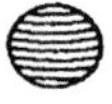 2) Gestalt, Psychodrama, and Redecision Group Therapy

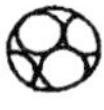 3) Behavior Management, Overeaters Anonymous, Smoking Cessation, etc.

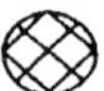 4) Interactional Group Psychotherapy, T-group, and Yalom's Model

Chapter 3

Preparing the Chemically Dependent Person for Group

Once it is determined that the chemically dependent individual is in need of treatment, it is inevitable that he or she will be placed in a psychotherapy group. This is an event that is rarely, if ever, questioned in the alcohol and drug treatment field. Group psychotherapy, for reasons that are not always clearly articulated, is the predominant mode of treatment in all alcohol and drug treatment programs. Every inpatient unit, day hospital, and aftercare program has group psychotherapy as an integral part of its treatment regimen. Other than the patient's involvement in a twelve-step program, it is hard to identity another treatment modality used more frequently in the treatment of addiction. Despite the predominance of its use, little attention is given to the importance of preparing patients for entry into a psychotherapy group. This is unfortunate because entry into a psychotherapy group can be quite difficult and anxiety-provoking for the prospective patient. Many addicted patients who would otherwise profit from group psychotherapy are unable to benefit more completely from treatment because they cannot manage the initial anxiety that group psychotherapy always triggers. Because twelve-step programs are viewed by some as a form of a group therapy in which its members enter without preparation, many treatment personnel in the alcohol and drug field do not appreciate the importance of pre-group preparation for their prospective group members.

Pre-group preparation for the chemically dependent patient takes on added complications because of the acute state of withdrawal and toxicity that accompanies the addicted patient early in treatment. Their level of cognitive impairment and chemical-induced emotionality make it difficult, and in many cases impossible, for them to respond appropriately to psychological levels of intervention. Entering a group is difficult for anyone. It can be overwhelming for a person in a state of acute crisis who is also in the throes of the early stages of withdrawal. Rarely do addicts and alcoholics enter treatment without a crisis precipitating it. Most are coerced into treatment by disgruntled spouses, employers, a punitive legal system, or a life-threatening medical complication. Add to this that their first introduction to group and treatment is usually in an institutional setting, and it is no small wonder that they are unable to be appreciative, grateful, and receptive to the well-intended efforts of the staff to help them. It is doubtful that an alcoholic or addict wakes up one fine morning and announces, "Wow, I feel great today, its wonderful to be alive, I think I'll go check myself into that hospital treatment program for 28 days!"

While many theorists and practitioners of group psychotherapy recognize the need for preparing prospective group members before they are placed in a group because groups are so difficult to enter and evoke so much anxiety, little attention has been paid to the special circumstances of the addicted patient. There is a substantial body of research and clinical experience that provides helpful and practical guidelines for accomplishing this task, but most of the recommendations that are presented are made for a non-addicted population entering outpatient treatment. While these recommendations have a great deal of merit and are generalizable to addicted patients, they overlook the considerable levels of acute neurological impairment that are present in most alcoholics and addicts early in their abstinence. Chapter 8 will provide an overview of the research that addresses this issue. For now, it is enough to know that the level of impairment is usually severe enough, in most cases, to warrant the opinion that most addicts and alcoholics will look and sound better than they actually are. They will be able to follow only the most concrete, simple, and rudimentary interventions or suggestions. This is a fact that must not be overlooked in the early stages of treatment.

Fortunately, the importance of preparing patients for entry into other contemporary forms of group psychotherapy has not been overlooked by Yalom et al. (1967) and others (Rutan and Stone, 1984; Agazarian and Peters, 1981). While the issue of patient preparation is a controversial one, there has been substantial research in this area. It is important to understand the implications of this research and how pre-group preparation affects group members who are entering a group for the first time. The results from Yalom's and others' experiences in this area yield important information that can be helpful for the group leader who is about to embark on the difficult task of leading a group consisting entirely of alcoholics and addicts.

RECOMMENDATIONS FOR ENTRY INTO A THERAPY GROUP

While no one method has been universally accepted, Rutan and Stone (1984) recommend that preparation must accomplish the following:

1. Establish a preliminary alliance between patient and clinician;
2. Gain a clear consensus about the patient's therapeutic hopes;
3. Offer information and instruction about group psychotherapy;
4. Deal with the initial anxiety about joining a group;
5. Present and gain acceptance of a contract.

ESTABLISH A PRELIMINARY ALLIANCE

Entering a group is stressful and it is very helpful for new group members to have at least a minimal alliance with the group leader. Most patients will experience group therapy as the most difficult form of psychotherapy to begin. Having an alliance with the group leader, however brief this alliance may be, will minimize the impact of this difficulty.

As Sigmund Freud (1921) succinctly pointed out many years ago, groups promote regression. Members entering group for the first time are forced to experience and handle powerful emotions triggered by issues related to survival, rejection, and acceptance. Group members must determine how they are to survive in the group and discover who is likely to attack or support them. They must adapt to the unknown demands of the group and learn which behaviors will lead to acceptance and which behaviors will lead to rejection. If the group is a particularly unstructured situation, as it is in dynamic group psychotherapy, clues regarding how to proceed are minimal. Through trial and error, members must orient themselves to discover which behaviors or interactions will work and which will not work. The ambiguity of such a situation produces regression, and the degree of regression is idiosyncratic to each particular member. While the group leader can expect group members to regress in such an unstructured situation, the way the group members respond to this regression is unpredictable.

With a group of alcoholics and addicts in the early stages of their withdrawal from chemicals, techniques that promote regression can have detrimental and, in some cases, even catastrophic consequences. Alcoholics and addicts handle stress poorly. They rely on their previously maladaptive styles of coping–namely the ingesting of chemicals into their body–if they are forced to deal with ambiguity too early in their recovery. Only after they have learned more adaptive ways of coping should they be required to handle regression in group. The group leader must understand and appreciate that a relapse can sometimes be fatal for a group member. All interventions that have a potential to increase the likelihood of drug and alcohol use should therefore be used sparingly. Consequently, any measures the group leader can take that will prevent regression during the early stages of recovery should be initiated and maintained.

While it is impossible to establish a true working alliance with a potential group member in one interview, much anxiety or fear can be reduced if the effort is made. A one-time meeting, however brief, can enhance the group member's transition into a group, thus increasing the possibility of more responsiveness to treatment. There are different recommendations on how many individual sessions are needed when introducing non-addicted patients into a weekly outpatient therapy group. The realities of time and economics sometimes dictate that this be accomplished in a single session. If the pre-group preparation is done well, this will be enough in most cases. The realities of institutional settings make it more difficult and sometimes impossible for the group leader to have time to prepare each member before they enter group. Since most addicts and alcoholics are initially introduced to group in some form of institutional setting (hospital, day-treatment program, outpatient program, etc.), it is rare that time is allowed for a group leader to meet with individuals before they show up in their group. If possible, a ten or fifteen minute meeting prior to the start of group would by better than nothing. Sometimes, these introductions and preparations can be incorporated into an agenda round format (see Chapter 10).

One method for minimizing regression in group is to establish an alliance with group members before they enter group. An alliance with the group leader will decrease the likelihood of a relapse occurring because of the intensity of the feelings that are triggered by the regressive pull of the group. An alliance is especially important if a group member has had no prior psychotherapy experience. It is the patient who has never been exposed to individual or group psychotherapy who is most likely to prematurely drop out of treatment.

Implications for Research Findings

A study conducted at a major university reported that 70 of 198 patients dropped out of therapy after less than five visits, even though their therapists felt they could benefit from further treatment (MacLeod, 1968). Yalom and Rand (1966) report similar findings in another study that found one-third of all patients beginning group therapy dropped out unimproved after the first dozen meetings. This was contrasted with another study that found those patients who stayed in a group for fifty meetings were more likely to show clinical improvement. All of this suggests the importance of managing the first few meetings with newly acquired group members. It has been reasoned by MacLeod (1968) that the awkwardness of the management of the early hours of treatment was the most significant factor contributing to premature dropouts and treatment failures. If you cannot keep the patient in treatment, there is little chance they will have the opportunity to improve. He further suggests that

> the best technique for avoiding unfortunate instability in the treatment situation has always been focus on the development of a therapeutic alliance or relationship as promptly as possible, that is immediately. The focus on the development of a therapeutic alliance means that the patient and the therapist become acquainted actively as real people in a real current experience. The therapist should not attempt to present himself energetically as a transference object, such as by adopting a blank screen model. (1968, p. 402)

MacLeod concludes that any technique which is going to interfere with the development of the alliance or create significant additional frustration or anxiety in the early stages of treatment should therefore be used sparingly.

GAIN A CLEAR CONSENSUS ABOUT THE PATIENT'S THERAPEUTIC HOPES

Anyone who has worked with alcoholics or addicts on a sustained basis knows that they all possess a much-desired but equally unreachable goal. Each wishes to be able to take drugs recreationally and to drink normally. This is a goal they can never attain and the sooner each addict and alcoholic realizes and accepts this, the less progress will be impeded in treatment. Admittance and acceptance of this limitation is in fact the first step of Alcoholics Anonymous. While some may argue that controlled drinking is a feasible option for some alcoholics (Sobell and Sobell, 1973b), research in this area is certainly inconclusive. The risk of relapse and the associated possible consequence of death is too important an issue to be debated academically. Within Alcoholics Anonymous, an alcoholic is somebody who, by definition of their alcoholism, cannot drink normally. Tell a group of eight alcoholics that there is a statistical probability that one of them may return to normal drinking and each alcoholic in that group will believe he or she is the one exception.

While abstinence should be the primary goal of treatment, especially for an alcoholic or addict just beginning treatment, this does not imply that other goals should be ignored. Vernon Johnson (1973), in his classic book, *I'll Quit Tomorrow,* outlines two explicit goals for alcoholics entering psychotherapy groups.

> The purpose of this paper is to discuss the assumptions and techniques we are using in conducting group therapy. To begin with, let's look at some of the similarities within our group. In addition to our alcoholism we all have two things in common. First, before we came to the point of seeking outside help, we each tried our own *do it yourself* program in an effort to change ourselves. The second similarity is that we all failed. A basic assumption of group therapy is that a major reason for this failure is that our most determined efforts can't change what we can't see, and that there is a great deal that we are not seeing clearly.
>
> For this reason our *goal* in group therapy is:
>
> To discover ourselves and others as feeling persons, and
>
> To identify *the defenses that prevent this discovery.*
>
> While change is the ultimate goal, our immediate purpose is to see more accurately what needs change. This requires seeing ourselves–*discovering ourselves*–at a feeling level.
>
> In examining our purpose one of the things that stands out is our emphasis on feelings. We stress feelings for several reasons. First of all, our behavior in the past has been so opposed to our value system that considerable feelings of remorse and self-loathing have been built up. It appears that we have accumulated a pool of negative feelings and walled them off with a variety of masks or *defenses that prevent this discovery.* This began with mild disapproval of ourself, then growing remorse, and finally a deep self-loathing. Statements such as: "I'm no damn good!" or "The world would be better off without me," reflect these negative feelings and attitudes. It is important to be in touch with these in order to take the First Step of the Alcoholics Anonymous Program where: "We admitted that we were powerless over alcohol–that our lives had become unmanageable."
>
> Being in touch with the hostile feelings we have toward ourselves and the sense of helplessness and hopelessness that accompany them, make the First Step a moving description instead of simply an abstract theory. We *feel* the *powerlessness* and the *unmanageability.*

> One of the important functions of the group is to help us identify the defenses that prevent this discovery. (Johnson, 1976, pp. 118-119)

Group psychotherapy from this perspective requires a focus on feelings. The group leader will soon learn that, unlike non-addicted patients in group, chemically dependent individuals are completely out of touch with their feelings. A seemingly simplistic intervention such as, "What are you feeling right now?" will produce a startling effect. As a group leader, you will soon discover that these addicted individuals do not know how to identify and interpret their feelings. They must learn how to accomplish this task, because addicts and alcoholics who do not learn to understand their feelings will undoubtedly relapse. Chemically dependent individual must be led to understand that the management of their feelings is an essential requirement for the attainment of abstinence and recovery.

Ernest Kurtz (1979) views Alcoholics Anonymous as teaching alcoholics that they cannot attain what all alcoholics unrealistically strive for, and that is unlimited control of their feelings. The alcoholic's addiction to alcohol is, for Kurtz, related to the alcoholic's misunderstanding and denial of the spiritual. "The active alcoholic was attempting to attain the spiritual, the unlimited, by means of the material. He was trying to achieve a *quality* of living by the mere adding up of quantities of or experiences with alcohol" (p. 208). The quality of living pursued by the alcoholic was confused with the spiritual because it involved a claim to the absolute, i.e., complete control of feelings, which is a striving to reach beyond the limits of human finiteness. Only God or the absolute has total control of feelings and AA set as its task to teach the alcoholic that he or she was *Not-God.*

> The alcoholic attempted to achieve by the drinking of alcohol what reality would give only by living as fully human. Reality does not grant to humans *absolute* control over moods and feelings; emotions are meant to be a *response* to reality, and mainly to realities outside the self. *Absolute control* over emotion, in the sense of absolutely autonomous self-determination of moods and feelings, involved a claim to unlimitedness, and so a claim beyond any human. (Kurtz, 1979, p. 209)

Treatment from this perspective requires that alcoholics learn how to identify and accept the limitation of their feelings if they wish to maintain true sobriety. Consequently, the group leader must gently encourage alcoholics, and addicts, to understand the futility of a position that demands they either feel good all the time or avoid feeling bad at any time. Feelings are there for a reason. As Kurtz indicates, emotions allow us to judge reality and our relation to reality. Emotions tell us when we are really happy and when we are acting against the values we truly hold internally.

Once abstinence from drugs and alcohol is maintained for at least a year, more explicit personal goals can be established by the patient. AA, NA, and CA encourage their members not to make any significant changes (i.e., divorces, job transfers, etc.) until their first year of sobriety is achieved. These twelve-step programs intuitively know what neuropsychological research has just begun to prove empirically. Alcoholics and addicts, because of their drinking and drug use, suffer from deficits in their cognitive processes that make abstract reasoning difficult. While their level of impairment is subtle, it is detectable with tests sensitive to its assessment. Chapter 8 will deal with this issue in more detail. For now, it will suffice to say that once sobriety is maintained for at least a year, many of the goals that are desired by non-addicted patients can be initiated and negotiated with less danger of relapse.

OFFER INFORMATION AND INSTRUCTION ABOUT GROUP PSYCHOTHERAPY

Because a group will rapidly evoke intense feelings in chemically dependent patients, it will be important to help them feel grounded by giving them specific and concrete information about how groups work. Once they know what to expect, group members will be able to respond to the group more appropriately. There are a number of ways this can be accomplished.

A. Give the new group members reading material that explains the structure and rationales of group psychotherapy (Gauron and Rawlings, 1975).
B. Didactically explain to them what they can expect in group and how best to put the group to their advantage (Wogan et al., 1977).
C. Some group leaders have presented group members with an opportunity to view a group session behind a one-way mirror (Wogan et al., 1977).
D. In some cases, prospective group members have been given audiotapes of a "good patient's" participation in group. This was done in the hopes that new members would model their behavior after the "good patient" (Truax and Wargo, 1969).

All the studies cited here showed similar results suggesting greater improvement after three months among patients who were prepared ahead of time than among those patients who entered a control group without preparation. While there was no evidence to suggest that any format led to fewer dropouts, there was a general agreement indicating that group norms are shaped more quickly in the direction of a therapeutic group environment as a result of group member preparation.

Yalom sought to answer the question concerning the benefits of preparing group members for group. His query was prompted by his understanding of the crucial importance of early meetings in shaping the future course of group. Yalom had discovered that group norms established early in the life of a group tended to persist, outliving even a complete turnover in the group population. Consequently, Yalom reasoned that the establishment of healthy group norms early in group would be beneficial to the functioning of the group. Yalom was also aware that there was a cost involved in preparing members for group. Arguments, especially by psychodynamic-oriented group therapists, suggested that any technique that interfered with the development and resolution of transference and transference distortions should be used sparingly. Since preparing members for group might interfere with this process, it was judged that group treatment would be impaired. It was essential that the group leader enhance the development of transference in group. Enigma and ambiguity on the leader's part would facilitate transference, and the therapist should do nothing, such as preparing group members, to interfere with this process.

Yalom's answer to this argument was that the benefits of preparing patients for group far outweigh the costs. Primarily, preparing group members enhanced the development of the other important curative factors operating in group. Yalom also felt that transference is a healthy organism; it will still manifest itself despite the organizational activity involved in the group members' preparation.

Yalom's Controlled Study for Preparing Patients for Group Therapy

Yalom et al.'s 1967 study required a twenty-five minute preparatory meeting for new group members. Subjects for this study were randomly assigned to one of two conditions: those prepared for group in the manner to be discussed and those randomly assigned to groups without preparation. The twenty-five minute preparatory meeting was designed to attain three goals:

1. Enhance the new group members' faith in group therapy and increase the positive expectancy that group would be helpful.
2. Enhance the attractiveness of group and develop cohesion.

3. Direct the group members toward the confrontational, here and now interaction within the group. Yalom placed the greatest emphasis on this topic during the preparatory session.

In order to accomplish these three goals, Yalom had each of the new group members presented with five sources of specific instructions:

1. A theoretical basis of group therapy was discussed with an emphasis placed on the interpersonal theory of psychiatry.
2. A rational description of group was presented.
3. The expected effectiveness and results of group treatment were outlined.
4. Sources of possible stress within group were identified.
5. Members were instructed to discuss their feelings with other members in the group.

Theoretical Basis of Group Psychotherapy

Each prospective group member was presented with a brief history of the evolution of group therapy. It was explained that group first gained value because of economics. More people could be treated at less expense. However, group members were clearly told that group therapy had now evolved to the point that it was a very sophisticated and unique form of treatment that could justify itself on its own merit. In fact, group therapy is often the treatment of choice. In many cases, it has been found to be more effective than individual treatment. The remarks during this introduction were aimed to instill faith in group therapy as a mode of treatment and dispel any notions of group therapy being an inferior or a second-class approach to treatment.

Rational Description for Group

Sullivan's interpersonal theory of psychiatry was briefly presented. Everyone was reminded that a universal concern for people was their difficulty establishing and maintaining close, gratifying relationships with others. Members were reminded that they may have wished many times to clarify a relationship, to be honest with another about their feelings, both positive and negative, while being able to get honest feedback on how others perceive them. Group therapy was described as a hall of mirrors–a place where they could discover how they affect others, how others perceive them, and how they, in turn, are affected by others. Since the general structure of society does not permit such interactions to occur, group could be viewed as a social microcosm where honest interpersonal interaction was not only permitted, but encouraged.

Effectiveness of Group Psychotherapy

Group members were cautioned that group therapy could be a difficult endeavor for them to undertake. While starting in a group was not often easy–in fact, they were warned that it could be quite stressful working directly on their relationships with other members in the group–they were assured there would be tremendous carryover to the "real world." Members were instructed that if they were willing to honestly work through, resolve, and clarify their relationships with other group members, this would lead them to discover pathways to more rewarding relationships with others outside of group.

Sources of Possible Stress Within the Group

All prospective group members were reminded of how stressful and difficult it could be to be honest with others in the group. They were forewarned that, at times, especially during the beginning of group, feelings of puzzlement and discouragement could be expected. They were warned that they might question how the group could possibly help them or their situation. At other times, it might not be apparent to them how working on group problems and their interpersonal relationships with the other group members could be of value in solving problems that led them to join the group in the first place. Puzzlement and discouragement should be expected, and they were urged not to follow through with their inclinations to drop out of group. It was often difficult for people to risk revealing themselves honestly, and they should be aware of their tendency to withdraw emotionally. They were told that they may want to hide their feelings or may allow others to express their feelings for them. This, in turn, could lead to concealing their alliances with others from the group and its leader. There were a number of different emotions that they might expect to occur. Annoyance and frustration at the group leader for not giving more direction to the group was common. Many members might direct this frustration toward the other members and wonder, as Yalom et al. said, "How can the blind lead the blind?" (1967, p. 418). Even when group members are unaware of anxiety and nervousness, they were told these are common emotions during the beginning of group. While everyone fears attack and rejection for appearing foolish, it is essential that these fears be gradually worked through. On the other hand, members were given the reassurance that group is not a forced confessional and that they can set their own pace in self-disclosing.

The Encouragement of Group Member Interaction

Group members were repeatedly instructed that the way group would be most helpful for them was if they would be honest and direct with the other members and the group leader. The open sharing of feelings as they are occurring at this moment was emphasized continually by Yalom. This, the members were instructed, was the core of group therapy. Trust often took time to develop in group, and they were reminded that people have different rates of developing trust. While it was essential that trust, safety, and cohesiveness be established, they were encouraged to view group as a forum for risk-taking. As learning and risk-taking progressed, they were encouraged to try new types of behavior.

Results of Preparing Group Members for Group

Yalom et al.'s 1967 study failed to have any significant effect on group members' terminating therapy early or dropping out prematurely. A number of studies since that time have generally supported Yalom's findings indicating that pre-group preparation has little effect on group members staying in group. However, Yalom et al.'s study does show evidence that preparation of group members does enhance the members' faith in group and that those groups with prepared members engaged in interaction more quickly. Consequently, groups composed of prepared members are spared the initial stage of uncertainty and move more quickly into the basic task of group. Personal benefit and improvement is attained more quickly when compared to groups composed of unprepared group members.

Special Problems in the Preparation of the Chemically Dependent Individual

There is one unique aspect involved in preparing the chemically dependent person for outpatient group therapy that is usually not necessary for non-addicted members. Most alcoholics and addicts have at some time during their addiction attended meetings of Alcoholics Anonymous, Cocaine Anonymous, or Narcotics Anonymous. In some cases, prospective members may be very active currently in AA, CA, or NA. These individuals should be encouraged to continue their participation in these organizations. It would be important to inform them that the psychotherapy group is not designed to treat their addiction or be a substitute for the peer-oriented (AA, CA, and NA) program. Rather, the group can support or complement such peer-oriented programs. In some cases, if the person does not have enough sobriety, group therapy may be contraindicated, especially if the group leader is unfamiliar with the treatment format of these programs.

If it is judged that the prospective group member can benefit from group therapy, the group leader will have to give clear instructions that the therapy group does not operate like an AA, CA, or NA meeting. This is especially important if the group member has never been in a therapy group previously and has been active in AA, CA or NA for years. Confusion between the twelve-step format and group therapy can hinder both forms of treatment. Understanding the difference between peer groups and professional therapy groups is not as crucial for the member who has three years of sobriety as it is for the newly recovering individual with only two weeks of sobriety. Individuals with a few years of recovery under their belts are usually more equipped to handle the adjustment to the change in treatment format. Newly recovering addicts or alcoholics are in a highly charged emotional state and are more easily confused and threatened by their misunderstanding of the differing demands each modality makes upon them. Transmitting this information can be helpful and in some cases crucial.

Both professionally oriented groups and peer-oriented groups (Alcoholics Anonymous, Cocaine Anonymous, Narcotics Anonymous) should be considered active treatment groups designed to facilitate recovery and abstinence from alcohol. A critical difference exists, however, between the professionally oriented and peer-oriented group. The professionally led therapy group emphasizes the use of specific behavioral and psychological prescriptions and techniques that are applied to a global, generalized, symptom reduction effort. In comparison, the AA format focuses on a specific, regimented approach addressing one specific, component of recovery (i.e., abstinence).

The core content of the professionally oriented group should consist of the attempt to facilitate gradually increasing introspection and compliance through the use of group confrontation, discussion, and education. In contrast, the peer-oriented group is almost entirely supportive, fostering a degree of dependence on the acceptance of a specific and limited treatment approach focused entirely on compliance and abstinence from alcohol and drugs.

Treatment Characteristics

In order to gain a more comprehensive overview of the content of each treatment group, a projected list of similarities and differences between the two treatment groups is presented. Divergent and common elements are listed in Table 3.1 and Table 3.2, respectively.

TABLE 3.1 Divergent Elements

Peer-Oriented Group (AA, CA, NA)	Professionally Oriented Group
1. Treatment goal will focus specifically on abstinence.	1. Treatment goals will be individually determined by the person, which requires that social, psychological, physical, and drinking-related behavior be examined and evaluated.
2. Emphasis on the "how" of abstinence and recovery.	2. Emphasis on the "why" of abstinence and recovery.
3. Opening of group with readings of the AA "Big Book" and the Twelve Steps of Recovery.	3. Development of group cohesiveness and traditional group processes.
4. Structured use of life histories dealing specifically with personal history of alcoholism and recovery.	4. Verbal reports of general progress without notation and rigid format.
5. Didactic format by group leaders to impart AA principles.	5. Mobilization of group support and feedback.
6. Emphasis on the first four steps of AA's traditional twelve steps with less emphasis on feelings and emotions.	6. More emphasis on group discussion of feelings and emotions.
7. More democratic group leadership with members taking a more active role in the group discussion.	7. More traditional role of group leader in the group process.
8. Group discussion focused on ways to remain abstinent.	8. More confrontation and exploration of resistance.

These specific treatment procedures should be developed and monitored in their application throughout the course of treatment in order to ensure that the treatments offered (professional vs. peer [AA]) are both clinically meaningful and discriminately different. In this way, maximum benefit can be realized by the group leader by contrasting different types of therapy with the identifiable characteristics of certain alcoholics and addicts.

TABLE 3.2. Common Elements

1. Group discussion.
2. Correct misconceptions about addiction.
3. Impart information on addiction and need for compliance.
4. Formulation of treatment issues.
5. Group support at beginning.
6. Aim to reduce patient complaints and behavior that interfere with alcohol and drug abstinence.
7. Attempt to involve and change family environment.
8. Search for continuing causes of abstinence difficulties.

DEAL WITH THE INITIAL ANXIETY ABOUT JOINING THE GROUP

Most people are quite anxious about joining a group. The group leader should encourage the prospective members to talk about their anxiety in group and reassure them that all individuals entering group will be sharing these feelings. Instruction should be given that it will be helpful to discuss such feelings during the initial hours of the group.

However, alcoholics and addicts pose some unique problems for the group leader when it comes to the issue of pre-group anxiety. The group leader will find that pre-group preparation with this population will result in anxiety being manifested in one of two extreme manners. With alcoholics and addicts who have a propensity for acting out behavior (i.e., sociopathic features, repeated difficulty with the law, etc.) and illicit drug abuse (i.e., cocaine, heroin, marijuana, amphetamines, etc.), the group leader will find that their anxiety is usually kept out of their awareness. With those alcoholics and addicts who have a propensity for a more isolated existence (i.e., agoraphobic features, fear of crowds, etc.) and more licit drug abuse (i.e., prescription medications like Valium and Librium), the group leader will find that their anxiety is much more in their awareness because it is extremely high and often incapacitating. Each particular set of patients has to be approached differently when preparing them for group.

With group members who have more characterological features and whose anxiety is more unconscious, it would behoove the group leader to raise the anxiety to their awareness before they enter group. If their anxiety remains unconscious, there is a greater chance that they will react in group the way they deal with all situations that produce anxiety in the "real world"–namely, by acting out. Such group members must learn that membership in a group means expressing feelings verbally and not behaviorally. Once they become aware of their anxiety and agree to express such feelings verbally, they must be encouraged to realize that anxiety is universal. Such an awareness will reassure them that they are not less of a person just because they experience fear or discomfort.

Group members who have fewer characterological features accompanying their addiction are more likely to have a history of anxiety disorders (i.e., panic attacks, phobias). Their use of drugs and alcohol is often an attempt at self-medication. As they become increasingly alcohol- and drug-free, their anxiety may actually increase. Entry into a group will be especially difficult for this population of addicted individuals. Reassurance, support, and enhancement of their inadequate defensive process is a must if they are to survive the initial entry into a therapy group.

Complicating this process even further is a mismatch that often exists between the more socially and economically disadvantaged addict's or alcoholic's attitude toward treatment and the middle-class staff's expectations of them in treatment. As Heitler (1976) indicates in a review on addiction and the socially disadvantaged, "lower class patients are the most likely to be unsophisticated, unpracticed and even grossly misinformed about psychological kinds of treatment and to bring an array of values, life styles and expectations of therapy which clash with the working orientation of [the] traditional psychotherapist." Verinis (1995) agrees when he suggests that these types of patients require "immediate concrete solutions and direct interventions" (p. 96). My own research with Native American alcoholics (Flores, 1985) suggests that one reason why this population has such a dismal recovery rate for addiction is the disparity between Native American values and the values of the therapist or treatment staff. All of this suggests that sensitivity to social, economic, cultural, and educational differences must be applied when preparing the addict or alcoholic for group therapy.

Research and clinical opinion about the alleviation of initial anxiety during pre-group preparation with prospective group members who are *not* addicted sheds some light on issues that should be addressed with the chemically dependent individual. Agazarian and Peters (1981) list four common fears that may be stimulated by entry into a therapy group:

1. Confidentiality of personal information.
2. Rejection by the group.

3. Embarrassment over revealing intimate information to other group members.
4. Pathology of others.

Confidentiality of Personal Information

Agazarian and Peters (1981) write,

> Prospective group patients often worry that information presented in group sessions will "leak" and get back to someone who knows them in the outside world. They can be assured that this has not proved the case in the past and that such an event is not expected to occur in the future. If time permits associations to this worry can be explored with the patient. Most important is to encourage the patient to raise this concern with the group where it is always a therapeutically productive issue. (p. 189)

Confidentiality is always a concern for alcoholics and addicts. Many who enter an aftercare group or outpatient group may not feel it necessary to discuss it as an important issue because of their exposure to the required anonymity of twelve-step programs. However, this issue needs to be addressed even if the group leader has to force the topic into discussion. Confidentiality should not be assumed because many alcoholics and addicts have engaged in embarrassing, humiliating, and, in some cases, even illegal behavior while under the influence of alcohol or drugs. Confidentiality needs to be assured. Members should be told that they will undoubtedly talk about their experiences in group with friends and family, but that they should do so in such a manner that they do not talk specifically about or reveal the identities of the other members.

Worries About Rejection by Group Members

> Worries about rejection by group members are best dealt with by helping the worrier to link up his present fear with painful experiences in the past via his associations. Again, the patient should be reminded that this may well be a useful group-related issue for him to discuss with the group. (Agazarian and Peters, 1981, p. 189)

The issues raised by Agazarian and Peters will be similar with a chemically dependent population. Despite the fact that addicts or alcoholics, while drinking or taking drugs, might act in a way that indicates that rejection is of little concern to them, they have a tremendous need to be accepted and approved of by others.

Fear of Being Embarrassed

Agazarian and Peters (1981) suggest,

> Fear of being embarrassed in front of group members should be handled in much the same way as fear of rejection. In addition, the information already given about the way a group operates through sharing and honest feedback is helpful in letting the person know that he will not be alone in revealing his intimate thoughts and feelings. (p. 189)

Embarrassment and shame are crucial issues for addicts and alcoholics. As Kurtz (1979) suggests, chemically dependent individuals suffer from tremendous feelings of shame. Their self-esteem is very tenuous and, as a rule, they possess extremely intropunitive superegos. Consequently, even the smallest transgression will drive them to punish themselves in an overly sadistic and harsh manner. On the other hand, any indications that others may perceive them as loathsome or shameful will lead them to act out in a defensive and provocative manner. They cannot tolerate others perceiving them as they feel or perceive themselves. Many alcoholics and addicts need affirmation from others to help alleviate their painful feelings of shame and embarrassment.

Fears Concerning the Imagined Pathology of Others

> Fears concerning the imagined pathology of as-yet-unseen fellow group members are quite likely to be projections, the defensive nature of which is not conscious to the patient. Such fears may be expressed as fear of mental contamination (Foulkes and Anthony, 1973) or as doubts about what "a bunch of sickies" can do for the patient. Exploration of free associations is one avenue of relieving this kind of concern. Another is by telling the patient that these are people like himself who share many of his anxieties and concerns; such information helps him to approach the projective nature of his fears. (Agazarian and Peters, 1981, p. 186)

Usually, alcoholics and addicts are much more accepting of others' shortcomings and limitations. Because they have experienced such dreadful feelings and emotions during their numerous intoxications and withdrawals, they can readily accept such conditions in others. However, most alcoholics and addicts have tremendous fears that underneath their addiction, others may discover that they are either "crazy," perverted, or loathsome. They fear the truth will finally emerge and people will see them as they really are. Consequently, it will be important to reframe any of their concerns about their pathology and place it within the disease model. This will bolster their self-image until they are able to identify with the other members in the group and learn that their fears are universally shared.

PRESENT AND GAIN ACCEPTANCE OF THE CONTRACT

Presenting and having a group member accept a contract before entering a therapy group is the most crucial contributing factor to a successful outpatient therapy group. Unfortunately, its importance is often ignored and too little time is spent on training group leaders in this preparation process. For many addicts and alcoholics entering an inpatient treatment program under coercion or distress, it is impractical, and in some cases impossible, to get a working contract established. Since it is neither feasible nor desirable to adjust treatment goals to meet the specific preferences of each individual, abstinence should always be the primary goal of treatment. Newly entering inpatients are rarely asked, or in any condition to decide, if they will agree with the goal of the treatment unit at the hospital. Most would prefer to receive treatment without having to go through the difficulties that a therapy group demands. Consequently, they have little choice in their contract at this time. This is the way it should be. Nevertheless, it would still benefit the group leader to actively engage the new group members in the process of understanding the requirements and demands that the therapy group will impose upon them.

Inpatient and outpatient therapy groups pose different and unique problems for the group leader. Chapter 8 will address the differences that a group leader will have to negotiate when conducting an inpatient group. The suggestions to be presented here are most suitable for an aftercare group or an ongoing outpatient group.

Rutan and Stone (1984) outline seven elements that they feel are essential in the contract for an ongoing, open-ended therapy group. They feel the group members should agree:

1. To be present each week, to be on time and to remain throughout the meeting.

2. To work actively on the problems that brought them to group.
3. To put feelings in words, not actions.
4. To use the relationships in group therapeutically, not socially.
5. To remain in the group until the problems that brought them to the group have been resolved.
6. To be responsible for their bills.
7. To protect the names and identities of fellow group members.

(Rutan and Stone, 1984, pp. 114-115)

Rutan and Stone view the contract not so much as a formal written document, but rather as a verbal agreement regarding the ground rules for group. The ground rules provide the foundation for a productive and safe therapeutic environment and should be mutually agreed upon before a member enters an outpatient or aftercare group. In order to ensure an understanding of the group rules, I give each incoming member a written description of my eleven ground rules for group. Figure 3.1 is a copy of these ground rules.

The group leader will learn that the establishment of a clear contract and the understanding of the ground rules of group will prevent many of the difficulties that usually emerge in group. Managing the boundaries of group is one of the most important elements of an effective group. It helps establish the therapeutic environment (cohesion) and allows the other curative factors to be set in motion. Furthermore, the contract allows the group leader to use its violations as a way to understand the various resistances, character traits, and transferences that take place in group.

FIGURE 3.1

An effective group takes a lot of work and faith to develop. These eleven ground rules and accompanying notes have been prepared to help new members in a psychotherapy group understand conditions that are essential to a successful group.

1. *THE GROUP CONTRACT.* To help you benefit most from your group experience, you will agree to:

   A) Talk about the issues and problems that prompted you to join the group.
   B) Tell the emotionally meaningful stories of your life.
   C) Verbally communicate your immediate thoughts and feelings about yourself, the group leaders, and the group members.
   D) Take an equal share of the total talking time.
   E) Agree not to leave the group before you complete or resolve what you came to the group to address.

2. *CONFIDENTIALITY.* Each member of the group agrees that they will not reveal the identity of any other member of the group either by name or identifying material. Group members would not feel free to be completely open with their most intimate feelings if they thought they would be talked about outside of the group.

3. *CONTACT BETWEEN GROUP MEMBERS OUTSIDE OF GROUP.* There is no ground rule prohibiting such contact; however, any contact should be shared within the group. This keeps cliques from forming, which, if they did, could damage the integrity of the group as a working unit. It is important to remember that it is more beneficial to keep the group relationships therapeutic rather than social.

4. *SUBGROUPING.* When a subgroup of two or more members get together to talk about the group and how they feel about different members, they often keep this information to themselves. Consequently, important information that needs to be shared between group members is withheld. This eventually inhibits the potential for self-awareness and growth that can occur from this feedback when given directly within the group. In addition, subgroup members behave differently in group. Typically, they protect each other and do not give each other the feedback each needs. Therefore, it is imperative that talk outside of the group be brought back and discussed within the group.

5. *NO SEXUAL CONTACT BETWEEN GROUP MEMBERS.* The members agree that during their membership in group no sexual liaisons will be formed. This freedom from sexual liaisons facilitates an intimacy between group members that, in turn, provides a basis for growth and change. Thus, the trust necessary for openness and problem-solving can develop.

6. *NO HITTING OR DAMAGE TO THE OFFICE.* Anger is to be expressed verbally rather than physically. As with any other emotions, anger, freely and appropriately expressed, can form the basis for insight and growth.

7. *NO DRUGS OR ALCOHOL.* No one is to come to group, at any time, under the influence of alcohol or drugs.

8. *GRADUATION VERSUS TERMINATION FROM GROUP.* When members begin thinking about discontinuing psychotherapy, they are expected to discuss this in group, prior to making their final decision, as freely as they have discussed other feelings. *Graduation* from group therapy is a time of joy and sharing, which has been thought out and discussed with the group. On the other hand, group members may make a decision to *terminate* at a point in therapy when they are beginning to face some critical issues that they are attempting to avoid by leaving the group. The input of other group members is extremely valuable at this point. While no one needs the permission of the group to discontinue psychotherapy, it is in the spirit of growth that leaving the group will be discussed in the group.

Members are to give at least four weeks notice prior to graduation. Terminating group without notice has a detrimental effect on the group and is likely to represent the continuance of the same problem behavior for which you came to the group in the first place. This time also allows for good-byes and the resolution of any unfinished issues between members. Consequently, each group member agrees to allow other group members to participate in their decision to leave the group.

9. *ATTENDANCE.* Regular attendance and punctuality enhance the value of the group for each member. Such cohesiveness creates a climate of work, support, and success. In the event of a member's inability to or decision not to attend a session, a telephone call to this effect is expected. Group will begin and end promptly at the designated times. Group members will agree to be in group at the time it starts and stay until it finishes.

10. *COMMITMENT.* Members are allowed to join the group only if they are willing to make a six-month commitment. This agreement ensures that the group process will not be disrupted by members "dropping in" for one or two sessions and then dropping out of the group. This agreement also ensures that the person who joins the group will be making enough of a commitment to benefit from the group.

11. *CHARGES.* The rate for group psychotherapy is on a per session basis. The billing continues at the same rate even when members do not attend the group, i.e., when they take vacations or are ill. The reasoning is that members are being charged for slots that are reserved for them. It is their responsibility as to whether and how they choose to use this time. *Each group member agrees to pay their bill completely before the end of each month.*

Chapter 4

Interactional Group Psychotherapy

Irvin Yalom has written two excellent texts on group psychotherapy. The first, initially published in 1970 (the second edition came out in 1975, the third edition in 1985, and the fourth in 1995), deals primarily with the application of outpatient group psychotherapy to a non-addicted population. The second text deals almost exclusively with the application of inpatient group psychotherapy with psychotic patients primarily in an acute hospital setting (1982). Since it is Yalom's first text that provides the theoretical underpinnings for his approach to group psychotherapy, this chapter will concentrate on his contribution to group psychotherapy as it is outlined for an outpatient setting in his 1970 text. However, even this text devotes relatively little space and time to Yalom's theoretical rationale for conducting a group in his prescribed manner. Many group psychotherapists, while acknowledging that Yalom's 1975 text provides the reader with the best practical "nuts and bolts"'directions available for conducting an interactional group, criticize him at the same time for being atheoretical and ignoring the philosophical foundations for his approach to group psychotherapy.

This criticism is unfounded if one makes the effort to trace Yalom's link with Harry Stack Sullivan's (1953) theory of interpersonal psychiatry. A clear understanding of Sullivan's basic tenets will shed much light on the reasons why Yalom advocates that a group be led in the manner he describes. Jerome Frank's influence is also paramount in Yalom's approach to group psychotherapy, although Yalom, to my knowledge, has never acknowledged this relationship in print except in a cursory fashion. One only has to read through Yalom's list of curative factors in group (i.e., Instillation of Hope, Altruism, Universality, and Existential Factors, etc.) and see Jerome Frank's (1961) thesis concerning the anthropological aspects of persuasion and healing heavily influencing Yalom's recommendations. Later in this chapter, an interpretation of Yalom's theoretical foundations and the ways in which Sullivan's and Frank's work reflects and influences Yalom's approach to group psychotherapy will be presented.

First, however, Yalom's description of the "basic plumbing" of group psychotherapy and the basic task of the group leader will be explored. The material presented here is not intended to be original and is only a condensed presentation of Yalom's own work in chapters five (there are two chapter fives in his second edition) of his 1975 text. The interested reader is encouraged to explore this chapter in more detail if they wish to go to the original source of the information presented here.

YALOM'S BASIC TASKS

A group leader essentially has three major tasks within Yalom's model of group psychotherapy. These tasks are:

1. Ensure the physical survival of the group.
2. Build a group culture and establish therapeutic norms.
3. Teach and model for the group members the here and now work in the group setting.

The task of ensuring the physical survival of the group involves those efforts that go into establishing and maintaining a group. It is usually easier to predict which members will drop out of treatment than it is to predict which members will succeed and benefit from group psychotherapy. Yalom urges the group leader to spend more time on preparing members for groups than on perfect casting. Managing the boundaries of the group and preparing the members for group is dealt with more thoroughly in Chapter 3. The current chapter will be devoted primarily to describing Yalom's recommendations for the other two major tasks of the group leader and how the accomplishment of these tasks plays a major part in the success of a psychotherapy group for the chemically dependent individual.

Building a Group Culture and Establishing Therapeutic Norms

Once a group is a physical reality, group leaders must turn their energy toward shaping the group norms and group culture into a therapeutic social system. This will in turn set in motion the curative factors (see Chapter 15) that for Yalom are crucial to the group's effectiveness. Unlike in any other kind of group setting, the group members must feel free to comment on the immediate feelings they experience toward each member and toward the leader of the group. In order for this type of atmosphere to manifest, the group leader must steer the group members in the direction of establishing six essential group norms. They are:

1. Honesty and spontaneity must be encouraged and sanctioned.
2. A high level of involvement on the part of all group members must be ensured.
3. Self-disclosure of each member must be established in an atmosphere of what Yalom describes as "reciprocal vulnerability."
4. The desire for self-understanding must be instilled and encouraged in each group member.
5. Nonjudgmental acceptance of other group members' shortcomings, personal failings, and individual indiscretions must be established.
6. Dissatisfaction with the self must be experienced and a desire to change the behavior that is related to this dissatisfaction must be encouraged.

Most group leaders would agree that these are desirable norms to establish and maintain. But the question that ultimately must be asked is, How are these tasks to be accomplished? The answer is a simple one that is found within the realm of behavioral modification and reinforcement theory. A group leader must:

1. Establish and reinforce norms that are healthy and functional.
2. Avoid, ignore, and extinguish norms that are unhealthy and dysfunctional.

The therapist, within Yalom's perspective, is to build an atmosphere and climate for change. The group leader is an engineer and the group is a laboratory for the investigation and understanding of the interpersonal difficulties that each particular member brings to the group. Only when the group culture is just right can the group be used as a vehicle for changing each member's maladaptive behavior.

Therapists have at their disposal two readily available tools or methods for shaping the norms of the group. First, therapists are technical experts who hopefully have a better understanding of the dynamics and development of behavior, both maladaptive and adaptive, than the group members. With the benefit of their professional training, therapists have more access to pertinent information that will help them readily identify pathological behavior and determine what is healthy adaptive behavior. Second, group leaders, because of the special options available to them within a psychotherapy group, have the advantage of operating as "model-setting participants."

Technical Expert

What does Yalom mean when he refers to the leader as technical expert? The leader of a group is automatically assigned certain characteristics by the group members because of the already established role that the leader possesses in the group. For example, for many group members, this role may be the benevolent guardian and for others, it may be seen as the authoritarian autocrat. While many forms of group psychotherapy (i.e., Tavistock) are primarily interested in the group members' transference reactions to the assigned characteristics of the group leader, Yalom is most interested in the interaction of group members and the building of a therapeutic group culture. Consequently, Yalom advocates that group leaders use the weight of their authority and experience toward the establishment of the norms that are necessary for a highly functioning therapeutic group. Transference and transference distortions toward the leader will always emerge and these distortions can be explored later when it is more advantageous for the leader to do so. While these transference distortions are judged by Yalom to be of therapeutic importance, they are secondary to the establishment of a proper group climate and the assurance that group members not be forced into a regressed posture too early in group.

Yalom therefore suggests that the group leader use his or her assigned role as technical expert to convince the group members to interact with each other rather than direct their energies toward interacting with the leader. One way Yalom convinces members to behave this way is by appealing to their reason. This is primarily accomplished by the preparatory first session that each individual is required to attend before they are placed in group (see Chapter 3).

However, even with the best instructions and detailed preparation, the group members will continue to direct their attention and energy toward the group leader. Yalom therefore suggests far more subtle reinforcing techniques to combat this difficulty. For example, the group leader can compliment members in the group who volunteer comments to other group members. Just a simple comment such as "good feedback" gives the other group members a clear message that interaction and feedback between group members is a norm in the group that is actively encouraged. The group leader can also become more direct about his or her desire for group member interaction by repeatedly asking why the group members do not direct their comments to each other while in group. A group leader can also wonder aloud why comments are being directed only toward him or her and ask the group in a general way why they refuse to speak to each other. Refusing to answer questions, either directly or indirectly, is another means of establishing group member interaction. Nonverbal behavior is yet another valuable tool that often encourages members to speak directly with each other. For example, the group leader can shift his or her body away from a group member who is only speaking directly to the leader and thus give the clear message that the leader is not interested in a leader-centered group. Transferring a member's gaze from his or her own eyes to another member in the group frequently results in the eye contact being established between the two members, thereby encouraging dialogue between them instead of limiting the exchange to the leader and a group member. Group leaders thus have as their task the responsibility of teaching the group to interact with each other rather than just with the leader. This is a task that is not accomplished easily and requires that the leader use his or her assigned role of technical expert to repeatedly give the group and its members the message in many different ways, both direct and indirect. Only by the leader's constant effort to teach the members that they must direct their energies toward each other can the climate be set for running group psychotherapy within Yalom's described and recommended fashion.

THE MODEL-SETTING PARTICIPANT

As Yalom suggests, leaders shape norms, not only through explicit or implicit social engineering, but through the example they set with their own interpersonal group behavior. It is from this perspective, the position of the therapist in the therapeutic setting, that the role of the group therapist is most radically different from the role the therapist in individual therapy. Yalom's description of group leaders as model-setting participants raises some very important issues regarding the leaders' neutrality and transparency about their own feelings, attitudes, and behavior while engaged in a therapeutic relationship with members in a group setting. In order for a therapy group to fulfill its potential, it requires that the group discard the social norms that dictate most interpersonal interactions. For example, we are frequently taught as youngsters to be polite and not mention anything that might offend another individual, even if the topic or behavior is blatantly obvious to all concerned. Successful group psychotherapy requires that members try new behavior and take risks in their interaction with other group members. The best way for this to be accomplished in group is for the members to observe the group leader's behavior and on some level internalize and model this behavior. Consequently, what the leader says is not as important as what the leader does. Or, as frequently reported in Alcoholics Anonymous, "You must learn to walk your talk." AA members, for example, are keenly aware of those participants in the AA program who talk a "good program," but do not follow through (walk) with what they say should be done or what they say they will do. In a similar way, how leaders deal with their own anxiety, anger, and frustration is a clear message of how these emotions will be dealt with in the group by its members. In short, as Marshall McLuhan frequently stated, "The medium is the message."

What the leader does and his or her presence as a person in group is far more important than what the leader says. An example will help illustrate this point. Martin Buber (1963), a Jewish theologian and existential philosopher, has written exclusively about the Jewish mystical movement of the Hasidim. In the Orthodox Jewish tradition, for example, it is believed, as it is in most orthodox disciplines, that only those ordained and chosen are allowed to interpret the scriptures. Within the orthodox teaching, individuals went to see the religious leader for advice, guidance, or the answers to their particular problem. Much like traditional medical care and orthodox views in psychotherapy, patients went to their doctor for the diagnosis, interpretation, or advice on how to change or alleviate their suffering. This was not the case with the Hasidic movement. Nor is this the case with Alcoholics Anonymous or the humanistic Third Force movement that emerged during the 1960s as a reaction to orthodox forms of psychotherapy. This change in perspective reflects a common position of both the modern-day religious revisionists and the contemporary forms of psychotherapy. The central issue is the difference between the traditional authoritarian view of the interpretations of the scriptures and the reformation movement, which required the active participant of the disciples, who were encouraged to discover God or Truth for themselves. The Gnostic movement of early Christianity, which advocated that disciples find truth for themselves, is another example of the shift in perspective. A popular song during the 1960s by John Prine captured the spirit of that era with the lyrics, "Move to the country, buy me a house, learn about Jesus by myself," which encouraged a personal responsibility in the search for personal understanding rather than relying on blind faith. The personal interpretation of spiritual truth is also exemplified in Alcoholics Anonymous in its reaction to traditional medicine and authoritative forms of psychotherapy in the treatment of addiction. This is the message that Martin Buber sought to give his readers in his interpretations of the Hasidic teachings. Within the Hasidic tradition, for example, the religious leader–the Zaddick–taught by example rather than by exhortation. Nothing is esoteric from this perspective. Everything is simple and all persons of faith can grasp the simplicity of the teaching for themselves. The Zaddick was not a scholar or seat of religious reason and wisdom. Much like the model-setting participant that Yalom writes about in his text, the relationship is the crucial factor. The personality of the teacher takes the place of the doctrine. He *is* the teaching. As a disciple of the Zaddick said, "I did not go to my Zaddick to learn Torah from him, but to watch him tie his bootlaces."

How much and what of themselves leaders choose to share must be carefully determined, however. When Yalom writes of the group leader's transparency, he is not suggesting that the leader bare all and "let it all hang out." Such an all-or-nothing approach is certainly doomed to failure and is usually destructive to the group and its members. Honesty for honesty's sake is a burlesque. Group leaders must temper how much of themselves they reveal and weigh that decision against how honesty and transparency on their part will benefit or hinder the group. Group members must learn this basic premise about honesty, and the group leader should be cautious in allowing members to hide behind truth in their destructive attacks on other group members. "I'm just being honest" is never a good excuse for viciously attacking or inflicting pain upon another. As Ernest Kurtz (1983) says, "Honesty with bad intent is worse than a lie." Group leaders must learn to balance their honesty with responsibility. Consequently, the decision on how transparent leaders will be while conducting their groups should be determined exclusively by the evaluation of whether their sharing of this information will help or hinder the group and its members. Group leaders must never forget that the group is not there to use for their own benefit or therapy. The question that always must be asked by group leaders before they honestly reveal themselves is whether the group and its members will be helped by the leader's openness at this moment. An illustration will help clarify this point.

> Bill, a recovering alcoholic with three years of sobriety, revealed to the group early in his fourth meeting that he had sexually molested his six-year-old daughter while in the midst of an alcoholic blackout three years earlier. Bill had not intended to reveal this information to the group, and its revelation had been prompted by another member talking openly and honestly about his guilt over past deeds he had regretted doing while intoxicated. Bill's revelation to the group hit like a bombshell and it was obvious by his own withdrawal and presentation that he had gotten carried away by his feelings and had opened up more of himself to the group than he had intended. Some of the group members, themselves children of alcoholic parents who had sexually abused them when they were youngsters, were especially stunned by a mixture of anger and embarrassment stirred in them by Bill's confession. As it became more apparent that the group

> was lost in their confusion about a way to respond to Bill, the leader, rather than let them struggle needlessly with their uncomfortableness, decided to share her own feelings about Bill's revelation. The leader stated, "Bill, I've been touched by your willingness to share such embarrassing and painful information with the group. It clearly indicates you have grown to trust the others in here to be willing to risk as much as you have. I know for myself, it brings up a mixture of feelings regarding my own father's molestation of me. I don't know if I would have been able to show the courage you have in sharing this, but I'm glad you took the risk." Quickly following this feedback from the group leader, other group members began to share similar feelings with Bill, helping him work through and resolve a great deal of guilt and self-condemnation he had been harboring for years. This incident also gave a clear message to the group and its other members. The deepest and most feared secret could be shared in this group and they would not be condemned, judged, or rejected. By choosing to respond as she did, the group leader avoided a possible disastrous situation in group that could have been destructive to Bill as well as destructive to the group's therapeutic climate.

Once the group's positive acceptance of Bill's sharing of his secret was experienced by him and the other group members, the group leader could now steer the group to explore the more negative reactions in a structured and guided fashion. After the group had integrated this experience and reached a positive resolution, the group leader could give the group more freedom and less direction in exploring its reactions if a similar situation should occur again in the future. The group, because of the leader's decision to take an active and directive role in the shaping of a positive norm, did not have to struggle needlessly through a difficult developmental phase before it was stable and cohesive enough to do so.

The leader must also model nonjudgmental acceptance and appreciation of each member's individual strengths and weaknesses. An interpretation or confrontation that is appropriate after the group has developed cohesion might be totally destructive and devastating to the group that is still in the early stages of development. For example, leaders do not want to give the message that it is unsafe to reveal secrets in the group. This certainly could have been the case with Bill when he spoke about his sexual molestation of his daughter. A group member, after a period of prolonged silence in the group, may choose to finally reveal a secret. Leaders have a choice in the type of response they make. They may respond with a statement that is interpreted as, "Why haven't you told us this before?" In contrast, leaders have the option of producing a totally different effect if they respond instead with a statement that says, "It appears you now trust the group enough to share this with us." The message to the group members in the first instance is more likely to evoke a response in which he or she fears, "Oh, hell, I'm sitting on a secret and if I tell it now, I'll get jumped on. I had better keep quiet." In the second instance, the group has learned it is safe to talk about any subject in the group and they can do this when they are ready, without having to fear condemnation or retribution from the leader or the other group members.

INTERPERSONAL HONESTY AND SPONTANEITY

Group leaders also have the task of modeling interpersonal honesty and spontaneity. This is essential unless the leader wishes to run the risk of having a group that is leader-centered and one-dimensional (all loving or all angry). However, honesty and spontaneity must be balanced with responsibility. Yalom utilizes Victor Frankl's comments on the social problems of the United States to illustrate this point when Frankl suggested that the Statue of Liberty on the East Coast should be balanced by the Statue of Responsibility on the West Coast. The freedom of honesty and spontaneity becomes possible in a therapy group only when it is tempered by a sense of responsibility. Group leaders must always balance their decisions in group on a narrow ridge between complete, spontaneous honesty on one side and controlled, structured responsibility on the other side. Martin Buber, whose writings have had significant influence on Carl Rogers and countless other theorists, has written extensively about the narrow ridge that exists between the exact, structured world of science and the chaotic, inexact world of religion and spirituality. Buber's writing reflects his belief that the psychotherapist must be not only an authentic person in his or her own right, but a person who lives in the "holy insecurity" of knowing there are no absolutes in the world. Buber's concept of the narrow ridge is the key to understanding the edifice upon which his philosophy of the I-Thou relationship stands. It is through this position of denying absolutes that Buber sought to express his personal view on understanding and knowledge.

> I have occasionally described my standpoint to my friends as the "narrow ridge." I wanted by this to express that I did not rest on the broad upland of a system that includes a series of sure statements about the absolute, but on a narrow, rocky ridge between the gulfs

> where there is no sureness of expressible knowledge but the certainty of meeting that remains undisclosed. (Buber, 1955, p. 184)

For Buber, the narrow ridge represented the balance between the chaos of uncertainty and the exactness of certainty based on the belief of absolute knowledge. Buber saw difficulties in each extreme position. Believing that one has absolute knowledge leads to dogmatism, grandiosity, and loss of spirituality. Believing in the other extreme leads to chaos, nihilism, and hedonism. Understanding Buber's narrow ridge opens the door to interpreting his concepts of the I-Thou relationship, the abyss, and the "holy insecurity" of his existential philosophy. It also robs group leaders of the comfortableness that comes from having pat formulas and concise answers to their patients' problems and dilemmas.

As a practicing psychotherapist and a person who spends the majority of my professional time with patients in individual and group psychotherapy, I am constantly forced to come to grips with this struggle each day in my life as I anticipate the arrival of my next appointment. I always feel the anxiety, some days greater than others, of the anticipation of the meeting with the individual. What will be demanded of me this day? Will I respond as another person to the call of this person? I struggle with my desire to control the therapy hour, to provide answers, pat formulas, and concise information because I fear what may be demanded of me when I take the risk of meeting another person in a unique and uncertain situation. I know I would find comfort in these formulations, but I realize that I must walk Buber's narrow ridge between spontaneity and control. I must assure myself and confirm myself anew of the faith in the meeting of two souls and allow the dialogue between us to take its course.

Psychotherapy, as it should be practiced, demands much, perhaps more in some cases than the therapist can give in a given situation. The demand upon the group leader is such that few individuals may attempt to venture into the world of sick souls with their whole being, as Buber so aptly illustrates:

> In certain cases, a therapist is terrified by what he is doing because he begins to suspect that something entirely other is demanded of him. Something incompatible with the economics of his profession, dangerously threatening, indeed, to his regulated practice of it. What is demanded of him is that he draw the particular case out of the correct methodological objectification and himself step forth out of the role of professional superiority, achieved and guaranteed by long training and practice, into the elementary situation between one who calls and one who is called. The abyss does not call to his confidently

> functioning security of action, but to the abyss, that is, to the self of the doctor, that selfhood that is hidden under the structures erected throughout training and practice, that is itself encompassed by chaos, itself familiar with demons, but is graced with the humble power of wrestling and overcoming, and is ready to wrestle and overcome thus ever anew. Through his hearing of this call erupts in the most exposed of the intellectual professions, the crisis of its paradox. In a decisive hour together with the patient entrusted to and trusting in him, he has left the closed room of psychological treatment in which the analyst rules by means of a systematic and methodological superiority and has stepped forward with him into the air of the world where self is exposed to self. (Buber, 1964, p. 395)

Such a stance on the part of group leaders requires that they relinquish their need to be perceived as perfect. Group leaders must be willing to accept and admit their fallibility. Some examples might illustrate this position more clearly.

> It is the fourth meeting of a psychotherapy training group and one group member confronts the group leader, accusing him of being controlling, dominating, and remaining aloof during the previous group meetings. This is the first confrontation of the group leader and there is a moment of stunned silence while the rest of the group members sit on the edge of their chairs waiting to see how the group leader will respond to this attack. The group leader chooses quickly to ask if this is the same way the young woman viewed and responded to her father. The group member, caught by surprise and somewhat relieved for the opportunity to diffuse the conflict between her and the group leader, quickly acknowledged that this was true and began, at the leader's encouragement, to explore her feelings toward her father and their relationship. While the group leader's interpretation was a correct one, for these were qualities her father possessed, the group member was also accurate in her perception of the group leader, since he was indeed aloof and controlling. It was more in the service of his own needs and fears that the group leader quickly moved the group member to explore her past relationship with her father. It allowed the group leader to take the heat off himself, while promoting the attitude of his own infallibility. Rather than retreat so quickly into the there and then with this young woman, the group leader would have been of more therapeutic help to his group and this woman if he had allowed her full access to her feelings and perceptions of him. After these feelings were explored completely in the here and now, the group leader could have then

guided the woman to understand why she had such a strong reaction to someone who possessed such traits, especially if that person was an authority figure.

By adopting such a here and now strategy, the group leader would be giving the group members the message that he is not perfect, that he does possess traits that are not always completely admirable, while demonstrating that he could accept such shortcomings in himself and was willing to acknowledge them to another without fear or defensiveness. Group members would subsequently learn a powerful message. They don't have to be infallible, and they, as well as others, can have certain faults without it affecting their capacity to have a happy and meaningful relationship with another person. They could also learn that the leader could be confronted and that confrontation could be resolved in a constructive manner.

Another example of a group leader's acceptance of his or her own fallibility and its subsequent positive effect on the group process is illustrated by a Gestalt group that was led by Erv Polster.

Once while I was in a training group he was conducting, Erv had become embroiled in a group member's difficulty reaching a decision regarding a marriage proposal he was reluctant to make to his girlfriend. Erv, operating from a Gestalt framework, had guided this man to list all the reasons he had for marrying this woman. After being repeatedly encouraged to understand better why he was refusing to marry her, the group member finally responded to Erv that he felt Erv was behaving like a Jewish mother who was trying to marry him off to this woman. Erv, somewhat stunned by his remark, stopped and asked why the man felt this way, whereupon the group member proceeded to outline all of Erv's encouraging statements. Erv, after a moment of contemplation, laughed and said, "You know you're right!" The work was promptly completed and the group laughed along with Erv in admiration for a man who could admit he was wrong and change his thinking when given evidence that illustrated the incorrectness of his position. This was a valuable learning experience for all of the group members.

ESTABLISHMENT OF THE GROUP NORMS

Now that the question of how the group leader goes about establishing the group norms has been addressed, the group leader must come to recognize which norms he or she wishes to establish.

First and foremost is the establishment of the norm of the self-monitoring group. If this is not addressed, the group will become leader-centered, dependent, and passive. The group leader must channel his or her energies toward steering the group to reflect on and evaluate itself. Yalom gives an example on how the group leader might respond after the group has struggled with a half hour of superficial chatter or has been monopolized by a group member who has rambled on in a nonproductive fashion. Yalom suggests that the group leader direct the group to reflect on itself by posing questions to its members regarding their passivity. For example, the group leader could say, "I see a half hour has gone by and how has the group gone today? Are each of you satisfied with its direction and content? If not, why haven't you said anything? What could you have done differently? What stopped you from taking action? How do you rate the group so far today on a scale from one to ten? How would you rate your own participation on the same scale? What could have caused a higher rating or what is it you could have done yourself to get the rating higher?"

Each question and statement posed here would have prompted the group to examine itself. The aim of each of these questions is to shift the evaluation function from the leader to the group.

THE NORM OF SELF-DISCLOSURE

While self-disclosure is crucial to the development of a healthy functioning group, the group leader must allow the group members to set their own pace. However, the group leader must at the same time encourage others in the group to talk about themselves. The group only goes as far and as deep as its most guarded and defended member. The members in a group will self-disclose up to a point, and then wait for the other members to join them in the atmosphere of "reciprocal vulnerability." The most guarded members of a group, usually holding back because of their fears of the other members' possible reactions to their sharing, will have to be gently encouraged to talk about their secrets sooner or later when they are ready. They must be told, however, that the longer they wait, the more difficult the sharing will become. The big secret, and every group has at least one member who has at least one big secret, is like a spider web with the secret at the hub and all conversations resembling threads that may run to that hub. The more the group members fear revealing the big secret, the more restricted they will be in their conversation about other subjects because they will fear this conversation may connect to the thread that leads to the hub at the center of the web where the big secret lies.

Yalom reminds his readers that the group is not a forced confessional and that members should never be coerced into revealing their big secret. Most members fear the reaction of the group and their catastrophic fears and beliefs should be explored before they reveal or self-disclose. This can be accomplished by a very simple, yet effective technique, which Yalom calls Metadisclosures–disclosures about the disclosure. For example, group members may suddenly freeze up after talking freely for a time in group and may even openly say that this is a subject they cannot talk about any further. The group leader, rather than forcing the issue or retreating to submissiveness, can ask the group member the nature of their catastrophic fear if they were to disclose. "What do you fear will happen if you were to talk about this subject with the group? Who do you fear will react the strongest and who do you believe will be the most accepting? What is the worst thing that could happen if you did share this information with the group?" All of these questions are geared to get group members to explore their resistance. In Gestalt terminology, this is defined as going with the resistance and is frequently the essence of Gestalt therapy. Group members are encouraged to explore the fears, both rational and irrational, surrounding their reluctance to self-disclose. The group can go even further with the theme of Metadisclosures by asking the group member how he or she feels about not being able to talk about this subject with the group and asking if the group member's feelings of isolation are painful or familiar. The issue of the feelings surrounding these fears becomes the focus of the work with the group member and is usually much more important and meaningful than the very secret itself he or she feared to disclose. In fact, group leaders must be cautious in their exploration of the group member's resistance to self-disclosure since a damaging norm would be established in the group if the group member were seduced into a premature self-disclosure. The sense of safety and trust in the group might be seriously damaged if the group leader gave lip service to the group members' right to protect themselves from premature self-disclosure and then proceeded to seduce members into revealing themselves before they were ready to share their secrets.

Metadisclosures can also be used after members have revealed their secrets or disclosed parts of themselves in group. A group leader can ask group members what it was like sharing their secret with the group. Group members can also be guided to explore their fears with each particular member in the group, allowing them to modify their catastrophic belief system and realize they are not as terrible or as loathsome as they believed. As a group leader, I would respond to a group member who has self-disclosed for the first time by reinforcing the risks they have taken and encouraging them to verify the invalidity of their expected fears. For example, I might say,

> Mary, you have taken an important risk today by sharing this information with the group and I am happy to see you now trust us enough to share such a painful experience. I know you fear condemnation from the other members because your parents were so critical and demeaning of you. I would like you to remember the responses you have heard from the other group members today and understand they do not think less of you because of what you have said. To the contrary, if you looked around at their faces, you will see more caring and understanding than was there previously in the group before you shared this information. Your fear of rejection and self-disclosure has led you to build a wall around yourself that has resulted in you keeping others away, creating the very rejection and criticism you feared the most.

Yalom's concern is more with the process of disclosure than with the context of disclosure. His model is much more focused on the working through of previously inhibiting fears and the evolving climate of acceptance of feelings in the group. This is the key to Yalom's model. The climate and atmosphere takes precedence over the interventions, confrontations, and exploration of the members' resistance and expressions of feelings.

Once a disclosure has been forthcoming, a member should never be punished for disclosing. Most importantly, do not permit dirty fighting in the group between its members. Frequently, in the heat of a confrontation, one member may use material that is sensitive to another member in his or her attack on that member. For instance, in the case of Bill, who had revealed to the group his molestation of his daughter while he was in an alcoholic blackout, a group member may have used that material against him during a confrontation and shouted, "What right have you to criticize me, at least I never molested my children!" At this point the leader must "stop action," interrupt the conflict quickly, and say, "Something important has just happened in group." Ask the offended member about his or her feelings and ask the other members whether they have had similar experiences of having their disclosures used later in a punitive manner against them. Encourage other members of the group to talk about their own reactions to the conflict between the two individuals. Point out to the group how this attack will make it difficult for others to reveal themselves. Explore how this conflict will affect the group and its willingness to be open and honest in the future. It is the leader's task at this time to ensure that the group realize that self-disclosure will be honored in the group and that the leader will take precautions to prevent the punitive use of previously disclosed material. Dirty fighting will not be allowed in the group.

This is important for many reasons. Individuals usually fear being authentic and real. Most people, especially alcoholics and addicts, do not want to take an authentic stance in life because of their fear of rejection or disapproval. It is all right if you reject me or dislike me because of what you think I am. But if I am real and you get to know me and then you still reject me, this is much more frightening and painful. Consequently, we all use impression management in our interactions with others. We try to decide what will get us approval and act in that way. The difficulty with such an artificial approach to life is summed up best by Kurt Vonnegut's statement, "You have to be careful what you pretend to be, because you may wake up someday and discover that's what you are."

In group, the task is to get people to risk being real with each other so they can learn that they can be loved and accepted for what or who they are rather than what they do or how they act. This allows them to reverse their introjection (You wouldn't like me if you really knew me because I'm bad). A group that encourages honest self-disclosure and is accepting of that self-disclosure permits individuals to understand the way their introjections interfere with their ability to be nurtured and enjoyed by others. Group members will learn eventually how they shut themselves off from meaningful relationships and the ways their negative self-images lead to continued poor choices of lovers and friends. They also learn through this awareness how they contribute to their difficulties. Being authentic with others will lead to a corrective emotional experience that will allow them to create a true sense of self and enhance their self-esteem. Group conducted from this perspective allows reparative work on each person's sense of self. The aim of treatment is to get at the individuals' internal messages, self-evaluations, and the ways they condemn themselves. If they are encouraged to be more genuine in group, they will begin to feel less deceptive and less false and will eventually take an authentic stand in life. At this juncture, they will learn the crucial message, "I am worth something if I am real."

PROCEDURAL NORMS AND ANTITHERAPEUTIC NORMS

Optimally, the more unstructured, unrehearsed, and freely interacting the group remains the more effective the group will be. However, group leaders must be cautious in determining how unstructured and unrehearsed the group is to be. If they are not active and directive enough, the group can degenerate into a number of antitherapeutic norms. Such norms can be easily established and are often difficult to extinguish if left unattended for too long. Some of the more common and troublesome antitherapeutic norms that can be established by a group are listed below.

A. *Take turns format.* The group will devote the entire meeting sequentially to each particular member. The first person to speak will, for instance, become the focus of the entire session. Groups can have enormous difficulty shifting the focus from one member to the next. This can become especially troublesome for two reasons. First, it enhances premature self-disclosure. The group member elected to be the focus of the group session will succumb more and more to the mounting group pressure, leading the overwhelmed member to reveal more than he or she had been prepared to share. The person can be emotionally raped. The second danger is that it will enhance the other group members' anxiety as they realize their turn in group will be due next. The anxiety and the fear of the hot seat may become so great that a member may drop out of group rather than face his or her turn next week.

B. *One-topic format.* The group can establish a pattern of devoting the entire session to the first issue or topic presented. An unspoken rule against changing the subject matter may be established, with sanctions being erected without the open acknowledgement of such sanctions.

C. *"Can you top this" format.* A norm can be established in the group where members will only reveal or self-disclose if the material is more personal and emotionally charged than the last member's disclosure. The group can develop what Yalom describes as a "spiraling orgy of self-disclosure." The group must learn that the subtle, often unobvious pattern of their behaviors is a far more potent source of conflict for them than the "spilling of their guts on the group floor."

D. *The group can become so tightly knit that it can become hostile to new members.* If the leader is not careful, bringing new members into the group can cause conflict resulting in the new member being denied group acceptance. Preparing the group for new members is a task that must be addressed cautiously. Chapter 11 will address the pitfalls that must be avoided when bringing new members into group.

E. *Leader-centered group.* The group can become unchallenging of the group leader. Their needs can become subservient to those of the leader and the group will become leader-centered and dependent.

F. *One-sided experience.* The group can become one-dimensional, all loving or all attacking. Real intimacy will be avoided and the group may establish norms that do not permit the full range and expression of feelings and thoughts.

IMPORTANCE OF GROUP

The more important the members consider the group, the more effective the group will become in their treatment. Group leaders must appreciate the importance of this position and reinforce this belief in whatever way they can. A group's survival requires two elements: (1) structure or purpose and (2) commitment. Group leaders must define the structure and purpose of the group before it starts. Once the group sessions are in progress, group leaders must give members the message that the group is the most important event in their lives. Group leaders accomplish this by being punctual and informing members well in advance of their concern at being absent from one of the group sessions. Leaders constantly address other members' absences, requiring them to let the group know well in advance the reasons why they are not going to be present for a meeting. If leaders are thinking about the group between sessions, it behooves them to speak about these thoughts with the group members. This sharing of thoughts between sessions helps instill a sense of continuity between the sessions. Encouraging this continuity helps the group work through issues from one meeting to the next. Group leaders should aim to make connections whenever they can in group. For instance, if one group member presents an issue in group which is similar to that presented by another group member, the leader might say, "This sounds very much like what John was working on two weeks ago in group." Noticing the withdrawal or change in affect of a group member can be helpful if this is traced to some previous interaction in the group. For instance, the group leader might comment to a withdrawn member, "I've noticed, Mary, you've been quiet in group since you and Joan had the disagreement two weeks ago."

Members as Agents of Help

As Yalom advocates, the group functions best when members appreciate the valuable help they can provide one another. The group must learn to diminish its reliance on the leader as the only source of help. Reinforce whenever possible the mutual helpfulness of group members. Comments that group members have found helpful can be easily elicited by the simple question, "You've gotten a lot of feedback on this issue, Bob, what has been the most helpful?" If members wonder out loud in group if they are too selfish, respond by asking, "Ken, there are many people who know you well in here, why don't you ask them?"

These norms, once established, must be constantly maintained. This requires the monitoring of behavior that could undermine these norms. For instance, one group member may respond to another with the statement, "Joe, you have no right to say that to him; you're worse than he is." The leader should intervene quickly at this point saying, "That's not my experience of you, Joe. While we all may have similar problems, your comments are usually helpful." Ask the other group members at this time about their perceptions of Joe. Is it true that he is helpful or destructive? Once this matter is settled, the group leader can address his or her comments toward the attacking group member: "It seems the rest of the group perceives Joe differently. Is there something else regarding your feelings toward Joe?"

Yalom defines the role of the group leader as being active and directive. His suggestions are not the nonjudgmental mirroring or clarifying comments typically associated with the tasks of the therapist in individual therapy. The importance of norm-setting in group takes precedence over the other aspects of the group leader's role within Yalom's model. It is vital that the group leader establish, maintain, and develop norms that will allow the therapeutic process to unfold in group. Once these norms are set, the group leader can turn to the third basic task of the therapist, which is defined by Yalom as the activation and process illumination of the here and now.

THE HERE AND NOW ACTIVATION AND PROCESS ILLUMINATION

What is the task of the group leader from this perspective? The group leader must ensure that the group members focus their attention on their immediate feelings and thoughts toward the other group members, the group leader, and the group itself as a whole. The immediate events in the group take precedence over the events in the past or current life of each member outside of the group. The events in the here and now within the group become the primary focus of the group leader.

Why does Yalom advocate such an approach and what are the advantages of a here and now focus? Because, such a therapeutic stance will facilitate the development and stark emergence of each member's social microcosm. Group leaders will not have to prompt members to talk about their interpersonal conflicts, doubts, or fears. These issues will all emerge within their interactions with the leader and the other members of the group. People who alienate others will alienate their fellow members in group. Individuals who are taken advantage of by others will allow themselves to be taken advantage of by others in the group. Those members who cannot handle anger will experience this difficulty in group when anger is expressed. The idiosyncratic, psychological Achilles heel of each individual group member will emerge for all to see in the demonstration of his or her behavior in the here and now of the group process. The group, from this viewpoint, is a laboratory, a social microcosm where members will act out in the here and now (rather than talk about it in the there and then) their particular idiosyncratic conflicts.

Once group leaders are aware of what they must accomplish in order to set in motion the curative group process, the next question concerns how this task is accomplished. This approach is ahistoric and de-emphasizes both what has happened outside the group and past individual experiences. The here and now is the power cell of the group and it is composed of two layers: (1) content–the current feelings experienced by group and its members; (2) process–the reflective examination and clarification or process illumination of what has occurred sequentially. Consequently, Yalom's model requires two steps. First, the content of the experience must be understood. The experience of the immediate occurrence of events must be realized and recognized by the group and its members. Secondly, the sequential process of events must be understood. The group must reflect back upon itself and understand the content of its own transactions. The group, therefore, must transcend the pure content of its experience and reflect back on the process that led to that event. Process, for example, examines the reasons Joe responded to Mary and not to Bill at this particular time in this particular manner. Why does Lucille pick only the men to respond to when there is a question asked and why does she not respond to the members of the group who are the most helpful? Why does Sharon make a broad, general statement such as, "I trust everyone" at the time when Sandra is talking about her fears of being judged? These questions exemplify the process illumination that Yalom encourages the group leader to constantly monitor. Adherence to this posture is justified on the basis that psychopathology is ubiquitous in interpersonal interactions. A single interpersonal transaction is representative of a larger pattern of behavior. It gives the group leader a peek at the whole.

The understanding of the here and now requires the self-reflective loop. Within this illustration, the group reflects back on the content of the here and now experience. It is largely the group leader's task to steer the group to the self-reflective loop so that it can understand the process (or the what and why) of a particular experience. The group becomes aware of this process by the leader's commentary on the process. Consequently, it is the leader's responsibility to make process commentary so this potential can be actualized. (See Figure 4.1.)

Process commentary, in turn, requires understanding the metacommunicational aspects of a particular message. As Yalom writes,

FIGURE 4.1

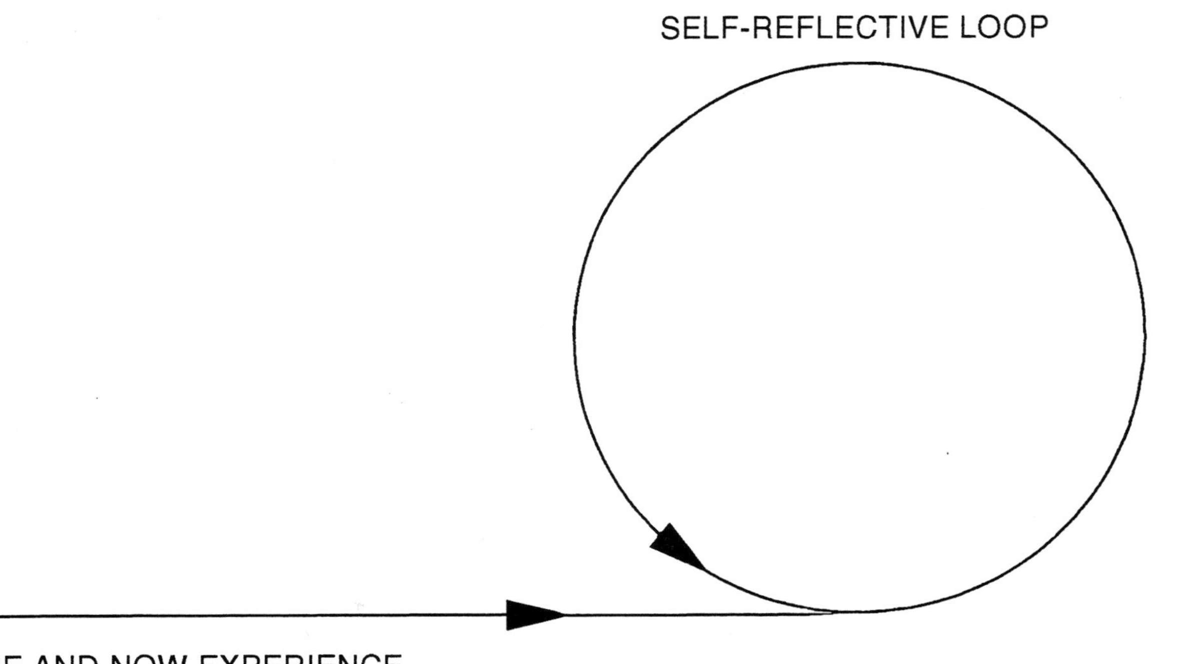

> Metacommunication refers to communication about the communication. Compare for example, "Close the window!" "Wouldn't you like to close the window? You must be cold?" "I'm cold, would you please close the window?" "Why is this window open?" Each of these statements contains a great deal more than a simple request or command, each conveys a metacommunication–a message about the nature of the relationship between two interacting individuals. (1975, pp. 122-123)

The group leader is forced to understand why this group member is making this statement to this person at this time in this manner. Process concerns itself with the how and why of an interpersonal communication. Yalom gives some excellent examples of process illumination in his text. For instance, Yalom reports that a student asks a question of the lecturer, "What was the date of Freud's death?" After the lecturer replies 1939, the student says, "No, it was 1938." As Yalom says, a question ain't a question if you already know the answer. Why did the student ask a question to which he already knew the answer? Presumably to either demonstrate his knowledge or embarrass the lecturer. Process illumination in group involves the same principle. The leader must constantly monitor the sequence of such transactions, noting when and to whom they are directed.

Yalom gives another example:

> Early in the course of a group therapy meeting, Burt, a tenacious, bulldog-faced, intense student, exclaimed to the group in general and to Rose (an unsophisticated, astrologically inclined cosmetologist) in particular, "Parenthood is degrading!" This provocative statement elicited considerable response from the group, all of whom possessed parents and many of whom were parents, and the ensuing donnybrook consumed the remainder of the group session. (1975, p. 123)

Examined only on the content level, the members engaged Burt in a debate about parenthood. Examined from a process level, this interaction is rich in inferences about Burt and his transactions with the group and its members. The group leader can ask himself a number of questions about the process of this transaction: (1) Why was Burt's message actually directed at Rose, who is more emotional, nonintellectual, and has many children? (2) Why is Burt so intolerant of nonintellectuals? (3) Why did Burt attack Rose so indirectly? (4) Why did Burt provoke the group and set himself up for a universal attack?

As Yalom suggests, any of these observations could be correct as each represents an aspect of Burt that must be explored and examined in the course of therapy.

Therapists' Techniques for the Here and Now

The process illumination can only occur if the group leader keeps the focus of the group in the here and now. This can be a difficult task, since the group, in numerous and subtle ways, will always attempt to shift the focus away from the immediate into the there and then. Whenever an issue regarding an outside event of the group is raised in the group, group leaders must think in what way this issue may be related to the unspoken and often unconscious stirrings of the group and its members. Group leaders must ask themselves how this material applies to the present and how this event can come alive in the here and now.

An example will help illustrate this point:

> In the first meeting of a psychotherapy training group, Tom begins the group by requesting some help from the group members regarding his difficulty with his roommate. Tom proceeds to talk in detail about his lack of trust with his friend and his fear of speaking openly with his roommate about the issues that have led to his distrust. The group first responds by giving Tom advice and eventually by relating their own difficulties with friends who have failed them in the past after they had entrusted them with sensitive information. The group leader at this point commented about the importance of the issue of trust and asked the group if this was a fear they shared in regard to the group and the members in the group. The group quickly shifted its focus from the there and then issue of trust and began to explore their feelings of trust in the here and now with each other. A rich discussion ensued that resulted in a deepening of the interchange between the members of the group and their fears of others' reactions if they were to trust them with the open and honest expression of their deepest fears and feelings. Once this topic of trust shifted to the here and now, it consumed the remainder of the group session. Before ending the meeting, the group leader asked Tom if his problem with the roommate had been properly addressed. Tom admitted that his roommate wasn't really the issue and he realized that his concerns were actually with the group.

Tom's revelation illustrates an important principle of psychotherapy. The question that group leaders must constantly ask themselves is why, out of all the material that patients can talk about, have they chosen the particular topic that they have at this particular time? There has been a myriad of important events in the individual's life since the group session. Why, out of all of the events in the last week, had Tom chosen the issue of trust and his fear of talking openly about his distrust? While Tom was not conscious of the reasons he picked the topic of his friend, unconsciously the material had been triggered by the similar atmosphere of fear and distrust in the group. These issues, trust with his roommate and trust in the group, were parallel concerns in Tom's life. The group triggered in Tom an emotion that was associated with his roommate. He picked the topic that was most salient to his consciousness, but was secondary to the real current issues in the here and now. The group leader must learn to keep a third ear to such parallel talk. Drawing parallels between events that the individual chooses to bring up for discussion in the here and now will allow the group leader to gain a peek at the possible unconscious material that lies repressed below the surface.

Fundamental to this therapeutic technique is the recognition of the importance of unconscious factors in all forms of communication. This position holds that an extremely important component of emotional dysfunction exists entirely outside the awareness of the individual, finding expression only in disguised or encoded form. At the heart of this approach is an understanding of the individual's unconscious communications—his or her encoded or disguised messages. It is therefore essential for the group leader to appreciate and be capable of fully applying the kind of listening process that allows the group members' unconscious expressions to be properly decoded and understood for their most significant meanings. Ronald Langs (1976) has outlined an intricate model that he calls the listening process or the communicative approach. Langs encourages the therapist to differentiate between the manifest content and the latent content of the individual's message. The manifest content is the surface aspect of the individual's associations. Such communication is direct, immediate, and self-evident in what the person says and means. The latent content is that which is not self-evident within the surface content of the person's message, but is contained in a disguised or encoded theme. The group leader's task is to decode this latent message and make it manifest. Since the material is often presented in a disguised form (e.g., Tom's concern with his trust of his roommate), the group leader must listen for the individual's derivatives. *Derivative* is a term originally coined by Freud and is used to imply that the manifest content (i.e., Tom's distrust of his roommate) is derived from the latent image (i.e., Tom's fear and distrust of the group).

Therapists and group leaders have difficulty working with and decoding derivative expressions for a number of reasons: (1) Most people prefer to work with that which is self-evident, directly on the surface, and relatively easy to manipulate; (2) It is a human tendency to treat the indirect–anything that cannot be directly seen, touched, immediately understood, and readily manipulated–as though it were nonexistent. The idea that surface material contains latent meanings and impressions not immediately discernible is a concept alien to many therapists; (3) Perhaps most importantly, individual's derivative associations often contain highly emotionally charged and compelling encoded perceptions of the therapist's errors, personal difficulties, and failings.

Even the most skilled therapists can fall prey to their own unconscious avoidance of these derivatives because they may contain confrontive and critical content. An excellent example of such an instance involves a skilled group psychotherapist who was presenting a national training workshop to a large contingent of nurses in a rural community setting. The trainer possessed excellent credentials from a highly respected psychoanalytic institute and had a thriving practice in which group psychotherapy was an integral part of her practice. Her all-day workshop was split into two segments. The first half contained an excellent didactic presentation on psychodynamic group theory, and the second half involved a demonstration experiential group composed of volunteers from the audience. It was during the experiential component of the presentation that the group trainer succumbed to her unconscious efforts to avoid derivative associations because of their highly charged emotional content. The group resisted her efforts to get them to move from the opening theme, which concerned their anger, frustration, and alienation with orthodox and fundamental religion. Since the majority of nurses attending the conference were from small, rural towns in the South, they had had more than their share of experiences with fundamental religious beliefs that were impractical and not applicable to their lives.

What the group trainer failed to appreciate was the effect her excellent didactic presentation had had on her audience. Her emphasis on Freud, psychodynamic theory, and long-term psychotherapy, with its associated emphasis on making the unconscious conscious, had evoked feelings of frustration similar to the ones they felt in relation to their experience with the fundamental religious teachings in their life. Their inability to apply such fundamental principles of religion in a practical way in their own lives was the manifest content of their message to the trainer. The derivative of this message was triggered by their latent, unconscious feelings of frustration related to the impracticality of applying Freudian principles of long-term psychotherapy to short-term treatment facilities with patients who were not particularly psychologically minded and lived in small, rural towns in the Deep South. As an observer sitting safely in the audience, I had little problem decoding the group's message to the trainer. Yet, the trainer, herself a very competent group therapist, was unable to hear the frustration being expressed latently because it evoked her own unconscious fears of attack and criticism.

Derivatives can be interpreted and deciphered in many ways. A group leader need not wait for group members to speak before drawing a hypothesis about their personality organization and possible behavior. Since all behavior is determined, derivatives and latent content are present in many forms. For example, a fellow colleague, interviewing a prospective group member, noted upon meeting the woman for the first appointment that she had been working diligently on a large book of crossword puzzles while in the waiting room. She was so preoccupied with the book, which she had nearly completed, that she had not noticed the therapist had entered the room to invite her into his office. She was so intensely engrossed in her crossword puzzle that he had to speak her name twice before she was able to respond to his call. As they walked together toward his office, the therapist thought to himself, "I wonder if this woman is into word games." The therapist was proved right, as the patient spent the majority of the therapy hour in a rambling discourse of her ideas and thoughts, hiding her feelings behind a rigid defensive structure of intellectualization, rationalization, and isolation of affect.

Here and Now Activation: Techniques

More important for group leaders than mastering any technique, is fully understanding the strategy and theoretical foundations upon which all effective technique must rest. Group leaders must discipline themselves to think predominantly in the here and now. They must move the focus from the outside to the inside and from the general to the specific. Each topic presented must prompt them to ask the questions: "How can I relate this to the group?" "How can I make this come alive in the here and now?" Such a focus is the power cell of Yalom's model. It is the theoretical stratagem that is the heart of his approach to group psychotherapy. If Yalom's strategy is followed, group leaders will not have to worry about repetitious monotonous group sessions. Group members will not put the group leader and their fellow members to sleep with abstract ramblings in the there and then about events that occurred six months to six years ago. Their histories, difficulties, and patterns of behavior will come alive in the here and now. Once the right atmosphere is established, group leaders will have a dynamic and alive laboratory for the exploration of human interactions and transactions. Keeping the here and now activation alive can be accomplished in a variety of ways. One method for fulfilling this task requires that group leaders take all there and then comments concerning individuals or events outside of the group and shift these issues into the here and now, exploring the ways these comments might relate to members presently in the group. For instance, a patient might begin to talk about a past hostile confrontation with his father. He could be asked, "Who here in group might evoke similar feelings in you?" Since the presenting complaint concerns a father, the group leader should be cautious for possible transference issues. Such a statement may also reflect the group member's attitude toward the group leader. Another group member might complain of her domineering sister, admitting there are many things she would like to tell her, but which she holds back because of her fear of the sister's reprisal. Turning this woman's there and then concerns into the here and now, she could easily be asked if she has held back saying certain things to the members of the group because of similar fears of reprisals and if she would be willing to share some of these feelings with them today. A group member may comment that he has become aware that his tendency to stereotype people has caused him numerous difficulties in his relationships in the past. Instead of exploring how these difficulties have manifested in the there and then, the group leader could ask him if he would be willing to tell the group members the way he has stereotyped each of them. Not only would such an intervention activate the interaction between the group members in the here and now, it would give members some important feedback on their perceived effect on another group member.

If a group has degenerated into cocktail party chatter and one group member comments that he doesn't think the group is taking its purpose seriously, the group leader could ask the individual if he would be willing to identify those members who do and those members who don't take the group seriously. Someone may complain that the group is too nice and everyone avoids conflicts. Asking the group member to identify the "leaders of the peace and tact movement in group" will activate the group into a rich source of interaction. Sometimes, even something as simple as asking one member to use "I statements" and speak directly to the other members can turn a dull, lifeless monologue into an exciting, alive dialogue.

Each of these illustrations suggests various ways group leaders can move the group into a here and now activation. In all of the examples, the leader had the option of asking a group member to respond to the group or another group member in either a provocative or supportive manner. Asking a group member to identify the most friendly, least threatening, most supportive, or most involved member will certainly require a different type of risk and invoke a different type of response than if a group member were asked to identify the most angry, least supportive, most uncaring, or least involved person in the group. Depending upon the group leaders' decisions and their line of inquiry, they can either build a group culture that is supportive or a group culture that is confrontational. Since both positions are required for a highly functioning therapy group, leaders do not want to sacrifice one position for the other. However, their decisions should be guided by the group's stage of development. If the group has not yet developed trust and cohesion, it would not be stage-appropriate to ask members to risk provocative confrontations. Stage-consistent interventions would require the group leader to encourage members to respond to the rest of the group in a way that would reduce regression and hostility. Later, after group trust and cohesion has been established, the leader could prompt the group members to risk more provocative positions when it is less likely to disrupt or threaten the group's existence.

Group leaders should also be aware that the neat, exact world of theory and purity of technique often fails to thrive in the harsh world of reality. Most addicted patients have never read Irvin Yalom and don't understand that they are supposed to respond in the "right way" to the group leader's noble efforts to help them see the error of their ways. Therefore, the group leader should be prepared to expect a claim of equality whenever he or she asks a group member to identify another group member as a possible source of interpersonal stimulus. Statements such as, "I trust everyone in the group the same. I like everyone here in the group equally" are never true. Don't ever believe it! No one in a psychotherapy group feels the same about everyone else. Each person in group is different and triggers a whole array of responses from the other members. Careful exploration of group members' responses to these differences are powerful sources of self-understanding and personal growth. While the group leader should never believe such claims of equality, neither should he or she always actively confront such a position. Rather than raise the group members' resistance, the group leader should encourage the members to explore their reactions to particular group members. This can be accomplished by gentle prodding. "Sure, I know you trust everyone in group, but if you had to pick someone you trusted more than others, who might that be? Would you be willing to take a few seconds and look around at each person's face and see who might trigger this feeling within you?" Such encouragement is not intrusive and most members will have feelings brought to their awareness by looking into the eyes and faces of their fellow group members. On those rare occasions when individuals are so defensive or resistant that they cannot or will not respond to such a suggestion, ask them how they would feel doing the exercise. Ask the other group members to respond with their own feelings in regard to the exercise. Almost always, this will bring forth a rich source of material from the other group members. Some may respond in disbelief that someone could feel absolutely the same about everyone. Others may respond in empathy to the anxiety such an exercise would trigger in them if they were required to take such a risk.

Sometimes, a group leader can choose to "just" encourage an isolated group member to make some genuine contact with another person in group. True intimacy and relatedness can be a powerful curative experience for individuals who have led their lives in false, contrived, and inauthentic interactions. "Healing through meeting" is a phrase coined by Martin Buber to emphasize the importance of true authentic dialogue in a person's life. Buber has written extensively about our need for human relatedness. Each of us possesses a primal need to be heard and listened to by another. Often it is enough just to know our cry has been heard and we are not alone in our isolation and suffering. In many cases, an individual's cry cannot be answered and, at these times, a response is not required or necessary. Buber described this phenomenon of the human condition as a cry that wants to be heard, but not answered. An example will help illustrate this position.

> Mary had sat quietly in group for more than three months, responding only to give support or encouragement to the other group members. Recently, she had begun to ask the group for advice concerning "my many problems." She was married to an alcoholic and had joined the group because she had become increasingly despondent over her husband's repeated failures to maintain sobriety for any length of time. Their six-year marriage had been marked by vacillating periods of multiple job losses, DUI arrests, and public humiliations intertwined with periodic episodes of relative success and stability which only lasted long enough to instill in her a false sense of hope that maybe this time, things would be different. As Mary talked about her isolation and despondency, the group began to respond to her as they usually did–namely, by giving advice endlessly. Mary's passivity and despondency usually evoked such responses in others and prevented her from mobilizing her own resources when confronted with difficulties that required important decisions. Stopping the group's feedback, the group leader asked Mary if she would be willing to look around the room and pick out one person she felt best understood her situation or her feelings at this moment. The group leader had chosen to intervene because he

> did not want the group to shift into their typical "let's give Mary advice and tell her what to do" mode. Rather, the leader hoped to have Mary connect with one person who might truly understand her position and her pain. After some initial claims that she felt everyone in the group understood her equally, Mary finally chose Sally, a woman who had refrained from giving her advice. Sally had been empathically connected with Mary because she had experienced a similar situation in her life. Sally proceeded to describe her own feelings at this moment, relating how difficult it was for her to make decisions, which often resulted in her feeling immobilized. As Sally shared more of her own difficulties, Mary began to acknowledge more of herself, talking about her rage at her husband and her need to take a stand with him. Mary's experience of herself was deepened by her identification with Sally, which was made possible because Sally had understood and really heard Mary in a way that Mary had not experienced before.

Fostering empathic understanding between group members and helping individuals connect with each other are two of the group leader's primary goals during the early stages of a newly developing group. The leader need not always ask group members to respond to each other in such a direct fashion. This can be accomplished by simply watching other group members' nonverbal responses and reactions as someone else is speaking in group. A knowing look, eye contact, a nodding head, or a subtle change of expression are clues that someone in group has empathically connected with another. The group leader need only give permission or encouragement for this empathy to be shared. Such a stance helps cohesion to develop in group, and one must always remember that unless cohesion is established, none of the other curative factors in group can be set in motion. Cohesion is enhanced as group members learn to share, relate, and feed each other in a caring way. Martin Buber illustrates the importance of people feeding each other in a story about the Baal Shem Tov, the first Zaddick of the Hasidic mystical tradition.

> When the Baal Shem Tov was a young rabbi, he prayed that God would someday show him the difference between heaven and hell. Shortly after his prayers, he had a dream one evening as he slept in which God ushered him into a large room where a group of starving people circled a great round table. Although there was an enormously large bowl of delicious, nourishing, warm stew in the middle of the table, all those who sat around the table were depleted, undernourished and emaciated. So large was the table that the bowl of

> food remained more than an arm's length away from each of them. Even though long wooden spoons were tied to each of their hands, which allowed each of these individuals to reach the food at the center of the table, the length of the spoon prevented them from reaching their own mouths. In spite of an abundance of food and nourishment in the room, each was suffering from starvation. The young rabbi was deeply saddened by such a sorrowful sight. Starving people, all who could see, smell and reach the food with their spoons, were unable to feed themselves and get the nourishment they desperately needed and craved. This is hell, God sadly told the young rabbi. God then proceeded to take the young rabbi to another room. Here, the scene appeared much the same as the first. A great round table with an abundance of food and people sitting around a circular table with giant spoons tied to their hands. Only here, instead of sadness and starvation, each person was well-nourished, healthy, happy and well-fed. The room was alive with merriment, laughter and happiness. Although the spoons were still too long to allow this group to feed themselves, they could easily reach across the table to feed each other. This is heaven, God said to the young rabbi, and the difference is that here people feed each other instead of trying to feed themselves in isolation.

So it is with group psychotherapy. Group members are encouraged and permitted to feed each other. None has to sit in isolation suffering from emotional malnourishment. Group leaders have many ways they can encourage members to "feed" and interact with each other. Each of the previous examples are only a few of the possible activating techniques available to group leaders. But it is important to remember, the techniques presented are only intended to illuminate the underlying principle of Yalom's format for group psychotherapy and are not intended to be ends in themselves. Rather, such techniques are to be used judiciously in the leader's efforts to establish a group culture that is curative and alive. As Yalom says:

> Remember that sheer acceleration of interaction is not the purpose of these techniques; if the therapist moves too quickly, using gimmicks to make interactions, emotional expression and self-disclosure too easy, he misses the whole point. Resistance, fear, guardedness, distrust, in short everything which impedes the development of satisfying interpersonal relations must be permitted expression. The goal is not to create a slick-functioning, streamlined social organization, but instead one which functions well enough and engenders sufficient

> trust for the unfolding of each member's social microcosm. Working through the resistances to change is the key to the production of change. Thus, the therapist does not want to go around obstacles but through them. (1975, p. 140)

INTERPERSONAL THEORY OF BEHAVIOR

After group leaders have steered their group into the here and now focus, they must next direct their energies toward the goal of helping members understand their behavior and the impact they have on others. Yalom outlines a systematic approach for understanding the process of personal impact in group and how each group member's interpersonal process within the group will reflect his or her general behavior and problems outside of group. By exploring in detail this interpersonal process, Yalom aims to answer the question of how process illumination of the here and now interaction leads to change. Before examining Yalom's outline, it would be helpful for group leaders to understand the theoretical foundation upon which Yalom's group edifice stands.

Although Yalom does not formally identify himself as a Sullivanian, he does acknowledge the importance of interpersonal learning in groups. He repeatedly makes reference to Harry Stack Sullivan and suggests presenting a brief explanation of Sullivan's interpersonal theory of psychiatry to every patient before he or she is placed in group. Therefore, understanding Sullivan's key concepts will provide the reader with a better understanding of Yalom and his approach to group psychotherapy.

SULLIVAN'S INTERPERSONAL THEORY OF PSYCHIATRY

Obviously, a comprehensive explanation of Sullivan and his interpersonal theory of psychiatry is beyond the scope of this chapter. The interested reader is referred to Yalom (1975) and his recommended references for understanding Sullivan. In order to comprehend the importance of Sullivan's influence on Yalom, it is necessary only to appreciate the four basic tenets of Sullivan's theory. Sullivan contends:

1. Personality is almost entirely a product of a person's interaction with others.
2. As human beings, our need to be closely related to others is basic.
3. As a young, developing child, we seek the approval of others and avoid their disapproval.

4. Eventually, the concept of the self (self-dynamism) is developed based on our perceived approval or disapproval by others.

If one fully understands the significance of these four basic principles of Sullivanian theory, one can appreciate the basic aim of Yalom's approach to group psychotherapy. If we are a product, for better or for worse, of our interactions with others, what better way to understand our strengths and weaknesses than to go to the source of our behavior—our interactions with others. However, merely observing our interactions with others misses the significance of the potential for change that exists within a psychotherapy group. Yalom utilizes three other principles of Sullivan's theory in his attempt to mobilize the group to bring about change in an individual's life. These three key concepts are:

1. *Parataxic distortions.* We all possess a proclivity to distort our perceptions of others. Here Sullivan refers to our tendency to relate to others, not on the basis of the realistic aspects of another, but on our perceived distortion of interpersonal reality. These distortions are determined and influenced by our interpersonal needs.

2. *Self-fulfilling prophecy.* In Sullivan's language, our interpersonal distortions tend to be self-perpetuating and lead to a self-fulfilling prophecy. For instance, an individual who possesses a concept of his self (self-dynamism) as disliked and inadequate may, through selective inattention, incorrectly perceive others as harsh and rejecting. More important, the person may gradually develop traits and attitudes such as defensiveness or servility that actually lead others to relate to him as he expects.

3. *Consensual validation.* This concept refers to Sullivan's emphasis on the importance of peer relationships in an individual's psychological development. As children we develop "chum relationships," which cause us to examine and compare our perceptions with others with whom we identify. Through these comparisons, we become aware that our friends or chums often see things differently than we or our family. Perceptions that were distorted become invalidated. As Sullivan says, "Parataxic distortions are modified primarily through consensual validation." If Mary perceives Jim as attacking and hostile while the rest of the group perceives him as supportive and kind, Mary will be forced to come to terms with her distortions of Jim. Perceptions that are not validated by the consensus of others lead to internal psychological shifts.

Understanding these three concepts helps explain Yalom's goal and purpose of group. As Sullivan advocated, the aim of psychiatry is the study of the process that goes on between people. Symptomatology becomes translated into interpersonal behavior, and the group leader observes and treats the interpersonal problems accordingly. From this view, a mental disorder is not statically embedded in a person. Instead, psychopathology is considered to be anchored in a dysfunctional system and interaction. These dysfunctional interactions are perpetuated by distortions within that system. Individuals carry their scripts and play their own assigned roles based on their unvalidated perceptual distortions of themselves and others. These scripts are constantly re-enacted within the larger framework of our personal relationships with others in our life. We become unwitting actors in a play whose plot we do not understand. From this perspective, the freedom of appropriate interchanges pertaining to reciprocal impressions, feelings, and observations within the context of the group situation becomes the medium from which awareness, validation, and change become possible. The goal or cure of treatment becomes the modifying and altering of these interpersonal distortions, thus enabling individuals to experience more satisfying lives based on the mutual realistic aspects of their interpersonal relationships. This is achieved for Sullivan when their sense of self is expanded to the point that they are known and perceived by others in the same manner that they perceive or know themselves. Or in Rogerian terms, there is congruence between their sense of self, their behavior, and how others perceive them. For instance, a person who perceives herself as loving and caring, but who acts hostilely and aggressively toward others while being perceived by others as aloof and unsupportive is in a distinct state of incongruence. Consensual validation from the group brings these three aspects of individuals' lives into sharp contrast: (1) their sense of self; (2) their behavior; and (3) their impression and effect upon others. Such a focus will allow them to see the lack of alignment and congruence in their lives.

Operating from this theoretical context, the group leader is encouraged by Yalom to follow a complex task that consists of several stages.

1. Members must recognize what they are doing with other people.
2. Then, they must appreciate the impact of their behavior on others.
3. They must, in turn, understand how their behavior influences others' opinions of them.
4. Eventually, they must decide whether they are satisfied with this interpersonal style.
5. Inevitably, if they decide to change, they must exercise their will to change.
6. Finally, the group and its leader must help the members solidify this change and generalize it to the outside.

Each of these stages that Yalom outlines must be facilitated by the specific cognitive input from the group leader. Eventually, Yalom feels the group must take over the leader's role as the only person responsible for the process observations of individual behavior in the here and now of the group interaction. This is an important role that the group must adopt because it is the series of process comments that allows the group members to change. The group leader can help initiate this process of change by escorting the group through this sequence:

1. *Here is what your behavior is like.* Through feedback and, later, through self-observation, patients learn to see themselves as others see them.
2. *Here is how your behavior makes others feel.* Members learn about the impact of their behavior on the feelings of other members.
3. *Here is how your behavior influences the opinions others have of you.* Members learn that, as a result of their behavior, others value them, dislike them, find them unpleasant, respect them, avoid them, etc.
4. *Here is how your behavior influences your opinion of yourself.* Building on the information gathered in the first three steps, patients formulate self-evaluations; they make judgments about their self-worth and their lovability (Recall Sullivan's aphorism that the self-concept is largely constructed from reflected self-appraisals.) (Yalom, 1975, pp. 154-155)

Each of the basic premises that Yalom outlines can be a powerful stimulant to change. Knowing and understanding, as Yalom indicates, are often not enough to produce change. Consequently, Yalom's four premises address what in his later writings (1980) he comes to identify as the key issues in his approach to existential psychotherapy. These four premises parallel Yalom's four ultimate concerns that form the foundation of his existential position–Responsibility, Death, Isolation, and Meaningfulness. As Yalom (1975) writes,

> The therapist's goal is to guide the patient to a point where he accepts one, several, or all of the following basic premises:
>
> 1. Only I can change the world I have created for myself.
> 2. There is no danger in change.
> 3. To attain what I really want, I must change.
> 4. I can change, I am potent. (p. 157)

Responsibility–Only I Can Change the World I Have Created for Myself

Each person who enters a group starts off on equal ground with all the others members of the group. Each person is in one sense given a clean slate, or as Yalom writes, "Each person is born together in the group." Each member shapes his or her own position, destiny, and life space in group. "Each in the deepest sense of the concept is 'responsible' for this space and for the sequence of events which will occur to him in the group" (Yalom, 1975, p. 153). If group leaders do their job correctly and build the appropriate group culture, group members will learn that their new life space within the group is safe and predictable. Since the group is a place that allows the learning and trying of new behavior, group members will eventually come to realize that it is not because they cannot change that they continue to suffer, but because they will not change. With this understanding, group members are forced to realize they are responsible for what happens to them. If they are to change, only they can accomplish this task for themselves.

Death–There Is No Danger in Change

Psychopathology, from Yalom's existential position, is rooted in the failure of individuals to transcend their death anxiety. Even if they understand they are responsible for their position in the world, they will frequently fail to make the decisions necessary for change. The obstacle to this change is fear–fear that one may fail. This is an inferred position that Yalom defines as "You behave as if you feel there were considerable danger that would befall you if you were to change. You fear to act otherwise lest some calamity befall you" (Yalom, 1975, p. 158). The group leader's task is to detoxify the discomfort that stems from the belief that change is dangerous. We fear change and responsibility. We continue to engage in self-defeating behavioral patterns even though we may be aware of their dysfunctional nature because our anxiety cements us rigidly in our position. This is the very theme of Erich Fromm's classic book, *Escape from Freedom.* It is essential that group members explore the fantasies of calamity which they expect to befall them if they should change. As the unrealistic aspects of these expectations are desensitized, they will be able to proceed in small increments of change and, more important, learn that there is no danger in change.

Isolation–To Attain What I Really Want, I Must Change

The group leader must understand the payoff or secondary gain that individuals obtain from continuing to engage in behavior that is counter to their best interests. Usually, such conflicts between the way people behave and the way they want to be are the result of conflicting desires that cannot be satisfied simultaneously. These conflicts are frequently the result of infantile needs that get played out on an unconscious level because of the terrifying fears associated with the dread of isolation and adulthood. Yalom writes,

> Another explanatory approach which many therapists take to deal with the paradox that patients persist in behaving counter to their best interests is to consider the payoffs of their present behavior. Though the behavior of the patient sabotages many of his mature needs and goals, at the same time it satisfies another set of needs and goals. In other words, the patient has conflicting motivations which cannot be simultaneously satisfied. For example, a patient may wish to be able to establish mature heterosexual relationships, but at another, often unconscious, level he may wish to be nurtured, to be cradled endlessly, to assuage castration anxiety by a maternal identification, or, to use another vocabulary, to be sheltered from the terrifying freedom of adulthood.
>
> Obviously, he cannot satisfy both sets of wishes: he cannot establish an adult heterosexual relationship with a woman if he also says (and much more loudly), "Take care of me, protect me, nurse me, let me be a part of you."
>
> The therapist attempts to clarify this for the patient. "Your behavior makes sense if we assume that you wish to satisfy the deeper, more primitive, more infantile need." He tries to help the patient to understand the nature of his conflicting desires, to choose between them, to relinquish those which cannot be fulfilled except at enormous cost to his integrity and autonomy. Once the patient realizes what he "really" wants (as an adult) and that his behavior is designed to fulfill opposing growth-retarding needs, he gradually concludes that "to attain what I really want, I must change." (Yalom, 1975, pp. 159-160)

Relationships, whether they be with a group, the group leader, or another person of significance, have a tendency to produce an emergence of infantile expectations and needs. Dependency, the wish to be loved and coddled, as well as the infantile fears of abandonment and rejection, are heightened in any close interpersonal relationship. Those infantile needs and frustrations that have become problematic for individuals become unique characteristics of their personality. These unique sets of infantile needs will manifest in the group as they would in any significant relationship. The group leader's task is to force group members to modify their needs by understanding that such needs are infantile wishes that are no longer useful in their adult life. They must instead learn to tolerate in awareness the tension occasioned by these unfulfilled needs.

Hans Strupp (1978) sums up this position precisely when he writes,

> (the patient) must take action to satisfy it, abandon it, or modify it. What the therapist no longer permits him (the patient) to do is to use the relationship with a significant person for the purpose of expressing his need in symbolic or disguised ways. The therapist says in effect: if you want me to coddle you, baby you, protect you, love you, you must experience the feelings associated with these expectations in my presence and as directed toward me. This is predictably painful but cannot be helped. Once you have undergone this painful experience, you may realize that your expectations were (a) anachronistic–that is, they may have been reasonable in childhood but no longer useful; (b) unrealistic–that is, as a mature independent adult I cannot possibly coddle you, and, if I did you would be appalled by it and reject it or; (c) based on gross misperceptions of the current situations as well as that prevailing in your childhood, we must understand these distortions. What I will not allow you to do is to act as if you did not have these expectations of me while at the same time expecting me to fulfill them. This is what Freud meant when he said that a conflict must be raised to awareness and fought out on that level. (p. 15)

What Strupp and Yalom are addressing is the conflict that all of us experience in all of our interpersonal relationships. It is important for the group leader to understand that the gratification of these infantile needs is ultimately unproductive for the members. Once they get what they think they want (based on unrecognized, unfulfilled, infantile wishes), they will reject it because it does not fit within their self-definition of the healthy functioning that is expected of a mature, independent adult.

Meaninglessness– I Can Change; I Am Potent

Only when individuals understand the true context of their behavior will they be able to develop a sense of personal mastery and meaning in their lives. Understanding the meaning of our behavior moves us from a position of being driven by frightening, unknown forces to a position of control and mastery. We are the riders instead of the ridden. To offer an explanation ("a because") for their behavior allows individuals to attain the true existential position of authenticity. It also allows them to develop a system by which they can order the events in their lives in a coherent and predictable pattern. Life has meaning for them. They are as they are now because of events in their life that helped shape their perceptions of the world.

As Scott Rutan says, "Our patients come to us with solutions, not problems" (Rutan, 1983). As group leaders, we must not lose sight of the fact that what we see as therapists is a child's normal and even at times creative adaptation to a maladaptive situation. As Sullivanian theory indicates, children are shaped by their interpersonal environment and interaction with others in their life. If there is a conflict between the growth inclinations of the child and the interpersonal demands of the parents, growth will be compromised for security. Robert and Mary Goulding (1979) share similar sentiments in Redecision Therapy. We all make early decisions on how we are to survive in our world based on the information we have available to us at the time. Unfortunately, children are often forced to make early decisions based on erroneous information before they are cognitively and emotionally capable of such decisions. They hold on to these decisions unconsciously even after the circumstances that led to their position have changed. For example, "If I tell you how I truly feel, you will reject me. So if I am to survive with you, Mother, I will have to act as I think you want me to act." Helping individuals understand their position in life and how they came to hold this position will give them a sense of mastery and meaning in their life. They will not be bound to the past and will have the freedom to change in the future. As one group member announced, "I didn't like myself because I used to think I was to blame because of the way I was. Now that I understand why I am this way, I now feel I deserve more from my life."

Such an existential stance in group is summarized by Yalom's statement on will.

> The concept of will provides us with a useful construct in understanding the procedure of process illumination. The interpretive remarks of the therapist can all be viewed in terms of how they bear on the patient's will. The most common and simplistic therapeutic approach is an exhortative one. "Your behavior is, as you yourself now know, counter to your best interests. You are not satisfied, this is not what you want for yourself. Damn it, change!" The expectation that the patient will change is simply an extension of the moral philosophical belief that if man knows the good (i.e., what, in the deepest sense, is in his best interest), he will act accordingly. In the words of Aquinas: "Man, insofar as he acts willfully, acts according to some imagined good." And, indeed, for some individuals this knowledge and this exhortation is sufficient to produce therapeutic change. To be sure, this is often the case for individuals who change as a result

of some short-term experiential group. However, patients with significant and well-entrenched psychopathology generally need much more. (1975, p. 157)

EXAMPLES OF YALOM'S HERE AND NOW FOCUS

Some clinical examples will help illustrate Yalom's suggestions for the sequence of process comments which lead the group member to change.

> An experiential training group consisting of eight Masters-level counselors at an inpatient alcohol and drug treatment unit met weekly for ten sessions. The first session was dominated by three members. Chuck, a hostile, confrontational, recovering addict with over five years of sobriety spoke angrily about the hospital and the general incompetence of his program director. He spent much of the group time ruminating about whether he should return to school because he saw little hope for the situation changing. Betty, a hysterical recovering addict and nurse with four years of sobriety spoke endlessly about her fears surrounding her participation in the training group. She felt overwhelmed by others and feared they would find out how really unstable she was. Shirley, a psychiatric nurse who was clinical director on the ward, spent the remainder of the group time reassuring Betty and calming Chuck. Her responses were exclusively supportive and she had assigned herself the task of assuring the group that things would somehow work out okay. Shirley also devoted some of the group time to expressing her concern about Ann, an MSW on the unit who was unable to attend the first group session because of an unexpected emergency at home. Shirley went to great lengths to assure the group that Ann would be there next week. At the start of the second group session, Ann was indeed present, but remained quiet and withdrawn during the didactic lecture portion of the day. This part of the training group was geared toward presenting theory and the trainees were encouraged to ask questions about the experiential portion of group, which was conducted at a different time. After the didactic presentation was completed, the group proceeded to the group room where the experiential portion of the group was to be held. Midway through the group session, Ann suddenly arose from her slumber and began to attack the group leader and the group members, demanding to know "What are the group norms in this group?" Her outburst caught the group by surprise

and interrupted Betty, who again was in the midst of hysterically sharing with the group her fears of overwhelming others. The rest of the group responded in an uproar, with Chuck leading one half of the group in an attack on Ann and Shirley leading the other half in their attempts to be understanding and supporting of Ann.

By now, the group leader has a vast amount of data accumulated in his observance of Ann, Betty, Chuck, and Shirley. There are a number of important questions that he must start asking himself before he can lead the group members through Yalom's sequence of process illumination.

1. The Group Members Must Recognize What They Are Doing with Others in the Group

Does Ann realize how she is excluding and distancing herself from the rest of the group? Is Shirley aware of her tendency to rescue and take care of others in the group? Betty is overwhelming others with both her premature self-disclosure and her demands not to be rejected by the group members. Does she realize that her constant pouring forth of such strong feelings so prematurely creates the very impact on others that she fears most? Chuck seems oblivious to the impact that his anger has on others. Is he aware that the only feeling he can show is anger?

2. They Must Appreciate the Impact of Their Behavior on Others

Ann must come to realize how she affects others with her sudden demands and criticisms. Does Chuck realize that, other than Betty, the rest of the group turns away from him and does not respond to his constant show of anger? Is Shirley aware that her readiness to support everyone leads some individuals to constantly take from her and give very little in return? Betty needs to realize her hysterical presentation leads others to treat her in a patronizing manner.

3. They Must Understand the Influence Their Behavior Has upon Others' Opinions of Them

Ann must come to realize that her sudden outbursts of anger lead others to avoid her and perceive her as an angry woman who cannot be trusted. Chuck needs to be aware that his constant show of anger results in others viewing him as a critical and uncaring person. Betty must learn that her fears create the very impression she wishes to avoid. Others do see her as easily overwhelmed and question her stability. Shirley does not understand why everyone comes to her with their problems and why they are reluctant to give her the same support she gives them. She does not realize her tendency to take care of others leaves her one-dimensional in their eyes. They see her as a giver and someone who does not want to take.

4. They Must Decide Whether They are Satisfied with Their Interpersonal Style

Is Ann satisfied with being excluded by others? Is Chuck comfortable with his "angry-man-against-the-world routine?" Does Shirley want to shed her image as a rescuer? Is Betty gaining something by appearing unstable and easily overwhelmed? Often, the answers to such questions are not as obvious as one is led to believe. Yalom cautions the group leader to be aware of the difference between primary task and secondary gratification, and the dynamic tension between the two.

The primary task defines the reason individuals entered group or sought help. They wish symptom relief, be it freedom from suffering or improvement in relationships. However, as Yalom points out, an individual's presentation in group is rarely this simple and it will usually become more complicated as the group continues. Usually, the primary task changes considerably after a person enters group because of the secondary gratification that arises in group.

Yalom describes this dilemma:

> in each instance the patient has given priority not to the primary task but to some secondary gratification arising in the group; a relationship with another member, an image which he wishes to project, a group role in which he is the most sexually desirous, most influential, most wise, most superior. (1975, p. 147)

The group leader must constantly ask himself if the group member's behavioral presentation is a conflict between the primary task and the secondary gratification of the group. Is Betty's hysteria a way of getting group attention and support? Does her style of relating prevent her from assuming unwanted tasks of responsibility? Does Chuck like to portray the angry man routine because it is an image that he wishes to foster in order to prevent others from seeing the weak and frightened side of himself? Is Ann's attack on the group really an attack on the group leader? Is her attack a misguided attempt to demonstrate to the group that she is skilled in group therapy and that she wishes to let them know she understands group norms? Members frequently join groups so they learn the skills necessary to "out mental health" others. Is this part of her secondary gain?

5. Now, They Must Exercise Their Will to Change

In his book, *Existential Psychotherapy*, Yalom cites a Japanese proverb that states, "To know and not to act, is not to know at all" (1980, p. 286). This proverb illustrates the importance of members putting into action the insight and understanding they gain through psychotherapy. As Yalom suggests, if group members fail to act on this newfound knowledge, it will do them little practical good. The group leader must know how to utilize the group to facilitate change and action. Bob and Mary Goulding's (1979) unique perspective on psychotherapy can be of assistance in getting reluctant members to change. Bob Goulding views psychotherapy as being in many ways like a chess match between the patient and the group leader. There is a part of the patient that wants to get better and a part that wants to defeat the therapist. It is this part that the therapist must combat and "win over" if change is to be initiated. Goulding cautions the group leader to be aware of the "first con" that the group member presents. The "first con" is usually presented by the group member in the form his or her language takes and it is represented in such key words as "try, need, and can't." "Needs" are "wants" and "can'ts" are "don'ts" in Goulding's perspective. He requires group members to change the verbal presentation of their problem with the substitution of the words "won't" for "can't" and "want" for "need." Such a substitution magnifies patients' resistance and minimizes their helplessness. They must realize they don't change because they are unwilling to risk the change. "Try" is also viewed as an indication of helplessness and resistance. Members in Bob Goulding's group soon learn that the mention of the word "try" will result in appearance of the famous "try bell." Bob keeps a cow bell tucked within easy reach of his chair. Upon mentioning the word "try," Bob will ring his bell with vigor and delight. Through this medium, the group members become acutely aware of their reluctance to "try" and change their behavior.

An example of a beginning group of inpatient alcoholics meeting for the first time illustrates this dilemma.

> In anger at the staff's insistence that he start attending Alcoholics Anonymous meetings, one group member spoke about his dissatisfaction with the organization. Despite the fact that he had relapsed repeatedly and this was his second hospitalization for his alcoholism, this man could not understand why he was required to attend AA

> meetings. In a forced and dramatic presentation of his desperation, he pleaded his case by stating, "I've been trying to find an AA meeting I like, but I can't, and I don't think I need it." Encouraged to change his statement to "I won't find an AA meeting and I don't want one," he became more aware of his passive resistance to these requirements and realized that his relapses were due to his unwillingness to change rather than the result of the failure of the staff, the hospital, AA, or some compelling force in the universe.

The Gouldings' position on words such as "try," "can't," and "need" illustrate their insistence that people take full responsibility for themselves and not delude themselves into acting as if they have no power when they actually do. However, the Gouldings' stance on language bears further examination. Dealing with language alone, as the Gouldings know, does not necessarily result in powerful changes of will and power. Forceful, charismatic therapists can induce compliance and adaptive responses. A great deal of what occurs in therapy, if the therapist isn't careful, can be compliance and may just be surface structural rearrangements that do not affect deeper issues. The Gouldings are quite aware of this problem and stress constantly that decisions should be made out of a free-child ego state and not out of the adaptive-child ego state.

Yalom (1995) illustrates this point succinctly in his most recent book. Drawing on Faber's (1966) distinction between two different types of will, Yalom criticizes current psychological thought because it places an exaggerated emphasis on conscious will and has failed to fashion a succinct, workable definition of will, which adds to the confusion of what will is exactly.

Faber's first realm of the will (and it is here that Yalom feels that Faber has made his most important contribution) is not experienced consciously during an act and must be inferred after an event. Yalom and Faber are suggesting that important choices are not consciously experienced as choices. Most of us are not able to predict the consequences of the choices that we consciously make or how these choices will bind us to some destiny in our lives. There is, however, a second realm of will that is a conscious component and is experienced during an event. "I will do this to get that. If I stop eating I will lose weight, etc." Yalom suggests that these two realms of will must be approached differently in therapy. He writes,

> The second realm (conscious) of will is approached through exhortation and appeals to willpower, effort, and determination. The first realm is impervious to these enjoiners and must be approached obliquely. A serious problem occurs when one applies exhortative

> second realm techniques to first realm activities. For example, I can will knowledge, but not wisdom; going to bed, but not sleeping; eating, but not hunger; meekness, but not humility. (1980, p. 299)

Yalom is addressing a very crucial issue that William James and pragmatists struggled with years ago. James argued that there was no objective truth in the world. Truth, for James, was determined by utility. Truth is what works! James proposed that individuals act themselves into a new way of thinking rather than think themselves into a new way of acting. Act as you want to believe and you will soon believe how you act. James' influence on Alcoholics Anonymous is well-documented and his pragmatism is one of the important reasons this program enjoys the success it does. AA members are told to change their behavior first and their thinking will follow. Similarly, this is the same principle that operates within the Gouldings' insistence on producing behavioral change. Confucius, in fact, proposed this axiom over two thousand years ago: "I hear and I forget, I see and I remember, I do and I understand."

6. Help Them Solidify Change and Generalize to the Outside

The group leader must also be cognizant of the magnitude of the power of reinforcement that exists within the group. When group members change some aspect of their behavior, no matter how trivial or small, this change should be acknowledged by the group. Bob and Mary Goulding frequently lead the group in cheers and applause when group members report even an insignificant change in their lives. The group that only spends its time on dredging up pain, anger, and resentment is missing a crucial part of its curative process and is not fulfilling its potential as a powerful change agent in a person's life. Laughter and encouragement used creatively in the group lubricate the creative process and can be powerful forces in helping members put their insight into action.

Through the process of illumination, the group members will gradually deepen their awareness of their behavior and the impact their behavior has on others. They will also learn the consequences they suffer because of the impact they have on others. Yalom outlines the sequence of process illumination in four steps:

1. *Here is what your behavior is like:*
    A. Every time someone shares feelings in here you:
        1. rescue them
        2. laugh or make a joke

3. get angry (i.e., When someone doesn't agree with what you say, your jaws tighten, you clench your fist, you glare and your voice gets louder.)

2. *Here is how your behavior affects my feelings about you:*
   A. I get annoyed at you for always rescuing.
   B. I get hurt that you laugh at my feelings.
   C. I become frightened and I don't want to share my thoughts or feelings honestly with you.
3. *Here is how your behavior influences my opinion of you:*
   A. I don't think you're really sincere because you have to take care of everyone.
   B. I don't trust you and your laughter.
   C. I think you must really be an uncaring SOB and I don't want anything to do with you.
4. *Here is how your behavior influences your opinion of yourself:*
   A. The very reason you came to group was because you were dissatisfied and angry with yourself because you didn't have any friends or a satisfying long-lasting relationship. You viewed yourself as someone who must be unlovable and despised the fact you were alienating everyone around you. Do you want to continue this behavior that is causing you so much difficulty and, most importantly, are you willing to change? (Yalom, 1995)

Yalom's model for group psychotherapy brings the members painstakingly through each of these sequences. Group members must realize what their behavior is like and how this ultimately leads to their dissatisfaction with themselves and their life. Yalom's model can be summarized as a sequence of change based on fourteen basic assumptions:

1. All of us are influenced and shaped by our interpersonal relationships, and we all share our own interpersonal world based on our early relationships.
2. Group psychotherapy can provide a corrective emotional experience of the distorted or disrupted interpersonal relationship that occurred early in our lives.
3. Group psychotherapy acts as a social microcosm of our interpersonal world.
4. Group psychotherapy is a vehicle for the study of interpersonal relationships.
5. Through the process of consensual validation and self-observation, group members become aware of the parataxic distortions involved in their interpersonal relationships.

6. Via feedback from the group leader and other group members, individuals can learn to appreciate the impact of their own behavior in regard to how others think and feel about them and how this influences their own opinion of themselves.
7. Given this increased awareness, the members learn that they are responsible for the reality, not the fantasy, of their interpersonal relationships.
8. Given this kind of responsibility, the members learn that they alone can change their own behavior.
9. Most important, such awareness is positively correlated with the amount of affect (feelings) experienced by individuals. Adversely, the more intellectual this experience, the less the learning and the less the correlation with change.
10. Change is a direct function of motivation, involvement in the group, the rigidity of the interpersonal character structure, and interpersonal style. Consequently, the more motivated, more involved, and less rigid the individuals, the more chance there will be for change in their behavior.
11. Such changes in group may spur changes in other interpersonal relationships. The amount of change is dependent on the amount of self-analysis and feedback individuals receive from other members in the group.
12. The irrational fears connected with change will be overcome, and such changes will not result in the basic fears of loss of individuality, death, abandonment, and engulfment.
13. Over time, the social microcosm of the group results in outside behavior becoming honestly present within group and the new learned behavior being exported eventually to the outside world. The behavior within the group and outside of the group becomes more congruent.
14. Eventually, an adaptive procedure develops internally, first within the group and then eventually generates to the world outside of the group. Group members practice their new learned group behavior outside of the group and return to the group with this experience and change in their behavior over time. Distortions begin to be diminished. The members' capacity for developing healthy relationships increases. Eventually, their anxiety decreases and their self-esteem increases to the point that they feel freer to be themselves. The increased positive response of other group members to the exposure of themselves leads to an increase in self-esteem and self-confidence. A cycle of exposure of one's true self, risk-taking,

and increased self-esteem eventually leads to a more autonomous and conflict-free individual.

INTEGRATION OF MODERN ANALYTIC APPROACH

Yalom's model of interactional group psychotherapy is one of the most widely applied approaches to group treatment (Dies, 1992). Part of the reason for its popularity is that it is a relatively simple, practical, and straightforward approach to group therapy that is easy to comprehend and teach. His text is well written and easily understandable. All the basics for conducting an effective group are clearly defined. His model is also easily adaptable and this is why so much emphasis has been placed on its description. However, no single model can be everything for everyone. Consequently, other alternative but complementary approaches need to be examined. Yalom's basic model is still the preferred approach for early and middle stage recovery issues. However, this model lacks the complete comprehension necessary for treating chemically dependent individuals through the later phases of their recovery. As it becomes more evident that the characterological features associated with chemical dependency must be modified if long-term recovery is to be achieved, a more extensive theoretical formulation must be posited to address all of the diverse dynamics that are likely to manifest in extended group therapy. Since the changing of one's character takes more than a few months of treatment, a more extensive and inclusive model of group treatment is needed to supplement Yalom's recommendations. The proper treatment of one's character often takes years of psychotherapy. AA and the other twelve-step programs intuitively know this and recognize that the removal of character defects requires many years of working the program. Louis Ormont's modern approach to group treatment is one model that addresses long-term treatment more thoroughly while still being compatible with Yalom's theoretical position.

The unexpected discovery of the similarities that exist between their respective positions was made while I was watching these two esteemed practitioners serve on the same panel of senior group therapists presenting contrasting theoretical views on representative group therapy events at the 1992 American Group Psychotherapy Association (AGPA) conference in New York City. After the panel, and the audience, viewed a videotape of Dr. Yalom conducting a demonstration group, the members of the panel presented critiques and offered contrasting recommendations based on their observations. They also provided alternative interventions that reflected each of their different theoretical positions. As a result of the lively, and sometimes provocative, debate that ensued among the panelists, it soon became evident to those of us present in the audience that Dr. Ormont and Dr. Yalom were strongly aligned and that they shared many similar sentiments and opinions about what they believed were necessary and important elements in effective group psychotherapy. An important question emerged as a result of the surprising mutuality that these two esteemed group practitioners shared while they were defending their theoretical positions with the other panelists. How could Irvin Yalom, a self-proclaimed existentialist influenced by Sullivanian theory, and often openly critical of classical psychoanalytic theory, be so aligned with Louis Ormont, a group psychotherapist heavily influenced by psychoanalytic theory and a self-proclaimed modern psychoanalyst?

It is important to explore and contrast each of their views on group psychotherapy in an attempt to better explain and identify the commonalities that exist between them. Hopefully, this endeavor will lead to a more thorough understanding of the convergent elements that exist in their respective approaches to group psychotherapy. Further, it is hoped that such an attempt at synthesizing and integrating each of their theoretical positions will lead to a more complete and cogent theory of group psychotherapy in general and interpersonal group psychotherapy in particular. This is an important undertaking in light of the immense popularity of Dr. Yalom's writings, lectures, and theories on group psychotherapy, and the extensive influence they have on the general public and the professional community (Dies, 1992). This popularity exists despite the frequent criticism his classic text, *The Theory and Practice of Group Psychotherapy*, elicits from many respected group theorists who judge his model of group psychotherapy to be either atheoretical or an assortment of techniques in search of a theory. While his book is often praised as providing the most pragmatic "nuts and bolts" information for the uninformed or new group therapist, it is thought by some to be in need of more organized theoretical direction. Hopefully, Louis Ormont's firm theoretical grounding in modern psychoanalytic theory can provide some needed theoretical support for some of Yalom's recommendations. Examining in more detail the similarities and differences in their respective approaches to group treatment can help establish a firmer theoretical foundation for interactional or interpersonal group psychotherapy. The synthesis of their views on group psychotherapy will possibly provide a more expansive view of Yalom's theory and furnish some clarification, elaboration, and alternative explanations for his recommended strategies.

As is often the case, the more competent and experienced practitioners of all forms of good psychotherapy share many similar attitudes and approaches, even though they often use a very different language to explain what, how, and why they do what they do (Frank, 1978; Bergin, 1971). Not only is their language often different, but the theoretical rationale for its application may at times be diametrically opposed. Despite this, what may appear controversial or oppositional in theoretical explanations may in actuality be quite complementary when seen in action or investigated retrospectively. Yvonne Agazarian and Anne Alonso (1993) made a very similar discovery when they were trying to explain why their sometimes divergent views on group psychotherapy produced similar results despite their different interpretations and explanations about the same phenomena in group treatment.

It is hoped that the same might hold true if Yalom's and Ormont's views on group psychotherapy are critically examined and compared. Not only might there be a clearer understanding of their respective approaches to group treatment, but such an investigation might also lead to a more thorough exploration of interventions and strategies that will prove to be helpful in all forms of group treatment.

Shared Similarities

While watching Dr. Yalom and Dr. Ormont support each other's views on what they advocated as essential and crucial elements in effective group psychotherapy, it became apparent that there were numerous issues upon which they were passionately joined. Foremost among these are the following:

1. The importance and significance of the here and now in group;
2. The proposed and required activity level of the group leader to ensure active participation of all group members;
3. The necessity of establishing a cohesive group or community where emotional communication is valued over intellectual communication;
4. The establishment of therapeutic norms that require active participation by all group members in accepting responsibility for the group and all of its members' participation; and
5. The lack of emphasis, and at times a total disregard, for the use of group-as-a-whole intervention.

While Yalom has written more extensively and prolifically on these issues, Ormont has earned a reputation among senior AGPA members as being one of its most highly respected practitioners of group psychotherapy–a group leader who makes abstract theory come alive in the actual practice and art of the group therapy experience. While Ormont has also written extensively on group theory and has recently published an excellent book (1992) on the subject, he does not share the same recognition, outside of AGPA and New York City, that Yalom does. Despite their diverse backgrounds and different theoretical orientations, they prove to be quite complementary to each other in terms of their strategies, interventions, and approaches to treatment in group.

Here and Now

There is probably no single theorist on group psychotherapy who has emphasized the importance of the here and now more that Irvin Yalom. Consequently, his name has become nearly synonymous with the use of the here and now in group psychotherapy. Contrary to how it may appear at times, Yalom did not "invent" the concept; rather his emphasis on its importance helped firmly establish its obvious significance. Any competent, well-trained group leader knows the value of the here and now in group. All experienced and effective group leaders, whatever their theoretical orientation might be, constantly emphasize and guide their groups to operate in the here and now because they know this is where the action takes place. Perhaps, as some critics claim, Yalom does at times overstate his case and the importance of the here and now. However, it might also be true that the here and now would not be so obviously important to us all if Yalom had not pushed this concept under our noses so frequently and reminded us so thoroughly of its vitalness to group therapy.

Many other theorists acknowledge the significance of the here and now to group. For instance, Malcolm Pines suggests the here and now can come in many different shapes and forms. The therapist's creativity and ability to recognize the many different ways it can exist or be evoked is crucial if it is be experienced by the group and its members. The group must learn how to respond to it and not retreat from it when it is manifested. The multidimensional ways it can exist and be recognized is dependent upon group leaders' theory, skill, knowledge, experience, and courage (Pines, 1992). All of these attributes are necessary if therapists are going to be able or willing to leave the comfortableness and certainty of their well-trained professional role that is firmly grounded in their theoretical framework and go out and meet the group and its members in the spontaneity and uncertainty of the moment. The here and now, Pines suggests, is always being created; it is not just there waiting to be discovered. It is more likely to be created between the leader and the members in the group when the group leader is able to use his or her own creativity and the depth of his or her own feeling to help the group members engage each other on the true, honest, and intimate level in the reality of the here and now.

Yalom has long described the here and now as the power cell of group and calls it the "key concept of group therapy" (Yalom, 1985, p. 28). He suggests that the group leader must ensure that the group members focus their attention on their immediate feelings and thoughts toward the other group members, the group leader, and the group itself as a whole. The immediate here and now events in the group must take precedence over the events in the past or in the current life events of each member outside of the group. The events in the here and now within the group become the primary focus of the group leader. Yalom emphasizes this because he believes it will facilitate the development and stark emergence of each member's social microcosm. Both Alonso (1985) and Rutan (1983) say the same thing more cleverly when they point out that "Group members will not have to talk about their problems in group, they will have them."

The idiosyncratic psychological Achilles' heel of each individual group member will emerge for all to see and experience in the here and now of the group process. The group, from this perspective, becomes a laboratory on interpersonal behavior where members will experience and act out their idiosyncratic conflicts or their repetition compulsions through their interactions with each other. All members will have a chance to access and experience their internal world, which contains the introjections and the repressed, denied, and dissociated elements of self and object representations that frequently get projected onto others. The stark emergence of each member's internal world will be played out in the repetition compulsion on a level that he or she can experience and eventually own and master, since it cannot be denied or disavowed because the group, through the group therapist's leadership, will not allow it to go unnoticed for long. As Ormont suggests in his book, it is rare for people to have the opportunity to reflect on themselves and their behavior. A group conducted along the lines that Ormont and Yalom suggest will allow each member this opportunity. Ormont writes,

> This is the subtle value of group treatment and certainly one that I did not myself see or appreciate for years. It is that people can make instantaneous readings of themselves, catching and labeling momentary feelings that are important in their psyches, but that in daily existence are typically gone before they can be captured.
>
> The power of group to do this kind of in vivo work is sweeping.
>
> There are people, perhaps the majority, who go through life with only subsensible, unconscious intimations of what they are really

> feeling; they sense the existence of crucial, activating emotions. If only they were to stop themselves at pivotal instants, to "freeze frame" their emotional life, so to speak, at the proper moment, then they could pinpoint these dynamic actuating forces within them—these feelings that motivate them and color their whole existence. (1992, p. 38)

Unlike Yalom, who is a self-proclaimed existentialist, Ormont takes a less radical stance on the here and now in group. Like any well-trained modern psychoanalyst, he views the past as always coming alive in the present, usually through the activation of transference distortions and the group members' resistances to aggression, intimacy, and spontaneity. While Ormont said he "vehemently agreed" with Yalom on the importance of the here and now in group, he added that the here and now was not just important in itself, but that it was important because the here and now was the arena that allowed resistances and transferences to be activated. True to his psychoanalytic heritage, Ormont views the activation, identification, and subsequent treatment of resistance and transferences as the cornerstone of psychotherapy. Ormont knows, as any good analyst knows, that the internal world of the individual comes alive in the here and now interactions of the group. The past, as it is projected into the here and now, is always triggered or activated by the actuality of the immediate moment. Consequently, the interpersonal transferences and resistances that result from this provide the therapist with a window to individuals' past as well as their current life. The closer the therapist stays to the consensually validated here and now data, the more likely the group member will be unable to refute it. But the opportunity for all in the group to see the past recreated in the present provides far more important information.

Such a stance in therapy is not unique or new; every well-trained therapist shares this belief. However, Ormont and Yalom put a special twist on this topic because they both emphasize the investigation of resistance as it is evoked interpersonally. Drawing on the influence of Harry Stack Sullivan, Ormont writes,

> the interpersonal analyst saw resistances as expressing not just the patient's past but his or her ongoing dealing with others. Harry Stack Sullivan pointed out that resistances are an artifact of the given personal relationship. Someone may invoke resistance in one person, but not another. For Sullivan, even repression was interpersonal. (1992, p. 121)

Ormont, like most modern psychoanalysts and self-psychologists, sees pathology as the result of self-defeating defenses or resistances that are erected against transference wishes, shame, guilt, and fears of oedipal and pre-oedipal retaliations. He views these defenses as necessary, though maladaptive, attempts at self-preservation that are the consequences of unmet developmental needs.

This is why Ormont encourages the group leader to invite individuals' resistances and transferences. He wants them to come into full bloom in the group. The group members will naturally resist this. Their insistence on the use of the past and the future is a protective device that serves to ward off the anxiety and emotional stimulation of the immediate present. Ormont's emphasis on the immediacy of the moment is reflective of his immediacy principle and is very similar to Yalom's concept of the here and now. However, Ormont's immediacy principle is more expansive because it carries an implicit requirement of emotionality in its presentation and does not limit the extent of the content to the group. Unlike Yalom, Ormont does not discourage talk of the there and then. He recognizes that it is vitally important for group members to be able to tell the important stories of their lives. However, if these stories are communicated in a remote or detached and intellectual manner that is emotionally deadening to the group and its members, the group leader's task is to bring this to the individual's and the group's immediate attention. Ormont, like Yalom, is very aware that all individuals possess a potential to deaden their experience in life or water down the drama, tragedies, and excitement of their existence.

Yalom and Ormont's position on this issue is very similar to that of the late Polish novelist Jerzy Kozinski (1977), who believed it is essential that people be fully aware and in touch with the personal drama of their own lives as well as the personal drama that is being played out by each individual who crosses their path. Failure to do so means we are shortchanging ourselves and not being true to our existence. This is very close to describing what existentialists such as Heidegger, Buber, and Sartre mean when they write about existential guilt. We are existentially guilty of not fully experiencing Being in the purest ontological sense if we do not get in touch with how we are all playing out our own personal drama with the rest of society serving as a background for this drama. We owe it to ourselves, and as group leaders we owe it to our group members, to prompt, prod, and encourage them to take more responsibility for living authentic lives. Sartre cautions us not to live in "bad faith." Heidegger warns us to remain *das man* and avoid the deadening security of the crowd or herd mentality. Buber takes this position even one step further in his philosophical anthropology when he proclaims we can never live authentic lives in isolation and only truly know ourselves in relation to others.

In order to take full advantage of the potential for the group to come alive authentically and emotionally, the group leader needs to discipline him or herself to think predominantly in the here and now. He or she must make every attempt to find ways to move the focus from the outside to the inside and from the general to the specific as it applies to the group. Each topic presented must prompt the group leader to ask questions: "How can I relate this to the group? How can I make this come alive in the here and now?" Such a focus is the power cell of Yalom's model and Ormont's immediacy principle.

Interaction Between Group Members

No two group therapists place more emphasis on the importance of group members interacting and responding to each other than Yalom and Ormont. Their strategies and reasons for this may not be exactly similar, but they both require it of their individuals and a group is always a here and now event. In fact, the immediacy of two or more people directly responding to each other is so intertwined with the here and now that it is often impossible to separate these two concepts.

Yalom has repeatedly identified interpersonal input, output, and learning as the cornerstone of his approach to group therapy. He wants a high level of involvement from all group members where honesty and spontaneity are encouraged and sanctioned. Nonjudgmental acceptance, self-disclosure, reciprocal vulnerability, and the desire for self-understanding are crucial elements of the "therapeutic norms" he tries to establish in group. Heavily influenced by Harry Stack Sullivan's interpersonal theory of psychiatry, Yalom has drawn upon Sullivan's concepts of Parataxic Distortions and Consensual Validation to help construct a model of group psychotherapy that is guided by the principles inherent in interpersonal relationships and interactions.

Leszcz (1992), coming from an interpersonal perspective that is heavily influenced by Yalom, discusses the "critical importance of interpersonal relationships as a window through which the therapist is best able to access the internal world of the patients in the group" (p. 43). Ormont, theoretically grounded in modern analytic concepts, shares similar sentiments. Object relations theory has taught us that introjected self and object representations carry with them intense affect and that these internalized introjections contribute to a person's propensity to project his or her internal world onto the external world (Ogden, 1982). Through the power of projective identification, individuals are likely to coerce, induce, or provoke others in the external world to be unwitting contributors to the individual's internal struggles and expectations. This becomes a life script, a self-fulfilled prophecy, and an unconscious contributor to the repetition compulsion that fuels or drives individuals' interpersonal interactions in such a way that their external world begins to conform or fit to their internal expectations and experiences. In a paradoxical way, a perverse sense of comfort results from the familiarity of the experience, which serves to satisfy the need or drive for consistency in their life.

Ormont suggests that since such an approach to group treatment is likely to result in an overwhelming array of stimuli, it would be impossible for the group leader to try to attend to it all. Instead, Ormont recommends that the group leader pay special attention to two phenomena above all others:

1. How the members express new feelings toward one another.
2. How they evolve their emotional relationships.

To help the group leader best accomplish this task, Ormont has coined a phrase to help clarify a crucial therapeutic strategy that can be utilized by the group leader. The concept is called *bridging*. Ormont describes bridging as "any technique geared to evoke meaningful talk between group members, to develop emotional connections where they did not exist before" (1992, p. 15). Properly used, bridging will enliven the group, decrease detachment, and enhance emotional intimacy between group members. This requires the group leader to keep a persistent focus on the interpersonal transactions in the here and now of the group and to intervene when such transactions are not happening.

Such a position requires the leaders to be very active at times. However, the activity level of the group leader is directly related to whether the group members are relating well and disclosing to each other on an honest, open, and emotional level. If this is happening, the group leader does not interfere and tries to play as little a role as possible. The art and the skill of competent group leadership is to know when to be silent and when to be active. This also requires the group leader to know when the emotional, commutative communication is missing or diminishing. The therapist must be able to use his or her own emotional reading as a tool, a kind of emotional "Geiger counter" that will detect when there is an absence of direct emotional communication and quickly signal the therapist to investigate what might be prohibiting the group members from truly engaging each other.

At these times, the group leader's activity is predominantly directed toward getting people to communicate their immediate thoughts and feelings with each other as quickly as possible. An arena where spontaneity and immediacy are established is more likely to leave the group and its members with a profound sense of authenticity and actual experience that can only come if there is total involvement of each member with the others on an emotional level. Ormont strongly believes that the affect level is the only way you can keep people truly involved and participating in group. Communication through feeling is necessary if any true characterological change is to occur. The power of a group is only unleashed through the freeing of emotions and when a person gets into "the emotional anvil" of the group experience. Ormont is protesting against the tendency of the more classically trained therapists to place too much emphasis on interpretation and intellectual understanding. Much like Fromm-Reichman, he believes, as May previously said, "The patient needs an experience not an explanation" (May, 1983, p. 158).

An example will help clarify this point.

> At the beginning of an ongoing outpatient psychotherapy group that had been meeting once a week for over a year, Betty revealed that she had just learned that her worsening physical condition might require surgery and that her employer was eliminating her job since her deteriorating health prevented her from performing her duties at work. As the rest of the group sat stunned and shocked by the callousness of her employer's decision to terminate her employment, Betty expressed anger at what she called their betrayal, adding "I thought these people I worked with cared about me." After the group leader had given Betty enough time to vent some of her frustration about people not caring, the group leader asked her if she felt people here in the group cared about her right now. Betty responded quickly with a yes, but also added that she felt most apprehensive about Tom, who was one of the least demonstrative and less verbally supportive members of the group. Tom, somewhat taken back by her comment, added that since everyone else had so clearly voiced their concern and outrage at her unfair treatment by her employer, he felt his comments would "just be redundant and of little consequence." A number of the group members, who had previously been on the receiving end of Tom's apparent apathy, turned on him, accusing him of being aloof, callous, and indifferent. After observing the group escalate its attack on Tom for a while, the group leader intervened to prevent Tom from being scapegoated, since it was apparent that Tom had now become the group container for undesirable and disavowed feelings. The group leader, staying with the theme of not caring, asked the group, "Doesn't anyone in the group care that Tom is not being given the freedom to either not express himself or express feelings that are unpopular or different?"

Pete, who had been quiet up to this point, quickly responded to Tom, saying that he did care that Tom be able to talk honestly about his feelings even if it was an unpopular feeling like not caring. With another nudge from the group leader requesting that people own their projections onto Tom, two other group members joined his subgroup admitting that they too had difficulty expressing their feeling of caring because they had come into the group tonight preoccupied with their own conflicts and stress. Free from containing the all bad split and regressive collusion of the group to care for Betty, Tom was able to speak up after a few minutes, protesting to the group that "In fact, I do care a lot for Betty!" He then went on to add that his wife and closest friends were always accusing him of the same thing (being distant and unresponsive). Tom attempted to explain his position further, telling the group that it has always been difficult for him to show or demonstrate his interest in or caring for others because he believed it wouldn't make any difference or be of any consequence if he did. At this point, Andy confronted Tom further, saying "I hear what you're saying, but you look like you just don't give a shit when anybody talks to you!" After Andy spoke, a look of awareness came over Tom's face as he told the group that he just recalled a continual argument he used to have with his mother as a child about his father's lack of caring for him. Tom remembered screaming at his mother, "Dad just doesn't look like he gives a shit when I talk to him!" His mother would always defend his father, telling Tom, "Your father cares even if he doesn't show it." At this point, Andy followed up Tom's statement by telling him, "Can't you see what you're doing. You are becoming just like your father and that's scary because that's my biggest fear, to become like my father."

If group members are allowed to stay detached with statements such as "I wonder" or "I think," they will analyze, comment, and say what they think, but they will not be emotionally involved. Ormont wants to create a sense of community, "a crucible where feelings are exchanged." He stresses that this is far different from an atmosphere where learning, education, and even intellectual insight are given priority. Ormont believes that many individuals do not respond to interpretation and must be approached and influenced through feelings and actions. They must be given an experience, and this experience is most likely to be created if the members in the group are interacting with each other in the immediacy of the moment. As Ormont writes, "Always we want our members to interact, for the sake of group fluidity, and there are times when unless they do, a group will absolutely fall apart" (1992, p. 17).

Cohesion versus Community in Group

Yalom has repeatedly placed special emphasis on the value of cohesion in group psychotherapy. He has included it as an essential component of his twelve identified curative factors and has given it special status by indicating that, while cohesion may not be a curative factor in itself, it is crucial that it be established quickly because without its existence, none of the other eleven curative factors can be properly activated. Parallels have been drawn between the importance of a working alliance in individual therapy and the establishment of cohesion in group therapy (Flores, 1988, Leszcz, 1992). In most cases, treatment will be greatly impeded if proper attention is not directed toward its maintenance. However, cohesion in group is not, as Scheidlinger (1983) suggests, to be confused with adhesion. While it is crucial to establish a therapeutic community, this does not mean that the leader should create a support group atmosphere where emotional consensus is required and only positive feelings toward one another are permitted. Anything that prohibits the group members from the freedom to experience and express some of the more troublesome emotions like aggression, envy, and fear will lead to a one-sided and unrealistic group experience.

Ormont's concept of a therapeutic community shares some similarities with Yalom's views on cohesion. However, Ormont's description of the cohesive unity inherent in his concept allows for a more expansive and better integrated view of cohesion. This is one of his more valuable contributions to the model of group therapy and helps solidify the interpersonal approach to group psychotherapy because it adds the final cornerstone to the three essential elements of Yalom's model:

1. The here and now,
2. Interaction between group members,
3. Cohesion or the establishment of a therapeutic community.

Ormont strongly believes that if group leaders orchestrate the right mixture of emotional involvement and communication between all members of the group, they will harness an important source of therapeutic power and effectiveness. Ormont says that if the right atmosphere is created, "these people will understand themselves better together as a consensual mass than they ever would with interpretation or singular insight" (1992). They will have the potential to put something more together as a unit if they are an integral part of a working community. If the therapeutic community is established correctly and operates as a dynamic, active whole with individuals fully participating on an emotional level, the group members will stick together and learn more from each other than they ever could from a single individual. Uncompromising acceptance, honesty, and commitment will be the result if the therapist keeps everyone involved.

The emphasis on the immediacy of emotional communication is what distinguishes modern group analysis from the earlier methods of classical analysis. The aim of Ormont's approach is to utilize all of the members as players. If the group members are encouraged to talk about their feelings and reactions to one another, Ormont believes they will profit far more than if they talk only about themselves or their problems.

As Ormont writes,

> A successful group moves forward as a whole. If the analyst does include all the members all the time, he will find to his delight that before long, the group members themselves will assist the cohesiveness of the group. They are quick to feel any disturbances in its intactness. They are alert to stragglers, to those who are not contributing, and thus every member becomes part of the organism that is a successful group. (1992, p. 14)

Establishment of Therapeutic Norms

If the group leader is able to keep the group members interacting with each other as a working community and if this interaction includes all members fully participating on an emotional level in the immediacy of the here and now, the group members are more likely to have a better awareness of the benefits that can be derived from their participation in a group that is fully connected and engaged. Yalom, in particular, feels that one of the primary tasks of the group leader is to teach the group and its members what a good group session is like. Teaching them does not mean telling them what to do; it means orchestrating the opportunity for each member to have an authentic, emotional experience in group, one that leaves the members impacted by each other in a way that allows them to learn from the experience the difference between an actual encounter and an abstract explanation. If this can be accomplished, Yalom believes that the group will become self-monitoring. A self-monitoring group is more likely to be autonomous and responsible for itself. One primary method for accomplishing this end is for the group leader to be a source of identification and modeling for the group members. Yalom's description of the leader as a "model-setting participant" outlines the different and sometimes unique skills that are required of a group leader. In a similar fashion, modern analytic descriptions of the therapist as "participant observer" have an obvious influence on Ormont as he suggests that the group leader is sometimes required to present herself or himself as a real object for the group members. The group leader's presence in group at times requires that he or she be more than a detached, uninvolved observer who makes comments on group process.

Yalom's description of the group leader as a model-setting participant raises some very important questions regarding the leader's stance on neutrality and the level of transparency of self. As Dies (1977) and Leszcz (1992) suggest, transparency does not mean that the therapist should be transparent with all of his or her feelings and reactions. Norm Neibergh (1993) reminds us the transparency exists on two levels. It involves the therapist's personal history and his or her availability of self as a real person. The former is hardly ever appropriate, and the latter is sometimes required under certain conditions. Transparency needs to be utilized judiciously and should serve only the interests of the group members and never the group leader's own personal needs or self-aggrandizement. The group leader needs to develop the skill of distinguishing between reactions and feelings evoked by the group and the feelings that he or she brings to the therapeutic setting. Leszcz, writing about the therapeutic use of transparency, says, "It is the therapist's task to find palatable ways of saying unpalatable things in order to help the group move beyond the perimeter of engagement into actual engagement (1992, p. 54).

Ormont has written extensively on the importance of group leaders' ability to utilize their own feelings in helping decode, identify, and evaluate the presently denied group experience. As Ormont says, "The worst therapists are those out of touch with their feelings or in bondage to them to the degree that their feelings dictate their performance" (1992, p. 52). While Ormont stresses that as therapists, we should be able to differentiate between the objective and subjective countertransferences induced in us by our patients, he also emphasizes that it is crucial to remember it is our sensitivity and our own humanity that is our most precious instrument of treatment.

Staying detached from our potentially rich emotional life not only robs us of our most valuable instrument of treatment, it also can create a dangerously false illusion of emotional availability. As Ormont suggests, if the group leader is constantly staying detached emotionally, utilizing interpretations that rely on intellectual awareness, the group members will model themselves after him or her. Ormont is attempting to bridge the gap between the couch and the analyst's chair by emphasizing the impact that therapists, as detached experts, can have on a group or individual. At times, therapists need to make themselves available as "real objects" who actively evoke the potential for a real relationship and personal exchange in the here and now. Ormont cautions that therapists can reinforce patients' detachment by becoming one more person in a chain of important or powerful individuals who have pretended to take an interest or pretended to be emotionally available to them. It is more potentially destructive in such a scenario if patients, too, must pretend that the therapists' interest is real. In truth, both patients and therapists know on some unconscious level that the therapists responses are determined more by the therapists' definition of their role than by the feelings that the patients arouse in them. Laing (1972) has identified this dilemma by cleverly referring to it as "the absence of the therapist presence," or the more destructive experience of "the presence of the therapist's absence."

Successful group psychotherapy requires that the members feel free to try new behaviors and take risks with each other in group. Establishing the right group atmosphere for this to unfold requires the proper orchestration of cohesion, honesty, immediacy, emotional involvement, and interaction between group members. One major avenue for accomplishing this task is to give group members the opportunity to observe the group leader's authenticity and emotional involvement.

Group-as-a-Whole

Any competent, interpersonal-oriented group therapist knows that the dynamics of the group have a tremendous impact on individuals' feelings and behaviors in group. It is impossible not to be affected by the regressive pull and the emotional contamination of the group climate. Developmental stages do dictate the pace of the group and contribute to the members' actions, resistances, defenses, and transference distortions. None of this can be denied or avoided. Even though Yalom and Ormont spend less time addressing these issues in their writings, they do not fail to appreciate their significance. But rather than emphasize and focus on these phenomena, they suggest more emphasis be placed on the real authentic relationships, or the lack of them, that exist in the group. Unlike most group-as-a-whole approaches, their approaches do not focus on this unless group-as-a-whole resistances start to impede or interfere with the interactions between group members.

As any competent group leader knows, group-as-a-whole interventions are helpful when the group becomes stuck or embroiled in Bion's basic assumptions (1961). However, as D. G. Brown (1985) has convincingly argued, basic assumptions can be iatrogenically introduced or encouraged by the presence of an unavailable or passive group leader who inhibits or does not promote genuine human emotional contact. Any environment that recreates a pathological similarity to a dysfunctional family is likely to produce dependency, pairing, or fight-flight group resistances. Any gathering of three or more people that does not permit true intimate contact is likely to induce a basic assumption reaction in this gathering. Any time difficult feelings in a relationship are disavowed or denied expression, the group and its members are likely to regress to a more primitive state of emotional functioning.

Ormont and Yalom advocate a more active involvement on the part of group leaders any time they witness the potential for basic assumptions to develop in group. As Ormont writes, "Instead of being passive and waiting for the members to see what they are doing, as classical analysts often do in individual analysis, we do not simply wait for the resistance to emerge, we bring it to the fore, using group members to help us" (1990, p. 7).

Group-as-a-whole interventions are not ignored, especially when the group has colluded to avoid an emotionally charged subject. Rather, the intervention is applied in a way that still keeps the focus on the interpersonal exchange of the group members. For example:

> In the early moments of a session of an ongoing therapy group that had been meeting for a number of years, Fred, a relatively new group member, began to speak about his mixed feelings toward the group and its different members. He felt close to some and others evoked feelings of hostility and fear. As he continued to direct his very courageous and honest responses to other members in the group, he confessed that establishing and maintaining close, intimate relationships with people was extremely difficult and threatening. Other group members joined him, revealing that they too had mixed feelings about others in the group that resembled their personal conflicts outside of group. Suddenly, in the middle of this important exchange, Steve, one of the more boisterous and aggressive individuals in the group, began to speak of similar difficulties with his ex-girlfriend and "took off" on a five-minute monologue about the inherent difficulties that exist in all relationships. The group leader, using herself as an emotional barometer, noticed that she was becoming more detached and deadened as Steve continued his soliloquy and that the group began to settle back into a more comfortable chatter about relationships rather than continue with their feelings about each other. Seizing the opportunity, while Steve was pausing to make a point, the group leader looked at three of the more de-

tached members in the group and said "I hope you three and the rest of the group appreciates what Steve is doing for the group at this moment. After giving the group a few seconds to ponder what in the world she was talking about, the group leader continued, "He is helping everyone flee from the uncertainty of the emotional exchange that was occurring here in the group and escape to the safety of the events that exist outside of the immediate relationships here in this group right now." Following the statement, the group began once again to deal with the anxiety inherent in their own relationships with each other.

CONCLUSION

Yalom and Ormont share many important differences that have not been elaborated upon in this chapter. The aim was to investigate and emphasize their similarities in the hope of identifying convergent elements in both men's theories that might provide a more complete and cogent rationale for interpersonal group psychotherapy. Yalom has rightfully been given most of the credit for constructing a systematic approach to group therapy that emphasizes a focus on the interactions among group members. Ormont has a great deal of innovative and creative perspectives on this approach to group therapy, even though he would never identity himself as a Sullivanian or an interpersonal theorist and is firmly grounded in modern psychoanalytic theory. It is enriching and exciting when two different theoretical perspectives contribute similar views on the same subject. Ormont's descriptions of the immediacy principle, bridging, and the establishment of a therapeutic community share important complementary perspectives with Yalom's concepts of the here and now, interaction, and cohesion. Both men advocate that the leader take an active role in creating an emotional climate of participation that is much more experiential than cognitive. Both men write eloquently and at times passionately about the importance of creating an authentic experience for their group members.

Critique of Yalom

Before ending this chapter on Yalom's interactional model of group psychotherapy, it is important to remember that there are many other excellent approaches to group therapy that differ from this model. Ormont's modern analytic approach is one that nicely complements Yalom's model while not radically altering his basic premise and recommendations. Later in the book, other alternative perspectives will be presented that give special attention to the later-stage requirements for the successful treatment of the addict and alcoholic. Object-relations theory and self-psychology in particular have a wealth of useful recommendations for treating the characterological features that almost always accompany addiction.

In closing this chapter on Yalom, it is important that his basic model be explored and understood. This is especially true for the novice or beginning group therapist. Whenever I think in terms of Yalom's model and other creative group therapists, I immediately conjure up memories of the great masters: Erv Polster, Bob Goulding, Louis Ormont, Fritz Perlis, Anne Alonso, Scott Rutan, and Yvonne Agazarian. Each is known for going beyond the norm or the accepted to create and develop revolutionary forms of group treatment. Yet, before they became masters in their own right, each was first a student of fundamentals.

This is a rule that certainly applies to all creative forms of art. Picasso, for instance, is well-known for his abstract, cubist art, and his ability to break the fundamental rules in a creative fashion made him immortal. But a walk through the Picasso museum in Spain will reveal that his earlier sketches and paintings emphasized realism. His earlier work clearly demonstrates that Picasso had an acute mastery of traditional art, emphasizing detail, form, composition, contrast, and expression. His work demonstrates the axiom that applies in the case of innovation and creativity. You have to know the rules before you know how to break them. This is the same with group leaders. Before they can break the rules of group, they must know what these rules are. This is why it is so crucial for them to be well-grounded in one model or approach to group treatment. Once this model is established, group leaders are then free to break the rules in a creative fashion. Yalom's model, more than any other model, allows group leaders more freedom, because it teaches sound practical principles for group treatment, especially for the early stages of the type of group work needed for the recovering addict or alcoholic.

Chapter 5

Modifications of Yalom's Interactional Model

As research has rushed to catch up with the huge influx of alcoholics and addicts who began to enter treatment in the 1970s, it soon discovered that treatment strategies that worked for the non-addicted patient would not necessarily work for the addicted individual. Foremost among these strategical inadequacies was the increased use of drugs or medication by primary care physicians for the treatment of mental and behavioral disorders. While modern psychiatry was moving more and more toward defining mental illness as a biochemical disorder requiring pharmacological intervention, addiction treatment was heading in the other direction. Drugs and medication were not the answer; they were the problem! Since modern medicine and pharmacology did not have the answer for addiction, addicted individuals had to turn elsewhere for help and a solution for their disorders. This failure had previously lead to the revolution of the self-help movement and Alcoholics Anonymous in the 1940s. The psychological and medical community has still not completely recovered from this revolution and is trying to discover what role, if any, it has in the treatment of addiction.

The treatment of addiction demanded that the stereotypical medical model and all its inherent inadequacies be discarded, or at least reevaluated in the way it was applied to addicts and alcoholics. Not only were medication or drugs not the answer, individual psychotherapy, as it was practiced by the conventions of that time, was judged to be inadequate at best and destructive at worst. It was inevitable that group therapy should join forces with addiction treatment, for a number of reasons. Foremost among these was the parallel evolution of addiction as a recognizable and identifiable disorder with its own set of symptoms and dynamics and the legitimation of group therapy as an independent method of treatment with its own theory and rationale for its application. Just as addiction was demanding alternative methods of treatment, group psychotherapy was beginning to be recognized as a viable alternative for the treatment of mental and behavioral disorders. Even though group therapy gradually became the identified treatment of choice for addiction, the model upon which it was originally based was, for the most part, derived from the practice of outpatient psychotherapy with non-addicted patients. It was eventually discovered that the theoretical and practical considerations underlying outpatient group therapy with a non-addicted population were not always applicable to individuals suffering from chemical dependency. Eventually, the accepted principles of group therapy were gradually altered to meet the realities of treating the addicted patient.

It was reasoned that if group therapy was to be an effective tool in the treatment of addiction, it had to be linked as clearly as possible to a comprehensive theory of addiction and a practical concept for its cure or arrestment. This is where some of the research findings and the clinical recommendations of those who worked with addicted individuals on a regular basis began to shape the direction of treatment and group psychotherapy.

In the early 1970s, addiction treatment began to be a focus of outcome research. In an extensive review of 384 alcoholism treatment studies, Emerick (1974) concluded that while treatment of some kind is superior to no treatment, differences in professionally applied treatment methods did not significantly affect long-term outcome. His findings were corroborated by Stinson et al. (1979), who reported that "peer-oriented care" (Alcoholics Anonymous) or abstinence based and twelve-step-oriented treatment approaches were more successful in improving recovery than professionally oriented treatment approaches. These results were consistent with Strupp and Hadley's (1979) findings, which suggested that nonspecific factors in psychotherapy (e.g., therapist characteristics) may be more important than specific factors (e.g., techniques) in determining successful treatment outcome.

These research findings take on added ramifications when one considers the high degree of success that a peer-oriented self-help approach such as Alcoholics Anonymous (AA) has demonstrated in alcoholism treatment (Emrick, Lassen, and Edwards, 1977). This raises the question of what part, if any, professionally oriented systems have in alcoholism treatment when considering the fact that peer-oriented programs such as AA provide a simpler, more successful, and less expensive form of alcoholism treatment (Stinson et al., 1979).

Considering the implication resulting from these research findings, it became obvious that it would be beneficial to examine more closely the possible symbiotic relationship between professionally and peer-oriented treatment systems for addiction treatment. Wallace (1978b), Brown and Yalom (1977), and Cummings (1979) all had suggested that a close working relationship between the two would improve success in treatment. Add to this speculation the large number of alcoholics who had not responded well to the peer-oriented system of AA (Emrick, Lassen, and Edwards, 1977) and addiction treatment specialists began to see the possibility that each approach has something to offer and could complement the other as far as successful treatment outcome was concerned.

Smart, Schmidt, and Moss (1969) had recognized earlier that group therapy was considered to be "dogma" in the treatment of alcoholism, although there was a lack of adequately based clinical investigations regarding its effectiveness. They went on to conclude that at least in the United States, group therapy on the whole has been preponderantly employed for patients of the upper-middle class and seldom for those of the lower-middle class. Consequently, it was recommended that the currently accepted principles of group therapy needed to be altered to meet the realities and necessities of treating the addicted patient.

Too often, therapists with experience only in individual therapy or experience only with non-addicted patients were thrust into a group psychotherapy leadership role. Because group psychotherapy is difficult and requires a number of special skills, many groups led by untrained or poorly trained leaders did not fulfill their potential or may have had negative effects on patient recovery. It was obvious that a need existed for educating potential group therapists who were and would be leading groups composed of chemically dependent individuals.

TREATMENT CONSIDERATIONS AND GROUP THERAPY

Within the last few years there has been an increasing body of research and clinical experience that suggests specific ways group psychotherapy must be adapted to fit the specific needs of the addicted patient. Generally, there has been a growing consensus among those who regularly work with addicted patients in a group therapy format. Khantzian, Halliday, and McAuliffe (1990), Vannicelli (1988a), S. Brown (1985), Matano and Yalom (1991), and the author of this book (Flores, 1988) have provided extensive suggestions about the ways that proven group therapy strategies can be adapted and modified to address the unique problems and characteristics of the addicted patient. All agree that abstinence is a crucial, if not the most important element, in the substance abuser's recovery. All are supportive of chemically dependent patients' involvement in twelve-step programs while the patients are participating in group therapy. All of these authors operate from a group therapy perspective that usually includes an interpersonal approach to group psychotherapy that relies heavily on Irvin Yalom's (1975) theoretical model of interactional group therapy. In addition to Yalom's theory, most of them have also adopted many of the principles of psychodynamic group therapy with some modifications in technique that take into special consideration chemically dependent individuals' propensity to return to chemical use if their anxiety, shame, anger, and guilt is not modulated carefully. This is especially true during the early phase of treatment. The concept of optimal frustration is a necessary component of the group therapy experience and because of the importance of this concept in patients' treatment, it will be explored in more detail later in the book (Chapter 6).

While there are many unique features of addiction that the group leader has to be cognizant of when conducting a therapy group composed entirely of addicted patients, it is important the group leader be aware of the common curative forces that are available in any well-conducted therapy. Some of the following curative forces are especially important in the treatment of addiction:

1. Positive peer support and pressure for abstinence from alcohol and drugs.
2. Mutual identification and the opportunity for individuals to learn they are not alone or unique as they struggle with their compulsive obsession with chemicals.
3. The opportunity to better understand their own attitudes and denial of addiction by confronting similar attitudes and defenses in other alcoholics and addicts.
4. Experimental learning and exchange of factual information which conveys that abstinence is always accorded priority, enhancing the patients' acceptance of their identification as alcoholics or addicts.
5. Identification, cohesiveness, hope, and support are provided in a setting that is also structured and disciplined with clearly defined limits and with appropriate consequences that help substance abusers make the proper distinction between what they are responsible for and not responsible for.
6. Chemically dependent individuals are granted the opportunity to become more aware of how their interpersonal characterological style interferes with their ability to establish gratifying, healthy, and intimate relationships with others.

This last issue is especially crucial since it is rare to find substance abusers who do not have either a character disorder or enough character pathology to cause them consistent difficulties in their interpersonal relationships. Difficulties forming and maintaining healthy interpersonal relationships is especially important because the inability to establish healthy relationships is a major contributing factor to relapse and the return to chemical use. As Khantzian, Halliday, and McAuliffe (1990) write, "While it is the drug-taking that initially brings the person to treatment, it is the treatment of character that leads not only to giving up drugs but also to profound change in one's experience of self and the world. . . . Ultimately we view the treatment of character disorder as the road to recovery from addiction" (p. 3).

Prolonged experience treating substance abusers suggests that their inability to form mutually satisfying and emotionally intimate relationships with others leaves them forever with an internal vulnerability that repeatedly leads them to seek external sources of stimulation or gratification (i.e., alcohol, drugs, sex, food, gambling, pornography, work, etc.). Consequently, they are prone to substitute one addiction for another. Because of their character pathology, the relationships they do form are likely to be as destructive, obsessive, and addictive as the substances they were abusing.

As is frequently reported in AA, "Alcoholics don't have relationships, they take hostages." Because most substance abusers have extreme difficulty regulating their emotions and impulses, they require a substantial amount of support, gratification, and structure early in their treatment before they have enough ego strength to work through the character defects and structural defensives. Managing the intensity of their emotions (in order to prevent a relapse) while compelling them to look at and come to understand their self-destructive interpersonal styles is a delicate task that the group leader must achieve if substance abusers are to make the internal changes necessary to ensure both abstinence and healthy functioning.

Because of the many confounding and conflicting influences that the group leader must manage when leading a group composed of chemically dependent individuals, it is important that the group leader be well versed in the language and philosophy of AA and its associated twelve-step programs. Matano and Yalom (1991) strongly recommend that the therapist become thoroughly familiar with Alcoholics Anonymous language, steps and traditions for numerous reasons, one of them being the addict's or alcoholics's propensity to use AA as therapy resistance either because of deliberate avoidance or misperceptions about the program. As Matano and Yalom suggest, "It is important that therapists not permit misconceptions of AA to be used as therapy resistance and that they be able to harness the wisdom of AA for psychotherapeutic ends" (p. 269).

Many excellent therapists have been frustrated by AA's distorted view of them as "ignorant professionals" who have failed to help AA and its members in the past. Matano and Yalom outline some ways of establishing credibility while integrating AA philosophy into an interactive format. There are other excellent descriptions and interpretations of AA that will permit the group leader to gain a better understanding of AA from a more scientific, analytic, and psychological perspective (i.e., Flores, 1988a; Kurtz, 1982; Thune, 1977). Certainly, it would behoove the group leader who wishes to work with this population on a sustained basis to learn what AA has to offer professionals for better understanding and treating the chemically dependent individual.

EARLY AND LATER STAGE TREATMENT

To effectively manage the proper care and treatment of addicted patients in group, it is important to approach their treatment in two distinct stages. John Wallace (1978b) has previously described treatment of the alcoholic as a "time-dependent" process. Essentially, this means that a particular therapeutic intervention for a recently recovering substance abuser or alcoholic will be far different for someone who has managed to achieve several months or years of abstinence and sobriety. The way that the chemically dependent person is therapeutically approached in group will be determined by a number of factors. The patient's ego strength, character pathology, motivation, denial, and length of abstinence from chemicals are the most crucial elements that must be weighed carefully. However, the length of time since the substance abuser's last use of chemicals is easily the most important for a variety of reasons. Foremost among these is physiological evidence gathered from CAT scans, neuropsychological assessments, and other neurophysiological examinations, which reveal that most substance abusers are cognitively and psychologically impaired during their first few months of abstinence and are incapable of responding to anything but the rudimentary components of psychotherapy (Flores, 1988b). Another vastly important issue is the substance abusers' initial refusal to view their use of chemicals as a primary contributing cause to their behavioral and emotional difficulties. Complicating their destructive defensive process is their propensity to return to chemical use if their anxiety or depression is raised to unmanageable levels too quickly. The most difficult task in the early stages of therapy with substance abusers is counteracting their denial while encouraging self-disclosure and self-awareness and simultaneously keeping their anxiety at a tolerable level. However, a gradual shift from support, encouragement, and gentle confrontation to a position that eventually compels them to take a cold hard look at their character pathology and painful emotional past is necessary if true characterological and emotional change is to occur. Consequently, the group leader needs to know how to balance and manage this shift while addressing the different treatment strategies required for the early stage and later stage recovering substance abuser.

A case illustration may help explain the significant changes that can occur quickly if an alcoholic is accurately diagnosed and treated.

> Alice was a thirty-five-year-old Caucasian female who had been in outpatient treatment at a community mental health center for over five years. She had "worn out" six different therapists because of her violent outbursts and demanding, provocative behavior. She was diagnosed as a Borderline Personality Disorder, and none of the outpatient staff wanted to carry her on their caseload, so they referred her to an outpatient group at the clinic in the hope that this would help. As Alice attended her weekly group sessions, it became clear that her explosive tirades in group and difficulties outside of group usually followed severe or prolonged drinking episodes. Six months into treatment, the group leaders, who had a thorough background in addictions, began to point out these patterns in her behavior. Initially she rejected these comments, but eventually she started to respond more favorably after the other group members began to share similar observations. Unable to deny the consensual observation of the group, Alice succumbed to the opinion that she should stop drinking and seek treatment for her alcoholism. After completing a thirty-day outpatient treatment program, she returned to the group and continued to attend meetings at Alcoholics Anonymous. The change in her behavior in group was dramatic. She was able to tolerate other members' disagreement and proved receptive to feedback from others for the first time. Where previously she had reacted to disagreements by vehemently attacking others, she now was able to see alternative viewpoints. Her behavior change was so apparent that staff members who had treated her earlier began to make appreciatory comments about the potent effectiveness of her treatment in group. Little did they realize that her abstinence from alcohol and her involvement in AA allowed her to respond favorably to therapeutic intervention. In actuality, it was the proper diagnosis of her condition that led to the primary condition (alcoholism) being treated appropriately. Instead of committing the frequent error of

futilely trying to combat the affective storms produced by her addiction, the group leader required that she stop drinking and used the group to reinforce this requirement.

RECOMMENDATION FOR GROUP PSYCHOTHERAPY

Any use of group psychotherapy as a treatment regimen needs to be linked as clearly as possible to theory, both about group treatment and addiction. In treating alcoholics and addicts, a model of group treatment based on Yalom's (1975, 1985, 1995) interactional approach is recommended. Modifications in technique that will allow for the incorporation of modern analytic and self-psychology perspectives will also be necessary, especially in later stage treatment requirements. The application of technique should follow as closely as possible the guidelines laid down by Brown and Yalom's (1977) initial recommendations and later updated by Matano and Yalom (1991). Later stage recommendations by Khantzian, Halliday, and McAuliffe (1990) and Flores and Mahon (1993) should be employed once abstinence is achieved. A more thorough description of these later stage recommendations will follow in Chapter 11.

For now, the particular strategies and recommended protocol will be described. Consideration will be given to treatment as a time-dependent process as described by Wallace (1978b) and expanded by S. Brown (1985) in her description of recovery as a developmental process or model. Further consideration will be given to the tactics outlined by Cummings (1979) in his description of exclusion therapy and numerous other clinicians (i.e., Matano and Yalom, 1991) and researchers (i.e., S. Brown, 1985) who strongly recommend that abstinence be the primary goal of treatment. This interactional group model should be contrasted with a group established and run according to the guidelines of Alcoholics Anonymous and described both by Emrick, Lassen, and Edwards (1977) and Alibrandi (1978).

PROTOCOL

A brief description of the protocol for the group psychotherapy treatment strategy will be presented below.

The early stages of therapy should be patterned after Cummings' description of "exclusion therapy" (1979). Essentially this approach requires that the issue of drug usage be approached first and the client excluded from therapy unless he/she agrees to the goals of abstinence. Alcohol addiction should therefore be the primary focus during the early stages of treatment.

During the first two months of treatment, much of the group's time would be spent on the education of the disease concept of alcoholism and the development of what Yalom describes as group cohesiveness (1985). The group at this point would provide support and structure as Wallace recommends (1978b). Gradually the shift should be initiated to move the group from a support model to an interactional model as described by Yalom (1974). During this time, directive and active leadership required at this early stage (Wallace, 1975) should shift to allow the group members to take a more active and responsible role in the group process.

In most cases, the entire first six months of treatment would be spent on "just" maintaining sobriety with little or no active encouragement of personality modification (Wallace, 1978b). As Brown and Yalom (1977) suggest, group members during this period will not be encouraged to take a look at themselves beyond a rather shallow and superficial level. In one sense, the strategy requires that all therapeutic interventions occur at a slower pace (Brown and Yalom, 1977; Wallace, 1977b). Dynamics will not be explored in great detail until nine to twelve months of sobriety have been established (Brown and Yalom, 1977).

Much of the time throughout treatment should be spent on confronting the alcoholics' denial system (Wallace, 1975; Cummings, 1979). A heavy focus should be directed toward getting alcoholics to make a gradual recognition of their buried feelings. Usually, feelings of extreme guilt would be best dealt with by providing an overall simplistic cognitive structure of their illness (Wallace, 1975). The strategies that Wallace (1978) describes should be utilized to deal with alcoholics' "preferred defense structure."

Alcoholism treatment within this perspective should be viewed as a "time-dependent" process as described by Wallace (1975) and corroborated by Brown and Yalom (1977). Essentially this means that a particular therapeutic intervention for a recently drinking alcoholic may be entirely inappropriate for one who has managed to achieve several years of sobriety.

Wallace's recommendations for a therapy specific to alcoholism are as follows:

1. Alcoholics can be described in terms of preferred defense structure. This preferred defense structure (PDS) need not be cast in negative terms. In fact, it need not be construed at all in terms of the classical language of defense mechanisms. The alcoholic's PDS can be thought

of as a collection of skills or abilities–tactics and strategies, if you will–for achieving one's ends.

2. Therapy with alcoholics as it is currently practiced too often attempts to remove the alcoholic's PDS instead of utilizing it effectively to facilitate the achievement of abstinence. Therapeutic efforts that confront the alcoholic's PDS prematurely and too heavily will increase rather than reduce the probability of further drinking.
3. Recovery programs successful in producing abstinence, such as Alcoholics Anonymous, partially owe their success to the intuitive recognition of the fact that the alcoholic's PDS is to be protected and capitalized upon rather than confronted and radically altered.
4. Paradoxically, the very same defenses that the alcoholic used to maintain his or her drinking can be used effectively to achieve abstinence.
5. Equally paradoxically, the very same defenses that enabled the alcoholic to drink, as well as achieve abstinence, must ultimately be removed if long-term sobriety is to be maintained. However, in many cases such growth must take place over periods of time ranging from two to five years of abstinence. (1978b)

CORE TREATMENT PROGRAM

It is important to follow Pattison's (1979) recommendations and determine the population characteristics of the alcoholics to be treated if these difficulties are to be minimized. Moore (1973, p. 224) describes the typical alcoholic as an

> employed, or at least partially financially solvent patient, lower-middle-class and up, not necessarily very psychologically minded, not grossly psychopathic, but more likely an "essential" or "reactive" alcoholic. He or she may show considerable depression, is not significantly brain damaged, is more or less voluntary, probably still has or has just been separated from a family treatment, is covered by private funds or health insurance or is provided in a public clinic. In other words, I am talking about the bulk of our alcoholic population. While the public inebriate may attract a large part of our attention, he constitutes only an estimated three to five percent of the alcoholic population.

Next, it would be important to determine if there are any personality characteristics shared by the population described. Attempts at identifying personality variables consistently related to alcoholism have historically resulted in ambiguous and contradictory findings. Much evidence indicates that there are various personality types among alcoholics (Pattison, 1966; English, 1975). In spite of negative conclusions reached in their reviews, researchers have generally not concluded that the search for an alcoholic personality should be abandoned (Barnes, 1979). Wallace (1975) points out that the strength of a belief in something called an alcoholic personality is a direct function of the degree of involvement with alcoholics on a sustained basis. He defends his argument on the basis of AA intuitive knowledge derived from years of successful treatment of alcoholism. Thus, in the fellowship of AA, persons are said to be alcoholic in personality whether they are drinking or not, and the alcoholic personality can return at any time in the form of a "dry drunk." Furthermore AA recognizes the fact that many heavy drinkers are not necessarily alcoholic (Alcoholics Anonymous, 1960). On the other hand, Wallace feels that the concept of the alcoholic personality has not fared well among those whose acquaintance with alcoholics is merely passing or entirely academic.

Evidence suggesting shared post-alcoholic characteristics have significant implications for treatment. In an extensive review of the literature, Barnes (1979) suggests that it may be useful to break the concept of the alcoholic personality into two different descriptions–a post-alcoholic personality and a pre-alcoholic personality. There is a vast amount of evidence as presented by Barnes to suggest that there are a number of different personality measurements that can readily differentiate post-alcoholics from neurotics, psychotics, and non-alcoholics–MMPI, Field-Dependence, Internal-External, and the Eysenck Personality Inventory. While post-alcoholic personality measures are generally conclusive, those on pre-alcoholic identification have been found on only one longitudinal study conducted with the MacAndrew scale of the MMPI (Hoffman, Loper, and Kammeier, 1974). This pattern of findings suggests that the process of alcoholism itself may produce some changes that are common to all alcoholics. What is noteworthy for our purpose is the awareness of significant homogeneity among post-alcoholic personalities. Wallace (1975) agrees when he says, "It is more fruitful to think of the many commonalities apparent among alcoholics as common outcomes of alcoholism rather than as antecedent conditions." Furthermore, this seems to indicate strongly that alcoholics may be a rather homogenous group as a result of their disease.

THE ADDICTIVE PERSONALITY

While misconceptions about the addictive personality are legion, recent evidence suggests that the experience of addiction itself may induce characteristics common to most addictive individuals. While most of the research on addiction has been focused on alcoholism, it is recognized that many alcoholics have a history of cross-addiction and poly-drug abuse. Consequently, for purposes of brevity, the reader is asked to equate the two. A review of the literature suggests that there is little evidence for a pre-alcoholic personality; however, there is strong evidence for shared, post-alcoholic characteristics that have significant implications for treatment.

Much of the research on this topic revealed a consistent difficulty with dependency conflicts, and most studies painted a picture of a typical clinical psychopath or sociopath. However, there was one important distinction that was frequently overlooked and was illustrated by Button (1956), who stated, "The primary peak on the Pd scale and the secondary peak at D, superimposed upon a relatively 'neurotic' (as opposed to psychotic) profile almost in themselves tell the story of how the alcoholic sees himself; as an unhappy, tense, bitter person who somehow feels responsible for the many evidences of aggression and hostility he sees about him" (p. 271). Button goes on to quote Buhler and Lefever (1956) in pointing out a very important distinction. "Differing from the psychopath, the alcoholic escapes with a bad conscience." This position is also supported by Apfeldorf (1978), who suggested that the high scorer on the MacAndrew MMPI subscale is "bold, uninhibited, self-confident, and mixes well with others." Apfeldorf tells of carousing, gambling, playing hooky, and generally cutting up, yet the alcoholic or addict "is drawn to religion and uses repression, faith and inspiration to hold his impulses in check." This analysis suggests that the addictive personality is composed of many factors or components, including a lively or ready sociability, antisocial attitudes, religiosity, and guilt. Apfeldof felt it might be fruitful to attempt to accumulate an expanded item pool to explore MacAndrew's study and other profile composites of the MMPI because the picture painted by this content analysis has a striking similarity to issues of importance to AA. Superficially, self-centeredness, poor impulse control, and guilt are all of central importance to the AA treatment approach (Alcoholics Anonymous, 1955).

Constructing a consensus of a personality profile based on the aforementioned studies with the MMPI, we are left with the picture of an alcoholic as someone who is self-centered, immature, gregarious, frequently charming in a superficial manner, and expressing all the behavior typically associated with the narcissistic personality save for the tremendous guilt and shame that surface during his or her sober moments.

Most of the recent studies in the area of personality assessments related to alcoholism have focused on the isolated measure and differentiation between alcoholics and non-alcoholics (Tarter and Sugerman, 1976; Donovan and O'Leary, 1975). In accounting for the consistent findings that alcoholics are more dependent or external than other groups, research generally supports the predisposition rather than the consequence hypothesis. Essentially, the latter hypothesis views field-dependence and externality as consequences of drinking while the former hypothesis suggests that field dependence and externality are predisposing factors. Little research has been conducted to determine if there has been any suggestion of change over time. Researchers have generally been satisfied with accepting the conclusion that alcoholics may stop drinking but their cognitive functioning and basic personality will undoubtedly stay the same.

An initial study by Dahany (1977) suggests that this may not be the case. If Alcoholics Anonymous's criteria for recovery is accepted, that is, if alcoholics must make some change in themselves before they can stop drinking, the expected corollary would suggest that alcohol consumption ceases and some personality or cognitive change occurs. One plausible explanation for the growing interest due to these research findings is the strong evidence that exists for a relationship between control, dependency, and addiction. Dependency conflicts and cognitive styles could lead to, or be a result of, an exaggerated need to be in control as a consequence of conflicts in dependency needs. A corollary to this theory suggests that a change in alcohol consumption should result in changes on measures of dependency and control orientations (Danahy, 1977).

As a result of such plausible interpretations, a number of different measures for this general theoretical framework have been utilized in a wide range of empirical research. Most of the research has looked at the relationship of dependency and control to addiction. Utilizing the research of Witkin (Witkin and Oltmen, 1967) with field dependency and Rotter (1966) with Internal-External (I-E) locus of control, there has been conflicting evidence in the similarities and differences in alcoholics and addicts.

Although there has been some confusion in determining whether alcoholics are externally or internally oriented, there have been several possible explanations advanced to explain the unexpected discovery of an internal orientation among alcoholics. Goss and Morosko (1970) suggested two possible implications regarding the problem of alcoholism. One is that alcoholics believe that they can control their drinking, and the other is that they may also have learned that they have a readily available method for controlling their moods as well.

Oziel, Obitz, and Kerpon (1972) suggest that the passive-aggressive drinking and social behavior seen among alcoholics is the reaction of internally controlled individuals to resist manipulation by others who want them to stop drinking. Disterfano, Pryer, and Garrison (1972) question the common assumption that internal control is necessarily a good thing. They suggest that perhaps a "happy medium" between the low scores of alcoholics and the high scores of the general psychiatric population might be a better indication of psychological health. In view of the IE findings, Gozali and Sloan (1971) suggest that perhaps psychotherapy for alcoholics should be oriented more toward shifting control orientation from internal to external. This is what AA has always tried to do. The AA program stresses the admission of "powerlessness over alcohol" and giving up control to a "higher power." While this program cannot, of course, be said to have been proven right by the findings from the IE scale, it is possible that AA emphasizes a feature of the alcoholic personality that has therapeutic significance.

VALUES AND DEPENDENCE IN ALCOHOLISM TREATMENT

Addictive behavior and difficulties in interpersonal relations (Szasz, 1966) can be assumed to leave traces in an individual's value system. If therapy is to be successful, it may surely be manifested as changes or rearrangements of value priorities. Rokeach (1973) presents convincing evidence that values do exist as stable entities, can be easily assessed, are paramount in influencing a person's attitudes and behavior, and can be easily changed by effective psychotherapy.

Research has suggested the possibility that religious or spiritual elements of treatment, such as the "Higher Power" concept of Alcoholics Anonymous, may augment the recovery process. Jacobson and Ritter (1977) administered the Purpose in Life (PIL) test and the Allport-Vernon-Lindsey Study of Values (SOV) to a group of alcoholics in a thirty-day treatment program. They reported a significant change in scores when administered soon after admission and repeated again before discharge. They reported that contrary to expectation, significant correlations were found between scores from the second PIL Test and the Religious and Aesthetic scales of the SOV.

TREATMENT ISSUES

Homogeneity vs Heterogeneity

The research, then, suggests that alcoholics and addicts may be a rather homogeneous group as a result of their diseases. As Yalom points out, the likelihood of homogeneity within the group can be a detriment to the growth process. Heterogeneity for conflict areas and homogeneity for ego strength are two factors important for group composition (Yalom, 1975). Yalom feels that "homogeneous groups jell more quickly to become more cohesive, to offer more immediate support to the group members, to have better attendance, less conflict, and to provide more rapid symptomatic relief" (p. 261). This is often the situation that the therapist will find with an alcoholism recovery group. It would be wise to encourage the group to rally around the homogeneous problem of alcoholism at the beginning of therapy and use this shared concern to its greatest advantage. The group often consists of patients from different occupations and interests who at first share only their common conflict with alcohol consumption. Later, as abstinence becomes less and growth more of an issue, the therapist will often find that the group has a very diverse set of problems resulting from drinking. The therapist should also utilize *this* advantage to its fullest.

Passivity and Field Dependence

The work of Witkin, Karp, and Goodenough (1959), Rotter (1966), and Blane (1968) all points to the general consensus of alcoholics being more cognitively and psychologically dependent than non-alcoholics. This was also borne out in Brown and Yalom's experience (1977). They found that dependency or counterdependency was expressed behaviorally but that the alcoholic would emphatically deny all dependency. This observation is especially interesting in light of Donovan and O'Leary's (1975) research on Rotter's internal-external differentiation in alcoholics. Their results showed that alcoholics were either more external or internal than non-alcoholics.

Research applying Witkin and Oltman's (1967) field dependency/field independency theory has shown rather conclusively that alcoholics are more field dependent that non-alcoholics (Tarter and Sugerman, 1976). Brown and Yalom (1977) discovered similar patterns in their study. They interpreted this phenomenon as occurring because alcoholics were incapable of fully experiencing themselves from within. Many of their group members based their behaviors on external clues. "For example, they scan their environment, looking to others for direction, trying to determine what others expect. Through self-deception they convert these outside signals into a sense that they have actively made a choice. Yet, much of their behavior is not choiceful. They cannot turn their gaze inward to ask themselves what they want and then act accordingly" (p. 488).

Fehr (1976) considers these styles of alcoholics to manifest in passive-dependent behavior. Schiff and Schiff (1971) discuss the difficulties involved in treating patients with significant passive behaviors. The major treatment hurdle is the frequency with which passive patients discount and deny their problems. Typically, when they do recognize the existence of a problem, they will fail to see its significance in their lives. Even if they do recognize its significance, passive-dependent patients will often compound their situations by denying the solvability of their difficulties, leaving little hope for anything better in their lives.

According to Fehr (1976), alcoholics will rarely be able to recognize their real reasons for drinking, and even more often they will not view the excessive alcohol consumption as the significant problem in their lives. Rather than viewing alcoholics as people who do not want to stop drinking, it is better to conceptualize them as people who do not realize the possibility of alternate lifestyles. In contrast, neurotic patients frequently have identified their major difficulties before they even enter group therapy. Usually they are self-referrals interested in making some change in their behavior. As Fehr points out, the therapist in this situation is more of a consultant, whose job it is to listen and guide the client. The therapist usually attempts to limit his or her input and is likely to err in the direction of too much intervention. This is in contrast to work with the alcoholic, where the therapeutic error is more likely to be in the direction of too little intervention. The more directive and active the therapist, the more effective he or she is (Fehr, 1976; Johnson, 1973; Wallace, 1975).

Alcoholics in group therapy tend to support each other's passivity (Fehr, 1976). The group rallies around the subject of alcoholism and its causes and cures, endlessly debating the merits of Alcoholics Anonymous and covering many issues extraneous to the task at hand. Group members are notorious for their tendency to focus on themselves and each other as alcoholics rather than persons, thereby limiting the amount of genuine interaction among themselves. As such, there is relatively little in the early exchanges between group members that can be considered therapeutically productive (Fehr, 1976). It is important to realize that conventional group psychotherapy procedures, with their emphasis on the interaction between group members, should not be employed during the early phases of treatment because of their relative ineffectiveness with passive, dependent alcoholics. However, such group procedures should be introduced into the treatment plan as the members mature in their ability to function within the group.

Time Factors

The intelligent treatment of the recovering alcoholic must be viewed in terms of a long time-span. A particular therapeutic intervention for a neurotic may be entirely inappropriate for a recently drinking alcoholic and even for one who has managed to achieve several years of sobriety. Yalom asserts that even most non-alcoholic patients require approximately twelve to twenty-four months to undergo substantial change, although it is possible to resolve a crisis in a briefer period of time. It is best to interpret the immediate problem of alcoholic drinking as a crisis that must be dealt with first. AA and most alcoholism-directed therapeutic systems recognize that the first year of treatment is crisis-oriented and that it is not wise to push change too early in the recovery process (Alcoholics Anonymous, 1960; Chalmers and Wallace, 1978; Johnson, 1973).

The therapist may find that in some cases the entire first year of treatment may be spent on "just" maintaining sobriety, with little or no active encouragement of personality modification. Brown and Yalom (1977) address the importance of the time perspective in alcoholism treatment: "The therapist's patience and hope provide reassurance to patients who have frustrated and been abandoned by many would-be helpers. Continuing, unwavering commitment is required of the therapist; it is not the best setting for therapists who need immediate gratification of their needs to be healers" (p. 437).

In one sense, the therapist must recognize that in dealing with the alcoholic client, all therapeutic interventions occur at a slower pace. The therapist must move cautiously, realizing, on one hand, that conflict and anxiety are necessary for change, but on the other hand, that too much anxiety and conflict will frequently push alcoholics to cope with their situation by drinking. Yalom recognizes that, although alcoholics often desire change, they realize that they have so much to lose if they resume drinking that they will often resist engaging in the therapy process.

Structure

Another factor influencing this general reluctance to change has been described by Brown and Yalom (1977) as the rigid defense system of the typical alcoholic. "Members could recognize in one another the tendency to assume rigid positions which they labeled as black and white or all or nothing viewpoints." It is often the case that the alcoholic will exhibit a strong preference for certainty. Judgments of people, events, and situations are often extreme. Wallace (1975) agrees: "Perceived alternatives are few, consisting largely of yes-no, black-white, dichotomized categories. It is in this sense that the thinking is said to be all or nothing in character" (p. 23).

Because of this, Wallace feels that alcoholics prefer large amounts of structure and prefer that events proceed in a predictable and structured manner. Meetings of AA, for example, are among the most structured of social encounters. As Wallace (1978a) illustrated, a meeting in Southern California begins with a reading of Chapter 5 of the book, *Alcoholics Anonymous*. "Hence, for example, an alcoholic from Anaheim, sober for

10 years, attending three meetings of AA a week, has heard the same thing read 1560 times!" (p. 23, 1939). Brown and Yalom (1977) likewise suggest that it is important for the therapist to provide a support system on which patients can rely. "Thus, it was vitally important that members be assured that the group was ongoing and would always meet at the appointed time" (p. 442). This simple factor underscores the importance of the long-term therapy experience. Shorter group experiences, Yalom feels, cannot provide the necessary stable, continuous community needed for recovery.

The Denial System

Alcoholics can be best described in terms of their preferred defense structure, which includes the predominantly used mechanisms of denial, rationalization, projection, intellectualization, and minimization, (Wallace, 1975). Typically, this results in a group consisting mostly of alcoholics who have no idea what they are feeling and subsequently are operating from a distorted view of what is really happening to them. In accounting for alcoholics' apparent lack of understanding of the relationship between their drinking and their troubles, professionals conclude that alcoholics are using denial. Alcoholism is considered by many to constitute "a disease of denial" (Alcoholics Anonymous, 1939; Tiebout, 1953; Wallace, 1975). Rather than become angered with alcoholics' blatant refusal to acknowledge what they are feeling, the therapist must recognize that this is the very problem that must be reconciled slowly with supportive and patient understanding.

The most difficult task in alcoholism therapy is to lessen denial and encourage self-awareness and disclosure, while simultaneously keeping anxiety at a minimum. This means that the therapist must be content with a gradually deepening self-awareness rather than demanding sudden, dramatic breakthroughs. As Yalom (1975) clearly illustrates, "pipedreams" or "vital lies" are often essential to personal and social integrity (p. 216). He warns that they should not be taken lightly or impulsively stripped away in the service of honesty. Above honesty, the therapist has a responsibility to his patients and their tasks, which clearly should override any tendency to utilize techniques or confront for confrontation's sake. Moreover, the therapist must ensure a therapeutic context in which high levels of support are available as the client uncovers aspects of self and discloses these to others. Alcoholism therapy is best described as consisting of important choices and decisions in light of too much blame or too little responsibility, too much guilt or too much sociopathology, too much anger or too much compliance, too much denial or too much self-disclosure (Wallace, 1975).

Psychotherapy within this context differs from conventional treatment in that the therapist must constantly weigh each intervention, since too rapid or too much confrontation may result in alcoholic behavior. This situation must be tempered with gentle probing and the realization that, if changes do not occur, alcoholic behavior cannot be far behind. This theme will permeate the entire treatment process but ideally should become less of a concern the longer sobriety is maintained.

Therapy with alcoholics, as it is currently practiced, too often attempts to remove the alcoholic's preferred defense system instead of utilizing it to facilitate the achievement of abstinence. Therapeutic efforts that confront the alcoholic's preferred defense system prematurely will increase rather then decrease the probability of further drinking. Paradoxically, the same defenses that the alcoholic uses to maintain his or her drinking can be used effectively to achieve abstinence (Wallace, 1975). Equally paradoxically, the very same defenses that enable the alcoholic to drink and to achieve abstinence must ultimately be removed if long-term sobriety is to be maintained. However, in many cases, such growth takes place over periods of time ranging from two to five years of abstinence (Alcoholics Anonymous, 1955; Wallace, 1975).

ALCOHOLICS ANONYMOUS AND GROUP PSYCHOTHERAPY

Is a dual affiliation in both AA and group psychotherapy possible? Recent strategies have been developed addressing this issue. The leading theorists in the field all suggest alternatives, based on years of clinical experience, that enhance treatment success (Brown and Yalom, 1977; Cummings, 1979; Wallace, 1975, 1978b). Cummings (1979), for instance, in his description of "exclusion therapy," outlines tactics compatible with AA that require abstinence as the primary goal of treatment.

Alcoholics need enormous support to attain and maintain abstinence. Brown and Yalom (1977) were concerned that an interactional group (in which conflict as well as acceptance is necessary) would not be able to provide the total support needed for the recovery process, but resolved this problem by encouraging group members to obtain other help, if necessary, from Alcoholics Anonymous. However, they feared that the dual affiliation might hinder progress in the interactional group. At first there was some dissonance between the two as they had to bridge the gap between

AA and some alcoholics' stereotype of "ignorant professionals." This was resolved by pointing out to group members that AA and the therapy group serve very different, but equally necessary, functions in their recovery. There are things that AA can give their members that the group cannot and vice versa. The issue of dependency provides an excellent example. AA, by the nature of its format, tends to gratify dependency needs. New members are encouraged to rely on the other members, and on a "Higher Power" to remain abstinent. The therapy group, on the other hand, satisfies dependency needs only enough keep the patient in therapy.

Ideally, a solid, continuing membership in AA frees members to participate fully in the therapy group. AA can serve as a support system that helps the group members with their concerns about alcohol and also allows them to tolerate the frustrations of the therapy process. In fact, active membership should be encouraged, but the therapist must also be willing and able to counter misconceptions, prejudices, and distortions of fact about AA.

Wallace (1978a) contends that attendance at AA meetings is, in effect, a behavioral change program in that it advocates practical methods of achieving and maintaining sobriety. "Positive reinforcement (social recognition and status for staying sober), social modeling (the accessibility of role models and their behaviors for learning how to stay sober), desensitization (anxiety and guilt reduction through sharing of common experience, laughter and general merriment over past alcoholic behaviors, and a general atmosphere of social acceptance), and cognitive behavioral change (cognitive restructuring of self, behavior, and alcoholism) are aspects of AA that are most congruent with modern versions of behavior therapy" (p. 102).

Matano and Yalom (1991) support the integration of AA and other self-help groups in the treatment process and even go so far as to recommend that the interactional model be modified to incorporate and accommodate the language of these self-help programs. They write,

> Therefore if therapists are to be effective with the alcoholic population it behooves them to be thoroughly familiar with the AA traditions. There are two reasons for this: (1) to draw on the knowledge of AA and incorporate that knowledge into the therapy process and (2) to spot and prevent the misuse of AA concepts–that is, their distortion and utilization in therapy resistance. (p. 279)

As they go on to say, they do not believe that interactive group psychotherapy should be intended to replace AA's importance in the addict's or alcoholic's recovery. Rather, they recommend that "the group therapist actively enlist the aid of AA." Matano and Yalom also speak to the common misconceptions that both professionals and members of AA and other self-help groups have of each other. These misconceptions will be dealt with in Chapter 6, where a thorough examination of AA and its twelve steps and twelve traditions will be put forth.

A working relationship between AA and group therapy can enhance the recovery process. The recommendations set forth in this chapter should not only help in the treatment process; they should also help group leaders avoid many of the common pitfalls that confront every therapist when working with this difficult population.

Chapter 6

Psychodynamic Theory

Addiction can be explained and understood from many different perspectives. The disease concept just happens to be the one explanation that has the longest history and, more important, the most practical reasons for its utilization. It has been, so far, the only perspective that has had any long-standing pragmatic influence on successful treatment outcome and recovery. Historically, a multitude of alternative views have been presented from behavioral, spiritual, cognitive, transactional, phenomenological, cultural, sociological, biological, genetic, existential, psychological, and epidemiological perspectives. Many of these explanations have had much merit and plausibility. However, only one–the disease concept–has demonstrated any consistent benefit over any extended period of time in the treatment of addiction. In short, the disease concept has so far stood the test of time. New methods, with all their initial promise, excitement, and elaborate explanations, have faded faster than last year's latest pop-music star. This is not to imply that tradition and orthodox should rule the medical sciences. To the contrary, alternative explanations, especially those that either complement the pragmatic aspects of another perspective or, in the case of addiction, provide more subtle and thorough descriptions of the same phenomena, are crucial if the chemically dependent person is going to be helped more effectively in the future.

One such alternative explanation is the "self-medication hypothesis" of Khantzian et al. (1990). Building on the early theoretical observations and formulations of Kohut (1977b), Khantzian provides an alternative explanation for the addiction process that is not only compatible with the disease concept, but also expands it while providing useful and practical theoretical formulations that can enhance an addict's and alcoholic's treatment and recovery. The "self-medication hypothesis" has important implications for group psychotherapy. It not only helps expand an existing explanation of addiction, it also complements the way AA and other twelve-step programs treat chemical dependency. The self-psychology perspective provides alternative explanations for why twelve-step programs work as they do and how the curative forces in these programs have a direct relation to the strategies that need to be emphasized in group therapy when treating the chemically dependent individual.

In order to place this complementary relationship in its proper perspective, it will be helpful to understand how AA and other twelve-step programs evolved in their applications and why these programs have enjoyed the success that they have. In the past twenty years, numerous institutions and organizations have utilized the principles of the twelve-step program of AA as an attempt to deal with the increased alcohol and drug problem that has confronted our society. AA's internal integrity has been maintained while numerous attempts have been made to modify and adapt the principles of its twelve-step program to deal with similarities of other related disorders. Narcotics Anonymous, Cocaine Anonymous, Gamblers Anonymous, Adult Children of Alcoholics, Co-Dependency, Al-Anon, multiple eating disorders (i.e., bulimia, anorexia) and even Emotions Anonymous have all applied the principles of AA's twelve-step program to their different maladies with generally successful results. The question to be answered is, What is it that links these diverse conditions together so that they derive a common benefit from a similar approach?

Certainly, many of the curative factors (Universality, Instillation of Hope, Cohesiveness, etc.) that Yalom identifies (see Chapter 15) may be operating in the group treatment format that the AA program employs. The argument could also be presented that the principles of AA (i.e., honesty, personal evaluation, removal of character defects. the helping of others, etc.) could be helpful to anyone who applied these tenets to their life. While this may be true, such a statement misses the important relationship that exists between different types of addiction and personality variables. It is important to understand the similarities and common characteristics these addicted individuals share. Those familiar with AA know that many alcoholics stop drinking, rid themselves of their abundant interpersonal problems, and turn their lives around. Many abstinent alcoholics begin to enjoy life and go on to develop productive, healthy, successful careers and relationships. However, for every success, there is an equal number of individuals who are unable to remain sober and continue to act out their destructive patterns in a similar fashion with other obsessions and addictions. They suffer constant relapses and often end up substituting one problem (cocaine, heroin, marijuana) for another. Many become bulimic, overweight, or anorexic. Their eating becomes as compulsive and out of control as their drinking or drug use was. They become compulsive workers or gamblers or use sex just as they have used chemicals—to combat the emptiness, boredom, and depression that threatens to engulf them. They do not have a healthy sobriety and serenity escapes them. They become what AA terms a "dry drunk." They stop their alcohol use, but their personality characteristics do not change. Even the Big Book of AA recognizes that the AA program may not be for everyone.

> There are such unfortunates. They are not at fault; they seem to have been born that way. They are naturally incapable of grasping and developing a manner of living which demands rigorous honesty. Their chances are less than average. There are those, too, who suffer from grave emotional and mental disorders. (Alcoholics Anonymous, 1939, p. 58)

The questions regarding these individuals who continue to relapse and the reasons for their failures must be answered and understood. It would be tempting to write them off, saying that they are not ready "to get the program" or have not "hit their bottom yet." Father Martin, the lovable, leprechaun-like Catholic priest, abhors such an attitude. He is fond of saying, "Of course you are right when you say you can lead a horse to water, but you can't make him drink. But, you can sure make him thirsty!" Father Martin feels strongly that professionals must not take an uninvolved or neutral stance when working with alcoholics and addicts, but rather, they must find ways to increase addicts' and alcoholics' motivation for treatment. Certainly, one way to increase their thirst for treatment is to provide them with something that is nourishing and fulfilling. This requires an understanding of the special dynamics involved in patients who suffer from multiple addictions and frequently substitute one disorder for another. Understanding their condition will allow the professional to treat them in a way that will address the deficits that leads them to feel undernourished and dissatisfied.

CHARACTER PATHOLOGY AND ADDICTION

This brings us to the purpose of this chapter. Recent advances in the understanding of addiction have shed some new light on the perplexing problem of those "who may be too sick to get the program." Their sickness may be tied into a condition that can be described by a number of different terms–character pathology, personality disorder, structural deficits, or an uncohesive sense of self. *DSM-IV* (American Psychiatric Association, 1980) refers to these conditions as personality disorders. Psychiatric and psychoanalytic classifications of personality disorders are based on the repeated observation that patients who present symptoms due to maladaptively structured personalities fall into a small number of fixed groups, separated by similarities in the collection of personality traits. Furthermore, analytic exploration of descriptively homogeneous patients reveals broad similarities in basic conflicts and developmental experiences. Although these classifications are intended to discriminate among persons with personality disorders, they offer a useful framework for separating "kinds of people" in general. Personality disorders are distinguished from personality types, not by the presence of any definable pathological trait but by the inappropriate application of that trait in an individual's interpersonal relationships. People with personality disorders tend to see the unresolved dramas of their earlier experiences lurking in everyday life and react with rigid attempts to combat them in spite of inner disquiet or contemporary adaptive failure. In fact, the stress and regressive pull of illness often blurs the distinction between health and illness, and the general psychiatric classification has been used along with some of the common descriptive synonyms to outline the usual range of personality types encountered in psychiatric practice.

Indeed, if an alcoholic or drug addict does have a sociopathic, borderline, or narcissistic personality disorder, this patient is going to present with far more complicated treatment issues than the alcoholic or addict who does not suffer from character pathology. The relationship between addiction and character pathology has important implications for treatment. Schuckit has succinctly summarized the etiological possibilities that exist between these two conditions (1973). First, there are those who have character disorders and abuse drugs and alcohol because this is one common symptom of their personality disorder; second, the chemically dependent individual manifests character pathology as a consequence of primary drug and alcohol dependence; or third, there is a common shared factor that leads to both addiction and character disorders.

It is crucial to discern these three different possibilities in treating the addicted individual because what works with an alcoholic with character deficits will not work with a sociopath who is dependent on drugs and alcohol. In a study addressing this question, Vaillant (1983) feels that sociopathy and alcoholism have a complex and different multifactoral etiology. He concludes, "As soon as one disorder is present, the second becomes enormously likely" (p. 325). However, he contends that "in pre-morbid personality, the majority of alcoholics may be no different from non-alcoholics. On the other hand, sociopaths are very unhappy people with a poorly developed *sense of self* who seek to alter how they feel by abusing many kinds of drugs" (p. 325).

The understanding of what Vaillant calls "the sense of self" and its relationship to character disorders and addiction has reached important heights in the last decades. Two important contributing factors have led to this increase of competent professionals involved in the treatment and understanding of addiction and personality disorders. First, many physicians, psychologists, social workers, counselors, nurses, priests, and ministers have had to seek treatment for their own chemical dependency. They have learned what every addict and alcoholic has had to learn—they have had to stop their chemical use before they were able to make any substantial and long-lasting changes in their lives. Grand theories, insight, faith, and understanding had little significant impact on the arrestment and the alleviation of their dependency on alcohol or drugs. Their professional standing and education did not help them. Only Alcoholics Anonymous and the principles of the AA program allowed them to return to the world of the living and relieved them of their symptoms. The second contributing factor has been the serious investigation of alcoholism by a vast number of dedicated professionals who sought to understand this baffling disease the only way it could be realistically appreciated—by working with the chemically dependent individual. Numerous organizations of concerned professionals have emerged within the last decade. The Society of Psychologists in Addictive Behaviors (SPAD), The National Council on Alcoholism (NCA), The National Institute of Drug Addiction (NIDA), The National Institute of Alcoholism and Alcohol Abuse (NIAAA), The National Association of Drug and Alcohol Counselors (NADAC), The International Association of Doctors in Alcoholics Anonymous (IADAA), The American Medical Association (AMA), and The American Medical Association on Alcoholism (AMAA) are but a few of the more prominent organizations that have directed their energy in the last few years toward understanding alcoholism and drug dependency. Many professionals, either because of their own recovery from addiction, their association with colleagues who are recovering, or their involvement in these organizations, are more in touch with the realities of addiction than at any other time in recent history.

CONTRIBUTIONS OF OBJECT-RELATIONS THEORY AND SELF-PSYCHOLOGY

Within this change in professional interest in the understanding of alcoholism and drug dependence, there has been an emerging change in individual psychology within the last thirty years that has accumulated in the present-day object-relations theory of Otto Kernberg (1975) and the self-psychology of Heinz Kohut (1977b). Recent advances using standardized diagnostic approaches in psychiatry and a shift in psychoanalysis from a drive or instinct theory to a greater emphasis on adaptation and structural theory (ego and the self) have provided new findings and perspectives for explaining the relationship between psychological disturbance, interpersonal dysfunction, alcoholism, and drug dependence. Freud's concept of the private self, an intrapsychic structure that is self-contained and potentially perfectible has been replaced over time by the interpersonal determination of self that is influenced by our relationships with others. The internalized effort to be without shortcomings and to put up one's best front as a contained, enclosed, intrapsychic self (conflict theory) has been exchanged for a view that defines one's self as determined by one's desire to be with others as oneself, with all its imperfections and its shortcomings, while recognizing that others are independent, separate, and not there just to serve one's own needs and desires (object-relations theory).

Within this change in perspective, more emphasis has been placed on the effects of interpersonal relationships in determining a person's behavior and personality. Paralleling Martin Buber's anthropological question about what makes man unique, psychoanalysis and psychodynamic theory have arrived at a conclusion similar to that of Buber's. Humans are unique because they are defined by their relationships with others. Much like Harry Stack Sullivan's interpersonal theory of psychiatry, this viewpoint holds that we are a product of our relationships with others and that our sense of self is defined by the way we are perceived by others and how we perceive or distort our perception of others. Martin Buber (1955) summarizes this position when he writes,

> The fundamental fact of human existence is neither the individual as such nor the aggregate as such. Each, considered by itself, is a mighty abstraction. The individual is a fact of existence insofar as he steps into a living relation with other individuals. The aggregate is a fact of existence insofar as it is built up of living units of relation. The fundamental fact of human existence is man with man. What is peculiarly characteristic of the human world is above all that something takes place between one being and another the like of which can be found nowhere in nature. Language is only a sign and a means for it, all achievement of the spirit has been incited by it. Man is made man by it; but on its way it does not merely unfold, it also decays and withers away. It is rooted in one being turning to another as another, as this particular other being, in order to communicate

> with it in a sphere which is common to them but which reaches out beyond the special sphere of each. I call this sphere, which is established with the existence of man as man but which is conceptually still uncomprehended, the sphere of "between." Though being realized in very different degrees, it is a primal category of human reality. This is where the genuine third alternative must begin.
>
> The view which establishes the concept of "between" is to be acquired by no longer localizing the relation between human beings, as is customary, either within individual souls or in a general world which embraces and determines them, but in actual fact *between* them. (p. 203)

Buber's principle is that the development of this self is merely preparatory for true dialogic existence. We become what we are in order to be able to develop authentic real relationships with others. We therefore remain inauthentic or false until we are able to engage another in true dialogue. Nowhere is this principle more beautifully stated than in Buber's classic description of the I-Thou relationship (1960).

People often confuse the description of the I-Thou with the belief that it describes a mystical union with another in which two separate individuals unite as one. While this is somewhat true, it is not the most significant contribution to the understanding of relationships that this concept describes. Martin Buber was fond of saying an I precedes a Thou and the action takes place between the boundaries. By this, Buber wished to emphasize the importance of understanding one's separateness before entering into an I-Thou relationship. We must first be autonomous and independent before we can fully engage another. If we do not know our boundaries, we can lose ourselves in our relationships and confuse that which is ours with that which is not ours.

This is the theme that Heinz Kohut (1977b), Margaret Mahler (1979), and other object relations theorists are now addressing. Coming from diverse backgrounds and different perspectives, their theories, based on empirical observation (Kohut with adults and Mahler with children), are converging on an important and crucial understanding of the human condition. Can I be close to another without losing myself and can I tolerate really being alone? In Kohut's language, how does the individual develop a cohesive self that is authentic and not grandiose or false? We all have a basic drive to be loved and respected for what we really are.

This is an important theme in the treatment of addiction. Many alcoholics and addicts feel at their core that they are unworthy or defective in some way. Their chemical use is a way to combat their feelings of worthlessness and contributes to their false-self formation. Their grandiosity and self-centeredness is a defensive facade used to combat their feelings of fragmentation and incompleteness. Our worst fear (addicts and alcoholics do not have a lack of this type of trepidation) is to be rejected and unloved if we are real with another human being. Within this perspective, Martin Buber, the object-relations theorists, and Alcoholics Anonymous all have the same common goals of cure and treatment. Addicts and alcoholics must become real and authentic. They must learn that they will not be rejected or unloved just because of who and what they are. Eventually, they must come to realize that it is their behavior and actions that lead them to be rejected and uncared for. Once they realize what it is that they are doing that alienates others, they must change their behavior accordingly. Finally, they must recognize that they are separate, alone, and responsible for their condition and position in life. It is through this process of awareness and the establishment of healthy relationships that their structural and character deficits can be alleviated.

For better or worse, psychoanalytic and psychodynamic theory is the most influential and comprehensive theory of human psychological development and functioning that has been formulated to date. The change in focus from an intrapsychic model to an interpersonal model is significantly important. Such a shift in perspective has allowed the development of a theory of psychological functioning that explains more completely how similar developmental processes contribute to a wide range of diverse symptomatology. Within this perspective, all addictions (drugs, foods, gambling, sex, etc.) can be seen as relating to a characterological deficit of the self (character defects, poor impulse control, grandiosity, self-centeredness, etc). Such a theory has important implications for the professional working with the chemically dependent individual and can help the group leader make sense out of what was heretofore a seemingly unrelated collage of separated events in the addict's and alcoholic's life.

Kohut summarizes his position with a preface he wrote to a recent NIDA research monograph:

> The explanatory power of the new psychology of the self is nowhere as evident as with regard to these four types of psychological disturbance: (1) the narcissistic personality disorders, (2) the perversions, (3) the delinquencies, and (4) the addictions. Why can these seemingly disparate conditions be examined so fruitfully with the aid of the same conceptual framework? Why can all these widely differing and even contrasting symptom pictures be comprehended when seen from the viewpoint of the psychology of the self? How, in other words, are these four conditions related to each other? What do they have in common, despite the fact that they exhibit widely differ-

> ing, and even contrasting, symptomatologies? The answer to these questions is simple: in all of these disorders the afflicted individual suffers from a central weakness, from a weakness in the core of his personality. He suffers from the consequences of a defect in the self. The symptoms of these disorders, whether comparatively hazy or hidden, or whether more distinct and conspicuous, arise secondarily as an outgrowth of a defect in the self. The manifestations of these disorders become intelligible if we call to mind that they are all attempts—unsuccessful attempts, it must be stressed—to remedy the central defect in the personality.
>
> The narcissistically disturbed individual yearns for praise and approval or for a merger with an idealized supportive other because he cannot sufficiently supply himself with self-approval or with a sense of strength through his own inner resources. The pervert is driven toward sexual enactments with figures or symbols that give him the feeling of being wanted, real, alive or powerful. The delinquent repeats over and over again certain acts through which he demonstrates to himself an escape from the realization that he feels devoid of sustaining self-confidence and of sustaining ideals. And. . . . the addict, finally, craves the drug because the drug seems to him to be capable of curing the central defect in his self. It becomes for him the substitute for a self-object which failed him traumatically at a time when he should still have had the feeling of omnipotently controlling its responses in accordance with his needs as if it were a part of himself. By ingesting the drug he symbolically compels the mirroring self-object to soothe him, to accept him. Or he symbolically compels the idealized self-object to submit to his merging into it and thus to his partaking in its magical power. In either case the ingestion of the drug provides him with the self-esteem which he does not possess.
>
> Through the incorporation of the drug he supplies for himself the feeling of being accepted and thus of being self-confident; or he creates the experience of being merged with a source of power that gives him the feeling of being strong and worthwhile. And all these effects of the drug tend to increase his feeling of being alive, tend to increase his certainty that he exists in this world. (1977a, pp. vii-ix)

Kohut sees the source of addictions tied into the child's early experiences. However, he makes an important distinction between cause and cure. In the end, Kohut stresses the importance of the child's early relationships in determining both the cause and treatment of addiction.

> It is the tragedy of all these attempts at self-cure that the solutions which they provide are impermanent, that in essence they cannot succeed. . . . Whatever the chemical nature of the substance that is employed, however frequently repeated its consumption, however cleverly rationalized or mythologized its ingestion with the support from others who are similarly afflicted–no psychic structure is built, the defect in the self remains. It is as if a person with a wide open gastric fistula were trying to still his hunger through eating. He may obtain pleasurable taste sensations by his frantic ingestion of food but, since the food does not enter that part of the digestive system where it is absorbed into the organism, he continues to starve. . . . Thus, in asking the crucial questions concerning the factors in childhood which lead to the addiction-prone personality, we will say that, in the last analysis, and within certain limits, it is less important to determine what the parents do than what they *are*. (1977a pp. vii-ix)

If one is to truly understand the implications of object relations theory, one must understand the contributions of three figures: Margaret Mahler (1979), Otto Kernberg (1975), and Henry Kohut (1977b). Mahler is most noted for her work with the psychological development of normal children. Kernberg has contributed most to the understanding of borderline personality organization. Kohut is almost exclusively aligned with the understanding and explanation of the narcissistic personality disorder. Each has an important contribution to make to the understanding of addictive behaviors and all three are not always in complete agreement about specific disturbances. For instance, Kernberg sees many, if not all, narcissistic disorders as having a borderline personality organization. Kohut, on the other hand, views borderline pathology as a result of severe narcissistic injuries caused by an unempathic and uncaring other. What often appear to be severe borderline reactions and demands are actually the iatrogenic effects of an unempathic self-object. Mahler avoids such controversy and insists she is just describing what she observes empirically.

MARGARET MAHLER'S THEORY OF NORMAL DEVELOPMENT

After having spent most of her professional career studying severely disturbed children, Mahler turned her energies to the investigation of normal children and their mothers at the Masters Children Center in New

York. Beginning in 1959, she and her colleagues set up an observation room where groups of children could be watched as they interacted with their mothers, played with toys, or experimented with their opportunities for separation from their mothers. Children from four months old through four years old were participants with their mothers in the study.

From the mass of data gathered over the years, Mahler began to construct a picture of the normal sequence of stages in the process of becoming a person. In essence, Mahler was studying the phenomenon of the psychological birth of the child. Her work was placed in an object-relations point of view, which stressed the ego's primary object-seeking qualities. This is in contrast to traditional instinct theory in which objects are sought not primarily because of their relationship potential, but for the purpose of drive reduction. Mahler's work focused on the internalization of interpersonal relationships. She was concerned with how interpersonal relations determine intrapsychic structures and how these intrapsychic structures preserve, modify, and reactivate past relations. The implications that these internalized relations have in the development of psychic structure and addiction will be explored later in this chapter. First, an overview of Mahler's stages of normal development and a defining of terms important to her theory will be presented.

EGO PSYCHOLOGY AND OBJECT-RELATIONS THEORY

Before one can truly understand Mahler, one must understand her relationship to object-relations theory and ego psychology. The concept of the ego is an especially confusing one for those familiar only with Alcoholics Anonynous and the way its members apply the term in discussing one's recovery or lack of it. Within AA, ego is commonly used in the popular sense to indicate an individual who is self-centered and has an inflated sense of his or her self-worth. Freud's original use of the word ego had far different implications and the ego psychologists have applied this term in its intended technical meaning to explain the part of the psyche that serves the executive functioning (i.e., reasoning, decisions, defensive operations, etc.) of the personality. Henry Tiebout, an important historic figure from AA's perspective because he was one of the few psychiatrists who was an early supporter of AA and was also a friend and psychotherapist to AA's founder, Bill Wilson, struggled with differentiating the two different definitions that this term carried:

> This popular view of ego, while it may not have scientific foundation, has one decided value: it possesses a meaning and can convey a

> concept which the average person can grasp. This concept of the inflated ego recognized the common ancestor of a whole series of traits, namely, that they are all manifestations of an underlying feeling state in which personal considerations are first and foremost.
>
> The existence of this ego has long been recognized, but a difficulty in terminology still remains. Part of the difficulty arises from the use of the word ego, in psychiatric and psychological circles, to designate those elements of the psyche which are supposed to rule psychic life. Freud divided mental life into three major subdivisions: the id, the ego and the superego. The first, he stated, contains the feeling life on a deep, instinctual level; the third is occupied by the conscience, whose function is to put brakes on the impulses arising within the id. The ego should act as mediator between the demands of the id and the restraints of the superego, which might be overzealous and bigoted. Freud's own research was concerned mainly with the activities of the id and the superego. The void he left with respect to the ego is one that his followers are endeavoring to fill, but as yet with no generally accepted conclusions. (1954, p. 4)

Ego psychologists, starting with Harry Stack Sullivan (Yalom's unacknowledged mentor) have placed more of an emphasis on the individual's interpersonal relationships. Object-relations theorists have taken the work of the ego psychologist and sought to understand how individuals' external functioning was a representation of their internal perceptions and distortions.

> If, for example, an individual's repertoire of object representations is simply and primitively organized and contains a view of others either as all-giving or maliciously and sadistically withholding (what others have termed need-satisfying object relations), then the behavior of others will be selectively perceived and organized to yield only such behavior as includes these two primitive and extreme experiences. In contrast, if these internal "images" comprehend many aspects of others, including their empathy, intelligence, sense of humor, motives, etc., then there is within that person the potential for a much more differentiated and subtle experience of others (what has been termed object consistency). (Hatcher and Krohn, 1980, p. 300)

If individuals have external difficulties in their relationships with others, it has been questioned whether these difficulties are related to their internal mentalistic distortions. Object-relations theory is therefore a mentalistic psychology aimed at answering this question. It is more interested in looking at the inner lives of people. The term *object* is a technical one that signifies an individual's ability to carry around an accurate mental representation of another person in his or her mind, even when that person is out of sight. This ability to develop object constancy and have accurate, undistorted mental representations of others is an important developmental task that not everyone is able to accomplish. Mahler sought to understand the source of these distortions and the relationship between developmental arrest and object constancy. Her investigation into these issues led her to trace the origin of the ego or the self as it related to the early maternal relationship. Mahler provides an important view of what happens to the individual's psyche under the impact of personal relations in "real life." Kernberg sums up the implications of Mahler's work when he describes object-relations theory:

> What is object-relations theory? In essence, it is the psychoanalytic approach to the internalization of interpersonal relations, the study of how interpersonal relations determines intrapsychic structures, and how these intrapsychic structures preserve, modify, and reactivate past internalized relations with others in the context of present interpersonal relations. Object-relations theory deals with the interactions between the internal world of objects (the internalized relations with others) and the actual interpersonal relations of the individual. (Kernberg, 1970, p. 1)

Many years earlier, Fyodor Dostoyevsky intuitively grasped and elegantly described this concept:

> You must know that there is nothing higher and stronger and more wholesome and good for life in the future than some good memory, especially a memory of childhood, of home. People talk to you a great deal about your education, but some good sacred memory, preserved from childhood, is perhaps the best education. If a man carries many such memories with him into life, he is safe to the end of his days. And if one has only one good memory left in one's heart, even that may sometime be the means of saving him. Perhaps we may grow wicked later on, may be unstable to refrain from evil, may laugh at men's tears and at those people, who say as Kolya did just now: "I want to suffer for all men." We may even jeer spitefully at such people. But however bad we may become–which God forbid–yet, when we recall how we buried Llusha, how we loved him in his last days, and how we have been talking like friends together, at this stone, the cruelest and most mocking of us–if we do become so–will

> not dare to laugh inwardly at having been kind and good at this moment! What's more, perhaps, that one memory may keep us from great evil and we will reflect and say: "Yes, I was good and brave and honest then!" (1957, p. 87)

Freud also alluded to this when he stated, "A man who has been the indisputable favorite of his mother keeps for life the feeling of a conqueror, that confidence of success that often induces real success" (1921, p. 19).

To understand completely the development of internal representations, it is important to grasp the meaning of Mahler's work. It also helps to understand Piaget's research, which focused on the stages of cognitive development in children (Piaget, 1954). Piaget parallels Mahler in that he sees object constancy as an important stage in a developmental process. Place a ball in front of a six-month-old child and cover the ball with a blanket and the ball will no longer exist for the infant. Out of sight, out of existence. Pull the blanket away from the ball and behold, the infant is amazed at the magical appearance of an object that just seconds prior had not existed. Piaget discovered that it is only later in the child's cognitive development that the infant is able to keep a mental representation of the ball even when it is covered by the blanket. The developmentally advanced infant will then search underneath the blanket for the ball, knowing that even though the ball is out of sight, it still exists. The principle is the same for infants in their relationships with significant caregivers in their life. The child's ability to realize that the mother still exists even though the mother is out of the room suggests an important stage of object constancy, and, in Erik Erikson's terminology, a stage of basic trust has been achieved.

A couple of examples will help clarify this point.

> Once, while a friend was visiting our home, my son and I were in the living room with this woman, while my wife had gone to the kitchen in search of some refreshments. The visitor was an older woman who had been a friend of the family for years. Though uneducated and unsophisticated, she was a solid, no-nonsense woman who had been reared in the rural hills of southern Kentucky. My son, who was two years old at the time, was busy playing on the living room rug and had not noticed my wife's departure into the kitchen. In the process of searching for something in the kitchen, my wife quickly walked into the adjoining garage, allowing the screen door to slam behind her. My son, startled briefly by the noise, looked up from his toys, noticed his mother had left the house and quickly returned to his

> play, unconcerned about her absence. His reaction prompted this very stoic lady to firmly announce "That's a good boy!" Somewhat surprised by the suddenness of her complement, I thanked her before I asked what had prompted her statement. She replied "He didn't cry when his mother left the room. He's a good boy!"

Unknown to this woman, my son had not reacted in fright because he had developed object constancy. His mother could leave the room and, although she was out of sight, she would continue to exist for him because he was developmentally able to carry around a stable mental representation of her in his head.

> Once, while working as a psychology intern in a University Hospital outpatient clinic, I was assigned to provide psychotherapy to a woman who had a history of multiple psychiatric hospitalizations and numerous different diagnostic labels, of which borderline personality disorder was the one used most frequently. After approximately ten sessions, the woman gradually began to experience increased anxiety as the time of our weekly session neared its end. She would begin the session without discomfort, only to have her fears mount as she prepared to leave my office. Her anxiety increased to the point that she would feel compelled to call me by the time she had reached the lobby of the hospital seven floors below my office. Each phone call would result in the same expressed concern: "Are you all right, I just became overwhelmed as I rode down the elevator thinking that something terrible had happened to you." Once assured that indeed I was all right and that I was still here, she would quickly compose herself until the next week when she would repeat the same procedure upon leaving my office.

This thirty-five-year-old woman, unlike my two-year-old son, was developmentally arrested and had not obtained object constancy. While my son felt little panic and fear when his mother left his sight because he had successfully negotiated an important developmental stage, this woman was unable to carry a mental representation of me in her head once I was out of sight and consequently became overwhelmed by her fears that an important object in her life had been lost. Her anxiety was triggered by the thought of leaving my presence and increased to the unmanageable point that she had to telephone me to be assured I still existed. A steady and calm assurance from me was enough to quickly soothe her sense of inner turmoil and fragmentation.

These presentations represent two extreme conditions that may manifest as a result of interference in a child's developmental process. Before one can understand the implications that alcohol and drug use have in relation to an individual's developmental fixation, one must understand the different stages of normal development. Horner (1979) describes this process:

> Psychological health and psychopathology can both be understood in terms of the vicissitudes of object relations development and its associated organizing and integrating impact. This developmental sequence begins with the stage of normal autism at birth and proceeds through the process of attachment to the stage of normal symbiosis, which is symbolized by the undifferentiated self-object representation. From this point the child faces the developmental tasks of the separation-individuation process. This process is subdivided into the subphases of hatching, the practicing period, and the rapprochement subphase, and it culminates in the achievement of identity and object constancy. At this point the child, and thus the adult he will become, has a firm sense of self and differentiated other, is able to relate to others as whole persons rather than just as need satisfiers, and can tolerate ambivalence without having to maintain a split between good and bad object-representations with its parallel split between good and bad self-representations. He also has the ability to sustain his or her own narcissistic equilibrium or good self-feeling from resources within the self, which are the outcome of the achievement of libidinal object constancy that comes about through the transmuting internalization of maternal functions into the self. (p. 25)

For those unfamiliar with object-relations terminology, Horner's statement can be confusing and initially difficult to comprehend. Mahler's stages of normal development will be thoroughly presented so one can grasp the full implications of Horner's statement.

MAHLER'S STAGES OF NORMAL DEVELOPMENT

Mahler constructed a theoretical picture of the normal stages of development in the process of the child acquiring object constancy and thus achieving a formation of a stable self-concept or a cohesive self. For the process to be completed, two early forerunner phases are required, normal autism and normal symbiosis, in which the mother and infant mutually lay the foundation for the child's psychological birth or hatching. Four subsequent phases of the separation individuation process are required and the process of separation climaxes at or near the end of the third year of life. (See Figure 6.1.)

Stage I: Two Forerunner Phases–Attachment
1. Normal Autism (0-1 month)
2. Normal Symbiosis (1-4 months)

Stage II: Three Subphases of Separation Individuation–Hatching
1. Differentiation (5-9 months)
2. Practicing (10-15 months)
3. Rapprochement (15-24 months)

Stage III: Fourth Subphase–Object Constancy
1. Consolidation of Self and Identity

Stage I: Normal Autism

During the first month of life, the infant is encapsulated in a psychic orbit that serves as a stimulus barrier protecting the child from excessive outside intrusions. In effect, the autistic shell serves as a stimulus barrier and protects the infant against extreme stimulation or excessive environmental demands. The child has a relative disinterest in external reality because an infant's physiological developmental limitations restrict their psychological investment in the environment. This stage of normal autism, differs from secondary autism, where the child seems from birth unable to utilize his or her mother as an auxiliary ego; that is, the child shows no interest in relating to his or her mother, or to any person. Mahler describes the true autistic child as having

> an obsessive desire for the preservation of sameness; a stereotyped preoccupation with a few inanimate objects or action patterns toward which he shows the only signs of emotional attachment. As a consequence, he shows utter intolerance of any change in his inanimate surroundings . . . The primarily autistic child differs from the organic, as well as from the predominantly symbiotic psychotic child, by his seemingly self-sufficient contentedness–*if only he is left alone.* These autistic children behave like omnipotent magicians if they are permitted to live within, and thus to command, their static and greatly constricted segment of inanimate environment. (Mahler, 1968, p. 68)

Horner (1976) differentiates the early development process of attachment in a normal child from that of the autistic child when she writes,

FIGURE 6.1. Stages of Normal Development: An Overview of Margaret Mahler's Contributions

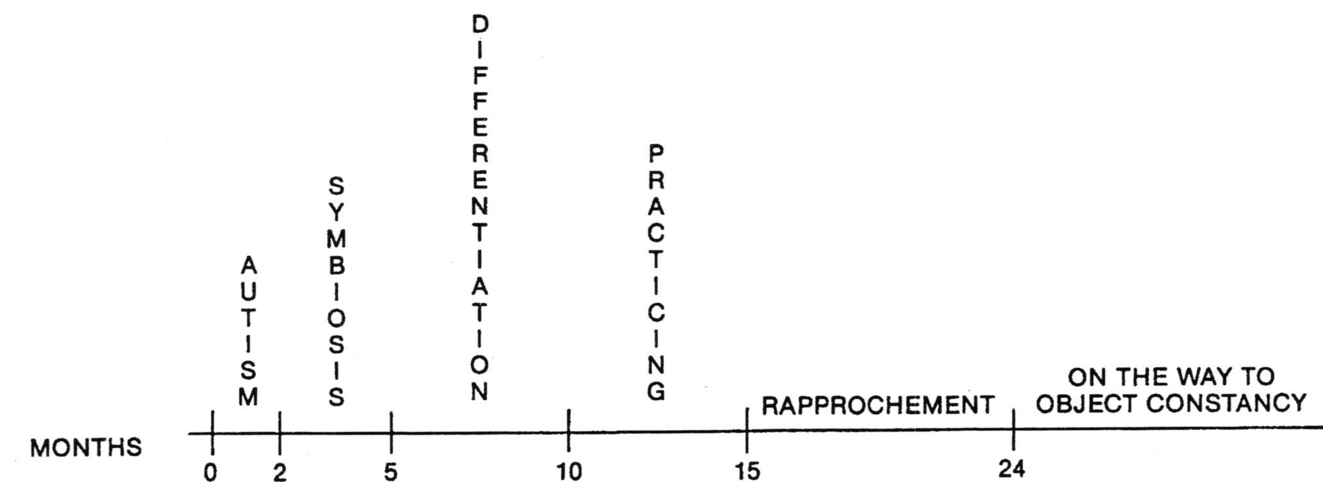

> At birth the child is in a state of what Mahler refers to as normal autism. Kohut (1977) who thinks in terms of the evolution of a cohesive self-structure, calls this same period the stage of the fragmented self. Mahler sees constitutional factors operating in childhood autism and comments on the fact that there is no anticipatory posture at nursing, no reaching out gestures, and no specific smiling response. What is lacking is attachment-seeking behavior, and thus the mother/child matrix that fosters ego development is nonexistent. Defensive or compensatory structure (Kohut, 1977) may allow for a higher level of functioning, but their failure would throw the individual back upon the core pathology.

The autistic infant remains fixated at this earliest stage of life and makes no move toward attachment. The absense of anticipatory posturing with little or no smiling and reaching out (attachment-seeking behavior) prevents the establishment of a mother-child matrix that usually fosters the infant's ego development. In situations where the environment is grossly pathological, disrupting the infant's basic organizational process, it is possible to force a retreat into secondary autism, although Mahler recognizes that constitutional factors play a far more important part in this process.

Normal Symbiosis–Attachment

By the second month of life, the infant becomes dimly aware of the mother as an external object. The infant begins to develop memory traces of the mother's face. The recognition of her face, based on past pleasant experiences, leads to a basic trust that relief of tension will regularly occur in her presence. However, the infant behaves as though he and his mother were a dual unity within a common boundary. From the infant's point of view there are really no boundaries between himself and his mother. They are one. At the height of this joyous period of his life, they are encapsulated in a symbiotic orbit. He cannot really comprehend that he and his mother are separate beings. The infant, through the process of attachment to a primary object, remains encapsulated in a symbiotic orbit. The infant also cannot differentiate between his own tension-reducing efforts and the mother's efforts made on his behalf. During these early months he internalizes his mother and uses her as a "beacon of orientation," engendering a basic sense of security, safety, and trust. The crude differentiation between object and self, good and bad, and pleasure and pain allows the symbiotic child to deal with painful experiences in the only way his limited cognitive defenses permit, by splitting the good and the bad, and projecting the bad outside of the symbiotic partnership. The primitive defensive process of splitting becomes critical in understanding the character pathology present in the adult borderline patient and will be explored in depth later in the chapter.

Crucial to this developmental phase is the infant's ability to attach itself to an external object. Horner describes the ramifications of the infant's inability to bond with another:

> At the most primitive level, failure of attachment may carry with it severe deficits in the early organization of the self. The failure to develop attachment and to achieve a satisfactory symbiosis because of environmental factors, such as institutionalization, may lead to the development of characteristic disturbances such as the inability to keep rules, lack of capacity to experience guilt, and indiscriminate friendliness with an inordinate craving for affection with no ability to make lasting relationships. The "affectionless psychopath" is also characterized by the failure to develop the affectional bond that goes with attachment.
>
> Another form of pathological attachment is attachment through the false-self organization. In this situation the real, core self has remained in a nonattached, non-object-related state. (Horner, 1979, pp. 28-29)

During the first five or six months of life, in the developmentally healthy child, there is innate attachment-seeking behavior to bring about a normal symbiosis. The earliest mental representations of self and object (the undifferentiated self-object representation) is characteristic of this stage. There is neither physical nor psychic differentiation. This brings us to the heart of Mahler's developmental work. Important during this time is the mutual selection of cues by mother and infant. Mahler writes:

> We observed that infants present a larger variety of cues to indicate needs, tension, and pleasure. In a complex manner the mother responds selectively to only certain of these clues. (1979, p. 18)

Mahler points out that this mutual cuing creates the complex pattern that becomes what Lichtenstein (1961) refers to as "the infant's becoming the child of his particular mother."

Bowlby (1958) emphasizes the degree to which infants themselves play a part in determining their own environment. Certain kinds of babies who tend to be overreactive or unpredictable make it difficult for the mother to provide good-enough mothering. But the mother is supposed to have a much larger role than the infant by the end of the first year, in the determination of the quantity as well as the quality of the transactions that occur between them.

The failure of attachment carries several deficits in the early organization of the self. There is a delicate and subtle interplay between constitutional and environmental factors that determines how this disturbance will manifest. Mahler and Horner have outlined this process in clear detail, and their schema will be briefly outlined.

1. The affectionless psychopath is characterized by the failure to develop the affectional bond that goes with attachment.
2. Disruption of attachment due to separation and loss may lead to a lifelong schizoid detachment. In this case, detachment is used as a defense against the frightening impact of object relatedness.
3. Another form of pathological attachment is attachment through the fake-self organization leading to narcissistic personality structure.

Stage II: Separation-Individuation Subphases

1. Differentiation

As strong as the child's yearnings for attachment are, the infant gradually begins to experience even more powerful urges to move away from the mother, to separate, and to explore. At four or five months, the infant begins to recognize that the mother who soothes, feeds, and reduces tension is separate. This is the beginning of the "hatching process." Hatching is the start of the infant's psychological birth and marks the beginning of the child's emergence as a separate individual free from the symbiotic attachment to a maternal object.

Failure to negotiate this developmental process results in an adult who becomes disorganized and suffers dissolution of the self when faced with object loss. The individual is unable to differentiate inner experiences from outer experiences, leading to confusion regarding what is me and what is not me. In the extreme cases, internal stimuli become confused with external reality, resulting in hallucinations and delusions. The enmeshed family, which is a breeding ground for schizophrenia, is an excellent example of the child's failure to separate from the parents' intrusiveness. The mother who sits in the therapist's office with her child and tells her daughter, "It's chilly in here, I feel cold, put on your sweater," is a clear indication of a family system where boundaries are not clearly set and feelings are not separately maintained.

2. Practicing

From approximately ten to fifteen months, the child's focus shifts from the mother to his or her own autonomous functioning. Locomotion, perception, and learning become self-motivated. Ego functioning, reality-testing, secondary thought process, and frustration tolerance leave a child with less reliance on external objects and the toddler begins to develop more self-reliance and autonomy. The practicing subphase shifts into high gear when the child begins to walk upright near the age of ten to twelve months. Now the child is truly physically independent, free to roam widely and proudly.

> Expanding locomotor capacity during the early practicing subphase widens the child's world; not only does he have a more active role in determining closeness and distance to mother, but the modalities that up to now were used to explore the relatively familiar environment suddenly expose him to a wider segment of reality; there is more to see, more to hear, more to touch. (Mahler, Pine, and Bergman, 1975, p. 66)

Toward the end of this subphase, the child begins to experience an inflated sense of omnipotence that is augmented by the toddler's feelings of his own magical power. He can stand, walk, climb, jump, and even speak. He truly believes he is the center of the universe! There is no stopping him now! Encouraged by his rapid, often spectacular growth in the last few months, the child is led to believe that the world is truly his oyster. Normal grandiosity and primary narcissism are healthy stage-specific developmental phases in the child's development. However, this inflated, omnipotent representation is the nucleus of the grandiose self that can be manifested as extreme self-centeredness or pathological narcissism in adult life if the child's developmental process is impaired by unavailable, intrusive, or uncaring self-objects.

Horner sees the development of a grandiose self as a result of difficulties experienced at the practicing stage of development. She writes:

> This inflated, omnipotent self-object representation is the nucleus of the grandiose self which obtains in cases of pathological narcissism, be it with the borderline patient or with the narcissistic personality disorder. Problems of subsequent development are related to the extent to which significant aspects of self are assimilated into the grandiose self structure and thus not available for conflict-free functioning or are otherwise kept out of the mainstream of normal maturation.

> When the autonomous functions are assimilated into a pathological grandiose self-structure, they are not available for achievements in reality that contribute to a healthy, reality-based self-esteem.
>
> The grandiose self may be a manifestation of structural pathology from this point of early development, or it may be recalled as a defense mechanism against the dangers of loss of self-esteem in a more evolved character. (Horner, 1979, p. 32)

Anyone working with alcoholics and addicts knows that self-centeredness and grandiosity are important treatment considerations. The implications of Mahler's research for the treatment of the alcoholic and addict will be explored at length later in this chapter.

3. Rapprochement

Toward the end of the toddler's practicing subphase, he becomes increasingly aware of his separateness from his mother and her separateness from him. At this time, the child is just beginning to confront the crisis of his second birth. While at the height of his omnipotent grandiosity, the young toddler bolts from his house in all his glory and speeds down the driveway to conquer his world and unexpectedly trips, tumbles forward, and scratches his knee. Suddenly, he is made acutely aware of his vulnerability and powerlessness, and invariably will face disillusionment. His knee hurts and bleeds. To make matters worse, his mother is nowhere in sight. The eighteen to twenty-four-month-old child is beginning to experience the rapprochement crisis.

He becomes distressed by the acute awareness of his separateness and helplessness. Frustrations persist in his mind and aggression becomes internalized. His experiences with reality have counteracted his overestimation of omnipotence. His self-esteem starts to be deflated and he is now vulnerable to shame. As he becomes acutely aware of his limitations, he undergoes a cognitive and affective decentering process. This occurs at a time when cognitive, motor, and emotional development bring about an awareness of the self that leads him to realize that causes and events exist outside of himself, independent of his needs and wishes. He suffers a loss of omnipotence and wishes to return to the safety of his mother.

The rapprochement phase becomes a period of contradictions. As the child becomes aware of his separateness, he develops strategies for preventing this awareness and maintaining close contact. Darting away behavior becomes pronounced as the child wishes reunion with the love object, but fears engulfment at the same time. The child's ambivalence about closeness and dependency is equally frustrating for the parent. The child has entered "the terrible twos" that all parents dread and bemoan. As one mother complained,

> I don't know what to do with that little bastard! He used to be happy away from me. Now, he cries for my attention and when I pick him up, he pushes me away. I don't know what he wants!

In developmental terms, the child is trying to assert his separateness and his selfhood. He may not know what he wants when he says "no," but he knows by saying "no" that he is separate from his mother. There will be confusion on the mother's part, as she tries to understand the child's frustration during this developmental process. This leads to a reemergence of the child's difficulty tolerating aggression in himself and others.

Monte summarizes the ramifications of this conflict for the child:

> From the viewpoint of ego development, the rapprochement phase may be crucial to the child's ability to internalize conflict and to reconcile clashes between an "all good" mother and an "all bad" one. The good mother is the person who has provided all pleasures, all securities, all warmth, and all companionship. In the symbiotic phase, this "good love object" was viewed as a part of self. But now the child's growing psychological sophistication confronts a serious conflict. Mothers unavoidably have their dark sides. Sometimes mother is a need-frustrator, or a pain-inflicter, or an indifferent and distracted caretaker, or, most painful of all her shortcomings, mother is sometimes absent altogether. For the child's newly developing ego, the "good mother" and the "bad mother" cannot be one and the same love object. She, who was once so long ago a part of me, cannot be bad; yet, undeniably, mother is not *always* good. If the good mother and the bad mother *are* one person, then I, too, must harbor some bad within me. That is not possible, for I am all good.
>
> Termed *"splitting"* of the ego, the rapprochement child may employ the defense mechanism of dealing with such contradictory love objects by treating them in all-or-none fashion. Thus, mother cannot be both good and bad simultaneously. There is a good mother, and there is a bad mother. The good mother is the love object that was internalized as part of the child's own narcissistic ego during symbiosis. The bad mother is externalized, projected to the outside world, outside me, where all pain-producing, threatening objects belong. (Monte, 1980, pp. 211-212)

Figure 6.2 outlines this development process and the difficulties that may emerge in the defensive operation of splitting.

FIGURE 6.2. Self-Object Development

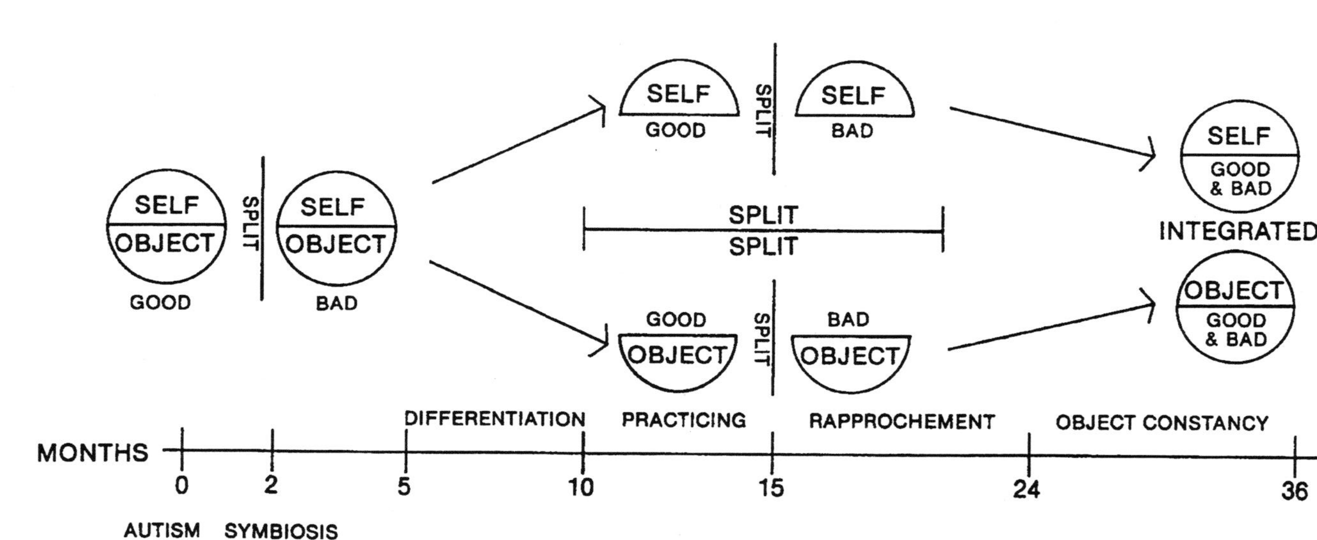

As described by Monte, object constancy involves the emotional acceptance of the idea that we are neither saints nor demons but whole people capable of both love and hate. By being able to unite or integrate such polar feelings, individuals confirm their sense of personal wholeness. When object constancy is weak, the only way to protect the good, cherished part of the self from the negative or undesirable aspects of the self is to force or split this off. As a result, it becomes impossible to appreciate the wholeness of the self or another. Individuals will simply get rid of others like unwanted objects if those others disappoint them. They will also fail to see the others' history of goodness and will only be able to recall the badness of the latest experience.

As the child resolves the rapprochement crisis with the help of a "good-enough mother," he begins to divest himself of his omnipotence without undue anxiety or shame and melds goodness and badness into an integrated whole. The child enters the last stage of object constancy, identity integration, and the development of a cohesive self. Mahler writes:

> By the eighteenth month, the junior toddler seems to be at the height of the process of dealing with his continuously experienced physical separateness from the mother. This coincides with his cognitive and perceptual achievement of the permanence of objects, in Piaget's sense. This is the time when his sensorimotor intelligence starts to develop into true representational intelligence, and when the important process of internalization, in Hartmann's sense–very gradually, through ego identifications–begins. (Mahler, 1968, p. 21)

Stage III: Object Constancy

Toward the end of the second year, and extending through the third year of life, the child is able to achieve a fair degree of emotional object constancy. Three major tasks are achieved:

1. Internally and mentally, such children are able to maintain an image of the mother even when she is not present. This sense of well-being comes from having internalized the good-enough mother and good self-experiences. The child can hold onto these positive images and function as a separate self, even if angry, frustrated, and alone.
2. Separation and individuation is achieved. Kohut, who thinks in terms of a cohesive self-structure, refers to this as a nuclear self being established. Kernberg sees this as a process through which identity integration is attained. Buber describes this as the develop-

ment of a separate I that is needed before a person is able to engage in an I-Thou relationship. The false-self organization or "as-if personality" of Winnicott would not prevail. In Sartre's language, an authentic self is established.

3. There is an enduring development of psychic structure. The final shift to well-secured separate identity ensures the capacity to regulate one's narcissistic equilibrium from the sources within one's self. In Kohut's language, transmuting internalization is obtained. Individuals are able to calm and soothe themselves and will not have to rely on external self-objects or external sources of gratification (i.e., alcohol, drugs, sex, food, excitement) to ward off painful affective states. Psychic structure has been adequately laid through the assimilation of maternal functions into self-representations. (See Figure 6.3.)

Figure 6.4 summarizes the developmental paradigm and is a modification from Horner's earlier presentation (1979).

As presented here, Mahler's research has important implications for understanding the relationship of addiction, development, and the establishment of psychic structure. Mahler's work focuses on the developmental and adaptational requirements children must negotiate during their first three years of life. Horner's schema (Figure 6.4) helps us understand the relationship of this developmental process to psychosis, character disorders, and neurosis. Mahler's theory of normal development has been summarized, starting with the earliest phases of achieving homeostasis and need-satisfying attachment, through subsequent phases of separation, individuation, and the capacity for mental representation (i.e., object constancy). Once a child has successfully negotiated these developmental stages, he or she attains what Kohut calls a cohesive self. Without the attainment of the psychic structure that is laid in the process of developing a cohesive self, there is a much greater risk for both character pathology and addiction.

Khantzian and Treece summarize this position in a statement that directly links structural deficits and addiction. They stress

> how optimal nurturance from the environment (as primarily represented by the mother) fosters adequate mastery of these phases by the infant, and leads to the development of stable ego structures and capacities to manage drives and object relations. To the extent that the individual is overly deprived or indulged In his/her development, varying degrees of ego impairment occur and drugs then come to substitute and compensate for the developmental defects and impairments. (1977, p. 73)

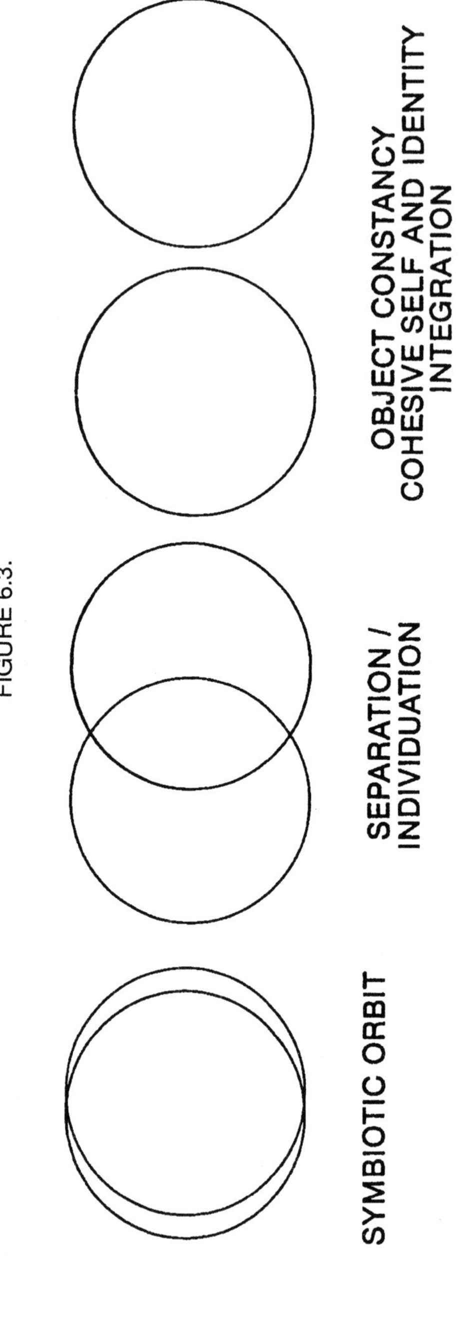
SYMBIOTIC ORBIT
SEPARATION / INDIVIDUATION
OBJECT CONSTANCY
COHESIVE SELF AND IDENTITY INTEGRATION

FIGURE 6.3.

FIGURE 6.4. Stages of Development of Object Relations and Associated Pathologies

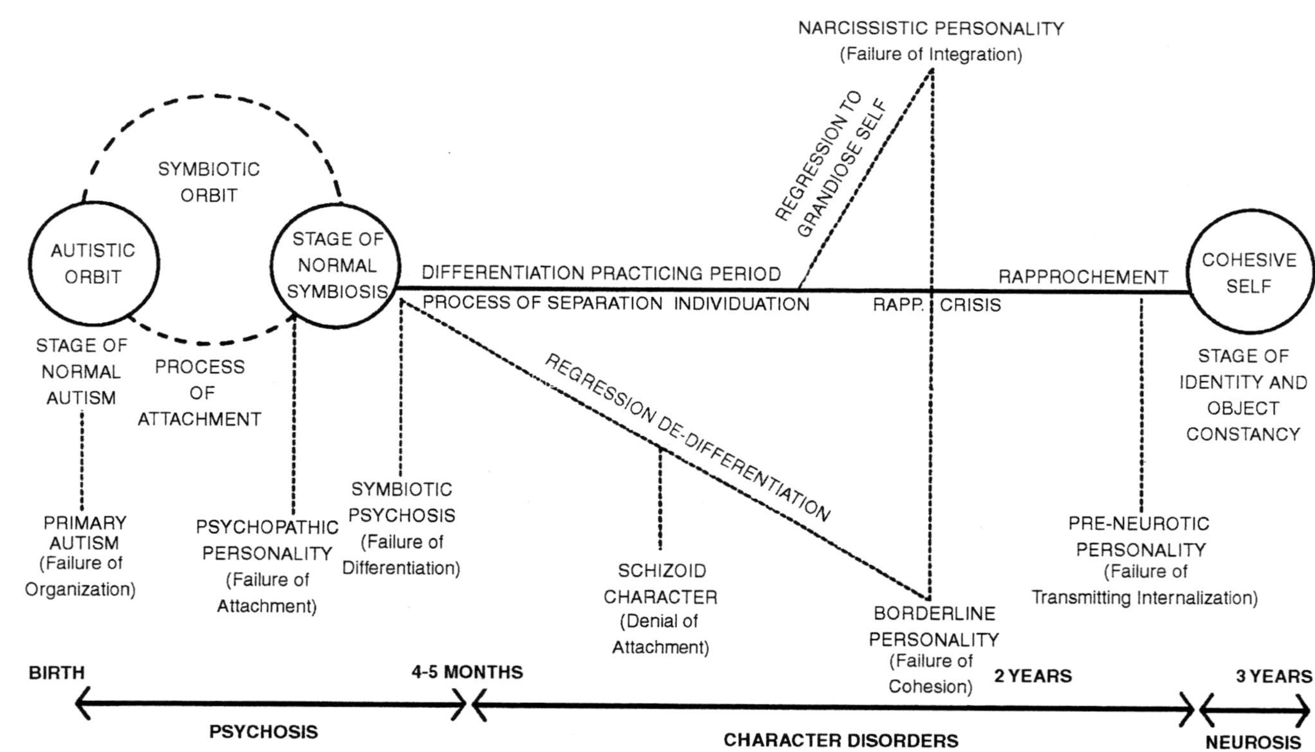

Adapted from A. Horner (1979)

Such a position clearly sets drug and alcohol dependence within the range of structural deficits commonly seen in character disorders. Khantzian sums up this position when he writes:

> Evidence has accumulated over the past two decades documenting a significant relationship between psychopathology and drug dependence. However, the etiologic connection or the relationship between the pathology and addiction has been less clear. Recent advances using standardized diagnostic approaches in psychiatry and a shift in psychoanalysis from a drive or instinct theory to a greater emphasis on adaptation, development and structural (ego and self) factors have provided new findings and perspectives in explaining the relationship between the psychological disturbances, dysfunction and the misuse of drugs.
>
> Although heavy reliance on drugs clearly produces psychological dysfunction and even psychiatric disorders, psychiatric and psychodynamic findings also suggest that substance abusers are predisposed to become dependent on drugs because they suffer with psychiatric disturbances and painful affect states. Their distress and suffering is the consequence of defects in ego and self capacities which leave such people ill-equipped to regulate and modulate feelings, self-esteem, relationships and behavior. (Khantzian, 1985, p. 1)

Considering the implications of this position, it is important to investigate Kohut's and Kernberg's descriptions of the narcissistic and borderline personality disorders.

BORDERLINE PERSONALITY ORGANIZATION AND PATHOLOGICAL NARCISSISM

The belief that typical personality traits establish themselves before the development of addiction is not universally accepted. However, Hartocollis (1964) presents evidence that these personality traits will be observed in formerly addicted patients after prolonged abstinence from alcohol, especially if these individuals have not received psychoanalytic treatment. Hartocollis' position is a clear example of the controversy that exists concerning the question of whether character pathology is the result or cause of addiction. In all probability, both positions are correct. Certainly, there are addicted individuals who present with a dual diagnosis of character pathology and addiction. There are also those individuals who present as if they were narcissistic and borderline due to the stress placed on their psychological system because of their alcohol or drug use. It will be important for the group leader to make a differential diagnosis because such a distinction has important implications for treatment. However, there are shared treatment recommendations, which suggest that the way Kernberg advocates treatment of borderline character pathology is very compatible with the treatment regimen recommended by Alcoholics Anonymous and those familiar with the disease concept approach to treatment. These similarities will be explored later in the chapter.

Hartocollis and Hartocollis (1980) sum up their position in the following paragraph, which emphasizes the deteriorating effect that alcohol and drugs can have on one's psychological functioning.

> . . . . alcoholics may for a long time manage to function in an apparently normal way. Narcissistic character traits, obsessive defenses, and a massive use of denial provide such individuals with a protective shield of self-deception, which isolates them from close personal contact with people whom they depend on but cannot trust. They feel empty and angry inside, very much like people with an "as-if personality," but so far as anyone else is concerned they are pleasant and function adequately. Gradually, however, as the cumulative impact of internal and external frustrations undermines the effectiveness of their protective devices, the level of their functioning begins to suffer, and, wishing to maintain their precarious emotional equilibrium, they resort to increasing amounts of alcohol, which has the power to reinforce denial, even though not performance, which continues to deteriorate, exposing further their borderline pathology. (1980, p. 99)

The fact that a person is addicted indicates that his or her primary defenses have been weakened on one level, yet strengthened on another. Drugs and alcohol become a substitute for a person whose basic mental mechanisms have lost their adaptive power. While drugs and alcohol provide temporary relief from psychic pain, their deteriorating chemical effect on the brain results in the use of more primitive defensive operations like denial, splitting, projective identification, and grandiosity. Secondary defenses are thereby erected within the context of the repression produced by alcohol and drug use, resulting in superficial, fragile, and maladaptive forms of reaction formation and obsessiveness. These defensive operations are attempts to shield the individual from the intolerable affects produced by loss of self-worth that leave them susceptible to frequent narcissistic injuries.

Such a developmental process can make the distinction between a narcissistic and a borderline disorder unclear. This problem is compounded by the fact that the distinction between the two conditions is not always clearly defined in the literature. In fact, a borderline patient for Kernberg is very likely to be viewed as a narcissistic patient by Kohut. Kernberg believes that a large portion of narcissistic individuals, if not all of them, share the same borderline personality organization.

Kohut, on the other hand, believes that many patients diagnosed as borderline are in actuality suffering from a narcissistic disorder of the self. The frequently cited behavioral pathology (i.e., rage responses, splitting, projective identification) of a borderline is the result of narcissistic injuries induced by the therapist's empathic failures.

KERNBERG'S BORDERLINE PATHOLOGY

Both Kohut and Kernberg have elaborated on how disturbances in early child development, especially around nurturance and dependency needs, lead to lack of identity integration and the development of a cohesive self. Although both have indicated that narcissistic and borderline pathology predisposes certain individuals to addiction, neither has systematically explored the relationship to addiction. Before that is attempted, a description of the borderline personality characteristics will be presented.

The *DSM-IV* lists criteria for the diagnosis of a borderline personality disorder. If five of the eight features are present, chances are strong that the individual may be suffering from the character pathology Kernberg describes. It also is important to discern whether these characteristics are the result of prolonged and excessive alcohol or drug use. Certainly anyone who has worked with alcoholics on a sustained basis will recognize these traits in most, if not all alcoholics, when they are acutely intoxicated. A schema (EAASSIII, PS) will be presented to help the group therapist understand these diverse characterological features.

1. *E.* Emptiness and Boredom; especially as these feelings relate to self and the lack of clear values and goals in life.
2. *A.* Affective instability; especially in relation to mood swings, impulsiveness, and unpredictability.
3. *A.* Anger; especially in the expression of intense anger and rage responses.
4. *S.* Stable Instability; especially in their interpersonal relationships, which are marked by a consistent history of intense, unstable relationships.

5. *S.* Self-Destructive; triggered by profound self-loathing and self-punitive superego development resulting in self-injurious behavior (i.e., suicide attempts, self-inflicted wounds, etc.).
6. *I.* Identity Confusion and Diffusion; a lack of identity integration.
7. *I.* Impulsiveness; especially in relation to acting out and alcohol and drug use.
8. *I.* Intolerance of Being Alone;
9. *P.* Psychotic Symptoms; capable of experiencing micropsychotic episodes from which they will quickly recompensate.
10. *S.* Superficial Adaptation; ability to relate on a superficial and social level.

Because many of these features and defenses are similar to the lower level defenses and features commonly seen in active alcoholics and addicts, many addicted individuals may be considered borderline, particularly in the way they respond to traditional psychotherapy. Most therapists from an object-relations viewpoint would fail to appreciate the impact that alcohol and drugs have on an addicted individual's behavior and would concentrate on the borderline personality organization in their treatment. Certainly in many cases, these issues must be addressed. However, the chances of successful intervention are enhanced if abstinence can be obtained.

Kernberg has specific suggestions for the treatment of borderline pathology that are significantly important because his approach does not conflict with that of AA. Specifically, Kernberg recommends supportive psychotherapy over insight-oriented psychotherapy or psychoanalysis. His suggestions are especially germane if they are applied after alcoholics or addicts have stopped their use of chemicals.

KERNBERG'S DESCRIPTION OF SUPPORTIVE PSYCHOTHERAPY

Kernberg says that supportive psychotherapy is preferred with borderline patients because they have such distorted images of others and do not possess a clear identity of their own selves (identity confusion). Their object relations are extremely poor and they have a tendency to split others into all good and all bad objects. They also cannot handle the regression that is produced by technical neutrality. Consequently, they require an active therapist who is going to confront and clarify their behavior (Kernberg, 1984).

Supportive psychotherapy has been criticized in the past because it has not been clearly defined. Many professionals look upon it as "Hertz rent-a-friend." Kernberg is well aware of this criticism and has outlined a treatment process that requires three components in its application.

1. Clarification and confrontation
2. Support–containing both:
   A. Affective components
   B. Cognitive components
3. Environmental intervention

Clarification and Confrontation

Psychotherapy with borderline patients requires an active therapist who will continually point out contradictions in the patients' behavior, especially differences between what the patients say and what the patients do. Little emphasis should be placed on the patients' past until the reality of the present is firmly established. Confrontation, however, does not mean angrily attacking borderline patients in a demeaning and critical fashion, since this will only narcissistically injure them and evoke primitive feelings of infantile rage. Rather, the contradictions in the patients' behavioral presentation must be clearly and firmly pointed out to them in a noncritical and supportive manner. The observed contradictions must be kept in the present because these patients have so much difficulty differentiating the past from the present. Before the past can be realistically explored, the present must first be made clear to them. Premature confrontations about the past will only lead to increased defensive distortions because they activate the patients' unresolved anger at injustices done to them in the past and raise fears that they will once again be disliked and rejected. Kernberg gives an excellent example of the detrimental consequences of premature confrontation with borderline patients.

> In the third session, the patient complained that Kernberg was angry, sadistic and controlling of him. At this juncture, Kernberg pointed out that the patient was describing him in the same terms and perceiving him in the same way that the patient had described his mother, namely as angry, bitter and unloving. "Could it be," Kernberg asked, "that you see me like your mother?" The patient readily agreed and added, "Yes, and it is my bad luck, after having such a mother, I get a psychoanalyst like this who treats me in the same manner." (Kernberg, 1983)

Supportive Psychotherapy

Kernberg's approach to psychotherapy for the borderline patient requires two components. The therapist must respond with both cognitive and emotional support. This does not mean the therapist only gives the patient a pat on the shoulder. Empathy, a key ingredient in a supportive approach, should not be confused with sympathy. Empathy, as Kohut describes it, requires being in tune with patients' feelings, both positive and negative. Affective and emotional support requires praise, encouragement, and a sharing of feelings. During the early part of treatment, borderline patients require an active therapist who will participate and interact with them. Cognitive support is also crucial. This requires giving patients advice at times, especially if it is directly asked for. It also means that the therapist will provide information that will help patients interpret their behavior and reality. However, Kernberg cautions against taking over too much control and evoking too strong of an idealizing transference. It is in this area of cognitive and emotional support that the group and AA provide an essential component to patients' treatment with less risk of compromising the therapist's position and the therapeutic relationship.

Environmental Intervention

Kernberg advocates that the therapist must actively intervene in patients' lives both inside and outside of the therapy hour. Outside intervention requires that the therapist talk with the family, school, or employer if necessary. Support systems (group, AA, etc.) must be established and encouraged. Kernberg believes this is crucial because patients could be destroying their lives outside of the therapy hour while the therapist methodically and painstakingly seeks to understand them. While this understanding of patients is a necessary and often slow process, it should not be accomplished at the cost of their outside lives just because the therapist does not want to compromise his or her stance of technical neutrality. Requiring borderline patients to attend AA meetings, calling their employers, and ensuring that they get to work on time are important steps in the treatment process that will allow the patients to survive as they gradually come to understand themselves and the meaning of their behavior.

Intervention is also required within the therapy hour. Acting out, both inside and outside the group session, must be curtailed. This requires limit-setting, confrontation, and clarification. Transference distortions must be identified and examined. It is crucial that patients be helped to understand the destructive ways they behave with the group members or the group leader that are parallel to the ways they behave with others outside of the group. Consensual validation from the group can be a critical component of recovery. However, Kernberg warns that external reality in the present must be clarified first before the past is explored. Kernberg gives an excellent example of intervention within the therapy hour:

> Kernberg described a patient who would smoke during the therapy hour, flick his ashes on the carpet and toss his cigarettes across the room in utter defiance of Kernberg's interpretations about his behavior. The man would agree with Kernberg's interpretations and respond with a big smile on his face, "Yes, I see how this is my way of showing disrespect for you and yes I agree this is very similar to my feelings toward my father." However, the patient's behavior did not change and he continued to toss his cigarettes across the room. The pleasure the man obtained from acting out was self-gratifying and consequently greater than his motivation to change. Finally, Kernberg told him he would stop the therapy sessions if the man continued to flick his cigarette and ashes on the floor of his office. At the announcement, the man promptly flicked his cigarette across the room. Kernberg stood up and asked the man to leave his office. The patient refused and Kernberg threatened to call security if he did not leave within twenty minutes because another patient was due at that time. The patient became enraged and told Kernberg, "This is not behavior suited for a psychoanalyst." Kernberg stood his ground and the patient left his office. The next session there was an affect storm in which the patient promptly tossed another cigarette across the room. Kernberg again required him to leave the office. The next session the patient did not toss his cigarette, but angrily attacked Kernberg for treating him in such a cruel and sadistic fashion. Kernberg explored the implications of this man's behavior in the subsequent sessions. Kernberg pointed out to the patient how he had provoked him to act in such a manner. In essence, the patient was told, "You are angry and cruel with me. You deny that you are angry and cruel; you treat me in a way that prompts me to be angry and cruel with you. Then you accuse me of the very behavior you deny in yourself." In essence, the patient's projective identification was interpreted. During this process, the patient remained reluctant to discuss the ramifications of his behavior. Kernberg had to repeatedly insist that their interaction be examined. Objections were continually put forth in a manner that would have resulted in compliance without understanding. "Look, I've stopped throwing my cigarettes across the room! Why do you insist on beating a dead horse," was an objection that would have

prevented this individual from understanding fully how his behavior had affected others. (Kernberg, 1983)

The key for Kernberg is the insistence that such an exchange be completely examined before it is dropped. Clarification needs to be completed or else the patient's experience would not have been integrated. In this case, this patient would have only perceived his interchange with Kernberg as another example of how people dislike him and treat him in angry and sadistic ways. Interpersonal distortions and object relations would not have been altered unless Kernberg had insisted on their examination and understanding.

Treatment from this perspective involves three key steps:

1. Clarification of their behavior. "This is what you are doing with me." Confront their distortions in a supportive, firm, and caring manner.
2. After they are completely aware of what they have done, gain consensual validation from the group and point out how they do this with others. Give them support, both cognitive and emotional.
3. Encourage them to act differently with others outside of the therapy hour.

NARCISSISTIC PERSONALITY DISORDER

Narcissism is frequently misunderstood by some as excessive self-absorption and self-love. In actuality, it represents individuals' attempts to create external self-presentations that are exciting, important, and recognized because they lack a firm sense of who they are internally. Woody Allen's movie, *Zelig*, is a clear example of an individual who lacks a solid core of identity and consequently succumbs to social and peer pressures (for conformity). Zelig is a chameleon. In the film, he not only acts and thinks accordingly with those whom he is around, but he actually begins to change his outward physical appearance to match theirs. In the company of obese individuals, he begins to balloon out in his appearance. With blacks, his skin begins to darken, and in the presence of orientals, his eyes become slanted. Zelig's life and his survival depends on his imitating and getting approval from those around him. While the movie can be viewed as a metaphor about social pressures toward conformity and loss of autonomy, the character of Zelig is an example of a severe personality disorder. More specifically, he represents the category of individuals commonly referred to as narcissistic personality disorders.

In order to understand such character pathology from a more objective perspective, the examination of the diagnostic criteria for such patients is in order. The *DSM-IV* lists eight features commonly present in the narcissistic personality disorder. It is important to note that while these characteristics are commonly seen features, they do not illustrate the complexity of narcissism as Kohut describes.

1. Grandiose Sense of Self-Importance; which often vacillates with strong feelings of unworthiness.
2. Preoccupation with Unlimited Sense of Power and Self; especially in relation to youth, appearance, beauty, and success. Needs to be seen with the right person and is fraught with envy.
3. Exhibitionistic Need for Constant Attention; desires admiration and recognition.
4. Cool indifference or rage and humiliation in response to criticism.
5. Feelings of Entitlement; expectations of others without reciprocity.
6. Exploitation of Others; without regard for personal integrity or rights of others.
7. Alternation from overidealization to devaluation of others.
8. Lack of Empathy; insensitive and unable to recognize how others feel.

Certainly, narcissism from this perspective is a pathological condition. Such individuals not only suffer enormous difficulties in their relationships with others and society at large, but they are usually intensely driven people who are deeply unsatisfied with themselves. However, Kohut views narcissism as having a much more complex set of dynamics. Narcissism, as defined by Kohut, is a compensatory structure established by individuals because of the deprivation they suffered as children. Narcissism is in many ways a self-preservative force responsible for helping children compensate for the continued narcissistic injuries suffered in a frustrating world and dysfunctional family system. Furthermore, it becomes an internal regulating system that allows children to adapt to an environment that is too insensitive to their struggle to recover from their lost sense of omnipotence. Kohut's view of narcissism therefore defines it as a driving force responsible for the establishment of the self, the enhancement of self-esteem, and the guardian for preserving the integrity of the self-concept. A major task of this force is to find meaning and give value to one's life.

Kohut goes beyond the *DSM-IV* in his description of the implications of narcissism for all of mankind. Kohut warns us that we all struggle with issues of narcissism. Not only do addicts and alcoholics have to guard against their tendency to be self-centered, grandiose, and easily offended, but we all have a propensity to believe we are the center of the universe. In this capacity, we can delude ourselves into believing we are special and unique while refusing to acknowledge our own mediocrity and limitedness. This is a theme that will be explored at length in Chapter 7 when the philosophical and psychological roots of Alcoholics Anonymous are investigated. For now, it will be enough to recognize that Kohut's explanation of addiction is important because it has a significant contribution to make in the treatment of chemical dependency and that it is a model which is in many ways highly compatible with AA. Kohut is attempting to get us to look at our self-centeredness and how our refusal to accept limitations in our lives not only leads to addiction, but to numerous other social, spiritual, and psychological difficulties.

Beyond the Ego: Kohut's Self-Theory

Heinz Kohut's work with patients whose central disturbance involved feelings of emptiness and depression is in many ways an extension of Margaret Mahler's observations concerning the roots of individuality in a child's development. Kohut found the need to extend psychoanalytic theory beyond its present concept of the ego so the patient's narcissistic vulnerability could be understood in terms of the patient's inadequately formed or damaged sense of self. Like Mahler, Kohut emphasizes the critical importance of the mother in permitting the development of internal mental structures for self-control and the eventual emergence of healthy individuality and separateness. Kohut emphasizes that a child's nuclear-self is formed during infancy and embodies the fundamental self-esteem, ideals, and ambitions of the child. The relationship with the mother allows the various agencies, drives, and conflicts of the mental apparatus to become unified into an integrated sense of self. However, the formation of the nuclear-self does not take place in relation to overt praise and rebuke. Rather, it is the empathic, nonverbal, intuitive responsiveness of the mother to her child's needs and the atmosphere she creates to validate healthy strivings that integrates or fragments the nuclear-self.

The nuclear-self is bipolar, organized around the two anchor points of ideals and ambitions. In his final book (Kohut, 1984), Kohut included a third constituent of the self, which involves the maturation of the alter ego or twinship needs. (See Figure 6.5.)

To help appreciate Kohut's (1977a) contribution to addiction and narcissism, an understanding of some of his key concepts is required. It is also necessary to examine many of the related contributions made by other object-relations theorists. Besides the work of Winnicott (1965), the theoret-

FIGURE 6.5.

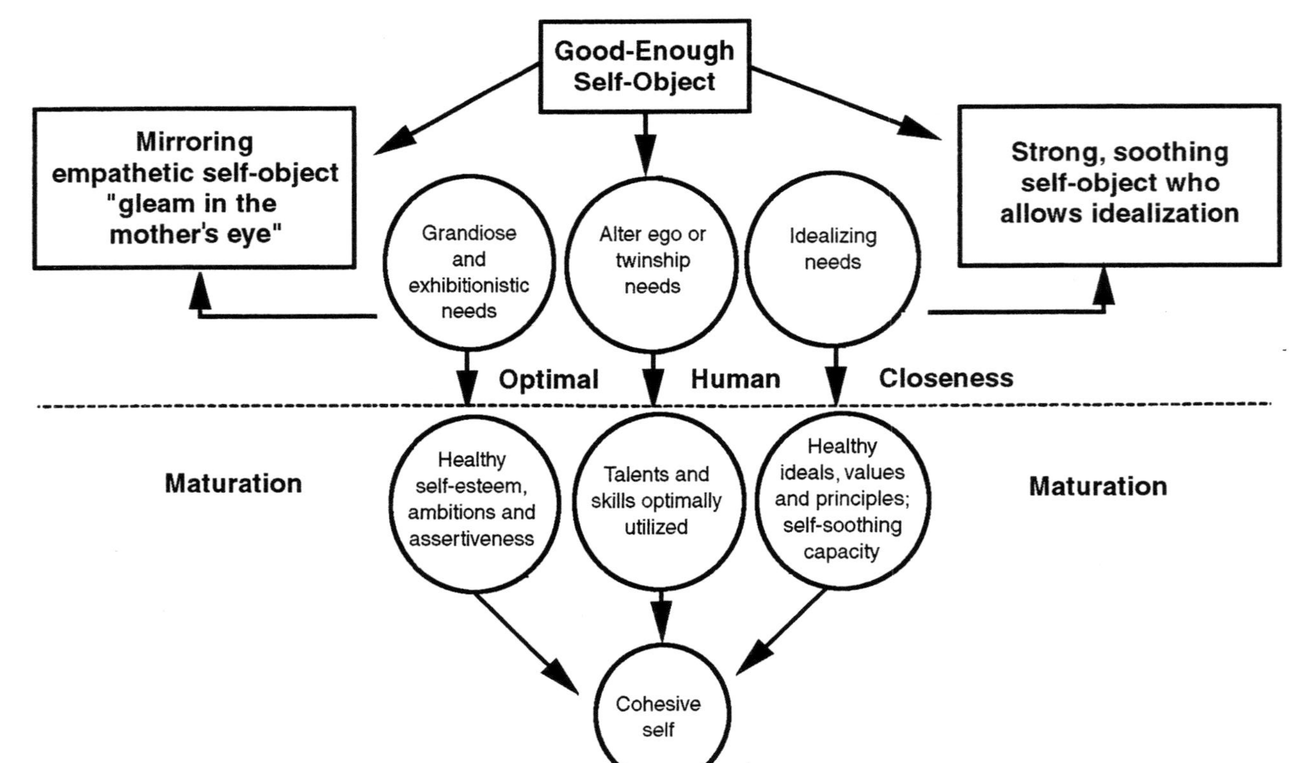

Adapted from E. Kahn (1985)

ical perspectives of Fairbairn (1952) and Guntrip (1971) have helped provide alternative explanations for personality and development that have important implications for addiction and its treatment. Listed below are seventeen key principles of object-relations theory.

1. An ego or self is present from birth.
2. Libido or instinctual energies are a function of or derived from the self and not the id.
3. There is no death instinct as Freud postulated. Aggression is not related to the id, but is a reaction to frustration or deprivation. In fact, there is no place for the concept of id within Fairbairn's theoretical view.
4. The self or ego and therefore libido or instinctual energy is fundamentally objects-seeking.
5. The original and earliest form of anxiety is experienced by the child as separation anxiety and is triggered by abandonment or failure of attunement.
6. Internalization of the object is a defensive measure originally adopted by the child to deal with frustrating and unsatisfactory aspects of the early parental figures.
7. The more frustrating and unsatisfying the early objects are in a child's development, the increased likelihood that these objects and their self-representations will be *introjected* and not just internalized.
8. Objects that are introjected always involve three related components: (A) Object-representation, (B) Self-representation, and (C) Affect related to the object and self-representations.
9. Two aspects of the introjected object (the exciting and the frustrating aspects) are split off from the main core of the object and repressed.
10. These two introjected object-representations are identified as the exciting (libidinal) or good object and the rejecting (antilibidinal) or bad object.
11. The self-representations are also split off in a similar fashion and are identified as the libidinal ego (good self) and the antilibidinal ego (bad self).
12. The main core of the internalized object, which is not repressed, is described as the ego-ideal.
13. Since the exciting (libidinal) and rejecting (antilibidinal) objects are collected by the original egos of the child, and owing to the fact that the repressed objects carry with them the collected self-representations of the libidinal and antilibidal egos, the individual is left

with a central core of the ego (central ego) that is not regressed, but acts as the agent of repression.

14. The resulting internalization of this situation leaves the original ego split into three parts. There is (A) a central ego (conscious) attached to the ego-ideal, (B) a repressed libidinal ego (good self) attached to the exciting libidinal object (good object), and (C) a repressed antilibidinal ego (bad self) attached to the rejecting antilibidinal ego (bad object).
15. This internal situation is the driving force behind what Fairbairn calls the basic schizoid position, which involves a true self that goes into hiding and remains detached from intimate human contact. A false-self (as-if personality) is constructed to deal with others in the external world.
16. Departing from Freud's drive theory, what was called the super-ego is identified as a tripartite structure consisting of (A) an ego ideal, (B) an antilibidinal ego, and (C) the antilibidinal object.
17. The antilibidinal ego (bad self), by virtue of its attachment to the rejecting antilibidinal object (bad object) adopts an uncompromising, hostile attitude toward all objects, even potentially good ones, and toward the libidinal ego (good self). Fairbairn came to call this self-representation the internal saboteur. It distrusts all promise of hope and especially potentially good objects whom it perceives might try to trick it into believing the promise is possible. It also attacks the libidinal ego (good self) for being stupid and gullible enough to believe the promise that it could be loved and for trusting that someone (libidinal object) could be loving of it without deceiving, abusing, or eventually rejecting and abandoning it.

Figures 6.6 and 6.7 are intended to be schematic representations of these seventeen positions that were outlined by Fairbairn and Guntrip. Figure 6.7 is intended to be a representation of a cohesive self with a healthy integrated psyche. Figure 6.6 is intended to be a representation of an uncohesive self that is dominated by the internal world of introjected self- and object-representations, which leave little psychic energy for authentic relationships in the reality of the external world. A false-self configuration rules its interaction with others, which results either in compliant or reactive (rebellious) behavior with others. Its core or true self remains minute and at times inaccessible to the central ego. Its internal world, repressed and unconscious, influences its interactions with others to the point that those individuals in the external world are gradually coerced or forced to comply with the internal realities of their inner experiences and expectations. Through the driving force of the repetition com-

FIGURE 6.6

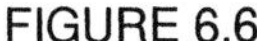

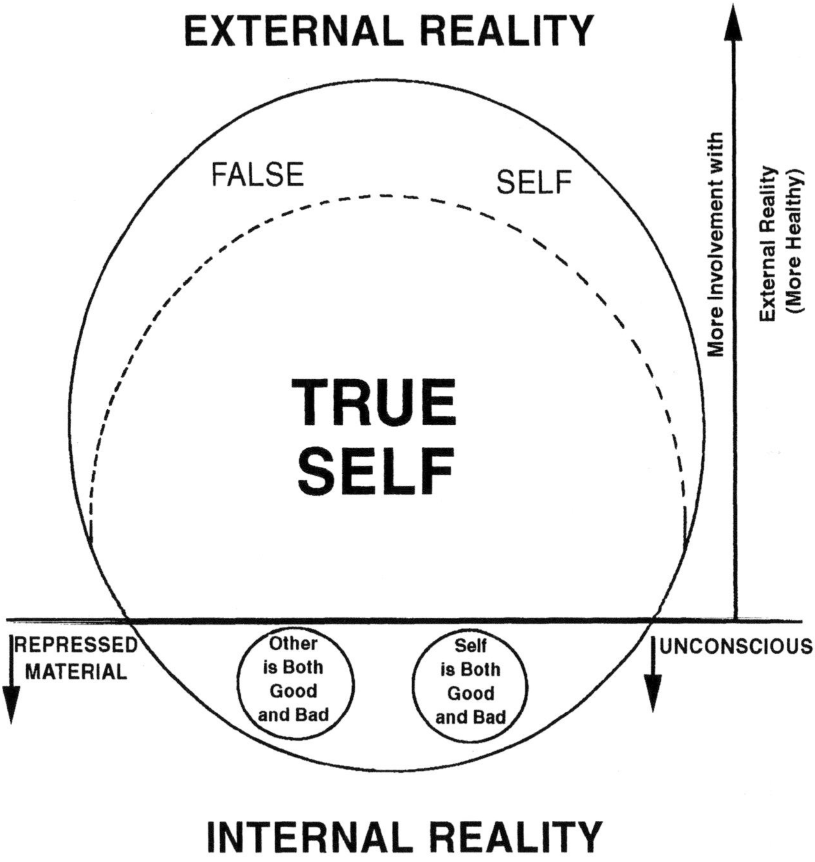

pulsion and the defense mechanism of projection-identification, the past continues to be repeated in the present, thus confirming all catastrophic expectations. Object choice (choosing people who are familiar to their internalized early objects) helps solidify this process. Paradoxically, even though this reenactment of the past in the present is painful, it produces some lessening of anxiety because it is familiar and removes the uncertainty of anticipation of the unexpected. "It has happened, just as I knew it would. I knew you would let me down and that I couldn't trust you."

Figure 6.7, in contrast, represents a cohesive self that has much less psychic energy tied into the past and introjected object- and self-represen-

FIGURE 6.7

EXTERNAL REALITY

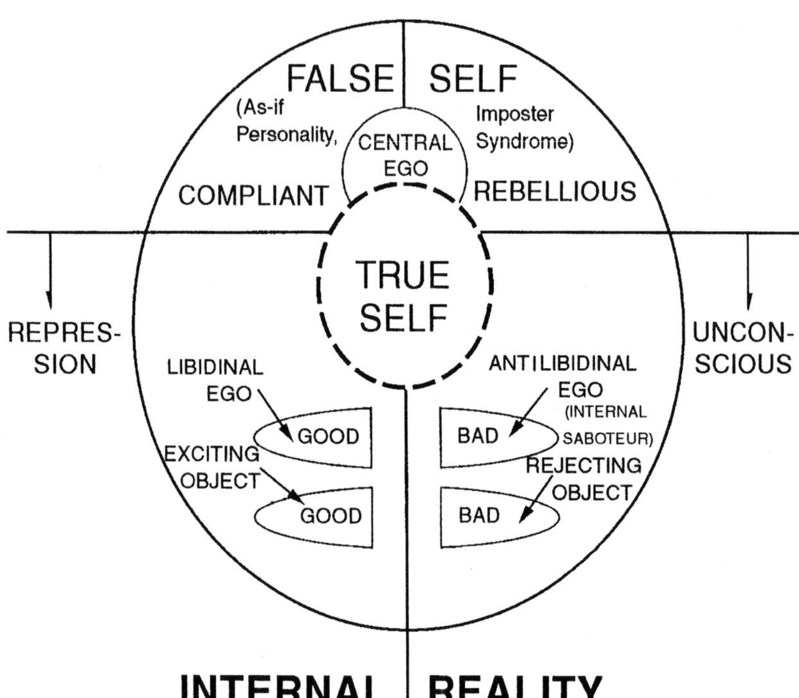

INTERNAL REALITY

1) Relationships are limited to idealize the fantasized other.

2) Feels unworthy, shameful, that their needs are sick and that their love can destroy. They are too needy.

1) Feels rejected and held in contempt by others.

2) Turns anger inward, attacks self and those that promise. Threatened by the possibility of hope.

tations. Many years ago, Freud drew the analogy of our psychic energy being very similar to that of an army. The larger our army, the more psychic energy we have available for authentic interactions in our external world. If, as children, we are forced to deal with an exorbitant number of conflicts and battles too early in our life, we will be forced to build a fort at each conflict and leave part of our army to man it. If we have to fight too many battles and consequently have to build too many forts, it leaves us depleted, with little psychic energy left for us as we continue to march forward in our life. The cohesive self has a much more accessible true self, and as the broken line in Figure 6.7 is meant to indicate, can easily influence and affect the self we choose to present to others. Such an individual has the capacity to present different aspects of him or herself as the situation dictates (e.g., social gathering, job requirements, conversation with a close friend, etc.), while holding onto internal consistency of the self. Less distortion occurs in interactions with others since the internalized object- and self-representations are integrated with good and bad aspects of each. Neediness and dependency have been worked through. The individual's internal life is no longer dominated by the pre-ambivalent infantile stage of dependency. The ambivalence of love and hate has been exchanged for a more mature stage of healthy dependency and the recognition that I, like others, am both good and bad.

Since the process of the internalization, or more correctly, the introjection of self- and object-representations, is such an integral part of this theory, an explanation of this process will be presented. The description is taken from an earlier article by Ogden (1983a). Ogden explains the foundation of the process when he writes,

> It is the thesis of the present paper that the internalization of an object relationship necessarily involves a splitting of the ego into parts that when repressed constitute internal objects which stand in a particular relationship to one another. This internal relationship is shaped by the nature of the original relationship . . . (p. 227)

Using more easily comprehended, nontechnical language in place of Ogden's more technically correct, but often obtuse and abstract language, the following sequence is presented to help clarify this process:

1. The child's early experience with a cruel, rejecting, critical, and cold mother shapes the nature of the internalized object relations.
2. The child, in order to manage the inherent difficulties of such an emotional assault, will repress the critical mother into his or her unconscious. The good aspects of the mother (good object) are split off from the

bad aspects of the mother (bad object). Not only is the bad object (critical mother) repressed, the self-representation (bad self) is repressed along with the intense emotional component of the relationship. The child is left with a bad object ("You are a terrible child"), a bad self ("I must be bad, I am a terrible child") and a self-representation that identifies with the internalized critical bad object ("I hate me like Mother hates me"). The idealized mother is kept conscious.

Ogden writes,

> To the extent that the "fit" between mother and infant is lacking, the infant experiences an intolerable feeling of disconnectedness and defends himself by means of splitting off the aspects of the ego which were felt to be unacceptable to the mother. These split-off portions of ego remain fixed in a relationship with the unsatisfactory aspects of the object. This part object relationship (split-off ego in relation to an emotionally absent or rejecting object) is repressed in order to master the feelings involved and in effort to change the object into a satisfactory object. . . . For example, the tantalizing qualities of the relationship and the rejecting qualities of the relationship become separated from one another in the infant's internal world. A significant aspect of the ego (the central ego) retains a relationship with the accepting and accepted qualities of the object (the good-enough mother [Winnicott, 1951] as opposed to the defensively idealized mother). (1983a, p. 230)

3. As an adult, the person has introjected inside of him or herself, an internalized object (critical mother and tantalizing mother), a self (bad child and good child), and an assortment of intense affects built on anger, rage, shame, and fear. Through the power of projective identification, these internal object relations lie dormant, ready to be activated by any close, intimate contact with objects in the external world.

4. The internalized object relationship gets played out with others through the use of projective identification. The person coerces objects in the external world to conform to the experience and expectancies of the internal world. Consequently, this "life script" gets played out or enacted by finding external objects (a cold, critical woman) that fit the internal object-representation (a cold, critical mother), or by coercing others to behave or treat them as is expected (i.e., in a cold, critical manner).

Ogden writes,

> projective identification is an interpersonal process in which one finds oneself being manipulated so as to be playing a part, no matter

> how difficult to recognize, in somebody else's phantasy. . . the person projectively identifying engages in an unconscious fantasy of ejecting an unwanted or endangered aspect of himself and of depositing that part of himself in another person in a controlling way. There is accompanying, real interpersonal pressure exerted on the 'recipient' of projective identification that is unconsciously designed to coerce him into experiencing himself and behaving in a way that is congruent with the unconscious projected fantasy. (1983a, p. 232)

5. Attachment to external bad objects (i.e., a cold, critical mother) is the result of the repetition compulsion and it is extremely difficult to release bad objects in the external world until internalized object- and self-representations are worked through or altered.

Ogden writes,

> resistance is understood in terms of the difficulty the patient has in giving up the pathological attachments involved in his unconscious internal object relations. . . . This tie is based on one's need to change the bad object into the kind of person one wishes the object were. . . . The second category of the bond to a bad internal object . . . takes the form of a crusade to expose the unfairness of, coldness of, or other forms of wrong doing on the part of the internal object. (1983a, p. 236)

6. The attachment to the tantalizing, internalized, split-off, good object- and self-representations is the collected bond that fuels the addictive process. The needy but undeserving good self-representation is not only a bottomless pit that can never be satisfied, but the tantalizing good object can never fulfill its promise of perfect love, acceptance, and complete nurturance without any limits or disappointments. The overindulgent, overgratifying, and inconsistent mother can be as damaging to the child's development as the cold, critical, and rejecting mother. In the former case, frustration tolerance is never internalized and impulse control is never mastered.

Ogden writes,

> one type of tie to a bad internal object is the attachment of the craving self to the tantalizing object. The nature of the tie to the object is that of the addict for the addicting agent and is extremely difficult to relinquish. (1983a, p. 236)

7. The antilibidinal ego (internal saboteur) becomes the repository of all the anger and rage that is accumulated around needing others (object

hunger) and the promise of hope and fulfillment. Not only does this rage get directed at the other (external bad object) who promises hope or love, it also gets directed at the self for needing and believing that things could be different. In the therapeutic setting, this would manifest with the patient not only resisting change, but actively attempting to sabotage it because any external change in behavior is a threat to internal object relations. Ogden writes,

> The object-component frequently maintains internal objectives by means of attempting to exert control over its object (i.e., control over the self-component of the internal relationship). The object-component may taunt, shame, threaten, lord over, or induce guilt in its object (the self-component of the internal relationship) in order to maintain connectedness with the self component. These efforts at control over the self-component become greatly intensified when there is a danger of the bond being threatened, e.g., by a more mature form of relatedness to the therapist that would make this internal, more primitive form of relatedness less necessary. (1983a, p. 238)

DEFINITION OF TERMS

Self-Objects: Self-objects are mental representations of others that we experience as part of ourselves. Expected control over them is closer to the sense of control that a mature adult would expect to have over his body and mind. In archaic forms, this control is expected to extend to others as if they were part of the self. There are two kinds of self-objects, mirroring and idealizing.

Mirroring Self-Object: Mirroring self-objects are objects who respond to and confirm the child's innate sense of vigor, greatness, and perfection. It is the gleam in the mother's eye as she is empathically in tune with the child's achievements. It is from this pole that the child's basic strivings for power and success emanate. Good-enough mothering results in the satisfaction of the child's healthy grandiose and exhibitionistic strivings. If these needs are adequately fulfilled, the child develops a healthy self-esteem with an appropriate sense of assertiveness and ambition. Failure of the self-object to optimally gratify the child's mirror-hungry needs results in individuals who need constant admiration, confirmation, and recognition from others because they are empty and cannot give this to themselves.

Idealizing Self-Object: Idealizing self-objects are objects with whom a child can merge as an image of calmness, infallibility, and omnipotence. If the child is presented with a strong, soothing self-object who allows idealization, he or she develops a capacity for healthy ideals, values, and principles. The child internalizes the calming, soothing qualities of the self-object and transmuting internalization is achieved. In contrast, children who do not have idealizing self-objects available are forever attempting to achieve a union with an idealized object, since in view of their specific structural defect (the insufficient idealization of their superego), their narcissistic equilibrium is safeguarded only through constant admiration, investment, and merger with a powerful other or ideal.

Empathy: Empathy is the mode of gathering data that allows the therapist to get a look at the inner mental life of people. Empathy is not just a useful way to gain access to the inner life of others; it is an attempt to experience others' feelings, wishes, hopes, and fears via vicarious introspection. The essence of psychotherapy lies in the therapist's protracted empathic immersion into the observed, for the purpose of data-gathering and explanation. Only after the others' experience is understood via vicarious introspection can it be explained. Scientific rigor is then employed in order to fit the observed and experienced data into a context of broader meaning and significance.

Optimal Frustration: Optimal frustration is the amount of anxiety, stress, or frustration infants can tolerate without detrimental effects on their ego, self, and development. Optimal frustration promotes growth and the development of psychic structure. Healthy personality development takes place under conditions of frustration that is not too long nor too intense. Just as too much or too little frustration in a given period can be an obstacle in a child's personality development, too little or too much frustration during psychotherapy can be an obstacle in the treatment experience.

Alter Ego or Twinship Merger: A firm self, resulting from the optimal interactions between the child and his or her self-objects, is made up of this third constituent in relation to the first pole from which emanate the basic strivings for power and success and the second pole that harbors the basic idealized goals. The core of the child's personality is determined by the tension arc in the intermediate area of basic talents and skills that is established between ambitions and ideals. This sector consists of the need of the self just to be like and with other people, a human among humans. Failure of the self-object during childhood development will result in individuals being unable to feel part of a larger whole. It will keep them alienated from their fellow humans and will prevent them from utilizing their talents and skills in a constructive manner.

Self-Object Transference: This refers to the revival of insufficiently responded-to childhood self-object needs in treatment and interpersonal relationships. (1) Mirror-hungry personalities thirst for self-objects whose confirming and admiring responses will nourish their famished selves. (2) Ideal-hungry personalities are forever in search of others they can admire for their prestige, power, beauty, intelligence, or moral stature. (3) Alter ego personalities need a relationship with a self-object that conforms to their own self's appearance, opinions, and values, thereby confirming the existence and reality of their own self.

Transmuting Internalization: It is in the matrix of a self-object environment that has responsive-empathic self-objects that a specific process of psychological structure formation develops. The nuclear self of the child is laid via the process of transmuting internalization. Structure building cannot occur without a previous stage in which the child's mirroring and idealizing needs have been responded to efficiently. Structure is laid as the consequence of minor, nontraumatic failures in the responses of mirroring and the idealized self-objects. These failures lead to a gradual replacement of the self-objects and their functions by the child's self and its functions. Self-regulating and self-soothing become internalized. It is the failure of transmuting internalization that leads the individual to seek externally (i.e., food, sex, drugs, others, etc.) what they cannot provide internally.

False Self: In the event that the integrity of the child's nuclear self is threatened, defensive or compensatory structures or a false self-organization may be established to prevent the self from further narcissistic injury. Such individuals develop an "as-if personality," frequently bolstered by a grandiose self that hides their "true self" from further fragmentation. Such a defensive process prevents them from nourishing their deflated sense of self because each success is attributed to the way they "acted" rather than the way they "really are." Consequently, they feel like "imposters" (i.e., imposter syndrome) who will eventually be discovered and exposed for what they really are.

The false self is a defensive function designed to hide and protect the true self. The false self accomplishes this by complying with environmental demands within five categories (Winnicott, 1965):

1. At one extreme: the false self sets itself up as real and it is this that observers tend to think is the real person.
2. Less extreme: the false self defends the true self. The true self is acknowledged as a potential and is allowed a secret life.
3. The false self has as its main concern a search for conditions that will make it possible for the true self to come into its own.

4. The false self is built on identifications and can take on chameleon-like properties.
5. The false self is presented by the whole organization of polite and well-mannered social constraints.

Ogden (1983a) gives an excellent and comprehensive description of Winnicott's false self contribution to object-relations theory:

> Donald Winnicott's major contribution to the development of a theory of internal object relations was his theory of multiple self-organizations functioning in relation to one another within the personality system. Winnicott envisioned the infant as born with the potential for unique individuality of personality (termed a True Self personality organization) which can develop in the context of a responsive holding environment provided by a good enough mother. However, when a mother substitutes something of herself for the infant's spontaneous gesture (e.g., her own anxiety over separateness for the infant's curious exploration), the infant experiences traumatic disruption of his developing sense of self. When such impingements are a central feature of the early mother-child relationship, the infant will attempt to defend himself by developing a second (reactive) personality organization (the False Self organization). This False Self vigilantly monitors and adapts to the conscious and unconscious needs of the mother and in so doing provides a protective exterior behind which the True Self is afforded the privacy that it requires to maintain its integrity.
>
> The False Self is not conceived of as malevolent; on the contrary it is a caretaker self that energetically "manages" life so that an inner self might not experience the threat of annihilation resulting from excessive pressure on it to develop according to the internal logic of another person (the mother). The dread of annihilation experienced by the True Self results in a feeling of utter dependence on the False Self personality organization. This makes it extremely difficult for a person to diminish his reliance on this False Self mode of functioning despite an awareness of the emptiness of life that devolves from such functioning. Functioning in this mode can frequently lead to academic, vocational, and social success, but over time, the person increasingly experiences himself as bored, "going through the motions," detached, mechanical, and lacking spontaneity. (p. 231)

Good-Enough Mothering: This is a term coined by Winnicott to describe the adaptive functioning of the mother that allows the child to lay down psychic structure as the result of optimal frustration. The good-enough mother does not gratify completely or traumatically frustrate the growing infant. Instead, she gradually diminishes her intuitive understanding for the sake of the child's furthering development and growing ability to tolerate frustration.

Application for Therapy–Corrective Emotional Expression

Refueling: During the practicing subphase, the infant ventures away from the mother; but as the child becomes fatigued, depleted, or anxious, he or she seeks to establish emotional contact with the self-object. The good-enough mother will allow emotional "refueling" without engulfing the child or pushing the child away in a rejecting fashion.

Splitting: As the infant begins to enter into the separation-individuation subphase, the symbiotic unit becomes split into four sets of images–good self, good object, bad self, bad object. The purpose of this split is to preserve the good images long enough for the infant to tolerate the awareness that "all good" and "all bad" images are the same person. Children are able to tolerate the realization that the "good mother" who feeds them is the "bad mother" who punishes them when they are bad. Developmentally arrested children, in order to protect themselves against the overwhelming anxiety produced by their inability to tolerate their mothers as both good and bad, will split their feelings into all-or-nothing or black-and-white images. Thus, their mothers cannot be both good and bad simultaneously. The child either internalizes and introjects the bad object into him or herself (i.e., I am bad, Mother is good) or idealizes the mother and projects the bad image onto the world (i.e., it is bad out there, I am good).

As a defense, Kernberg introduced the term "splitting" and defined it as an active defensive separation of the "all good" images from "all bad" images. Such a defensive process results in the individual being unable to keep a mental representation of an object as being capable of both good and bad images. Objects are idealized either as "all good" when gratifying or devalued as "all bad" when withholding. (See Figure 6.2.)

Projective Identification: This is a primitive defensive operation found in borderline personality structure. The purpose of the projection is to get rid of all bad internalized images by placing the images on others out there. Consequently, the outside externalized objects are perceived as bad (i.e., angry, threatening). An effort is then put forth by the individuals to control these externalized objects to prevent them from treating the individuals the way they fear they will be treated (i.e., attacked and controlled). Paradoxically, because of their suspicious defensive behavior, these individuals induce the very behavior in the others that they most dislike. They subsequently empathize and identify with this anger and feel confirmed in their belief that the objects out there are indeed bad (i.e., controlling and angry). Their suspicions become a self-fulfilling prophecy. Some examples will help clarify this important defensive process.

> A thirty-three-year-old cocaine addict became acutely intoxicated on cocaine and began to have fears that the people (police and the army) were after him. He proceeded to run down the street hiding behind mailboxes and telephone booths. Others, alarmed by his defensive, suspicious, and angry behavior, notified police, who began to pursue him. Upon perceiving police chasing after him, this individual's fears of being attacked and followed by others were confirmed. He consequently lashed out and attacked the police officers, justified in his beliefs that they were out to get him for no good reason.

> Ralph, a forty-two-year-old recovering alcoholic with five years of sobriety, was referred by his employer because of his constant arguments with employees at work. He performed his job more than satisfactorily, but because he created such distress in the office, he was about to be fired despite his excellent work record. After four group sessions, Ralph began to bitterly complain about the group leader's inadequacies. He insisted the group leader was not helping him and that the prices he charged for group sessions were outrageous and unfair. After the fifth session, he accused the group leader of looking at him in a disparaging way before he had entered the group session the previous week. He also accused him of reacting much more favorably to all the other group members and remarked that the group leader seemed to have a special dislike for him. Since this was completely untrue, the group leader explored this incident at length, eventually pointing out to Ralph that the way he (Ralph) was treating him was exactly the way he was treating all others in his life—namely, he would attribute to others (projection) qualities (anger, annoyance, criticism) that he possessed. He would then deny that he was treating them in this way and accuse others of behavior that was actually his own behavior (projective identification). The group leader was able to support his observations with a consensual validation from the group. Ralph, through feedback from the other group members, was able to realize an important defensive process that had led to many interpersonal difficulties in his life.

Transitional Object: This is Winnicott's (1965) concept that defines the infant's first recognition and choice of a possession that is "not-me." The possession is usually a blanket, a toy, or a teddy bear. The object usually facilitates the infant's recognition of separateness and soothes the child in the transition of becoming self-sufficient.

ADDICTION AS AN ATTEMPT AT SELF-REPAIR

In an attempt to explain the importance of self-psychology as a treatment approach, Howard Bacal wrote, "One simply cannot apply unmodified classical drive theory in the clinical situation and expect that the patient will feel understood" (1992, p. 56). In essence, Bacal is challenging what he describes as "a considerable discrepancy between what effective classical theorists preach and what they practice." This perspective has relevance for selecting the treatment approach when dealing with the chemically dependent individual. Bacal's criticism is reflective of his attempt to bring classical psychodynamic theory in line with the practicalities of treating the non-addicted patient. In a similar fashion, Khantzian has tried to do this for the addicted patient. It is no accident that both Bacal and Khantzian rely heavily on Heinz Kohut's self-psychology theoretical approach to accomplish this task because it offers a unique perspective, not only for addiction, but for all psychopathology. Self-psychology departs from Freud's classical drive theory with its emphasis on intrapsychic conflicts and moves the focus of attention to relationships and the age-appropriate developmental needs that were unmet and that led to arrested emotional development. Until this is repaired through the restoration of psychic structure, individuals will remain susceptible to seeking external sources of gratification because their internal self-structure is unable to provide this.

Addiction from this perspective is viewed as a misguided attempt at self-repair. Because of unmet developmental needs, certain individuals will be left with an injured, enfeebled, uncohesive, or fragmented self. Such individuals often look good on the outside, but are empty and feel incomplete on the inside. They are unable to regulate affect and in many cases are even unable to identify what it is they feel. Unable to draw on their own internal resources because there are not any, they remain in constant need (object hunger) of having those self-regulating resources met externally–out there. Since painful, rejecting, and shaming relationships are the cause of their deficits in self, they cannot turn to others to get what they need or have never received. Derivation of needs and object hunger leaves them with unrealistic and intolerable affects that are not only disturbing to others, but shameful to themselves. Consequently, alcohol, drugs, and other external sources of gratification (i.e., food, sex, work, etc.) take on a regulating function while creating a false sense of autonomy, independence, and denial of need for others. These attempts at self-repair can also take on obsessive-compulsive qualities (i.e., gambling, sexual perversions, masochistic-sadistic relationships), which only exacerbates their original difficulties. As Krystal (1982) suggests, addiction is an attempt at self-help that fails.

In his earlier work with narcotic addicts, Khantzian (1985) first recognized that opiates were the drug of choice for certain individuals because of their specific pharmacological effects. Opiate and heroin addicts prize their drug for its antiaggressive effects. It helps them soothe and calm their intense feeling of rage. Khantzian hypothesized that it isn't pleasure so much that addicts are seeking; rather they are attempting to regulate their emotional selves and escape, even momentarily, from the constant feelings of deprivation, shame, and inadequacy that dominate their lives. Drug addicts and alcoholics frequently describe themselves as "feeling as if I am always a quart low" or "It wasn't until I started using drugs that I felt normal." In his later work with cocaine addicts, Khantzian found that individuals who felt bored, empty, dead inside, or that life was meaningless were frequently drawn to stimulants. Later experience showed Khantzian that counterdependent, restricted, and inhibited individuals were likely to be drawn to alcohol and sedatives. Highly anxious and fearful people were most likely to become dependent on minor tranquilizers, while the more isolated and schizoid individuals were attracted to marijuana and the hallucinogens. As Khantzian (1982) wrote,

> . . . this self-selection is related to the distinctive psychoactive actions of various drugs . . . in the course of experimenting with different drugs, an individual discovers that the action of one drug over another is preferred. (p. 757)

While Khantzian's classifications do not fit in all cases with all individuals exactly as he describes, there is some merit in his observations. But more important, his self-medication hypothesis begins to point to addiction as the result of self-deficits and affect-deficits due to structural impairments that have affected the addict's or alcoholic's capacity for self-regulation. Chemically dependent individuals are in a sense acting as their own uncertified physicians to fix or repair what they are missing.

Khantzian and other psychodynamically oriented theorists (Krystal, 1982; Wurmser, 1978; and McDougall, 1989) began to draw on self-psychology and object-relations theory to help provide a more comprehensive and applicable theory of addiction. A growing consensus began to emerge that suggested four related problem areas that consistently manifest themselves with all addicts and alcoholics:

1. Self-esteem vulnerabilities that lead to the establishment of a false self with grandiose defenses to help combat overwhelming feelings of shame and humiliation.
2. Self-care failures.
3. The inability to identify, tolerate, and regulate their affect.
4. Difficulties establishing and maintaining healthy, mutually gratifying relationships that are not exploitive, controlling, sadistic, or masochistic.

SELF-ESTEEM VULNERABILITIES

Because alcoholics and addicts do not possess the internal structure necessary to combat their nauseous sense of fragmentation, anxiety, and failing self-esteem, they are drawn to external sources (i.e., alcohol, drugs, sex excitement, food, etc.) in their attempts to self-soothe and self-calm (i.e., transmuting internalization).

Kohut and Wolfe write,

> Individuals whose nascent selves have been insufficiently responded to will use any available stimuli to create a pseudo-excitement in order to ward off the painful feeling of deadness that tends to overtake them. . . . Adults have at their disposal an even wider armamentarium of self-stimulation–in particular, in the sexual sphere, addictive promiscuous activities and various perversions, and in the non-secular sphere, such activities as gambling, drug and alcohol induced excitement, and a lifestyle characterized by hypersociability. If the analyst is able to penetrate beneath the defensive facade presented by these activities, he will invariably find empty depression. (Kohut and Wolfe, 1978, p. 418)

In Kohut and Wolfe's view, the individuals' inability to obtain self-soothing via transmuting internalization is the reason they attempt to find relief from these tensions by the use of alcohol and drugs. It is the alcoholics' and addicts' inability to calm and soothe themselves that leads them to look for others to do for them what they are unable to do for themselves. Since their self-object needs and desires are distorted, they are continually disappointed in their relationships and the attainment of their goals. Seeking from the outside what can only be furnished from the inside leads to constant frustration and despair. Most alcoholics' and addicts' lives are dominated by a deficiency in which they experience themselves as being empty and deprived. They believe that if only another would supply them with this deprived "refueling," they could become whole and complete. They are inevitably disappointed, because as mature adults, they can no longer tolerate having these infantile needs satisfied in infantile ways. Consequently, they constantly battle to deny their sense of neediness. They become counterdependent and perceive others as rejecting and withholding. "If you loved me, you wouldn't disappoint me. Since I am disappointed, you don't love me." Their use of splitting, projective identification, and fear of closeness makes it impossible for them to obtain any satisfying relationships. They become resentful, disappointed people who do not understand the part they play in this process. Alcohol and drugs become their sole mistress and their only friend.

Narcissism Redefined

One of Kohut's primary contributions is a change in the way narcissism is conceptualized. Kohut legitimated narcissism as a normal, developmentally healthy, and age-appropriate need for object relatedness. From Kohut's perspective, narcissistic needs are not regarded as selfish, but reflective of a disturbance in the relationships between the self and its most significant others or self-objects. The classical drive theory regarded narcissism as selfishness or self-centeredness that reflected a stubborn insistence by an immature individual on having everything his or her own way. (This is a very similar description of what AA refers to when it speaks of the ego.) Kohut made the important distinction between healthy and unhealthy narcissism. Phase-appropriate, empathic responsiveness to the child's self-object needs is essential for the cohesion and development of the self and leads to healthy self-esteem. Without the idealizing or mirroring self-objects, a child is likely to grow up with a narcissistic behavioral or personality disorder. In either case, the individual is left without the internal structure necessary to manage the emotional injuries and disappointments that are sure to follow later in that life. As Bacal (1985) writes,

> the defects in the self produced by faulty responses of self objects lead this individual to establish what Kohut called transference like states, where he looks for self objects in his later life to provide him with the responses which he missed in order to repair the self. (p. 488)

From this perspective, Bacal is looking at relationships as attempts at self-repair much like Khantzian is when he posits that self-medication or the use of drugs and alcohol are attempts at self-repair.

Healthy self-esteem is the end product of sufficient age-appropriate responsiveness and parental emotional attunement. Healthy parental role models provide the other necessary component of idealization that leads to healthy narcissism, which is basic to emotional health and consists of a subjective sense of well-being and confidence in one's self-worth. A person who "feels" a balanced valuation of their importance and potential and can relate in mature ways to others will usually have a sense of meaning and know how they fit in the world.

In contrast to this, even though the majority of cocaine addicts and alcoholics appear to be very successful and are high achievers in their professional lives, those who work with these patients on a consistent basis are struck by how fragile their basic sense of self-worth has been. Despite their exaggerated striving for financial, physical, and intellectual success, their needs for approval and acceptance leave them consistently vulnerable to injury, rejection, shame, and humiliation.

Healthy and Unhealthy Narcissism

Self-psychology has consistently viewed healthy narcissism or mature narcissism as reflective not of the decrease of emotional investment in one's self but as reflective of a person's ability to establish mutually satisfying relationships with others in which giving and receiving are balanced. As Ornstien (1981) writes, "When . . . the self attains the capacity for becoming a relatively independent center of initiative . . . it is then also capable of recognizing the relatively independent center of initiative in the other" (p. 358). In the case of healthy narcissism, the person can hold a healthy respect for his or her uniqueness while at the same time being able to be in reciprocal resonance with the unique qualities and independence of another. Such a person can give as well as take and does not need to be one-up or one-down in a relationship.

In contrast, unhealthy narcissism, which manifests through narcissistic behavior or personality disorders, is seen in individuals who are incapable of true reciprocal mutuality in a relationship. They will either need to be one-down–where they idealize the other, or one-up–where they need the other as a mirroring self-object to furnish them with confirmation of their specialness. Mirroring self-objects are eventually devalued and held in contempt after they are used up. Once someone has lost his or her functional utility, he or she would be discarded like an old suit of clothes or traded in for a new model as one would do with an old automobile that is no longer stylish or efficient. Because individuals with a true narcissistic personality disorder are contemptuous and shameful of the less-than-perfect aspects of themselves, they cannot tolerate them in others.

Narcissism from this perspective ceases to be a source of healthy self-respect and self-esteem and becomes a defense—a false self or grandiose self that guards against painful feelings of shame and low self-worth. As Morrison (1989) and others convincingly argue, shame or humiliation is always the underbelly or the driving force behind a narcissistic defense. AA has long recognized that it is the individual's grandiosity, self-centeredness, and lack of humility that are the most difficult obstacles to overcome in addiction. Using technically incorrect terms drawn from psychodynamic concepts, they nevertheless capture the essence of the issues that must be addressed in recovery. Long before Kohut's self-psychology and the theoretical formulations of grandiosity and narcissism, early pioneers in the treatment of alcoholism such as H. Tiebout were writing in the 1950s about the necessity of ego factors and "surrender of the inflated ego" in alcoholics' recovery. In 1971, Bateson wrote about alcoholics' reluctance to relinquish their "false pride" as the biggest obstacle to recovery. While the terminology may be different, the basic premise is the same. Early theorists were recognizing that narcissistic features such as grandiosity were a primary corollary in the addiction process.

False pride, inflated ego, and grandiosity are consequently viewed as defenses against feelings of inferiority and inadequacy. As Tiebout (1954) suggests, one has to inflate oneself for a reason. If a person felt or believed they were enough, there would be no need for inflation of self or false pride. From this perspective, a sense of self-esteem, confidence, and pride would reflect healthy narcissism and imply that there would be no need for grandiosity. It is when individuals suffer from the absence of self-esteem that they are left with a set of intolerable affects often referred to as shame. Writing from a self-psychology perspective, Morrison (1989) sees that "the self's experience of shame is so painful that the narcissistic constrictions of perfection, grandiosity, superiority, and self-sufficiency are generated to eliminate and deny shame itself. . . . Shame, then, can be viewed as an inevitable feeling about the self for its narcissistic imperfection for failure, for being flawed" (p. 66).

Morrison and others view shame as the cornerstone of all psychopathology. To feel shame implies feeling exposed and having allowed others to have seen one's imperfections. Shame, by definition, requires that these imperfections remain hidden, not only from others, but eventually from the self. Embarrassment and humiliation are the inevitable results when individuals feel that they have left themselves exposed so that their badness, weakness, powerlessness, and neediness has been seen by others. On one end of the continuum are the shame-prone individuals who experience vulnerabilities and ordinary human shortcomings or failures as indictments that must be denied and avoided at all costs. At the other end are those individuals with narcissistic disorders who are so defended against their shameful imperfections that they convince themselves that they can do no wrong. They simply do not make mistakes! It is always the other person's problem or fault. In even more extreme cases, they are incapable of feeling healthy shame because they are so defended. Such individuals are essentially shameless. As Kurtz (1983) and Bradshaw (1993) point out, being shameless is far different than being guiltless. The latter implies innocence and indicates no wrongdoing. To be shameless indicates a very serious defect in character because individuals either lack or do not have access to the healthy internal signals of shame that help them set limits on the self and be respectful of the boundaries of others. Such individuals are susceptible to exhibitionistic and voyeuristic tendencies. In some cases, they can become sexually fixated, resulting in sexual perversions.

Figure 6.8 is intended to show the delicate balance that is inherent with healthy narcissism and healthy shame. When this balance is achieved, individuals have access to both sides of this continuum. When unhealthy narcissism predominates, as with narcissistic disorders, the narcissism takes on pathological aspects and the shame end of the pole is driven underground out of awareness. When individuals are dominated by their shame, the healthy components of narcissistic resources are unavailable to them and the shame takes on masochistic qualities.

The cycle of remorse, shame, and self-contempt that addicts and alcoholics experience the morning after an embarrassing evening of alcohol and drug use is what spurs the false promise to stop all drug and alcohol abuse and vow to never let it happen again. Alcohol and drugs are initially used to bolster the narcissistic defenses because the initial feeling of shame is such a prominent ones in the chemically dependent person's life. This attempt at self-repair only exacerbates the condition, partly due to its tendency to contribute to the rigidity of the defenses. When the inevitable backlash hits, the shame and remorse is so intense that alcoholics or addicts are forced to combat it with their only available resources, namely, alcohol or drugs.

From a self-psychology perspective, shame is the result of failures in early object relationships–either because of active, humiliating attacks or as a result of disruptions in empathic attunement by significant self-objects. Shame-prone people, as a result of compensatory defenses, are often excruciatingly ambitious and success-driven, responding to all failures as indictments and proof of their innate defectiveness. Shame can only be contained by constant achievements, grandiosity, or addictive-compulsive acting out. Exhibitionistic components of grandiosity reflect the need to be seen by others as powerful, independent, beautiful, and successful. The

FIGURE 6.8. Balance of Shame and Narcissism

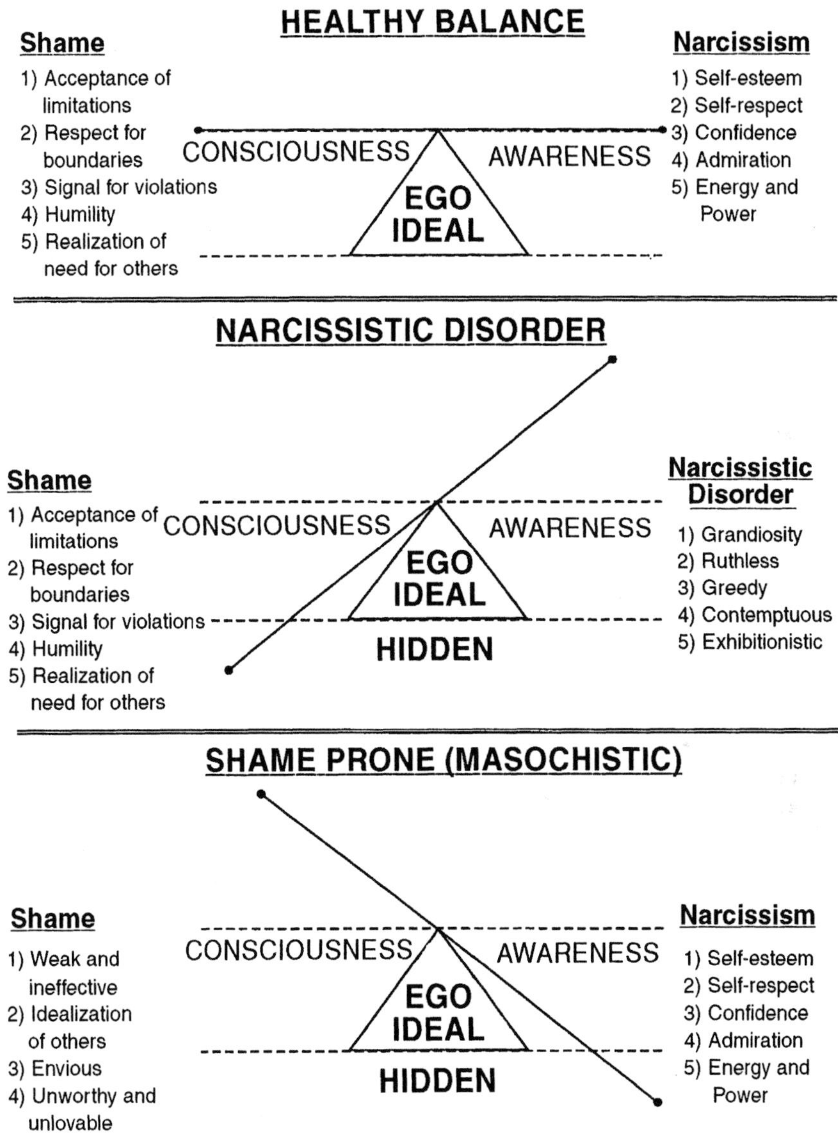

"showing off" of one's self is a defense that also distracts others from possibly seeing what is hidden (inadequacies, imperfections, and shortcomings). The narcissistic individual is like the magician in the circus sideshow, who is constantly employing sleight of hand as a distraction to get others to pay attention only to what the magician wants them to see so that they do not notice what is being hidden. Grandiosity as a defense should not be confused with grandiosity as a healthy component of psychic structure. As Bacal suggests:

> The one would reflect the sense of personal conviction of one's unique importance. This would be a self-percept that presumably arises out of optimal experiences of mirroring by self-objects. It is affectively toned in a healthy way. The other, which would be closer to the traditional notion of grandiosity, would reflect a self-percept that is inflated beyond what the individual would normally experience. This may properly be regarded as a pathological self state; and it is associated with a disavowed sense of low self-esteem. (1992, p. 72)

The relation between self-esteem, narcissism, grandiosity, and shame has tremendous implications for the treatment of addiction. Drugs and alcohol become such an intricate part of the grandiose defenses that it is impossible to separate them from one another. Once chemicals are no longer being used to bolster the grandiose self and its defenses, the narcissistic characterological features can then be dealt with more effectively. The shameful aspects of the self that were previously disavowed will surface, and until these are owned, acknowledged, and accepted, characterological change is impossible. Unless character defects are removed or characterological patterns are altered, the addicted individual will be continually vulnerable to relapse or prone to substituting one addiction for another. This is where self-psychology and the twelve-step philosophy join forces in explaining, understanding, and treating addiction. Both perspectives complement each other or furnish very similar recommendations for treatment even though their language is different. The resolution of shame and the treatment of disorder of the self will be dealt with more extensively in the chapters on AA (Chapter 7) and long-term treatment (Chapter 11).

Self-Care

Alcoholics and addicts are notorious for their self-destructive and self-defeating behavior. They essentially lack the ability to take care of themselves and protect themselves from self-defeating actions. Because chemically dependent individuals suffer with a deficient or underdeveloped ego capacity for modulating their feelings, they are often unable to tell when they are tired, sick, hungry, anxious, or depressed. Along with their history of substance abuse, they usually have numerous other notoriously poor health habits. Many smoke incessantly, do not exercise or overexercise, have poor dietary regimens, and demonstrate an almost complete inability to relax and enjoy themselves. Such disturbances in self-care also lead individuals to fail to be aware, cautious, worried, or frightened enough to resist or avoid behavior that is injurious or damaging. Because they were often poorly parented as children and since many come from alcoholic or dysfunctional families, they are poorly prepared to properly evaluate the consequences of risky or self-damaging behavior. They are constantly placing themselves in potentially destructive and painful circumstances. Unsatisfying and dysfunctional interpersonal relationships are the norm for them. Khantzian (1982) sees this inability for self-care as developmentally determined. Writing about Mahler and other developmental theorists, he contends, "They emphasize the importance developmentally of optimal parental nurturances and protection early in children's development for the establishment of this function, and how extremes of deprivation or indulgence have devastating consequences for the development of this capacity" (p. 589).

Affect Regulation

Whereas self-care limitations prevent addicts and alcoholics from guarding against continual self-defeating and dangerous behavior, they also suffer from deficits in ego functioning, which interferes with their ability to use their feelings as guides or signals in managing and protecting against the instability and chaos of their internal emotional lives. Alcoholics and addicts have a disturbance in the regulation of affect that manifests as "an inability to identify and verbalize feelings, an intolerance or incapacity for anxiety and depression, an inability to modulate feelings, activation, and initiate problems, and extreme manifestations of affect, such as hypomania, phobic-anxious states, panic and lability" (Khantzian, 1982, p. 590).

If development is undisturbed, feelings act as guides or signals for regulating one's behavior. Because alcoholics and addicts suffer from developmental arrest, they usually fail to differentiate or progress in the development of understanding their feelings. Consequently, they are unable to use feelings as signals or guides. As Khantzian states, "They suffer an ego defect in their stimulus barrier whereby they are either unable to identify affects, or their feelings are unbearable or overwhelming. As a result, denial or the effects of alcohol are used to ward off overwhelming feeling states in circumstances that would not be traumatic for other people (1982, p. 591). Such individuals are then unable to soothe or comfort themselves when distressed and become dependent upon an external agent to do so.

Dependency and the Self

The defect in the self leads to failures in ego-ideal formation. In Kohut's (1977b) schema, alcoholics and addicts have not adequately internalized the admired and admiring, encouraging, valued, and idealized qualities of their parents. As a result, they lack self-worth and suffer from chronic feelings of poor self-esteem. As a consequence of their inability to accurately evaluate themselves and judge their relationships, they greatly depend on sources outside themselves for approval and confirmation. Outside activities and the use of and dependence on others are attempts by alcoholics and addicts to feel good about themselves because they are almost totally unable to achieve this for themselves from within.

Kernberg (1975) stresses how the rigid and primitive defenses of these individuals lead to repression and dissociation of parts of the self. Alcohol and drugs can be viewed as an attempt to refuel the grandiose self and activate the all-good self-images and object images while denying the all-bad internalized objects. Krystal (1982) has suggested that because of these defensive operations, alcoholics and addicts are unable to experience their feelings unless they drink or use drugs. Chemical use thereby allows a brief and tolerable experience of such feelings.

Alexithymia

Alexithymia has been identified as a characteristic pattern indicating an inability to name and use one's emotions. Alcoholics' and addicts' inability to verbalize feelings leads to the somatization of affect responses. This results in them being confronted with sensations rather than feelings. Such physiological sensations are not useful as signals, but remain painful and overwhelming. Such painful affective states call attention to the uncomfortableness rather than to the "story behind the feelings." Such individuals are marked by their striking inability to articulate their most painful, bothersome, and important feelings. Many, if not all of their feelings are translated into somatic complaints about physical discomfort and craving. Alcohol and drugs are then used to block the affect, preventing the individual from interpreting and attending to the signal. Krystal (1982) sees this as also contributing to "a diminution in the capacity for drive-oriented fantasy. Thinking becomes operative, mundane and boring. The capacity for empathy with development of utilizable transference is seriously diminished" (p. 614). In short, alcoholics and addicts lose the capacity to enjoy themselves or others unless they are drinking or using drugs.

Anhedonia

Many alcoholics and addicts do not possess the capacity to experience joy, pleasure, or happiness. Drugs are virtually the only way they can obtain gratification and relief from distressful affective states. Krystal (1982) views this as a consequence of infantile traumatization resulting in a "doomsday" orientation, involving a constant dreaded expectation of the return of the unbearable traumatic state. Such individuals will then keep themselves very active for they fear slowing down, lest their expected catastrophe occur. Krystal (1982) writes about the importance of this in treatment:

> there is hardly any knowledge about how to help the patients to cultivate their capacity for pleasure and joy. This problem is an especially serious one in dealing with the alcoholic professional, such as the alcoholic physician. These individuals tend to present a combination of severe compulsiveness, "work addiction," and anhedonia underlying their problem drinking. The drug is often used to maintain a severe machine-like self-control regime. Many of these patients maintain for a long time a very high degree of success in their professional and business careers. Their "superb" adjustment to reality is actually part of the "operative" life style. (p. 615)

Affect Regression

Wurmser (1978) has constructed a heptad of specificity in compulsive drug use. The cycle of the addictive process involves seven steps and is always initiated by a significant acute narcissistic crisis (i.e., disappointment in self or a love object). This is experienced as an unbearable blow to self-respect that plunges the individual into a regressive spin. In succession, the individual experiences the following:

1. There is a sudden plummeting of self-esteem triggered by a "big letdown" from an expectation that may be justified, but usually greatly exaggerated.
2. The narcissistic injury produces an affect regression that cannot be articulated into words. The feeling is an uncontrollable, intense sense of rage, shame, or despair. Affect defenses are broken down and inadequate to contain internal feelings.

3. The affect disappears and a vague but unbearable tension remains. There may be a longing, a frantic search for excitement and relief. As a result of integrative dysfunction, there is an increasing dependence on externalization (i.e., drugs, excitement to self-soothe). Splitting occurs between observing and acting. More troublesome feelings are suppressed, massively denied, and disavowed. The individual fails to appreciate and interpret what he or she has experienced and perceived.
4. This development leads to desire for action, a search for an external concrete solution to the denied internal conflict. Aggression, excitement, and drugs (external objects) are acted upon so individuals can direct their affect outward away from internal uncomfortableness.
5. Aggression can now be dealt with by externalization. However, it is usually directed against the self (shame, humiliation) as well as being directed against others (violating social limits, transgressing boundaries). The reassertion of power by externalization requires the use of archaic forms of aggression.
6. Splitting of the superego occurs. As Wurmser (1978) writes, "The drowning man has commonly little regard for questions of integrity." Trustworthiness, reliability, and honesty are utterly irrelevant because despair has taken over. While commitments to others are acknowledged, they are treated with little importance.
7. The final point is enormous pleasure and gratification. The acute narcissistic crisis is temporarily resolved and the demand for the restoration of this blissful condition creates an extraordinarily demanding, unrealistic attitude on the part of individuals, which predisposes them to severe disappointment and thus to increased narcissistic vulnerability. This cycle is then complete and they are returned to the starting point of what Wurmser calls the "vicious cycle." Patients are back where they started with a much lower level of self-esteem and vulnerability.

Interpersonal Relations

Until substance abusers are able to form mutually satisfying relationships with others, they will remain vulnerable to addiction. There is an inverse relationship between individuals' capacity to form healthy reciprocal intimate relationships with others and their tendency to turn to drugs, alcohol, sex, food, excitement, work, and various other forms of compulsive distractions as substitutes for this need. As the object-relations and self-psychology theorists repeatedly contend, we are object-seeking animals from birth. We are driven innately to seek close human contact. To the degree that we are deprived of this or have an inability to accomplish this task we are emotionally sick or deficient in our psychological make-up. The much-quoted and often-seen bumper sticker that advocates "Hugs, Not Drugs" is a lot closer to the mark that we sometimes realize. This is not to imply that someone can be loved into health; this is a wish or fantasy that is unrealistic and is the force for co-dependency. Rather, a person's denial of a need for others is also a denial of being human. It often leads us to substitute things (i.e., drugs, alcohol, sex, food) for human closeness, warmth, and caring. Ernest Kurtz (1979) views the mutuality of AA–one alcoholic needing and helping another–as the cornerstone of the recovery process and the main reason why twelve-step programs are so successful. Isolation of one's self from the rest of humanity is one consequence of shame and the driving force behind addiction, since the use of chemicals enhances the denial, fuels the grandiose defenses, and keeps one isolated. Recovery reverses this process by requiring individuals to honestly admit to themselves that they do need chemicals ("I am an alcoholic") to survive and that the only hope for continual survival is to admit that they also need others. Figure 6.9 illustrates this process as Kurtz defines it. The denial of a need for others ("I don't need anyone") leads to the

FIGURE 6.9

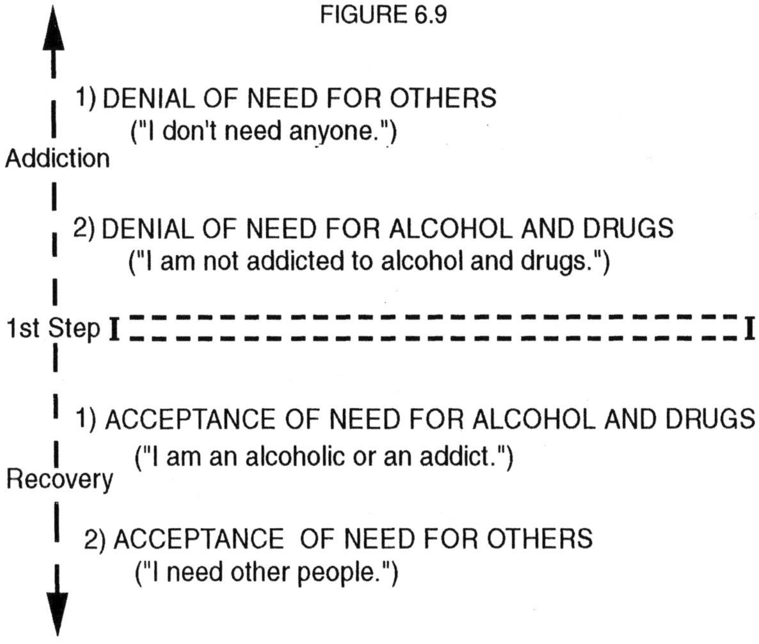

substitution of alcohol or drugs for human closeness and intimacy. As dependency and addiction become entrenched, denial of the dependency becomes salient ("I am not an alcoholic, I can quit anytime I want to"). Hitting bottom and breaking through denial reverses this process ("I am an alcoholic, I need to drink and cannot control it"). Eventually, recovery requires a recognition and acceptance of the original denial ("I do need others in my life"), and this forms the basis for the other eleven steps of the twelve-step program.

From this perspective, the first step of the twelve-step program is nothing more than alcoholics or addicts breaking through their denial of needing and admitting they are flawed. To be human is to be flawed and imperfect. From Kurtz's perspective, this is at the basis of original sin. To try to deny your imperfection is to be grandiose. It is the practice of idolatry to expect yourself to be only what God can be. Shame is what does in this grandiosity. It is the realization that we are naked and that we have sinned. We have eaten of the forbidden fruit of knowledge. Shame cannot be resolved alone by the acceptance of oneself as flawed; it also requires the acceptance from another who is also as flawed. From AA's perspective, the third step in this process requires individuals to take a "fearless moral inventory" of themselves as they are. It requires an honest appraisal, with no self-deception, that is done in the cold, stark, and harsh reality of mutual honesty. Nothing remains hidden. To stay sober and clean requires them eventually to admit that they need others and that they are imperfect. As they accept this in themselves, they will in turn need to feel it both from and toward others. Needing others and reciprocal mutuality will provide the foundation for continual recovery and mental health. The ways this is accomplished through AA will be explored in Chapter 7, and the ways it can happen in group will be explored throughout the rest of the book.

Chapter 7

Group Psychotherapy, AA, and Twelve-Step Programs

Despite the extensive utilization and immense popularity of the twelve-step abstinence-based approach for addiction treatment, this model remains surprisingly ignored and much maligned by many researchers. In a recent comprehensive and extensive literature review on addiction treatment, the twelve-step abstinence model or the AA disease concept approach was identified as the most widely used form of addiction treatment in this country (Miller, 1995). This fact was juxtaposed with another somewhat surprising discovery that, despite the wide popularity of this treatment approach, the twelve-step abstinence model has been largely and arbitrarily excluded from most previous reviews on addiction treatment. Attempting to explain this exclusion, Miller wondered if it was because of the limited number of studies conducted on this approach or if it had to do with methodological difficulties (no adequate control groups, self-selection bias, etc.) that rendered results which were judged to be unscientifically sound. Certainly, AA's requirement of anonymity for its members does not lend itself easily to scientific investigation and for obvious ethical reasons, an alcoholic could not be excluded from AA attendance in order to satisfy scientific rigor in research. However, Miller also asks if the exclusion from research reviews may be due to ideological differences between researchers and the twelve-step programs. He speculates that the "advocacy of a spiritual form of treatment contributed to the lack of scientific appeal and acceptance by the medical community" (1995).

Miller went on to conclude that this was somewhat surprising in light of a recent national survey of alcohol and drug (A&D) inpatient treatment centers by Roman (1989) that revealed an overwhelming reliance on twelve-step abstinence-based treatment approaches. The total sample consisted of 125 private, hospital-based, and free-standing treatment centers. Roman chose sampling regions so that the overall sample would approximate a representative composite of treatment programs across the country.

His responses were gathered from administrators, program directors, clinical supervisors, marketing personnel, and other employees (counselors, nurses, etc.).

Compared to the disproportionate amount of research conducted by professionals on nonabstinence approaches to addiction treatment, Roman's results were revealing. Ninety-seven percent of treatment program administrators reported that their treatment ideology was strongly influenced by the disease concept of alcoholism. The majority (95 percent) of administrators reported that their treatment program was based on the twelve-step program of AA. In addition 90 percent felt strongly that a treatment goal other than abstinence was unacceptable for any alcoholic or addict in their program.

Miller (1995), citing a survey conducted by Harrison, Hoffman, and Sneed (1991), reported:

> In an evaluation study a sample of an entire population of 8,087 inpatients and 1,663 outpatients was taken for assessment of effectiveness of the abstinence based treatment method. The contact rate was 70 percent at one year follow-up for 4,166 inpatients and 898 outpatients. The results showed that abstinence rates were strongly associated with attendance at continuing care and regular attendance at meetings of Alcoholics Anonymous post-discharge. (p. 8)

The findings of Miller's extensive literature review suggest that any serious attempt to treat alcoholics or addicts in group is going to require a thorough familiarity with twelve-step programs. Not only will it be necessary for group leaders to be able to speak the same language that their group members speak, it will help group leaders better understand addiction from their group members' experiential perspective. Countless other advantages can be derived from a thorough understanding and investigation of the program's philosophical and pragmatic applications. It can also enhance therapists' credibility as group leaders by helping them recognize when the principles of the twelve-step program are being used as a defense. The proper attainment of this understanding can only be accomplished if the evolution of the twelve-step movement is placed within its appropriate historical context. To understand twelve-step programs, abstinence, the disease concept and its relation to existentialism, shame, and self-psychology, a thorough comprehension of Alcoholics Anonymous is required.

MISCONCEPTIONS ABOUT ALCOHOLICS ANONYMOUS

As far as many professionals are concerned, Alcoholics Anonymous is a much-maligned, beleaguered, and misunderstood organization. A great many of AA's critics who write disparagingly of the organization do so without the benefit of attending AA meetings or familiarizing themselves with its workings on more than a passing, superficial, or purely analytic level. They fail to understand the subtleties of the AA program and often erroneously attribute qualities and characteristics to the organization that are one-dimensional and misleading and sometimes even border on slanderous. AA has been called by some a cult, a religion, ideological, unscientific, unempirical, and totalitarian (e.g., Jones, 1970; Tournier, 1979; Marlatt, 1983). Its members are said to be coerced into a regressive dependency that fosters servitude, compliance, and the surrendering of individual control to a higher power. Nothing could be further from the truth. Such a stance completely misses the point of AA. Fortunately, there are many professionals who have a much less narrow view of AA (e.g., Kurtz, 1982; Bateson, 1971; Barrett, 1985; Thune, 1977; Freimuth, 1994; Sollod, 1993; S. Brown, 1982).

Until recently, the relationship between professionals and self-help groups such as AA was predominantly one of mutual disregard and distrust, with the possibility of constructive interaction receiving scant consideration. At least part of this polarization stemmed from the fact that members of AA, before finding acceptance, help, and constructive change as a result of their involvement in the program, had unsuccessfully sought help from professionals. Many professionals, on the other hand, have found trying to work with alcoholics along traditional lines both frustrating and unrewarding. Both groups were equally dissatisfied in their interactions with each other. AA members viewed professionals as incompetent, uncaring, and distant. At the same time, professionals saw alcoholics as unmotivated, manipulative, and untreatable.

However, within the last decade or so, various developments have brought many professionals and loyal AA members closer together. It has been a common assumption that peer or mutual-help groups have always had grassroots rather than professional origins. However, as Lieberman and Borman (1979) have noted, there has, in fact, been appreciable professional input in the formation and encouragement of several self-help groups. This is the case with Alcoholics Anonymous, as can be seen if one takes the time to examine the historical roots of the twelve-step program. Alcoholics Anonymous' chief architect, Bill Wilson, had read William James's classic text, *The Varieties of Religious Experience* (1902) extensively, and James's philosophical position of pragmatism is a theme that runs throughout Alcoholics Anonymous's program of recovery. Wilson also had extensive correspondence with Carl Jung, and Jung's influence is strongly reflected in the spiritual emphasis of the program. Kurtz (1982) also notes that there are "profound parallels that exist between the AA insight and the animus of existential philosophy" (pp. 38-39). AA's philosophical and theoretical roots are diverse and they run deeply. The source of AA's influence will be explored in more detail later in the chapter. First, it is important to understand why AA has remained so misunderstood by countless professionals when the organization's sole purpose is to help suffering alcoholics and remain free of controversy (The fifth and tenth traditions of The Twelve Traditions).

While many dedicated professionals are aware or fast becoming aware of the importance of understanding and working closely with self-help groups such as AA, there are countless other professionals who have little desire or motivation to understand, much less learn from, these organizations. Lieberman and Borman (1979) point out that those professional contributors who work most closely with self-help groups share the distinguishing characteristic of having become disenchanted with the dominant orthodoxes of their respective fields of specialization in the treatment of addiction. Thus, professionals who have worked with alcoholics and addicts on a sustained basis have learned that more traditional, orthodox methods of treatment have not been of sufficient help. Therefore, the first form of "training" that has induced professionals to become interested in self-help groups such as AA has been professional defection from their prescribed ideological frameworks. Professionals in a refractory frame of mind were, in short, looking for better ways to help alcoholics at a time when alcoholics were trying to find ways to help themselves.

A related consideration is that many professionals have had to look for better help for themselves through AA because, in many cases, their own professional specialties had failed them. There are many physicians, psychiatrists, and psychologists who are members and staunch supporters of AA for the reason that it, alone, has provided successful help in the treatment of their own addiction. As Kurtz (1982) writes, "It is time to take Alcoholics Anonymous seriously" (p. 30). However, AA should not be understood only for its therapeutic success and social significance; it should be appreciated for its unique intellectual significance. AA is not given the intellectual respectability it deserves for a number of reasons. Kurtz sees this lack of appreciation tied to our culture's rejection of all existential philosophies that stress limitation and personal responsibility:

> AA is not generally accorded intellectual respectability because its core insistences on essential limitation and on mutuality as prefer-

> able to objectivity reveal it to be a counterenlightenment phenomenon antithetical to the central assumptions of self-styled "modernity." (1982, p. 38)

Thune (1977) expresses similar sentiments, but feels the misunderstanding of AA is due to the program's non-positivist, quasi-revivalistic, and transcendentalistic emphasis.

> It is no accident that the therapeutic program of Alcoholics Anonymous challenges the conventional medical, psychological, and sociological concepts of causation and that it ignores the findings and questions of specialists in these fields. Its roots lie less in the sciences than in such non-positivist, quasirevivalistic, transcendental efforts of the Oxford Group Movement. To attempt to understand AA on an analytic and positivist model obscures its uniqueness. (p. 75)

Kurtz (1979) and Thune (1977) are addressing a crucial issue in attempting to explain why many professionals still hold the belief that the integration of psychotherapy and twelve-step programs is impossible because their respective views and values are so divergent (Humphreys, 1993). Sollod (1993), for one, challenges the view that the values typically associated with twelve-step members and those typically fostered by professionals are examples of "immiscibility." Freimuth (1994) also disagrees, citing, "for example, sixty percent of AA membership has sought some form of psychological treatment" (p. 551). The similarity in values of what Bergin (1981) refers to as "scientific materialism" and "theistic realism" is just one example of a therapeutic psychological approach that recognizes that an irreparable chasm need not exist between the values of AA and the values of more scientifically oriented psychotherapists. Professionals wanting to work effectively with alcoholics and drug addicts must bridge this gap, and one way to accomplish this is to thoroughly explore the values and biases that they hold.

VALUES, SCIENCE, AND AA

The examination of values in science is not new. However, a scientist's own idiosyncratic experiences can distort the most objective of explanations and observations. For instance, Kuhn (1962) claims that while scientists may share many values, they will frequently differ in their application of these values. Usually, the judgment of the accuracy of facts is generally stable. However, the judgment of simplicity, consistency, plausibility, and so on will often vary greatly from individual to individual. In short, though values are widely shared by scientists and though commitment to them is both deep and constitutive of science, the application of values is sometimes affected considerably by features of the individual personality and history that determine the way these values will be applied and interpreted.

Reason versus Knowledge

The confusion over whether the scientific approach is a value-free one has been a recurring problem in the philosophy of science. Frank (1961) for one has tersely noted the insistence of researchers on examining value-laden behavior by scientific criteria in isolation rather than immediately involving cultural criteria. As Whitehead (1925) convincingly argues, the best way to advance beyond the culturally determined bias of reality is by abstraction. Whitehead credits the development of the science of pure mathematics as "the most original creation of the human spirit" (p. 19).

The more abstract the better, Whitehead argued, for it rids us of all our expectations and prejudices of reality. Mathematics is the mediating process between the abstract and the concrete. As long as you are dealing with pure mathematics, you are in the realm of complete abstraction, and to arrive at truth, divorced from bias, you need abstraction to treat objects in their complete uniqueness.

However, Whitehead warns that the indiscriminate use of abstraction is a major vice of the intellect and that the judicious use of reason is needed in its application. Here, Whitehead is reacting to the arrogant use of abstraction and is making an Emerson-like distinction between understanding and reason. Ralph Waldo Emerson viewed reason as a higher form of understanding because it allowed the intuitive feelings of the heart and sentiment to complement other perceptual apprehensions of reality (White, 1972). It is important to remember that Emerson and the Transcendentalists had an important influence on the Oxford Group Movement. Understanding alone, as Emerson, the Transcendentalists, and eventually the Oxford Group and AA came to realize, is incapable of comprehending the moral unity of our relationship with the cosmos because it is based on the knowledge limited by our five senses and thus presented to us as a distorted perception of reality.

Years prior to Emerson's development of his doctrine of moral sentiment as an alternative method to the attainment of knowledge, Kant (cited in White, 1972) had "solved" this problem for the Transcendentalists when he convincingly argued that neither our intellectual understanding nor our rational mind alone could lead us to any knowledge of what things are in themselves (Kant referred to this as *noumena*) or what we are in ourselves, since our understanding could not penetrate beyond the realms and limits of our possible experience (phenomena). Kant had shown that time and space were not empirical concepts derived from our experiences, but something "a priori," that is, imposed on our experiences to help us "make sense" of phenomena. Kant demonstrated that space and time are not what we perceive; rather, space and time are reflective of how we perceive. Our minds impose and organize phenomena into categories. Following Hume, Kant pointed out that what we come to judge as cause and effect is nothing more than "constant conjunction" or habit. It may be a useful and necessary habit, but nevertheless, it leads us to see or be receptive to what is familiar. We are then prone to miss what is outside of our expectations. The knowing mind is not a passive spectator, but an active agent. It does not just picture the world, it forms it. Because of the way our mind imposes structure on the objective world, we are subject to the same principles of causality. The noumena world of reality can never be completely understood by our rational mind alone. To escape this predicament, Kant appealed to practical reason or transcendental ways of knowing to help explain the supersensitive noumena world consisting of entities that are neither in space nor time and hence not subject to casual influences or dualities. Kant's aim was to define the extent and the limits of rational knowledge. He eventually appealed to moral sentiment or the heart as another way of knowing. As Kant wrote later in his life, "I had to limit reason to make room for faith."

Osborne and Baldwin (1982) express similar sentiments when they challenge psychotherapists to examine the limits of their perceptions of reality when providing psychotherapy to their patients. They suggest that much of psychotherapy involves a lateral shift from one state of illusion to another and that arrogance or certainty that their interpretation of reality is the only true reality is apt to create many unexpected difficulties not only for their patients, but for themselves. As Jacob Bronowski (1973) warned, "When people believe that they have absolute knowledge, with no test in reality. . . . this is when they aspire to the knowledge of gods." Knowledge and certainty must never be confused. This is a delusion that can have disastrous consequences. Watzlawick (1978) agreed that the most dangerous delusion of all is "the belief that one's own view of reality is the only reality (p. xiii). Indeed, as Osborne and Baldwin suggest, many professional psychotherapists may be caught up with patients in "the enactment of an illusion which is far broader than the client's problem" (p. 266). This is a very important issue because while many professionals can easily criticize AA's ideological base, they fail to examine their own perceptual bias with the same critical scrutiny. Closely tied to this process is the failure to realize that the conventional distinction between facts and values may be another illusion, reflecting "pseudo-objectivity based upon intersubjectivity" (p. 267). Or as Bixenstine (1956) contends, facts cannot be separated from values, but actually reflect a special class of values.

Self-deception is not limited to the alcoholic or the addict in denial, it is also present in any individual who gets caught up in the arrogance of certainty and a pride that prevents reason from examining its limitations. Reason without humility becomes self-deception. Sigmund Freud's (1910) development of the psychoanalytic method was originally intended to help us become more self-aware and honest with ourselves. He was acutely aware that we have a tendency to deceive ourselves and that our rational mind with all its elaborate defenses was the chief obstacle to overcome in this process. With Socrates, Freud urged, 'Know thyself." Psychoanalysis was built upon the foundations laid before it by the early Greek maxim You shall know the Truth and the Truth shall set you free. Above all, Freud set out to undermine our dishonesty with ourselves. Hans Strupp (1972) summed it up by saying,

> Unlike any man before him, Freud identified self-deception as a pervasive and universal human characteristic. Insight into our unconscious motivations through psychoanalysis is meant to pave the road for the kind of master and control Freud had in mind. (p. 40)

Unfortunately, Freud's cardinal article of faith becomes the frail human intellect, which is to serve as the only reliable guide on this discovery of truth. Alas, as Strupp points out, the intellect of rational thought may be as much an illusion as Freud considered religion to be. Unfortunately, Freud was following the path laid by philosophers before him who believed that human reason was capable of unlocking the secrets of the universe and thus offered humankind ultimate truth. But as Shestov (1932) warned, these philosophers only succeeded in chaining humankind to the power of *Ananke* (Reason), which they slavishly revere as a deity:

> Reason does without commandments, men will love it of themselves unbidden. The theory of knowledge simply sings the praises of reason but no one has the audacity to question it, and still less dare doubt its sovereign power. (p. 33)

Science versus Religion

Bergin (1981) for one argues that science has lost its authority as the dominating source of truth it once was. "This change is both reflected in and stimulated by analysis which reveals science to be an intuitive and value-laden cultural form" (p. 95). Bergin proposes that a science dominated by mechanistic thought and ethic naturalism has proved insufficient and something more is wanted, especially since the spiritual and social failures of many organized religious systems have been followed by the failures of nonreligious approaches. Bergin, like Bakan (1972), stands in opposition to the worshipping of the scientific method in place of God and condemns the notion of "methodolatry" in science. Nietzsche captured these same sentiments when he described Western culture's preoccupation with the scientific method as an example of religious idolatry that takes the form of individuals "grovelling before facts." Malcolm Muggeridge (1980) cautioned against the arid accumulation of knowledge when he said, "Accumulating knowledge is a form of avarice and lends itself to another version of the Midas story, this time of a man so avid for knowledge that everything he touches turns to facts; his faith becomes theology; his loves becomes lechery; his wisdom becomes science; pursuing meaning, he ignores truth." Seeking knowledge, without understanding its relation to truth, is not just worthless, according to Muggeridge, it is harmful. Muggeridge is not opposed to knowledge or science, but believes it "needs to be used in such a way that it serves God's purposes." By this, he means that knowledge applied without any relation to the spiritual or the emotional is sheer abstraction and alienates us from the authenticity of our experiences.

The distinction between religious and scientific criteria can be very subtle. Frank (1972), for instance, has facetiously drawn a comparison of the Catholic religion and his discipline, psychology, which he calls the Religion of Mental Health.

> The Mental Health movement resembles organized religions in some respects. Science is its theology and is followed by rituals like this conference in which various members of the priesthood read papers to their colleagues, who try to maintain an air of respectful attention. As a devotee of this religion, I would like to point out that, like all religions, it leads its adherents to ignore phenomena that are inconsistent with its cosmology. (pp. 242-243)

Whitehead is insistent that science meet this challenge and expand its paradigm to include intuition and emotion. Whitehead is thus protesting against the scientific Logos and the inhuman attitude of modern science, the mentality that reduces nature to a "dull affair, soundless, scentless, colourless; merely hurrying of material, endlessly, meaninglessly," (Brown, 1959, p. 316). Thus, modern science confirms Farenczi's aphorism: "Pure intelligence is thus a product of dying, or at least of becoming mentally insensitive and is therefore in principle madness" (Brown, 1959, p. 317). Whitehead agrees and writes,

> What is wanted is an appreciation of the infinite variety of vivid values achieved by an organism in its proper environment. When you understand all about the sun and all about the atmosphere and all about the rotation of the earth, you may still miss the radiance of the sunset. There is no substitute for the direct perception of the concrete achievement of a thing in its actuality. (p. 199)

Whitehead is therefore proposing the appreciation of the concrete as a way out of the labyrinth of abstract thought. Unlike Emerson and the transcendental beliefs that influenced AA, he does not radically appeal to sentiment as a higher form of knowledge. However, he does propose a need for the development of a more comprehensive acknowledgment of our relationship with the cosmos–one that avoids the confusion of the concrete with the abstract and draws upon more than what our frail intellect can offer.

Thus, Whitehead is not criticizing the scientific method itself but rather the "fallacy of misplaced concreteness." We are, Whitehead warns, in danger of losing ourselves in the abstract idealism of our own thought. We confuse the abstract with the concrete and then judge the abstraction to be real. The "scientific materialism" of "brute fact" cannot be applied as reality itself, for external objects exist, not in the sense of "simple location" (just there), but rather in relation. "Scientific investigation," Whitehead warns, "cannot speak of an entity without reference or relationship to the universe as a whole and its relationship to the entity" (p. 39). Whitehead recognizes that, although science claims it now has no need for philosophy, it has in fact carried one over from the Greek influence whether it realizes it or not. "A living science is impossible," Whitehead speculates, "and cannot exist unless there is a belief in an order of nature" (1925, p. 39).

PHILOSOPHY OF SCIENCE AND THE LIMITS OF RATIONALITY

American philosophy, in particular, has been characterized by its response to the challenge of modern science and the scientific method. As Morton White (1972) illustrates, there is a strong dualistic tendency deeply ingrained in American philosophical thought. This dualism has been manifested as a response of moral sentiment to science's challenges that knowledge is determined by experience or limited to analytical intent of meaning. Ralph Waldo Emerson, Jonathan Edwards, William James, and Charles Pierce have all spearheaded an appeal to some form of emotion, sentiment, or passion as a method of establishing knowledge that is fundamentally different from that associated with the scientific method. As James wrote, "Science can tell us what exists; but to compare the *worth*, both of what exists and of what does not exist, we must consult not science, but what Pascal calls our heart" (in White, 1972, p. 192).

Physics, in particular, has illustrated the far-reaching implications possible whenever a science has been able to unite itself with moral sentiment in its investigation. "Conceptual riddles," as Bronowski illustrates, "are solved in Quantum Physics by mathematical formulations only after being solved as mental riddles first. . . . and that requires not calculation, but insight, imagination–if you like, metaphysics" (1973, p. 363). Max Born indicated his support of this position when he confessed, "I am now convinced that theoretical physics is actual philosophy" (in Bronowski, 1973, p. 364). What he meant was that the new ideas in physics amount to a different view of reality. The world is not a fixed, solid array of objects out there, for it cannot be fully separated from our perception of it. It shifts under our gaze, it interacts with us, and the knowledge that it yields must be interpreted by us.

In trying to distinguish appearance from reality and lay bare the fundamental structure of the universe, science has had to translate the "rabble of the senses." Its highest edifices, Einstein has pointed out, "have been purchased at the price of emptiness of content" (in Barnett, 1948, p. 113).

Thus, gradually, scientists have been forced to abandon the ordinary world of our experience, the world of sense perceptions. In contrast to the edifice that John Locke and the rationalists had built in defining knowledge, scientists have arrived at the startling conclusion that since qualities exist only in the mind, the entire objective universe of matter and energy, atoms and stars, does not exist except as a construction of the consciousness, an edifice of conventional symbols shaped by the senses of man. As Barnett writes,

> So paradoxically what the scientist and the philosopher have called the world of appearance–the world of light and color designed by the physiology of human sense organs–is the world in which finite man is incarcerated by his essential nature. And what the scientist called the world of reality–the colorless, soundless, unpalpable cosmos which lies like an iceberg hidden beneath the plane of man's perception–is a skeleton structure of symbols. (Barnett, 1948, p. 137)

In our brief tenancy on earth, humans egocentrically order events in our minds according to our own feelings of past, present, and future. But except on the reels of one's own consciousness, the universe, the objective world of reality, does not "happen"; it simply exists. It can be encompassed in its entire majesty only by a cosmic intellect. While science tells us nothing of the true "nature" of things, it nevertheless succeeds in defining their relationship and depicting the events in which they are involved. "The event," Whitehead declared, "is the unit of things real" (1933, p. 198). By this he meant that however theoretical systems may change and however empty of content their symbols and concepts may be, the essential and enduring facts of life are the happenings, the activities, the events. For example, the principle of uncertainty indicates we cannot actually forecast the actual encounter of electrons. Thus, in a sense, the electrons are not "real" but merely theoretical symbols. On the other hand, the meeting itself is "real"–the event is "real." It is as though the true objective world lies forever half-concealed beneath the translucent, plastic dome of our consciousness and cannot be comprehended by our senses, only experienced by our being.

The principle of uncertainty asserts, therefore, that it is impossible with any principles now known to science to determine both the position and the velocity of any electron at the same time. For by the very act of observing its position its velocity is changed, and conversely, the more accurately its velocity is determined, the more indefinite its position becomes. Quantum physics thus appears to shake two pillars of old science, causality and determinism. By its admission of margins of uncertainty it yields up the ancient hope that science, given the present state and velocity of every material body in the universe, can forecast the history of the universe for all time. One byproduct of this surrender is a new argument for the existence of free will. For if physical events are indeterminate and the future is unpredictable, then perhaps the unknown quantity called "mind" may yet guide humankind's destiny among infinite uncertainties of a capricious universe.

It is here that Werner Heisenberg's Principle of Uncertainty startles us with its great simplicity. Bronowski exclaims it as a "profound idea, one of the great scientific ideas, not only of the twentieth century, but in the history of science" (Bronowski, 1973, p. 365). In one sense, it is a robust principle of the everyday. The fact exists that humans cannot observe nature objectively but inescapably take part in the processes we observe. Heisenberg's Principle, which states that there can be no physics without an observer, seems more and more to be primary among all physical laws. The answers to the mysteries of understanding the human condition seem to be at a point where science and religion, the rational and intuitive, reason and the heart all begin to meld.

LIMITS OF RATIONAL THOUGHT AND SCIENCE

The dialectical balance between knowledge as certainty and the uncertainty of existence as it is lived was not only the dilemma confronting social scientists and philosophers at the start of the twentieth century, it was also the lived experience of every alcoholic following the 1929 market crash and the Depression of the 1930s. Out of this climate of accumulated knowledge and the scientific method's promise of seemingly unending possibilities of mastering, controlling, and understanding the world was the actual experience of fear, doubt, dread, and uncertainty. While the disillusionment of the post-enlightenment period reflected society's coming to grips with the realization that the promise of science and rationality was not only limited, but deceiving, it also reflected the dilemma confronting those individuals who were trying to resolve their own personal conflicts between what their own reason told them and what they felt in their heart on a real, emotional level. Out of this emotional and intellectual atmosphere, existentialism, psychoanalysis, and eventually Alcoholics Anonymous emerged. An extensive and comprehensive analysis of the social, cultural, and intellectual climate that gave birth to the interconnectedness between AA, modern psychology, and existential philosophy is given by Ernest Kurtz (1979).

Describing the paradox of more becoming less, and how the confrontation between arrogance and limitedness was played out on a social level with existential philosophy and on a personal level with every practicing alcoholic, Kurtz writes:

> Twentieth-century American history is the story of four paradoxes of modernity that loomed ever more as contradictions plaguing first Americans, then all moderns. Increasingly, the very triumphs of rationalization and control seemed to reveal only the final impossibility of any ultimate rationalization and control. The thirst and quest for more rationalization and control, however, increased even as each success at them came to be perceived as increasingly empty. The fundamental modern endeavor, the very *identity* of modernity in modernity's own terms, revealed itself as inherently addictive; the striving always harder for the ever more that always satisfied ever less. (1979, p. 171)

Kurtz suggests that the dilemma confronting the existentialists was an anticipation of the dilemma that every alcoholic had to face. The existential writers, especially Sartre and Heidegger, were confronting the truth of human existence, which Heidegger called *Dasien*, as having been lost. The Hegelian dialectical idealism and the Cartesian cogito, with its futile quest for absolute objectivity and excessive emphasis on mind or thing over feeling or being, was the final wedge that split humans off from themselves. In a protest to both Hegel and Descartes, Sören Kierkegaard turned Descartes's famous credo "I think, therefore, I am" completely on its head when he countered with "I am, therefore, I think." For Kierkegaard, as for most other existentialists, being always precedes thought. Our over-investment in our thinking has come at the cost of our being in harmony with ourselves. The existentialists, in contrast to the growing trend of the rest of Western philosophy and the logical positivists, were intent on making a virtue of uncertainty. Existential writers were holding to the position that we do not know anything for certain, except, paradoxically, that we know we do not know. Martin Buber expressed similar sentiments when he wrote that knowledge always comes at the burden or the cost of knowing. By this, he meant that, unlike other living creatures, who are who or what they are unquestionably and therefore remain untroubled by the need to find meaning in their lives, we are doomed to know that we do not know and that we will never know. Despite this, Heidegger says, we must continue to always ask the difficult question, knowing we will never have a complete answer.

Addiction from this perspective implies a forced confrontation between our self-deception of unlimited knowledge, power, and control and the anguish, angst, fear, and dread that comes with admitting we do not know and that we are limited and finite. Kurtz, attempting to address this issue, suggests that viewing the disease of addiction as a metaphor for the human condition has much merit. Drawing parallels between AA and the classic Evangelical Pietistic position, Kurtz (1979) writes, "This ancient insight suggests that humankind exists in a state of being that is essentially limited, and that transcendence of this limitation requires first acceptance of it, then the embrace of salvation from it as coming from outside the individual self" (p. 202). Kurtz is suggesting that addiction is a process which reflects a condition that is also a metaphor for the human predicament. Any time we rely excessively on external sources of gratification or validation as means of determining our worth, giving us meaning, or providing us with happiness and pleasure without earning it by right actions and attitudes, we are attempting to control what we cannot ever possibly control. Addiction is coming to grips with our excessive arrogance, control, and demand for unlimited gratification. Addiction, the use of drugs and alcohol to bolster this arrogant control and illusion of not needing others, speeds up this inevitable process. It condenses our experience. It is for the MTV crowd, because addiction accelerates the inevitable confrontation between what we are trying to be and what we really are.

AA refers to this confrontation with our limitation as "hitting bottom." Others in the twelve-step program sometimes refer to it as spiritual emergency. The existentialists describe it as an existential crisis. Like AA, the existentialists recognize that this confrontation must ultimately be an individual one that is experienced alone, outside the confines of traditional definitions and restrictions of culturally approved institutions like the church or modern medicine. It is no wonder that the self-help movement would be the vehicle that would provide the direction for its development.

THE SELF-HELP MOVEMENT

Several forces have contributed to the self-help movement, of which AA is the earliest and best known. One factor is America's pluralistic ethnology; Americans are joiners who frequently seek a social identity through group affiliation (Dumont, 1974). The limited number of available professionals at the time who could offer help has also contributed to the self-help movement. During the 1930s, when AA was formed, there were fewer professionals available than there are now. Psychotherapy was also limited almost exclusively to individual therapy. Those professionals who were available continued to emphasize one-to-one therapy and underutilized the therapeutic potential of groups and peer influence, consequently failing to reach as many people as they would have if they had worked more with groups. Thus, professionals failed to meet the demands for service because they were too few in number and they did not utilize the more efficient and appropriate therapeutic strategies available for the disorders presented to them.

Even if the supply of professionals had been ample and these professionals had utilized the most efficient individual approaches to the kinds of problems dealt with in self-help groups, such groups would have continued to flourish for a number of other reasons. Two of the most important reasons are that self-help groups are inexpensive or free and peer influence is powerful.

This is especially true if the peer shares a similar problem. Identification, support, and sharing of common concerns are powerful curative forces. It was not until recently that professionals have come to understand the power of groups to maximize therapeutic gain. AA has intuitively recognized what Yalom and others are starting to take advantage of in an organized fashion. Peers are frequently more influential than professionals in producing behavioral change.

Psychological theory and research supports the clinical opinion that peers are a source of important influences. Peers have enormous influence on individuals during their childhood and adolescence (Muus, 1968; Patterson and Anderson, 1964). Peer influence is especially important in the early socialization of individuals (Hartup, 1970). Festinger (1954) has presented convincing evidence that individuals are most influenced by persons whom they perceive as like themselves. Gartner and Riessman (1984) agree when they write, "The strongest influences are those whom the subject sees as like himself. For example, in the statement of the old-timer at the AA meeting that he is an alcoholic, but obviously under control, the new member sees what he or she can become" (p. 21). Emrick, Lassen, and Edwards (1977) expressed similar sentiments when they wrote, "Resocialization may best describe the events and mechanisms occurring in peer-oriented residential treatment centers for drug addicts" (p. 121).

While peers powerfully affect individuals, peer groups do even more so. Research presented by Emrick, Lassen, and Edwards (1977) point to the influence of groups in providing individuals with social support, social identity, and social reality. Peer groups represent even more influence than groups not made up of peers. By definition, there is more of a basis for similarity in peer groups. In psychotherapy groups with peers, the similarity lies in the problem or issue that was the reason for the person joining the group. Common experiences and attitudes about alcohol and drugs yield more interpersonal attraction than when these commonalties are absent. Homogeneity of group members, as Yalom has clearly demonstrated, leads to more cohesiveness. Homogeneity and cohesiveness in turn yield greater influences of group members as well as greater uniformity of attitudes. Add to this the fact that people learn better and more readily from peers and are more likely to imitate peers, and there is ample evidence for why self-help groups like AA are so widespread and flourishing.

ALCOHOLICS ANONYMOUS: ITS HISTORICAL ROOTS

The usual birthdate assigned to AA is 1935, but the program has its origins earlier than that and started with its founder, Bill Wilson. To understand AA's history, you must understand William Griffith Wilson. A seemingly hopeless alcoholic who had made and lost two fortunes on Wall Street, Wilson was an intensely inquisitive man who had tried for years to control his drinking and had experienced repeated failures. Pushed to the point of despair and suicide, Wilson was visited by a good friend prior to what was to be Wilson's fourth and final hospitalization for his alcoholism. His friend, Ebby T., a hopeless alcoholic like Wilson, was miraculously sober. The friend revealed to Wilson that he had been led to salvation from his alcoholism after joining the Oxford Group Movement–an evangelically oriented group styled to recapture the pietist insight of primitive Christianity. Ebby T. had joined the Oxford Group Movement at the recommendation of Rowland H., a friend who had been treated by the noted Swiss psychiatrist Carl Jung. This young man, a talented and wealthy financial wizard, had attempted virtually every known cure for alcoholism and in desperation traveled to Zurich, Switzerland in 1931 to enter analysis with Jung. Shortly upon his return to the U.S., he promptly relapsed. Rowland H. was subsequently told by Jung that he was "frankly hopeless as far as any further medical and psychiatric treatment was concerned." Jung suggested that the only possible source of hope might be "spiritual or religious experiences–in short, a genuine conversion." He was cautioned, however, "that while such experiences had sometimes brought recovery to alcoholics, they were . . . comparatively rare" (Kurtz, 1979, pp. 8-9). As Ebby T. conveyed this story to his friend Bill W., it was presented with a Jungian insight and emphasis. Only later did this event have any significance for Wilson or AA.

Despite Ebby's efforts, Wilson did not remain sober. Wilson, however, did come to share this information with his doctor, William D. Silkworth. It was through the influences of these individuals (Jung, Silkworth, Ebby T.) that a series of events was set in motion that would eventually serve as a foundation for the AA program.

In *Alcoholics Anonymous Comes of Age* (1957), Wilson acknowledged the importance to AA of William D. Silkworth in helping to lay the foundation from which the disease concept of alcoholism was derived. More important, it was Silkworth who quoted William James's statement that "transforming spiritual experiences are nearly always founded on calamity and collapses" (James, 1902). In his book, Wilson describes the conversion experience he encountered while being treated for an especially severe case of depression and anxiety following his most recent drinking spree. By all descriptions available, he experienced what has been typically described in philosophical and religious literature as a mystical experience (Buber, 1960; Kaufmann, 1965; and Stace, 1966). Though not frequently articulated, Wilson's recorded descriptions share many of the common properties reported in such an experience, as they typically appear to transcend historical context and cultural influences. Typically reported is a flash of bright, blinding light followed by periods of euphoria, timelessness, serenity, and feelings of oneness with some higher presence. As Wilson wrote, "I now found myself in a new world of consciousness which was suffused by a Presence. One with the universe, a great peace stole over me"(cited in Kurtz, 1979, p. 20).

Wilson was almost immediately apprehensive about his "spiritual experience." Had he not been warned by Dr. Silkworth of alcohol-induced brain damage? It was only much later, at an AA convention in 1955, that Wilson set it down in print. He had been reluctant to recount this event, for he had discovered that it impaired rather than aided his credibility. There was nothing that he wanted to avoid more than the impression that AA was a bunch of drunks who had gotten sober because they had gotten religious.

When he had had a little time to reflect on this experience, Wilson began to test it. Discussions with his good friend, Dr. Silkworth, assured him that he was not mad, that conversion experiences sometimes were reported by "hopeless alcoholics" who had then turned around and recovered from their alcoholism. He referred Wilson to William James's *Varieties of Religious Experience.* In the years that followed, Wilson poured over James's writings. Much of the significance of James's writings was that it provided for Wilson a generalized discussion of the conversion experience. It was James's theory that spiritual experiences could have a definite objective reality and might totally transform a person's life. Some, but by no means all of these experiences, James believed, came through religious channels. All, however, appeared to have their source in pain and utter hopelessness. Complete "deflation at depth" was the one requirement to make someone ready for a transforming experience. "Deflation at depth," as any recovering alcoholic knows, is captured and expressed in AA terminology as hitting bottom.

Leuba (1896) and Starbuck (1899)–whose writings were frequently cited by James–addressed the conversion experience with specific clarity. Leuba emphasized this reversal and also pointed out that a second precondition to conversion is self-surrender. In fact, this is the first step of AA's twelve-step program. But Wilson was still apprehensive. It was not until later that Wilson was able to integrate his experience. Kurtz captures his struggle when he writes about Wilson's understanding of his experience through his reading of William James.

What Wilson got–or thought he got–from the book was to prove significant to the history of Alcoholics Anonymous:

> . . . Spiritual experiences, James thought, could have objective reality; almost like gifts from the blue, they could transform people. Some were sudden brilliant illuminations; others came on very gradually. Some flowed out of religious channels; others did not. But nearly all had the great common denominators of pain, suffering, calamity. Complete hopelessness and deflation at depth were almost always required to make the recipient ready. The significance of all this burst upon me. *Deflation at depth*–yes, that was *it.* Exactly that had happened to me.
>
> This was the substance of what Wilson had come to understand; also important was the meaning he found inherent in it, for his moment was–taken together with his "spiritual experience"–the third of the four founding movements of Alcoholics Anonymous. One-half of the core idea–the necessity of spiritual conversion–had passed from Dr. Carl Jung to Rowland. Clothed in Oxford Group practice, it had given rise to its yet separate other half–the simultaneous transmission of deflation and hope by "one alcoholic talking to another"–in the first meeting between Bill and Ebby. Now, under the benign guidance of Dr. Silkworth and the profound thought of William James, the two "halves, joined in Wilson's mind to form an as yet only implicitly realized whole." (Kurtz, 1979, pp. 20-21)

Wilson came to realize such dramatic shifts in personality are rare, but they do happen. Foremost among them are the phenomenon of conversion, such as religious conversions exemplified by the reports collected by William James and described in the case histories of Carl Jung. Similarly, Jung told Wilson that some cases of traumatic neurosis and relapse occurred after successful therapy and those occurrences represented shifts from health to neurosis.

Likewise, both Martin Heidegger (1963) and Karl Jaspers (1975) wrote extensively about situations that were capable of compelling individuals to make dramatic and drastic changes in their lives. Jaspers described these occurrences as "limit situations," conditions in which individuals would be confronted with the futility of their present mode or pattern of interacting. Limit situations, as Heidegger describes them, function as a catalyst for the evaluation and confrontation of one's existence. Anguish and despair (angst) were the necessary emotional components required to compel one to drastically alter one's awareness (Enlschlossenheit) and interaction with the world (Existenz).

Wilson intuitively recognized this phenomenon as the crucial component of his recovery process. Surrender is therefore the cornerstone of AA's twelve steps to recovery. Surrender usually refers to a state of non-assertion of individuality, of losing oneself in something else, but the difference as Angyal (1965) and AA apply it is momentous. "One submits to the alien and becomes diminished through submission, one surrenders one's isolation to enter a large unit and enlarges one's life" (Angyal, 1965, p. 107).

Years later Wilson began corresponding with Carl Jung. Jung's letters proved to be an important influence in Wilson's development of the AA treatment philosophy. It is important to note that Wilson's insistent drive to understand what he had experienced led him to struggle and resolve the psychological, religious, and spiritual aspects of what was later to become known as Alcoholics Anonymous. It was Wilson's desire to interpret and define this experience that later brought him in contact with the Oxford Group Movement.

Wilson wrote, "When the pupil is ready, the teacher appears" (cited in Kurtz, 1979). Such was the case because Wilson soon became involved with the leader of the Oxford Group Movement. The interchange that resulted was reciprocal, and soon the spiritual principles of the Oxford Group were to become the foundation upon which AA operates: (1) self-examination; (2) acknowledgment of faults; (3) restitutions of wrongs done, and above all; (4) constant work with others. The formulation of AA's basic tenets of character defects, restitution of harm done, and working with others can be directly traced back to the Oxford Group Movement, Ralph Waldo Emerson, and the influence of the Transcendentalists. The application of these principles would eventually lead to the development of the treatment modality that would soon be unsurpassed in the treatment of alcoholism and drug addiction.

AA–WHY AND HOW IT WORKS: AN INTERPRETATION OF AA

AA describes its organization as "a fellowship of men and women who share their experience, strength, and hope with each other so that they may solve their common problem and help others to recover from alcoholism" and adds that its purpose "is to stay sober and help other alcoholics achieve sobriety" (Alcoholics Anonymous, 1939). Anonymity is required to avoid the possible stigma of membership and possible ostracism of family and friends. Anonymity also ensures confidentiality, which permits free and candid discussion of problems and difficulties.

However, the cornerstone upon which the Alcoholics Anonymous philosophy is built remains the recognition and admittance that one has an uncontrollable drinking problem. The members of Alcoholics Anonymous do not pursue or coddle malingering prospects. They make it plain that if the prospects actually wanted to stop drinking, the members would anywhere, anytime, reach out to help them. The program will not work with those who only want to quit, or who want to quit because they are afraid of losing their families or their jobs. AA states that the effective desire must be based upon enlightened self-interest. Applicants must be fed up with the stark social loneliness that engulfs the uncontrolled drinker, and they must want to put some order into their bungled lives.

Alcoholics Anonymous is guided by its suggested "Twelve Steps." "Suggested" is the word to be emphasized, however, for there are no musts in AA except those that members set up for themselves. Basically, AA will demonstrate that alcoholics can be accepted and loved. Alcoholics who come to AA for the first time, strangers, rejected and lonely, are received as valued members of the human race worthy of being salvaged. Listening to members recount life experiences as dismal as their own, and then observing how they have overcome their drinking problems, alcoholics are filled with the hope that if the members could do it, perhaps they can also. They become motivated to try.

Alcoholics learn they must live one day at a time without taking a drink. By attending AA meetings and verbalizing problems, they strengthen their resistance to drink and gradually reconstruct their lifestyles to rid themselves of dependency on alcohol. The most crucial concept involves alcoholics recognizing themselves as individuals whose illness is an uncontrollable drinking problem; they must accept the tenet that becomes the foundation of their rehabilitation program: "Even one drink is too many."

Alcoholics, due to the nature of their illness, have established an elaborate denial and rationalization system. These psychological defenses that prevent the recognition and admittance of their illness are as much involved and intricately connected with their disease as alcohol itself is. Vernon Johnson (1973) sums up the dynamics of this interplay best:

> The primary factor within this primary condition, however, is the delusion, or impaired judgment, which keeps the harmfully dependent person locked into his self-destructive pattern. It must be met and dealt with first since it blocks his entering any therapeutic process at all. The alcoholic evades or denies outright any need for help whenever he is approached. It must be remembered that he is not in touch with reality. (p. 44)

AA acknowledges this need for recognition (it is the first of its twelve steps), and it can occur only when alcoholics have reached their crisis and at a gut level have surrendered to some Power greater than themselves. The spiritual and religious dynamics at the level of recovery cannot be overstated for alcoholics must confront themselves in their naked existence. The existential overtone to such a crisis is the central psychological factor of the recovery program. Alcoholics are asked simply to exchange the destructive dependence upon alcohol for a constructive Power (Steps Two and Three). The alcoholic's idea of what that Power may be is not important in AA. The important thing is for newcomers to recognize that they have not been able to manage the part of their life that has been affected by drinking. As alcoholics surrender they see that it is possible to risk being themselves, and they move consciously toward deepening their meaningful relationships with others because this will help them recover.

Once this gut-level surrender to some spiritual awakening is accepted, alcoholics must pay a personal cost. The dynamics of forgiveness and restoration are difficult concepts to acknowledge. The wrongs that have been done during the period of illness can never be completely reconciled. This process of reconciliation is part of the monotonous and painstaking road to sobriety. Regardless of what friends and neighbors may think, alcoholics do not necessarily feel happy to wake up in the morning facing life without a drink. Painful hangovers they have experienced previously may seem more tolerable than the gnawing fears and vague anxiety they now feel as they anticipate each day's activities.

The cost is one to be paid in psychological pain. The reward is the sense of forgiveness and the vitality of new interpersonal relationships. The goal to stop drinking is not a totally adequate one. A new way of viewing life, a new sense of self-worth and self-respect, and a new appreciation of one's responsibility and relationships with others are vital to sober living. Often a mature religious faith helps provide a new beginning and emotional help for the trying times facing every alcoholic.

Once alcoholics have a moral inventory of themselves (Step Four) with the aid of AA, they acknowledge these wrongdoings to their Higher Power and another individual (Step Five). They then restore and make amends to persons they have abused and, in general, clean up their past as well as they can (Step Nine). This catharsis is regarded as important because of the compulsion that a feeling of guilt exerts in the alcoholic obsession. The belief is that personal resentments have a strong influence on the push back to the bottle. Making a list of grudges (Step Eight) and resolving not to be stirred by them (Steps Ten and Eleven) are prerequisites to sobriety and the helping of other alcoholics (Step Twelve).

The AA approach is practical and is based on the idea that all problem drinkers at one time or another have gone at least twenty-four hours without a drink. So AA members do not swear off alcohol for life or for any other extended period of time. Alcoholics are made to realize that there is nothing they can do about tomorrow now. AA wants alcoholics to concentrate on staying sober today, during this twenty-four hours. Then when they feel the desire to take a drink, it is accepted simply as something that must be dealt with today. They are taught not to worry about tomorrow's craving but merely to concentrate on postponing taking a drink today.

Regular attendance at local meetings plays an important part in a life of sobriety. Group meetings and relationships provide the testing ground for new ways of dealing with one's emotions and with the problems of living. Alcoholics frequently accept confrontation and support from others who struggle with the same problems as they do, although they may reject similar responses from physicians, ministers, or other professional persons. AA is one of the most successful approaches to sobriety because it practices these principles. AA has the benefit of comradeship and shared problems coupled with the added asset of the emotional objectivity and personal understanding or personality dynamics that others provide.

But the general atmosphere of an AA meeting is one of gaiety and good fellowship. Generally, AA members take their alcoholism seriously, but not themselves. That is another important part of the recovery program.

PRAGMATISM: ITS INFLUENCE ON AA

Jacob Bronowski (1973), in defining the philosophy of science for the twentieth century, believed strongly that the key principle to any science is the idea that humans and the physical world are evolving. But this is not surprising; any freshman course in biology will teach you that. But, Bronowski emphasized the often-ignored fact that matter itself evolves. Matter and life are following the same pattern. This evolution is a process in which atoms build up into more complex structures. Evolution, as Bronowski explains, is the climbing of a ladder from the simple to the complex by steps, each of which is stable in itself.

Bronowski indicates that humans' intellectual evolution is also a process–a dynamic, changing view by which we advance slowly and painstakingly in stages. "Scientific, rational foundations are laid in man's ascent," explains Bronowski (1973). We build our theories and knowledge upon these foundations laid by others and arrive at a temporary stage in our evolution. Knowledge is never certain, and what we define as truth is not a determinate representation of the independently existing structure of things. Rather, our definition of truth is an intellectual construction, chosen from alternatives by reason of its economy and simplicity, which does not literally describe reality, but makes contact with it simply by furnishing instruments for predicting future observations on the basis of present ones.

Building on this perspective, William James (1907) came to the conclusion that truth is what pays or what works. James anticipated the phenomenologists and many of the existential ideas when he explained, "A true idea is a projected map of experience to lead one wherever one wants to go" (p. 37). The individual, according to James, verifies truth by experiencing the consequences of an idea. Truth is a means to the achievement by an organism of a vital end. Truth designates ideas that start ideas. Scientific theories, for James, are adopted simply because they work; their consequences are satisfactory.

Later in his life, James came to propose a form of Bergson anti-intellectualism. James eventually gave up his trialistic view of truth in which he felt knowledge was defined and coerced by experience (as in natural science), or coerced by analytic intent of concepts (as in pure science), or by free choice (as in moral sentiment) involved in religious and metaphysical beliefs. James exchanged this view for the one in which an individual judges a belief by its comparison to a whole stock of beliefs (metaphysics, logic, science, etc.). Similar to the phenomenologists, he proposes that the belief which balances itself between these whole sets of beliefs without disturbing the oldest and most honored beliefs was generally accepted as true for its survival value. James felt truth was a projected map of experience and that truth was synonymous with what was useful. Truth is pragmatic!

Of course, James was one of the primary proponents of the philosophical system called pragmatism. One of its chief tenets was that if something ceases to be useful, it will cease to be true. The notion of absolute truth functions as a limit point of investigation rather than any ultimate knowledge. What we expect, we find to be true. What is expedient is truth. Truth fits our needs.

John Dewey is another pragmatist who shared James' sentiments. Like James, Dewey had some arguments that closely paralleled many of Thune's propositions about AA. For instance, Dewey criticized the spectator and onlooker aspect of knowledge and claimed that thought was only one mode of action involved in any experience (cited in White, 1972). Dewey's organic theory of knowledge gave the view of man struggling with his world and its environment and that knowledge was derived from this experience of action with the world. Just as AA encourages recovering alcoholics to get involved with the program so they can expand their horizons of experience or dilate their constructs to pick up new elements, Dewey felt that too many theorists retreat from the world of chance into a safe world of abstract thought.

Certainly, this is an argument that many members of AA share in their criticism of professionals whose interest in alcoholism is purely academic or passing. Abstractly, their theories sound correct. But, when put to the concrete test of reality, these abstractions frequently fail to materialize. As Dewey says, many professionals are reluctant to leave the safe world of theory and engage alcoholics on a real concrete level because this type of meeting is too demanding. Many professionals compound this problem by confusing the abstract with the concrete or the real. For example, some professionals misinterpret the importance of technical neutrality in their treatment of alcoholics. Abstractly and theoretically, the principle of neutrality ensures that the therapist will be nonjudgmental and accepting of alcoholics, voicing neither pleasure nor displeasure with their behavior. The intent behind this principle is theoretically sound. It is best for individuals to come to their own decisions themselves, free from the influence and judgment of others. Theoretically, this is the way control is internalized. Such a stance also ensures against harmful dependency, idealization, and compliance. However, on a concrete, experiential, and "real" level, such a stance can be disastrous for an alcoholic. The excessive reliance on abstract concepts often leads many individuals to misinterpret the actual experience. Abstract understanding alone frequently comes at the cost of the experience of the concrete. The separation of the abstract from the concrete is an example of the dualistic split that permeates Western rational thought.

Throughout his life, Dewey had criticized the dualistic tendency of Western thought. He felt Western philosophy reflected an important and unexamined bias that has been carried over from the legacy of early Greek philosophical influence. "Spectator knowledge," as Dewey criticized, was judged superior by Greek philosophers because it differentiated the knowledge obtained by the ruler through passive contemplation from the knowledge obtained by the ruled, who were forced to labor as slaves in lowly, practical activities. Consequently, idealism came to be accepted as a higher form of knowledge. Dewey believed this was in actuality a retreat from the unpredictable world of action to the safe world of abstract thought. Therefore, knowledge obtained by the spectator or onlooker was judged by Dewey to be influenced by the fear of becoming involved in a mode of action and a reluctance to engage in the struggle of the experience of the world as it is. Agreeing with Will Durant and the AA philosophy, Dewey believed thought without action was a disease (Durant, 1926).

What AA and Dewey are criticizing is the association of the ego, abstract thought, and the dilemma of human existence, namely that knowledge is acquired at the cost of the burden of knowing. Buber especially accentuated the importance of differentiating the abstract (I-It) from the concrete (I-Thou). Buber emphasized the essential difference between the direct, mutual meeting, into which one enters with one's whole being and in full presentness, and the indirect, nonmutual relationship of subject and object. Buber felt we were in definite danger of losing ourselves in the abstract idealism of our own thought, an abstraction that has spirited Alfred North Whitehead (1925) to raise the question concerning the tendency for many to confuse abstract interpretations with concrete occurrence. Whitehead warns that the fallacy of misplaced concreteness is the common misconception of science.

The writing of Whitehead and James reflects a common principle that lies at the heart of AA's success. AA's insistence on "the event"–the real actual meeting of the alcoholic by another alcoholic–ensures that the concrete is not lost at the expense of the abstract. This orientation is clear in the oft-repeated AA mottos, "Vitalize, don't analyze," "Go to ninety meetings in ninety days," and "Take your body and your mind will follow." Such encouragement reflects James' recommendation that you should act your way into a new way of thinking rather than think your way into a new way of acting.

EXISTENTIAL VIEW OF AA

Kurtz makes a convincing argument that AA works because it parallels existential philosophy in a number of important aspects. Kurtz further states that AA has not been given the recognition it deserves as a movement of unique intellectual significance. When AA is examined in relation to its sources and origins, the program expresses many important existential themes. The first theme of all existential philosophies is the realization of humans' limitation of being. The first step of AA ("We admitted we were powerless over alcohol") requires the alcoholic to recognize and admit this essential limitation. Kurtz writes,

> We admitted that we were powerless over alcohol–that our lives had become unmanageable" (26, p. 59; 27, pp. 21-24). AA addresses itself not to alcoholism, but to the alcoholic. The First Step of the AA program focuses upon the alcoholic as one who is essentially limited. The acknowledgment "I am an alcoholic" that is inherent in

> the admission of powerlessness over alcohol accepts as first truth human essential limitation, personal fundamental finitude, at least for the alcoholic. (1982, p. 43)

Powerlessness over alcohol and the acceptance of one's limitation in relation to alcoholism serves as a prototype for the alcoholic facing and accepting other limitations of the human condition. The larger insight of AA is the wholeness of limitation, an insight that is required after alcoholics are able to accept the limitation that they cannot drink alcohol. Kurtz sums up this dilemma when he writes.

> AA borrowed and learned from diverse sources–William James and the Oxford Group, Carl Jung and William Duncan Silkworth. Its own continuing experience also significantly shaped the development of AA's thought. The concepts embodied in both terms of its name best briefly clarify that insight. The alcoholic, in the AA understanding, is one who finds himself in an utterly hopeless situation: obsessively-compulsively addicted to alcohol, he by definition must drink alcohol and so destroy himself. Although alcoholism is conceptualized by AA as by others as "disease" or "malady," the alcoholic does not have alcoholism–he is an "alcoholic." Therefore he cannot do what others, nonalcoholics, do with joyful impunity: non-obsessively-compulsively drink alcohol. Contained in the term "alcoholic," then, are the implications of utterly hopeless helplessness and essential personal limitation. (1982, p. 41)

Central to alcoholics' acceptance of limitation is the recognition that while they are vulnerable, they can only attain sobriety by exposing this vulnerability and accepting this limitation. This is the healing dynamic of AA–a mutual vulnerability openly acknowledged and shared with other alcoholics. Kurtz writes:

> "Not-God" means first "You are not God," the message of the AA program . . . The fundamental and first message of Alcoholics Anonymous to its members is that they are not infinite, not absolute, *not* God. Every alcoholic's problem had *first* been, according to this insight, claiming God-like powers, especially that of *control*. But the alcoholic at least, the message insists, is *not* in control, even of himself; and the first step towards recovery from alcoholism must be the admission and *acceptance* of this fact that is so blatantly obvious to others but so tenaciously denied by the obsessive-compulsive drinker.

> But Alcoholics Anonymous is *fellowship* as well as *program,* and thus there is a second side to its message of not-God-ness. Because the alcoholic is not God, not absolute, not infinite, he or she is essentially limited. Yet from this very limitation–from the alcoholic's *acceptance* of personal limitation–arises the beginning of healing and wholeness . . . To be an alcoholic within Alcoholics Anonymous is not only to accept oneself as not God; it implies also affirmation of one's connectedness with other alcoholics . . . The invitation to make such a connection with others and the awareness of the necessity of doing so arise from the alcoholic's very acceptance of limitation. (1992, p. 42)

Another important aspect of alcoholics' acceptance of the limits of the human condition is the requirement that they understand that they have limited control and limited dependence. They must learn the difference if they are to stay sober. Kurtz writes:

> The emphasis on control as limited, as neither absolute nor to be abdicated pervades the AA program. "You can do something, but not everything" runs the constant implicit, and at times explicit, message. AA members are warned against promising "never to drink again." They learn, rather, "not to take the first drink, one day at a time." They are encouraged to attend AA meetings, which they can do, rather than to avoid all contact with alcohol, which they cannot do. The AA sense of limited control is admirably summed up in its famed "Serenity Prayer": "God grant me the serenity to accept the things I cannot change, the courage to change the things I can, and the wisdom to know the difference." (1982, p. 53)

Hitting Bottom: An Existential Viewpoint

Such an acceptance of limitation requires more than an intellectual insight. Individuals will only give up their self-centered and perceived absolute control of the world if it is wrenched away from them and ruthlessly exposed with all its false assumptions and deceptive facades. Being confronted with such a realization engenders the dread, fear, and trembling of Kierkegaard, the angst of Heidegger, the *angoisse* of Sartre, and the abyss of Buber. Borrowing a term from William James (i.e., deflation at depth), AA refers to it as hitting bottom. Karl Jaspers, another existential writer, refers to it as "limit situations." These great philosophers share the common opinion that an emotional upheaval is required before individuals will truly question the core of their existential predicament. Not until this issue is addressed in the stark, naked light of existence will an individual want or be able to accept the limitedness of the human condition.

Albert Camus sums up this position most graphically when he challenges his readers to examine the authenticity of their lives. Like Sartre, Camus believes most of us are living our lives in "bad faith," hanging on to illusions because we do not want to face death, terror, and suffering in life. Camus felt that if we were brutally honest with ourselves, we would discover there are only two real truths in life. We are going to die, and after death, there is nothing. He further states that if we truly answer these questions without hanging on to our refusal to accept limitations in life, we will either kill ourselves or decide for the first time to truly live our lives authentically. We will become what Sartre calls "authentic." We will trivialize the trivial and prioritize the vital. We will no longer deny death and the limitations in life. By denying death, we ultimately deny life because the two are inseparable.

Needless to say, Camus's challenge is one that most individuals, alcoholics as well as non-alcoholics, fear accepting because of the suffering it produces. In most cases, alcoholics, pushed to the edge of their psychic abyss because of their alcoholism, have no choice but to address Camus's challenge. They literally must either die or change their lives by surrendering to the first step of the AA program. If alcoholics are able to meet this challenge and integrate this experience, they often lead more meaningful lives. Nietzsche, in his own iconoclastic style, captures this experience concisely when he writes, "That which doesn't kill you will make you stronger."

All philosophy and all the social sciences must deal with the problem of real human suffering. AA, at least, recognizes suffering as a necessary and a possibly positive part of life. Many other treatment modalities have failed to recognize the actual therapeutic aspects of mobilizing a patient's assets at the time of crisis, avoiding the consolidation of symptoms, and thereby making them more problematic. The ideal conclusion of suffering and treatment, to take a page from Viktor Frankl (1969, p. 713), is to give the individual a reason for his suffering, or in Logotherapeutic terms, the will-to-meaning, which gives the person's suffering meaning. Once suffering is viewed in a meaningful paradigm, it can serve as a growth process.

AA is addressing a very fundamental principle of treatment. Before individuals' resources can be mobilized for therapeutic change, they must experience a state of personal incongruence. Often, change does not occur unless their pain and suffering prompts them to initiate an honest assertion of their condition and behavior. However, suffering must be integrated into a personal, meaningful paradigm. People who suffer for no known reason become defeated, bitter, or demoralized.

Viktor Frankl's personal experiences during World War II vividly demonstrate this principle with stark realization. A Jewish psychiatrist who was arrested by the Nazis during the war and shipped to one of their most brutal extermination camps, Frankl had little reason to believe he was ever to leave the death camp alive. With each passing day, month, and year, he was repeatedly told by his Nazi guards that Germany was winning the war and he would never be released from prison. Experiencing only unbearable suffering, unmerciful death, and tragic losses around him, Frankl saw many of his fellow prisoners slowly give up and literally lie down and die. Frankl was able to eventually discern those who were about to die and those who would go on living. Those individuals who could not see any reason for their suffering were more likely to die because their life had ceased to have meaning. Frankl realized that those who had managed to put their suffering within some meaningful context through their faith, belief, or hope were the ones least destroyed and defeated by their pain and suffering.

In a less dramatic, but very similar fashion, AA members share "the kinship of common suffering." Within this context, recovery from alcoholism requires that people share their suffering with others who understand their experience. As Kurtz defines it, mutuality in AA is triggered by the sharing of common suffering. This, in turn, teaches the alcoholic "that to be fully human is to need others" (1982, p. 55). AA therefore provides alcoholics with a commonly shared explanation of their suffering. It helps alcoholics make sense of their affliction by providing them with a meaningful paradigm for their experience.

AA is in many ways an educational process that allows suffering to be integrated into a person's life in a meaningful way. However, AA is education of a unique sort. It trains alcoholics to be more self-aware and more honest with themselves. It also teaches them to achieve more adequate control over their primitive impulses and strivings; to be freer in expressing their feelings; to become more tolerant of human limitations; and to develop the ability to postpone, modify, and even forego gratifications whose demands previously seemed overpowering. Through education, alcoholics learn to accept that there are limits to unbounded joy in life. Like Freud, who once described the goal of psychoanalysis as transforming neurotic misery into ordinary human suffering, alcoholics are on the road to recovery when they accept the fact that they are limited in unbounded happiness as the rest of us.

This is not to imply that happiness and joy are an antithesis to therapy, treatment, and recovery. Rather, alcoholics must be taught not to suffer for the wrong reasons. Pain and suffering are a part of life, but so are joy and happiness. As the Buddhist religious doctrine teaches, it is ignorant craving that often produces suffering. This was a point made vivid in James Clavell's novel *Shogun.* After an innocent man had died because of Blackwell's ignorance of Japanese customs, Blackwell stood cursing himself and the world because of his anger at this man's senseless death. Speaking to his Japanese lover, Blackwell exclaimed the world was not right, that things like this should not happen. As he questioned whether he could continue to live with integrity in such a senseless world, his Japanese lover responded to his frustration, anger, and feelings of futility. Speaking from a very traditional Eastern philosophical position, she told him he was wrong and that the world was not senseless. Correctly, she reminded him that he was angry because of his refusal to accept the world as it was and his insistence on trying to make it into something else. Blackwell suffered as he did because he wanted the world to be different and because he wanted it to fit neatly into his self-centered, predetermined set of expectations.

There is a similar tradition in classical Buddhist doctrine that suggests that "useful illusions" serve important purposes for the disciple in religious training, as they do for the addict or alcoholic in recovery. Each needs hope and the promise that there is some meaning or reason for suffering. The search for a life free of suffering with absolute happiness is futile. As existentialists are so eager to remind us, there are only two absolute truths in the world, "people suffer and people die." Buddhist doctrine encourages us to recognize that it is our "nature as living beings to suffer and to die." While this is an inescapable truth, we must not suffer for the wrong reasons or succumb to nihilism and pessimism. We must, as the Buddhists encourage us to do, engage in the joyful participation of the suffering in the world. However, until newly recovering addicts or alcoholics are ready to face and manage the anguish of such a confrontation, they need something to hold to and to believe before they can relinquish all of their illusions. While seeking enlightenment, Buddhist students will learn when they are ready that the search was futile since they possessed the answer from the start. As T. S. Eliot wrote: "We shall not cease from exploration and the end of all our exploring will be to arrive where we started and know the place for the first time" (Eliot, 1943, p. 59).

The theme of searching and finding ourselves is parallel to Hermann Hesse's story of Siddhartha and complements Freud's goal of therapy as transforming neurotic misery into ordinary human suffering, or as Strupp puts it: "Therapy terminates when the patient accepts the fact that he is as unhappy as the rest of us" (1972, p. 31). Erv Polster (1981) expressed similar sentiments when he said, "We must learn to suffer without too much pain."

From this perspective, suffering is defined as individual's unwillingness to accept the world as it is and their insistence on making it fit into their own expected image. Thinking of this sort is a form of idolatry in which alcoholics use chemicals as a way of facing the world when the limits they face are found to be unacceptable. Alcohol and drugs become a way of denying unhappiness, suffering, and limitations. Through the process of their alcoholism, alcoholics disregard more and more the acceptable or normative pleasures that are usually earned in the areas of achievement, knowledge, friendships, good health, and well-being. Alcohol and drugs reward self-centeredness and hedonistic pleasure. Such an attainment of pleasure is akin to a cheap thrill and comes at the cost of the alcoholic's integrity and self-esteem. Pleasure must be authentically earned by a subtle and important interplay between values, beliefs, customs, ideas, and behavior that cause no harm to others. Alcohol and drugs are thrills cheaply purchased at the price of self-respect. Self-worth and self-esteem are gradually lost because the rules for socially accepted normative ways of attaining pleasure have been altered and compromised. Alcohol- and drug-induced highs are tricks (pleasure without purpose) played on the brain that come at the cost of self-esteem.

Treatment from this perspective requires the removal of cheaply purchased thrills and replaces them with authentically earned happiness. Integrity cannot be purchased. It is earned, and once earned, it is the antithesis of shame, disrespect, and neurotic misery.

Ernest Hemingway once defined happiness as getting your money's worth and knowing when you have gotten it. Hemingway's statement has relevance for the alcoholic's situation, wherein happiness purchased through the use of chemicals leads only to hollowness and loss of self-respect. It is important to note that Hemingway does not describe happiness as a bargain–something that you steal or get cheaply. Happiness is earned and comes at a cost. However, as Hemingway carefully adds, you have to know when you have earned it. Happiness purchased cheaply is hollow and leads to little sense of mastery. Essentially, it is unappreciated because it is not earned. Happiness attained without understanding is purchased at the price of self-respect. Schopenhauer expressed similar sentiments when he wrote, "What a person is contributes more to his happiness than what he has." Kant also summed up this position when he wrote, "Morality is not properly the doctrine of how we make ourselves happy; but how we make ourselves worthy of happiness" (cited in Durant, 1926).

Muggeridge (1980) warned that when mortal men try to live without faith or a belief in God, or in AA terms, a higher power, they will unfailingly succumb to megalomania or erotomania or both. Faith in God teaches us humility and without humility, Muggeridge cautions, we will continue to pursue excitement, pleasure, and the obsessive satisfaction of our appetites. In a state of arrogance, we will remain in danger of substituting pleasure for happiness and as Muggeridge so eloquently argues: "Happiness pursued cannot be caught . . . I think the pursuit is a misguided concept because I think the thing about happiness is that it happens–it comes to us. It comes to us mysteriously. Again, when our relations with God are harmonious." This is very similar to Bateson's view that addiction is the result of an individual becoming locked into a symmetrical (versus complementary or harmonious) relationship with alcohol and others that is competitive, combative, and controlling. As Bateson (1971) says, there is no self to control unless one is operating under the illusion that one is separate from oneself and others. Recovery is returning to harmony within oneself and adopting a complementary epistemological position. In Bateson's perspective, AA provides this new and correct shift in epistemology.

For the recovering alcoholic, the pursuit and understanding of happiness requires a shift in perspective. Unless this shift is made, the alcoholic will either relapse or suffer what AA calls "white knuckle sobriety." Many alcoholics do not make this shift in perspective. Those who attain serenity usually do, however. Serenity is a term commonly acknowledged as a desired aim and is actively pursued by AA members. Although it is often a misunderstood concept, the early Greek philosopher Epicurus captured it perfectly. Epicurus believed that pleasure is the only conceivable–and quite legitimate–end of life and action. "Nature leads every organism to prefer its own good to every other good. We must not avoid pleasures, but we must select them" (cited in Durant, 1926). Epicurus exalts the joys of tranquility rather than those of the senses. He warns against pleasures that excite and disturb the soul, which should rather quiet and appease. In the end, he proposes seeking not pleasure in its usual sense, but *ataraxia*–tranquility, equanimity, repose of mind.

Existential philosophy is profoundly pessimistic in one sense and optimistic in another. Existentialists generally believe that happiness can only be achieved once the individual gives up the illusion of unlimited happiness.

Ernest Becker (1973) describes this situation perfectly when he states, "I am talking to the cheerful robots. I think the world is full of too many cheerful robots who talk only about joy and the good things. I have considered it my task to talk about the terror and suffering in the world" (p. 36). The terror that Becker talks about is our refusal to deal with suffering and death. We must view these aspects realistically and not try to avoid them by only dwelling on the beautiful things in life. Becker defines this position nicely when he writes, "joy and hope and trust are things one achieves after one has been through the forlornness" (p. 36). Otto Rank (cited in Yalom, 1980) agreed when he wrote, "The dynamic evil is the attempt to make the world other than it is, to make it what it cannot be, a place free from impurity, a place free from death and suffering."

Many existential writers believe that in such a confrontation between the realistic acceptance of the world as it is and the self-centered demands for unlimited gratification, reason would prevail and the individual would choose more realistically between the alternatives–continued unhappy struggles with old patterns of expectations or authentic existence with expanded freedom of choice and responsible expression of drives and wishes. With Socrates, we are urged to "know thyself." In this fashion, AA members are taught to believe that the authentic existence advocated by the AA program holds the key to self-examination, self-knowledge, emancipation, cure, and eventual salvation.

To grow up, alcoholics must relinquish the paradise of limitless abundance and arrogance. They must learn to renounce, to work, to suffer, to postpone gratification, to become responsible, and above all, to take an active, responsible part in mastering their fate. AA has set out to undermine alcoholics' dishonesty with themselves. Unlike any other time in their lives, alcoholics must come to understand that self-deception is a pervasive and universal human characteristic. However, unlike the non-addicted, alcoholics and addicts cannot afford to deceive themselves, for self-deception inevitably leads back to a relapse. Alcoholics and addicts must be constantly reminded that they can delude themselves into believing they were living their lives independently, whereas, for the most part, their lives were lived for them by chemicals and the forces of which they were not aware, which they did not understand, and over which they had little control.

AA–HOW IT WORKS: A PHENOMENOLOGICAL PERSPECTIVE

As every student of existentialism knows, it was Husserl's student, Martin Heidegger (1963) who is generally recognized as the single most influential architect of the philosophical position now called existentialism. Husserl developed an investigative procedure called phenomenology that was intended to help the investigator get past, through, or around the presuppositions, assumptions, and abstractions that dominated science and Western philosophical thought. Heidegger, following Husserl, took this method and applied it with the intent of getting at the core of experience—the actual lived experience of the moment. He believed that examining the phenomena of our experience and existence, without permitting ourselves to be distracted by our analytic minds, would give us a less contaminated view of what it means to be truly human (Dasien). Unknowingly, Heidegger was attempting to arrive at a position that is similar to many aspects of Buddhist doctrine, which defines enlightenment as "the complete and pure awareness of the immediacy of the moment." In both cases, the attempt is to bypass the bias that is inherent in any method that wishes to analyze, explain, understand, or make sense of our experience.

Carl Thune (1977) took the phenomenological method and applied it in a penetrating investigation and interpretation of AA. From Thune's perspective, AA works because of its emphasis on members recounting their life histories at AA meetings. It is through the telling of their life histories that they are taught how to interpret their past in a way that gives meaning to the past and hope for the future. Thune, operating from a pure phenomenological framework, holds the position that the past never merely exists for anyone, whether they are alcoholic or not. Instead, the past is interpreted and created through the use of conceptual models. More significantly, "These models become models of and for the creation of the future, a future that is no more automatically 'given' than is the past" (p. 83).

Thune introduces the importance of life histories in AA when he writes,

> In a sense, then, one of the first lessons A.A. must teach new members is that their lives were incoherent and senseless as they knew them. Simultaneously, it must reveal the "correct" understanding and interpretation of the drinking alcoholic's vision of the world before a new member can accept the full benefits of the program—a program which offers a different coherence and meaning in their active alcoholic lives. In other words, according to A.A., not only do drinking alcoholics incorrectly perceive and understand the world, but they cannot even correctly perceive and understand their perceptions and understandings of it. Through therapy they must learn new methods for evaluating them.
>
> More abstractly it is not just a revised and now coherent vision of the world which A.A. offers, but one which has altered the relation between its components. For example, in their life histories members describe the drinking alcoholic's life as he understands it—going steadily 'down hill' or 'around in circles.' As long as drinking continued the future was merely a continuation of the past with the

present being but a moment in which that past was re-enacted. (1977, pp. 81-82)

The Life History: AA from a Phenomenological Perspective

One of the major tenets of phenomenology is the demonstration that the world and the self, rather than being automatically given in the order of things, are being constantly recreated as individuals proceed through life. Insight into individuals' lives then comes from an analysis of the world as they constructs it, in which they must live.

It is suggested by Thune that the nature, meaning, and experience of these constructions of the self and the world by alcoholics are subject to an ongoing process of reconstitution and redefinition, both in the process of becoming alcoholics and in the course of any successful treatment and recovery program. Central to this process will be the redefinition of the meaning and experience of alcoholism. Complementing this is the suggestion that alcoholism is better understood as in the terminology of AA: a defective mode of life (Madsen, 1974). The implication is that a treatment regimen directed at reconstitution and redefinition of self and world provides a better way to deal with alcoholism than a model holding it analogous to a physical disease or a bad habit subject to modification. This is AA's claim and lies at the heart of the success that AA has enjoyed.

Like most therapeutic systems, AA faces the twin problems of diagnosis and treatment. However, the program's analysis of these facets of the therapeutic process bears little relation to those of more "orthodox" Western medical systems (Thune, 1977). It is in the diagnosis and definition of alcoholism that AA parts company with many of the psychological definitions of alcoholism.

Objective diagnosis (an important and necessary component of scientific assessment in psychology) from a source other than alcoholics themselves is held irrelevant to the program. The success or failure of the program depends on whether individuals can diagnose themselves as alcoholics. It is this self-diagnosis that is the essence of AA's twelve steps to recovery. To paraphrase Laing (1969), alcoholics must come to understand that one does not have alcoholism; rather one is alcoholic.

In addition to the "physical allergy" to alcohol suggested by the disease model of alcoholism, alcoholics are held to possess an alcoholic personality described as immature and self-centered. They are spiritually sick, their naively egotistical and self-centered personalities preventing any but the most artificial and superficial relation to others or to a "higher power."

Within AA's therapy, the change needed to eliminate this mental and spiritual disequilibrium, which the program identifies as the heart of alcoholism, is more than just a shift in understanding of the essence of the self. It requires a sharing with others of one's past. From its founding, the life history has been a key element of AA practice and theory. In the life history, the members recount their experience and eventual control of alcoholism. In most cases, if the speaker was not a physical derelict at the time of his or her active alcoholism, the attempt is made to demonstrate that he or she was at least in a derelict frame of mind when drinking. And after accepting the program, many claim to have experienced "personality changes," which accompany a new understanding of themselves and their world.

The stories about their life histories are typically stereotyped and lead to the conclusion of the proper way to analyze and construct their past. Individuals' pasts are the means through which they attain control over their alcoholism. Through the stories, alcoholics come to understand their life as more intelligible; they view it within a different structure and logic than they had previously.

Unlike most medically oriented therapeutic systems, the real problem as AA analyzes it centers around helping alcoholics understand their basic "being" as alcoholic rather than as normal and non-alcoholic. It is AA's emphasis on the spiritually defective mode of being rather than a physical disability that provides the clearest expression of the belief that alcoholism is a defect of being. In many respects, AA invokes a spiritual or religious vocabulary in the absence of perhaps a more accurate but inaccessible philosophical-ontological terminology.

Alcoholism from the program's perspective is a total lifestyle or mode of being and action in the world within which misuse of alcohol is only one component, albeit the most important component. Elimination of drinking is an indispensable first concern, but it is just the first step before altering other important aspects of the overall defective lifestyle. It is not uncommon to hear AA members refer to someone who has stopped drinking but still maintains the defective mode of life as being a "dry drunk." The implication is that the alcoholic has given up alcohol but not the self-perceived construction of his or her self that is associated with the alcoholic lifestyle.

Whereas society has irrevocably linked alcohol to the alcoholic, AA insists upon their separation. As mentioned before, AA will argue that individuals are alcoholics whether or not they drink and that their behavior may be that of a typical alcoholic even if they have not had a drink for years. AA is therefore aware that many drinkers, even heavy drinkers, are not necessarily alcoholics (Alcoholics Anonymous, 1955).

Considering this orientation, it is not surprising that research claiming that alcoholics can be trained to drink socially (Sobell and Sobell, 1973b) strikes AA as absurd, since alcoholism from this viewpoint appears as a bad habit subject to correction through education. The chasm that seems to exist between AA and the scientific community evolved around the latter's attempt to place alcoholism in a research paradigm and its insistence on identifying personality variables related to its etiology. This controversy is not easily resolved. Highly qualified researchers have for years been unable to determine whether alcoholism is a physical or mental problem. The outstanding specialists in the field, however, such as Ruth Fox (1973), E. M. Jellinek (1960), and Marty Mann (1973) have all realized that alcoholism embraces cultural, psychological, and physical factors.

While there is a considerable amount of misunderstanding and controversy surrounding AA's approach to alcoholism, there is virtually none regarding the efficacy of AA as a treatment modality. The literature is replete with substantial evidence that supports the fact that AA really does work (Bourne and Fox, 1973, Bailey and Leach, 1965). The crucial question therefore is not whether AA works, but rather, why does it work? This answer has long escaped psychologists for a number of reasons. Part of the answer may be AA's transcendental and nonpositivist foundations, variables that do not lend themselves easily to scientific investigation. As Kuhn (1962) suggests, a scientific community can often become a closed system with communication limited to those with selected membership within that community. Under these conditions, it is understandable that professionals have generally been reluctant to leave their accepted scientific paradigm to investigate variables that do not fit neatly into its accepted and proven methodology.

Kuhn's discussion helps explain the reluctance of some professionals to accept AA as a legitimate treatment alternative. In light of Thune's phenomenological explanation of AA, it appears that much of their reluctance is due to their failure to shift paradigms when trying to understand and investigate AA. The problem, then, lies not with AA, but with the professionals for failing to expand their cognitive models of explanation so that AA is understood and examined in its proper light. Once this shift in perspective is accomplished, one may understand better Thune's conclusions about AA:

> AA's "treatment," then, involves the systematic manipulation of symbolic elements within an individual's life to provide a new vision of that life, and of his world. This provides new coherence, meaning

and implications for behavior. While the processes which have been discussed above clearly occurred in the groups investigated, the literature indicates that similar patterns exist in other AA groups. Indeed, any alcoholism treatment program must successfully demonstrate to the alcoholic that he is an alcoholic, or, more exactly, it must succeed in allowing the alcoholic to demonstrate this fact to himself. This seems possible only if the alcoholic himself can discover a new past to confirm what ultimately must be a self-diagnosis. I suggest that even in systems operating according to principles different from AA's, one of the therapeutic requirements is the presentation of a new model which defines self and world.

These suggestions, however, should not be taken as contradictions of the conclusions reached by other analytic perspectives. Rather, they are intended to provide phenomenological perspective which complements other perspectives such as those offered by medicine, sociology and psychology. It is the summation of these different but clearly complementary perspectives, rather than academic arguments over which is true or which is formally or logically prior, that will lead to a more complete understanding of alcoholism and the mechanisms of therapy. (1977, p. 88)

THE SELF-ATTRIBUTION OF ALCOHOLISM

Next to the importance Thune places on the telling of one's life story at an AA meeting, he views the constant introduction of oneself as an alcoholic as the next most essential component of the recovery program. Each self-proclamation of "I am an alcoholic" is a constant reminder to AA members that they are just a drink away from being the person they once were. This is a very confusing state of affairs to those whose interest in AA is only passing, superficial, or purely academic. They fail to understand the significance of this ritual. In fact, many critics take special issue with AA's insistence that all AA members introduce themselves as alcoholics. Individuals outside of the AA program interpret this as either degrading to the alcoholic or a constant negative reminder of the person's multiple shortcomings. They fail to understand how such a requirement can lead to anything but continual debasement and loss of self-respect. To the contrary, AA members who introduce themselves as alcoholics do so proudly, for they are conveying an important message to themselves each time they stand up and make such a proclamation.

The self-attribution of alcoholic conveys far more information for the alcoholic in AA than it does for the individual outside the program who defines him or herself as someone who once drank too much. The term "alcoholic" signifies everything (self-centered behavior, negative attitude, corrupt values) that sober AA members must guard against if they are to maintain a healthy sobriety. By constantly utilizing the self-definition of alcoholic, AA members automatically imply the opposite, which is everything a healthy, recovering, and sober member of AA must attain. AA members are thus reminded with each pronouncement of themselves as an alcoholic that they are just a drink away from losing what they have become, which is a person whose values, attitudes, and behavior is the direct opposite of that of an alcoholic.

Bill Wilson had expressed similar sentiment many years before when he wrote that within every recovering alcoholic there are two built-in authorities that the outside world could never understand. First, in the life of each AA member there still lurked a very real and ruthless tyrant represented by booze and all that was associated with it. The second authority, according to Wilson, was an inner voice. In talking with others, he would refer to it as a power, life-force, or any words with which the listener would be comfortable. In one sense, the recovering alcoholic is everything that the practicing alcoholic is not. This helps explain the failure of non-alcoholics to grasp how it is that one drink can cause alcoholics to slip back into their old behavior.

From this perspective, alcoholism is viewed as more than just excessive drinking. This is why AA believes that alcohol consumption cannot be curtailed without addressing and treating the rest of the alcoholic's personality disturbance. The difficulty professionals have with AA's treatment approach centers around the issue of the necessity of total abstinence. While many professionals continue to view alcoholism as a focal disturbance that could be eliminated or cut out as you would cut out a bad spot in an otherwise good apple, that AA views it as the primary issue that must be dealt with first. Abstinence from alcohol is the first step required for breaking the alcoholic style of living. Only after abstinence has been assured can alcoholics learn to focus on changing their characterological personality style.

Within this system, at any given moment, individuals are either healthy or unhealthy depending on which system is dominant. Drinking only encourages the unhealthy lifestyle to dominate the healthy potential within the alcoholic. As AA recognizes, alcoholics are isolated spiritually and can only relate to others on a superficial level. They cannot define themselves because their being is controlled and clouded by their drinking. Their alcoholism makes it impossible to relate to anyone or anything on a meaningful level. Because the fellowship of AA gives recovering alcoholics an identification with something greater than themselves, it permits a shift toward healthy relationships with others.

Angyal (1965) agreed with Thune when he suggested that alcoholics' new definitions of themselves do not cut them off from their past history, but changes their perception of their past. This is exactly what Thune says AA accomplishes in its recovery process. This is experienced through the alcoholics telling their life history. Angyal, however, addresses two other very significant issues that Thune omits. The first is the significance of denial and the second concerns relapse.

Angyal attempts to come to grips with the baffling process of denial so common to the alcoholic's recovery. Why is it that alcoholics are so reluctant to seek treatment? Why must they hit bottom before they will ever admit they have a drinking problem? Why is it that everyone else but the alcoholics will know they are alcoholics, and what is it that blinds them to what everyone else sees so readily? Having to admit that one has been at fault is not a calamity for a self-confident person, but it is for the alcoholic, in whose system compensatory pride is a crucial element and losing face is disastrous. The prospect of giving up the alcoholic lifestyle is experienced as a threat not to life but to the alcoholic's integrity. It is a self-betrayal to be resisted at all costs. Small wonder that when alcoholics' drinking is threatened, they feel that everything is falling to pieces, that they are about to drive into nothingness, that they are emotionally dying.

The second issue that Angyal addresses is the recovery process so necessary to AA's treatment approach. This involves two secondary issues. The first is the initial recognition of alcoholism and the second revolves around the typical problem of relapse, which is a constant concern for any recovering alcoholic. The first step in AA's twelve steps to recovery is the admittance that one is an alcoholic. Angyal writes, "To take responsibility, to acknowledge, simply and frankly, the part one has played, and is still playing, in all of one's actions and in one's self destruction. By one admitting this to another, the alcoholic discards his false front and moves beyond the confines of anxious secrecy" (1965, p. 118). This step forward cannot be made without some confidence that the alcoholic will be able to live differently in the future. AA gives alcoholics this model. When this has been accomplished, the next step is dealing with the guilt and shame. AA views the resolution of guilt and shame as an intricate part of the recovery process. The necessary components of resolving guilt and shame are in essence paraphrased in the last nine steps of the AA recovery process. Angyal writes, "There is only one way of dealing with guilt–to regret it. This means sorrow for the harm that was done and the constructive actions left undone; for chances that were never taken, for the adventures missed and perhaps no longer possible, for having short-changed those who loved or needed one and tried in vain to come close to be helpful" (p. 136). But more is required than regret in combatting shame. The removal of shame occurs only if the alcoholic gives up the alcoholic lifestyle, with a strong desire to live in a different way. Shame requires a change in a person's sense of self. This is accomplished more slowly and usually with more difficulty.

The resolution of shame depends on whether or not the alcoholic's insights and struggles will result in lasting changes of real consequence. This depends on whether the alcoholic identifies with the new emerging pattern of health, and redefines him or herself in terms radically different from the patterns associated with his or her self-concept. Angyal stresses the importance of this change in an alcoholic's life pattern: "Drawing on the reports of reformed alcoholics one finds that they differ from the short-lived conversions in that the habit was given up not merely because of its specific deleterious effects; a broader change of attitudes has rendered the habit incompatible with the dominant system" (p. 121). The AA member now feels that drinking is inconsistent with his or her self-definition as a rational and responsible being. As this process unfolds, the detrimental elements of shame diminish.

Angyal also makes an important distinction between the task of getting healthy (sober) and staying healthy (sober). He feels too little emphasis is placed on the latter. AA recognizes the danger of allowing the constructive orientation to get lost inadvertently and unnoticeably. The alcoholic pattern may reinstate itself through a series of small steps, and a long time may pass before the person realizes the change.

Therefore, it is crucial to alcoholics' recovery process that they avoid their past drinking situations. Through the process of their disease, alcoholics usually have isolated themselves from anyone who does not drink like they do. Continual contact with people to whom one had been tied in an alcoholic relationship represents a continual threat to new attitudes. These new attitudes may also wear off in routine dealings with people who assume that the patient's new conduct is merely a hypocritical pose.

Angyal suggests that the strongest protection against future relapses and the trait that AA deems essential to the alcoholic's development is the sense of humility expressed when alcoholics admit the "bankruptcy" of their former ways and discard their alcoholic compensations and pretenses. Angyal makes a final point in describing the change necessary before sobriety can be obtained: "It may sound exaggerated or outright false when a member of Alcoholics Anonymous, who has not touched a drop of liquor for years, still refers to himself as an alcoholic. Far from being insincere, this self-evaluation is literally true and is the best protection against relapses. When an alcoholic proudly proclaims that he 'has licked the habit for good' the time is not far off when he will go on a binge" (1965, p. 161).

HONESTY, DENIAL, AND THE NEED FOR OTHERS

The insight of AA and the philosophy of existential thinkers are identical in that both see denial and self-deception as the root of all human evil and the source of all alienation. The reversal of this trend requires alcoholics to face their need for others with uncompromising honesty. Kurtz (1982) sums up this process when he writes:

> According to the insight of AA, because of their essential limitation, human beings have needs. The denial of essential limitation usually manifests itself not directly, but in the denial of need. The alcoholic's denial of need is two-fold: his denial of his need for alcohol blends into and intertwines with his denial of his need for others. Early in the process of alcoholism, the alcoholic denies that it is his unmet, because insatiable, need for others that leads him to seek comfort or excitement in alcohol. "A few drinks" become more important than the people at a party, for example, as alcohol becomes a surer source of satisfaction than human interaction. Later in the process, after a few failures of "I can stop whenever I want to" (denial of the need for alcohol), the denial becomes again of the need for others: "Just let me alone–I can lick this thing by myself." (p. 73)

The concepts of honesty and mutuality advocated by Kurtz are crucial to understanding AA's recovery program. The interaction of both is essential for the healthy functioning of the individual. It is this combination that allows the individual to obtain the harmony necessary to function as an involved participant within the world. As existentialists suggest, an alcoholic in a state of isolation frequently suffers the manifestations of anxiety and alienation that determine the formation and actualization of the sweeping condition they refer to as an existential crisis. In a similar sense, the alcoholic is not part of the whole; he or she is uninvolved and has no real freedom to choose.

Of course, these are existential themes. Alienation and the inability or refusal to choose is characteristic of what Sartre calls "acting in bad faith." In a sense, authenticity, which is such a necessary part of an existential definition of health, is impossible for a person who is isolated from the world and him or herself.

Kurtz (1982) describes the struggle for authentic existence–to become and to be what one really is–as the most significant and meaningful event in any individual's life. This theme is also prevalent in most existential philosophy and existentialist Martin Buber addresses this very issue numerous times in his writings. He criticizes the collectivity of social thought that thickens the distance between human beings. Collectivity for Buber is the herd instinct or the "crowd" that alienates people, thus not allowing them to meet others in all their uniqueness. Buber, like Angyal, feels that our guilt lies in not fulfilling and recognizing our own potential and uniqueness. Martin Heidegger is right to say that we experience a primal guilt because of this situation. Real guilt, according to Heidegger, consists of the fact that the "existence is guilty in the ground of its being and the existence is guilty through not fulfilling itself"–not becoming what Heidegger calls "the one" (das Man) (cited in Buber, 1964, p. 390).

Buber anticipates Kurtz when he describes the importance of the I-Thou in determining a necessary state of human development. Like the AA program, Buber's concept of the I-Thou stresses the importance of one's involvement in something larger than one's self. Of course, the supreme I-Thou for Buber is the relationship that occurs when one experiences God on a personal level. However, Buber's I-Thou is more than a relation to God; it is that concrete experience of being in harmony with the universe. This meeting can occur whenever a person is open to the experience of true relating, whether it be with another person or some inanimate object. Even obscure meetings are microcosms of the supreme relationship. For Buber, relating to someone or something can be an experience comparable to being in touch with a spiritual power that unites the individual with the order of the cosmos.

Buber's genius was not his formulation of the I-Thou, for that was done by others before him. But it was Buber alone who placed at the center of a monumental corpus the task of pointing to the essential difference between the direct, mutual meeting–into which one enters with one's whole being and in full presentness–and the indirect, nonmutual relationship of subject and object, the I-It.

Like Angyal, Buber recognizes the necessity of autonomy or the ability to relate in the sphere of the I-It. Buber sees this separateness of the I in positive terms because it is the development of this I that allows the eternal Thou to be confronted with all its uniqueness. Therefore, the detached I is necessary in Buber's system for a number of reasons. Buber feels that a human being is more than just a rational animal. Animals, for Buber, do not need confirmation of their being because an animal is what it is unquestionably. Humans, in contrast, need to have a presence in the being of the "other." Consciousness, therefore, is higher because the element of choice is present. One human being, by his or her separateness of the I, can meet another human being as a Thou, in that both of them are able to recognize the paradox of their uniqueness and their similarity.

The parallel theme with Angyal and Buber is the importance they place upon a person being autonomous, yet capable of choosing *not* to control in order to become part of the dynamic whole. As Angyal emphatically states, "We are nothing in ourselves. We are a message which comes to life only by being understood and acknowledged by someone." Buber's therapist differs from the psychologist who clarifies by reference to his or her own self in self-observation, self-analysis and experimentation, relating what he or she knows from literature and observation. Buber's therapist instead must enter, completely and in reality, in the act of self-reflection in order to become aware of human wholeness. In other words, therapists must carry out this act of entry into that unique dimension as an act of their lives, without any prepared philosophical security; that is, they must expose themselves to all that can meet them when they are really living.

The implications for this in therapy are profound. Individuals in treatment are usually isolated and if they are to get in touch with that healthy potential in themselves it is necessary to understand their ability to engage in true mutual dialogue. That is why the actual meeting of two individuals can disrupt that spiral of isolation so prevalent in an alcoholic's life. Buber's emphasis in therapy has rested particularly on the healing-through-meeting process that is such an intricate part of true dialogue.

As Buber suggests, a crucial step in AA is self-transcendence, which involves embracing new relationships with others who are also recognized as essentially limited as we are. Such a shift in perspective requires a recognition that to be fully human is to need others. For alcoholics, this is no easy task. Kurtz feels this task is made more difficult for alcoholics because of the deep feelings of shame that accompany their alcoholism. In fact, Kurtz feels AA works because it is a therapy for shame. It is important to understand Kurtz's description of shame for it has many parallels to Kohut's description of the narcissistic personality disorder. Chapter 6 dealt exclusively with the relationship of object-relations, self-psychology, and character pathology to addiction and group psychotherapy. Kohut's description of these issues will not be repeated here, but it is useful to note the many parallels that exist between shame, as Kurtz describes it, and Kohut's description of narcissism.

AA: A SELF-PSYCHOLOGY PERSPECTIVE

Viewing addiction as a disorder of the self and narcissistic phenomena as the problematic expression of the need for self-object responsiveness helps provide an alternative explanation for why AA and other twelve-step programs work as they do for the chemically dependent individual. Self-psychologists hold many basic tenets that they believe are essential if narcissistic disturbances are to be repaired. Kohut viewed the narcissistic disorder as the expression of a reaction to injury of the self and regarded the experience of the bond between the self and the self object to be crucial for psychological health and growth. Kohut is implying that there is an inverse relationship between individuals' early experience of positive self-object responsiveness and their propensity to turn to alcohol, drugs, and other sources of gratification as substitutes for these missing or damaging relationships. Conversely, if they are to successfully give up these misguided attempts at self-repair, they must learn how to substitute healthy interpersonal relationships in which needs for self-object responsiveness (Mirroring, Merger, and Idealization) are satisfied in a gradual, gratifying way.

AA and other twelve-step programs accomplish this in a number of ways. First and foremost, AA provides a predictable and consistent holding environment that allows addicts and alcoholics to have their self-object needs met in a way that is not exploitive, destructive, or shameful. Because of unmet development needs, addicts or alcoholics have such strong and overpowering needs (Object Hunger) for human responsiveness that they feel insatiable and shamed by their neediness. Through their identification with other alcoholics and addicts, they come to accept in themselves what they could not previously because they believed their badness was unique. As one early recovering alcoholic said of his first experience in AA, "I told everyone all these terrible, horrible, and shameful things about myself and instead of being disgusted with me, everyone gave me their phone numbers." Acceptance at this level of emotional vulnerability can only be tolerated by addicts or alcoholics because they feel understood on a very basic, empathic level. Empathy and emotional attunement are not only the cornerstone of treatment for self-psychology, they are also the foundation from which chemically dependent individuals can begin to feel the kind of responsiveness and gratification they had been missing and were previously unable to tolerate in their lives.

AA, as a holding environment, also becomes a transitional object–a healthy dependency that provides enough separation to prevent depending too much on any single person until individuation and internalization are established. Gradually, alcoholics or addicts are able to give up the grandiose defenses (narcissism) and false-self persona for a discovery of self (true self) as they really are. In existential terms, the confrontation between what they tried to be and what they really are (not-God) results in them ceasing to live their life in bad faith (alcoholic) and become more authentic ("Hello, I'm Joe, a recovering alcoholic") with all the limitations that authentic life imposes on them. As infantile ways of getting one's needs met are gradually relinquished for more mature ways of establishing close human contact (removal of character defect by working the program), the alcoholic or addict is able to internalize more self-care and monitoring of affective states (transmuting internalization). The central issue in this process is the acceptance of one's self as one is, which requires dealing with shame about the self that was previously hidden.

Khantzian (1994) believes that AA is corrective for the alcoholic because the program is able to penetrate the narcissistic defenses of pride. The primary reason alcoholics suffer, according to Khantzian, is because they cannot control their drinking and they cannot control themselves. Unable to admit their vulnerabilities, they remain isolated, alone and cut off from others and themselves. What they need to do (admit their vulnerabilities to another), they cannot do because of the shame and their characterological grandiose defensive posture. AA works because once initiation into the program occurs, contact with others is sustained, and through continued interaction with others, alcoholics are able to alter the dysfunctional interpersonal style that up to now has dominated their life. Khantzian explains that only through this maintenance of contact with others can the disorders of the self be repaired. He identifies the four aspects of the disordered alcoholic as: (1) relation of emotions; (2) self-esteem or a lack of healthy narcissism; (3) mutually satisfying relationships; and (4) self-care. He agrees with Kurtz that it is shame that makes the engagement and contact difficult, if not sometimes impossible, for many practicing alcoholics.

AA: A TREATMENT FOR SHAME AND NARCISSISM

Kurtz (1981) says there are two different ways of feeling bad. One is guilt and the other is shame. For Kurtz, shame is a much more powerful and primitive emotion. Guilt implies feeling bad for something you have done. It is a violation of rules and its focus is on behavior and actions. I promised to pick you up after work and give you a ride home. I did not follow through with my promise, so I feel bad or guilty for something I have done. Shame is a falling short of a goal and concerns a person's sense of self and unworthiness. Shame strikes at the core of our being. Rather than feeling bad for what I have done, I feel bad for who or what I am. Guilt is repaired by a quantitative effort, redoing or correcting a behavior. Shame can only be repaired by quality—a re-being of what I am—and requires a conversion or a new sense of self.

From Kurtz's perspective, treatment for shame is a far more intricate and difficult process. Shame cannot be treated by talking about it. Shame can only be healed through vulnerability. We cannot get in touch with another's pain without getting in touch with our own pain. Therefore, treatment which not only allows alcoholics to learn that their own pain is not shameful, but allows them to connect and identify with another's shame and pain, teaches them that the sharing of pain can be healing. Alcoholics learn to accept in others those aspects of themselves of which they are ashamed. Before patients can be healed, they must learn they can be accepted as they are by another. This process is initiated by accepting those shameful aspects of the self in another.

Mutuality thus becomes the crucial aspect of therapy. This is why AA and group psychotherapy work while individual therapy frequently fails. Both AA and group psychotherapy allow for the breaking of the cycle of interpersonal isolation that is central to the establishment of shame. All alcoholics fear that they will be found out for what they feel they truly are or that they will be looked down upon and ignored. To expose one's real self is frightening. What is needed is confirmation from others through a process of reciprocal self-revelation. Embarrassment is the experience of a person exposing and getting in touch with the shameful parts of their his or her hidden true self. When alcoholics confront themselves, they are made aware of internal incongruence and their false self, defensive facade. Under the false self is fear and shame. Such feelings can only be resolved by the confrontation of this disparity and the continual confirmation from another, affirming that others are accepting of the exposed true self.

Shame involves exposure. It is triggered by a sense of being looked at and caught unexpectedly. Shame is enhanced by the exposure of self to self. Shame thus involves an experience of self being diminished. Typically, the self refuses to see itself. This is the basis of the alcoholic's denial and self-deception. Shame occurs when the self breaks through the false self, deceptive facade. In therapy, the self must be confronted as feared and seen as it is. For alcoholics who possess a tremendous fear of confronting their true-self, such an exposure of self requires courage as much as insight.

Kurtz (1982) draws some important parallels between the existential position of inauthenticity and the "false self" of Winnicott (see Chapter 6) and object-relations theorists. Kurtz describes how this false self-presentation originates:

> Sometimes, out of that terror, a person will dissimulate in his presentation of himself to others in an effort to quell the pain of separateness by winning approval and acceptance. To the extent that he does so, and succeeds, he will experience a queer, unnamable apprehension, becoming trapped in an uneasy state that he finds both painful and corrupting. (p. 61)

Kurtz sees the fear of exposure of the true self to others as the cause of dishonesty and self-deception. Once this habit of dishonesty has been set, it leads to the alcoholic's corruption.

> Whether from unwillingness or inability to tell the truth about who he is, such an individual knows himself in his heart to be faking. Not merely is he ashamed of having and harboring a secret, unlovely, illegitimate self. The spiritual burden of not appearing as the person he "is," or not "being" the person he appears to be–the extended and deliberate confusion of seeming and being–is by and large intolerable if held in direct view. Despairing of attaining the integrity he craves, the person turns to grasp at its illusion: since he cannot make public his private self, he commands his private self to conform to the public one. This choice beguiles to a loss of truth–not so much "telling" it, but knowing it. (p. 61)

Most individuals, alcoholic and non-alcoholic, are often unaware that they are false, unreal, and inauthentic. They know no other existence. They eventually come to believe their false self is real because without this defensive facade they have nothing. Their apprehension is therefore catastrophic when their false self facade is threatened. They will feel exposed to the shame and the fear of non-being.

It is here at the realm of the construction of the false self that Kurtz and the existentialists unite with Kohut and self-psychology in explaining the paradox of existence and recovery for the alcoholic. Kohut views narcissism as a defensive facade that is adapted because the true self is either fragmented, weak, or uncohesive. Exposing this unprotected true self to the world is a risk that must be avoided at all costs. Kurtz refers to this deep sense of worthlessness and embarrassment as shame and states this is a feeling that plagues every alcoholic. The alcoholic, in Kohut's view, is lacking a cohesive self and constantly seeks confirmation from others or a joining with a powerful other in order to bolster his or her self-esteem.

From Kohut's perspective, this is why AA is such an effective treatment program. Kohut defines narcissistic disorders as presenting with three types of transference distortions (see Chapter 6). They are either idealizing, mirror-hungry, or merger-prone. AA thus provides for them an idealized other (i.e., the AA program, the principles of AA, etc.) or goal that is concrete and attainable. If the alcoholics do what the principles of the AA program ask of them, they will get all the mirroring and confirmation they need. AA will accept them, no matter what they have done in the past and will always be there for them anytime they desire or need it in the future. AA is a constant "good-enough" mother that serves as a transitional object until the principles of the program are internalized. AA also provides idealized others (sponsors and sober members) with whom the alcoholic can merge. Merger with the idealized other serves as a container for the depleted self of the alcoholic. Those alcoholics whose need for confirmation is insatiable will be applauded by other AA members as long as they stay sober. Certain members of AA can take on "guru-like" qualities. They are then assured the mirroring upon which they thrive and they will do all that is necessary (sobriety) to ensure that this source of confirmation is never lost. At the same time, they will serve as idealized others for recovering alcoholics.

However, the danger for Kohut is that narcissistic individuals can come to believe that their false self is their true self. They can be deluded by their narcissistic and grandiose fantasies. Kurtz defines this process as the refusal of alcoholics to accept limitations in their aspirations. They are not only caught by their narcissism, but further corrupted by their own grandiosity.

The alcoholic's dilemma of wanting more and being satisfied with less parallels that of all human existence. As intelligent creatures, we all have the ability to conceive a state of affairs that does not exist at the present time. Through a vehicle called the mind, we can project into the future a set of circumstances setting into motion an action that will change the present. Consequently, we can plan, achieve, and create a state of affairs that would not have existed if we had not acted. We have the ability to affect others and make things other than they are. The more we achieve, the more we believe in our achievements. The more we believe in our achievements, the more we delude ourselves into thinking we are unique, special, and unlimited. We become mesmerized by our sense of our uniqueness and when we do this, we lose the edge that allows us to achieve, create, and improve our lives. We come to believe we are gods. We believe we have absolute control and lose the humility that keeps us from being ourselves.

Consequently, life contains a standing paradox. Humans are finite creatures on the one hand and infinite in their desires on the other hand. It is impossible to escape the influences of our successes. All of our achievements come at the cost of deluding ourselves into believing that we are special. Yet if we did not aspire to greatness, we would remain ordinary.

We are constantly reminded that there is a perfection beyond our grasp. Charles Frankel (1971) sums up this dilemma when he writes:

> No matter how men try, they cannot help but be caught up in local circumstances, a parochial outlook, and a personal, all-too-personal, self. There is bound to be egoism even in their highest flights of altruism; there is bound to be something personal, self-enclosed, and partisan about their thinking even when they believe they are being most objective. And yet despite the fact that men are captives of necessity in this way, they are also free. They cannot hold any point of view which is not relative, or have anything but a limited grasp of perfection. But they can know that there is a perfection beyond their grasp. They can see beyond their own local circumstances, recognize that some other point of view is possible, and believe that there is such a thing as impersonality and objectivity. In short, man is a creature living tensely between two worlds: one is the actual, limited world in which he lives, but from which he cannot help but feel alienated; the other is an ideal world for which he longs, but from which he is permanently excluded. To be disappointed idealists is the common and eternal fate of all men. Man's whole moral life requires him "to seek after an impossible victory and to adjust himself to an inevitable defeat." (p. 88)

The source of all our achievements is also the source of our wickedness and folly. Frankel's argument suggests that our vices and virtues have the same origins. Consequently, whatever human beings do is tainted. Our triumphs tempt us to forget our weaknesses and as our power grows, so does our pride and dogmatism. However, Frankel feels that if human beings could not see beyond the immediate future, they would not be goaded by their desire for something better, and none of their subsequent triumphs would be imagined. However, knowledge is acquired at the burden of knowing. Understanding is achieved at the cost of knowing that death and suffering are a part of life. Such understanding produces anxiety. This is what separates humans from animals. This is why we can never achieve the simple happiness animals experience because animals, unlike humans, are what they are unquestioningly. Frankel describes the existential dilemma that confronts every individual and that is the source of self-deception in the alcoholic:

> But anxiety is also the source of something else. It is the source of man's sinfulness. For the pain of anxiety drives men to try to escape it. They sink into sensuality in the effort to forget that there is anything beyond the immediate. They lose themselves in fanaticism in

> the effort to convince themselves that they have brought the Absolute to earth. They try to cut down their aspirations and fall into cynicism, or to inflate their powers and fall into pride and arrogance. In a word, they try to identify their own limited and relative powers with the Absolute. And this is the original sin. Sin is the narcosis of the soul; it is a perennial temptation to which men must inevitably succumb. (p. 89)

Original sin, as Frankel identifies it, is due to humans' eating of the fruit of knowledge. Purposeful thoughts lead man and woman to be banished from the Garden of Eden where they had shared the simple happiness of the animals who did not question their existence. It is thinking that creates in humans the split between the abstract and the concrete. Consciousness causes problems because it imposes a dualism where none really exists. Bateson (1971) describes this conflict in thinking as an error in epistemology left over from the philosophical heritage of Descartes, who created this split with his subject-object dualism. Alcoholics try to impose control where there is no possible control. No one can really control him or herself because there is not a "self" to control. The self is only an abstraction. Bateson sees this as an error in thinking (i.e., symmetry in Bateson's language) and being (i.e., epistemology). Individuals become caught in an internal battle and alcoholism becomes the battlefield, according to Bateson. AA asks alcoholics to give up the battle and rather than think symmetrically, they are urged to approach life in a complementary fashion. As Bateson says, AA urges alcoholics to give up the incorrect epistemology and consequently they will no longer try to do the impossible, which is to control themselves. Rather, they will accept themselves as they are. Kurtz (1982) sums up this position when he writes:

> Humane thinkers, those who study human phenomena, existentialist thought reminds, must eschew the imperative of control. Human beings, as human, are neither tools nor mere objects–for what is an "object" but another potential tool? The subject-object dualism that derives from Descartes has immeasurably increased human knowledge and control of things. Applied to persons, however, as the experience of AA within the field of alcoholism testifies, it is not only sadly lacking but tragically destructive. Subject-object dualism, with its demand for "objectivity" regards the attainment of truth as an act of conquest rather than of revelation. The dualistic style and approach thus do violence to humane values. Treating persons as things can only increase alienation. Such an approach thus fuels rather than cures alcoholism. (p. 47)

Chapter 8

Diagnosis and Addiction Treatment

Addiction treatment, never an easy endeavor, has become increasing complex and difficult over the last twenty years. Multiple factors have contributed to this increased complexity, the least of which is the growing increase in the use of drugs, licit and elicit, in this country. At one time addiction treatment referred almost exclusively to alcohol and the alcoholic, and in most cases, the alcoholic was a Caucasian male in his late thirties or forties. The increased utilization of illicit drugs such as marijuana, heroin, and cocaine, along with the rapid proliferation of the use of designer drugs by all members (men, women, adolescents, children) of society regardless of age, race, creed, socioeconomic status, and ethnic background, has complicated the treatment picture thoroughly. Added to this mix is the recent pharmacological revolution that has taken place in this country, which has brought with it not only the many benefits that pharmacology provides for the general population, but also an equal number of addictive and abusive uses of drugs such as amphetamines and tranquilizers. It is no wonder that addiction treatment specialists are caught in a labyrinth of contradictory and conflicting attitudes and recommendations for treatment strategies and approaches. Compounding this difficulty even further is the growing number of afflictions or disorders that are now referred to as addictions even though they have nothing at all to do with the ingestion or use of chemicals (gambling, sex, work, etc.). One final influential factor is the recent change in economic climate and third-party insurance coverage. Insurance companies whose mandate is to handle the reimbursement and financial aspects of care have themselves come under increasing competitive pressure to hold down costs and to market less expensive forms of addiction treatment.

Addiction treatment and chemical use does not occur in a vacuum. Neither can it be understood or explained outside of a societal and cultural context. Societal attitudes toward chemical use and its treatment are rapidly changing and this shift in attitudes plays an intricate part in the way addiction is treated and the reasons why the use of chemicals by individuals in our society is increasing. Specifically, our society has become a drug-oriented society. Whether the drug be illicit, such as heroin, or licit, unrecognized "non-drug" drugs such as nicotine and caffeine, the issue remains the same. We take drugs to perk us up, and we take drugs to calm us down. Beginning with the morning cup of coffee, through the midday aspirin, and ending with the evening martini, our culture has learned more and more to rely on drugs as effective means of helping us cope with the everyday stress of living. It is a well-supported opinion that the current increase in drug-taking behavior reflects a general cultural change in the direction of beginning to see drug use as an acceptable way to solve problems (Ray, 1972, Johnson, 1973).

There are a number of reasons for the increase in the number of drugs used in our society. In our generally affluent society, each individual learns early that science and technology will supply answers to problems once the problems are identified. Because of the present rate of social and technological change, the expectation of quick solutions to problems is now well ingrained in our culture. Drugs provide these quick solutions. The increase in drug use and misuse can be viewed as part of a rapidly developing biological revolution. One aspect of this awakening, of which we are in the midst, is the pharmacological revolution. One of the most interesting, but least studied, cultural changes is the use of psychoactive drugs for their effect on the mind, rather than on the body. We have moved from drugs to cure the body to drugs to cure the mind. For the first time, potent chemicals clearly labeled as drugs are being widely used by healthy people because of their social convenience.

This societal expectancy of an instant pharmacological answer to all our ills has been facilitated by the promise of drugs to solve most of our personal problems. The marketplace is replete with exhortations to use drugs to remedy a variety of uncomfortable situations. Such advertisements are not false, just misleading. Adding to these misconceptions of unrealistic expectations has been the medical profession's enthusiastic support for their consumption, prescription, and use. The physician's support has helped legitimize drug use in our culture by individuals who would not, under normal circumstances, tolerate its use. The issue becomes one of illusion, false assumptions, and failure to view drugs beyond culturally defined terms.

Due to these circumstances, our culture has become more lackadaisical about even acknowledging some drugs as drugs while at the same time showing increased alarm over the recreational use of other drugs. The discrepancy, in part, seems to be an indication of whether a drug's use becomes an ingrained part of society. Many individuals fail to see how a need for a cup of coffee, a smoke, a cola, or a beer is in any way related to drug use and abuse. The recent flow of antipsychotic, antidepressant, and antianxiety drugs from the hospital pharmacy to the home medicine cabinet is but a modern version of the acceptance of caffeine, nicotine, and distilled spirits as an intricate part of the American way of life.

Societal attitudes toward drug use as an acceptable and easy way to solve certain difficulties are also reflected in attitudes toward definitions and the treatment of addiction. What may be normal or acceptable use in one case may reflect misuse, abuse, or even addiction in another. The attitude toward drug use and the criteria one uses to define addiction dictate how, when, and in what way addiction will be treated. Certainly, the criterion confusion is one primary reason why there are so many conflicting recommendations and definitions of addiction. While some researchers (usually those associated within academic settings) view addition as a bad habit that must be altered, such as biting one's nails, others (usually practitioners who work with addiction in treatment settings) view it as a life or death disorder that has a multitude of spiritual, physical, and psychological ramifications. The former group often speaks of behavioral contingencies and cognitive reframing as treatment alternatives. Research is undertaken and articles are published addressing the importance of matching patient characteristics and attitudes with treatment methods. It is often recommended that brain-impaired addicts be asked to choose whether they prefer moderate use of chemicals or abstinence as treatment alternatives, much like someone who is asked whether they prefer their steak cooked medium-rare or well-done.

This is not to imply that alternative approaches to addiction treatment should not be explored. The point is that different societal and cultural attitudes toward drug and alcohol use reflect a similarity in attitudes toward treatment options and definitions of what constitutes an addiction. Certainly someone who moderately drinks, who has no prior history of social, legal, spiritual, marital, physical, psychological, or economic consequences as a result of drinking, and who asks for guidance or directions concerning his or her drinking should be presented other options. But how many of these individuals show up voluntarily seeking treatment? Not only does the issue of criterion differential have to be carefully evaluated, but the ethical consequences of applying treatment alternatives that have little practical value or have the potential for negative ramifications for an individual must be given cautious consideration.

A case vignette will illustrate this point:

> A twenty-two-year-old college senior at a local university sought an initial consultation with a therapist because of concerns about his

anger and depression. During the course of the initial interview, the therapist learned that his anger and verbal conflicts always manifested when he was either high on marijuana or out drinking with his buddies. This young man's depression usually followed his weekend episodes of "heavy partying." When questioned about the extent of his drug use, he denied it was any more or less than his "friends that he partied with." There were no other alarming signs of other substance-related problems like DUI, poor academic performance, etc. that would strongly support a diagnosis of addiction, dependence, or even abuse. He readily admitted, though, that his father, a very successful physician, was a recovery alcoholic who regularly attended AA meetings. When asked by the therapist if he had ever wondered if he too might be an alcoholic like his father, the young man admitted "the thought had crossed my mind." The therapist then suggested he might go to a few AA meetings and check it out, see if he identified or discovered for himself that he might indeed be an alcoholic like his father. The young man readily agreed, and when he returned for his next appointment later in the week, his mood had drastically changed. He had been to AA meetings every night since his appointment and decided to telephone his father and speak to him about these concerns. The young man continued his weekly therapy sessions and almost daily attendance at AA meetings until he graduated from college four months later. After graduation he left the city to pursue a job outside the state. Nearly three years later, upon moving back to the city, he telephoned the therapist to set up another appointment. Upon entering the office, he acknowledged that he was doing well and had successfully started a new job. Still sober and active in AA, he admitted that he had some gnawing doubts about his diagnosis and said the primary reason he set up this appointment was to question why the therapist had diagnosed him as alcoholic and he wondered if he should "try drinking alcohol again." He was somewhat alarmed and taken back by the therapist's reply that he (the therapist) had never diagnosed him as an alcoholic. He reminded him that the question had been, "Did it ever cross your mind that you might be an alcoholic?" and the suggestion was that he "check it out" by attending a few AA meetings. In actuality, he was reminded by the therapist that he himself had made a self-diagnosis. It took a few minutes for the young man to absorb this realization, then he said, "I don't think I'm an alcoholic anymore, what do you think I should do?" Without batting an eye the therapist replied, "Well, you could always check it out." Somewhat startled by this response, the young man admitted that the risk to discover if he was really an alcoholic by drinking again was too great. He had seen literally hundreds of people in the program return to the street or to drinking, and in every case the result was disastrous. By the end of the session, he concluded that the question of whether or not he was an alcoholic was not one he was willing to test empirically and that he could live with the doubt and uncertainty of whether his diagnosis was a correct one.

CRITERION DEFINITIONS OF ADDICTION

Any area of human behavior spans a complete spectrum from "normal" or "average" to "abnormal" or "excessive." Alcohol and drug use is simply another area of human behavior and as such covers a similar spectrum. Even within similar cultural or societal contexts, abstinence versus excessive alcohol and drug consumption can cover a wide range of acceptability. Nowhere is this more dramatically demonstrated than with Native Americans. Different tribes, even those who live practically next door to each other, such as the Pima in central Arizona and the Hopi who reside in an area just north of the Pima Indian Reservation, have extraordinary differences in the rates of alcohol consumption and alcoholism. While alcoholism is practically nonexistent for the Hopis, the Pima have rates of alcoholism that are four to five times that of the national average. Cultural attitudes toward acceptable levels of alcohol consumption appear to override any other factors defining what is normal or acceptable use of a drug.

"Normal" Use: As in all behavior, the term "normal" is culturally defined. For example, a drink (alcohol) or some marijuana taken at a social event is considered normal (or appropriate) behavior among many, but not all, social groups. Normal does not mean legal. Alcohol was illegal in the U.S. from 1919-1932; nicotine (cigarette smoking) was illegal in many states in the 1920s; marijuana is illegal now. Yet, their moderate use was (and is) considered normal among some groups despite their illegal status.

Abuse of Drugs: Abuse refers to the persistent administration of a drug for purposes (for kicks, to "escape," etc.) that are not medically indicated. The taking of morphine may be considered normal for relief of pain, but it would be considered drug abuse to take it for relief of depression. Some workers in this field describe another term, drug *misuse*. Here, the drug is used medically or therapeutically but inappropriately, for example, physicians who prescribe penicillin for viral infections (common cold), or people who (mis)use vitamin E to improve sexual performance.

Compulsive Abuse (Misuse): Compulsive abuse refers to behavior in which individuals feel that a drug is necessary to maintain their state of well-being. Examples are compulsive cigarette smokers who experience "nicotine-fits" when they haven't smoked for a while; and people who cannot face the day without their Librium, etc. The term *habituation* is sometimes used here.

Addiction: Addiction refers to a behavioral pattern of cultural abuse characterized by overwhelming involvement with obtaining and using a drug. The drug pervades the life of the user. This type of behavior differs from compulsive abuse only quantitatively. For example, a compulsive cigarette smoker might qualify for this category if cigarettes suddenly became illegal and the price went up to $50 a pack. In Germany after WWII, addicted smokers would trade food coupons or prostitute themselves for cigarettes.

Pharmacologists tend to avoid the word addiction because it is controversial and fraught with implications that have little to do with pharmacology. As a result, The Expert Committee on Drugs of the World Health Organization (WHO) coined the term *drug dependence*: a state of psychological and/or physical dependence (see definition below) resulting from chronic use of a drug. The nature of this dependence will vary from drug to drug, so the WHO Committee described several specific types of drug dependence: (1) opiate type; (2) alcohol-barbiturate (depressant) type; (3) amphetamine (stimulant) type; (4) hallucinogenic (LSD, etc.) type; and (5) cannabinol (marijuana) type. This system has at least three advantages: (1) It is flexible, that is, as people discover new drug categories to be abused, these can be added to the list; (2) In addition, it recognizes that dependence on one drug–alcohol, for example–will be quite different than dependence on a different drug, say marijuana. There is the possibility of physical and psychological dependence on alcohol. For marijuana, only psychological dependence seems to be possible, at least as far as can be ascertained at this time; and (3) The use of the term drug dependence shifts the emphasis from the user of the drug to the drug itself. The word *addiction* describes human (excessive) behavior; the term *drug dependence* describes properties or characteristics of drugs.

Tolerance

In addition to physical and/or psychological dependence, the phenomenon of *tolerance* often accompanies drug dependence. In tolerance, a given dose of a drug, after repeated administration (provided the administrations are not too far apart), produces a decreased effect. Another way of looking at it: a larger dose is needed to give the same effect as was originally obtained with a smaller dose. Not all drugs will produce tolerance, and any given drug will not produce tolerance to *all* its effects (see below).

Physical Dependence

This is an altered physiological state produced by repeated administration of a drug. The altered state necessitates the continued administration of the drug to prevent the appearance of a stereotyped syndrome (abstinence syndrome). Only some drugs have this property. This syndrome is characterized by rebound hypersensibility. Abstinence from the drug tends to produce the opposite effect of the drug.

Psychological Dependence

This condition, sometimes called *psychic craving,* can be brought about in some people by some drugs. It is a condition characterized by an emotional drive to continue taking a drug that the user feels is necessary for his or her well-being. The use of the drug is compulsive (compulsive abuse).

DRUG GROUPS

It is important to understand which group of drugs affect mood, behavior, and perception. The WHO Committee recognized that there are six such categories of drugs that are capable of producing dependence. It is important to note that different groups of people–pharmacologists, physicians, lawyers, narcotic agents, drug users, etc.–will have their own peculiar scheme of classifying drugs.

1. *Narcotic Analgesics:* These allay pain (or the anxiety concerning pain). In some people, especially those who develop dependence on these drugs, some of the more potent members of this class bring about a feeling of euphoria. Examples: morphine, heroin, meperidine (Demerol), methadone, codeine, etc.
2. *CNS Depressants:* These drugs depress a wide range of cellular functions in many organ systems in addition to the central nervous system. These drugs tend to allay anxiety and decrease tension. Examples: general anesthetics, alcohol, barbiturates, meprobamate, diazepam (Valium), etc.
3. *CNS Stimulants:* These drugs excite many organ systems in addition to the CNS. Many of these also induce euphoria. Examples: amphetamines, cocaine, caffeine, nicotine, etc.

4. *Psychedelics:* These cause hallucinations, altered sensory perceptions, and changes in mood and judgment. Examples: LSD, mescaline, psilocybin, etc. Many drugs in the above three groups can also produce hallucinations but cannot bring about the other effects reliably. (Examples: anticholinergics, amphetamines, narcotic antagonists, etc.)

5. *Cannabinols (Marijuana):* These are extremely difficult to classify. Some people put them in group 2 and others in group 4. They are quite unique in many ways.

6. *Antipsychotics and Antidepressants:* These are used to treat affective disorders. The effects of these drugs are unpleasant for most people and they are seldom abused. Examples: chlorpromazine, amitriptyline, etc. This group is *not* recognized as a dependence-producing group, although there are workers who report physical dependence for some of these drugs (see group 2).

DRUG DEPENDENCE AND THE DRUG GROUPS

Tolerance

Of these six groups, tolerance can develop to some of the effects of each group. There is some question as to whether or not tolerance can develop to the "high" of marijuana. Recent studies have shown that a reverse tolerance occurs with marijuana–it takes a smaller "dose" to get high. Tolerance will not develop to all the effects of a drug. It will develop to the analgetic and euphorigenic actions of narcotics, but tolerance will not develop to narcotic effects on the pupils of the eye (pinpoint pupils) nor to their effects on the gastrointestinal (GI) tract. A heroin user, for example, is always constipated when he is taking the drug.

Tolerance to the euphoric, analgetic, and lethal effects of narcotics is especially pronounced. An average individual would probably die if given 100 mg of morphine (10 mg is the usual dose therapeutically). Some chronic abusers of the drug have been known to take 4000 mg and do quite well. However, there is going to be some dose that will kill even the most tolerant individual.

There is less tolerance to the lethal effects of general depressants. An alcoholic might tolerate perhaps two times the blood concentration of alcohol that non-alcoholics tolerate. This is true of other depressants such as the barbiturates. An individual tolerant to a depressant will not be tolerant to a narcotic (unless he is also a chronic user of narcotics). However, he will be tolerant, to some extent, to all the other general depressants such as barbiturates, diazepam, etc. Analogously, a heroin user will be tolerant to all other narcotics, but *not* to alcohol, other depressants, amphetamines, or members of other drug groups.

Physical Dependence

At least two types of physical dependence occur, although in the past few years evidence for physical dependence on amphetamines and other CNS stimulants has been observed. There may be physical dependence on chlorpromazine, imipramine, and some other drugs (see below). The two well-defined types are: (1) the narcotic analgesic (or morphine) type, and (2) the CNS depressant (or barbiturate) type.

Abrupt cessation of narcotic administration to a physically dependent individual is followed by an abstinence syndrome described in texts (Ray, 1972). For heroin, the peak effects occur two to three days after withdrawal. The time course will be different for other narcotics. The syndrome, as bad as it sounds, is not regarded as life-threatening, and it can be ended instantly by the administration of any other narcotic. It cannot be ended by drugs belonging to other groups, such as amphetamines or barbiturates. This illustrates cross-dependence, the ability of one drug to suppress the manifestations of physical dependence induced by another and to substitute for the other in maintaining the physically dependent state.

The CNS depressants produce a kind of physical dependence that is more dangerous to the abuser and to society than that which occurs with the narcotics. For example, some studies show that 20 to 40 percent of males who were admitted to state mental hospitals were diagnosed as alcoholics. There are more barbiturate abusers than narcotic abusers; over half of automobile accidents resulting in death involve a drunken driver (Ray, 1972).

It was not widely realized, at least not in the U.S., that dependence to these depressants could occur until the late 1940s and 1950s when a group of investigators at the U.S. Public Health Service Center in Lexington, Kentucky did the conclusive experiments. Volunteers at the hospital were given as much alcohol as they wanted (average of about 4/5 quart of 100 proof alcohol per day) for about thirteen weeks. The subjects became quite tolerant to the effects of the drug, and then they were abruptly withdrawn from the alcohol. Within eight hours, they became nervous, weak, and apprehensive. Nearly all manifested tremors, perspiration, vomiting, diarrhea, and anorexia (loss of appetite). Two-thirds developed delirium, tremors (DTs) and hallucinations. Grand mal seizures occurred in about one-third of the subjects. The symptoms could be described as life-threatening.

Similar symptoms ensue upon sudden withdrawal of barbiturates or other CNS depressants from dependent individuals. The withdrawal symptoms caused by alcohol abstinence can be ended by barbiturates or other CNS depressants (cross-dependence) but not by members of other drug groups.

Psychological Dependence

Some, but not all drugs that act on the CNS, thereby affecting mood, behavior, and perception, will produce psychological dependence (psychic craving). However, drugs that affect the CNS but do not produce psychic craving will *not* be abused, even if these drugs cause physical dependence. In other words, it is possible to be *physically* dependent on a drug without being *psychologically* dependent. Certain narcotic antagonists, like nalorphine, have this property. Chlorpromazine and imipramine may also cause physical dependence, but these drugs almost never produce psychic cravings and are accordingly never abused. Obviously, the drugs most likely to be abused and most likely to dominate an individual's life are those that produce both physical and psychological dependence, such as alcohol, barbiturates, narcotics, amphetamines, nicotine, etc. With some drugs, psychological dependence seems to be the only factor involved in their abuse; marijuana and LSD are examples. These drugs do not bring about physical dependence as far as can be ascertained.

DEPENDENCE, TOLERANCE, ABUSE, AND ADDICTION

Most pharmacologists would agree that the core of the problem of why people become dependent on drugs lies in the user, not in the drugs. The reasons that people get "hooked" on drugs are primarily psychological and sociological (Ray, 1972), not pharmacological. Few people are accidentally hooked on drugs. Something in their personal make-up seems to predispose certain people toward drug abuse. Thousands of people have been chronically exposed to drugs such as morphine in hospitals and other settings and, even when physically dependent, evince no interest in continuing the use of narcotics after leaving the hospital. However, for a drug to be abused, it must have some desirable effect, and, in addition, drugs that produce tolerance and physical dependence are more likely to be abused.

Assessing an individual's level of involvement with a drug is crucial to determine if a person needs treatment and what kind of treatment is necessary. Is the person a recreational user, abuser, dependent, or addicted?

Many individuals go through a period of alcohol and drug experimentation in their life, where they have misused, abused, or excessively used chemicals. Not all of these people become dependent, and not all dependency leads to addiction. Drug and alcohol use often follows a predictable and identifiable pattern that can be categorized into four general areas.

1. Those individuals who experiment with drug and alcohol use and learn early how to control and modulate its use. These individuals, even though they may have had periods of heavy alcohol or drug abuse, were never really addicted.
2. Those individuals who learn later in their life that they cannot modulate it or control it so they stop either alone or with the help of a professional or a twelve-step program. These individuals are referred to as low-bottom alcoholics or addicts.
3. Those individuals who learn much later in life that they have to stop, but cannot or once they stop, they are unable to stay sober or clean and are plagued by constant relapses. They suffer constant losses and often require an outside consequence like cirrhosis of the liver or an intervention before they finally stop. Such individuals are referred to as high-bottom alcoholics or addicts.
4. There are individuals who never achieve any lasting sobriety or are able to stay clean. They often die from this condition or end up in the penal system because of their drug and alcohol use.

Within this last category, many of these individuals often have a dual diagnosis of appropriate primary mental disorder (i.e., schizophrenia, bipolar disorder, etc.), which in turn interferes with their ability to maintain abstinence for any length of time. Severe character disorders are other examples of conditions that often interfere with recovery. In the last few years, more and more evidence has been accumulated that suggests that the incidence of untreated sexual abuse is alarmingly high for female addicts and alcoholics. A preliminary investigation by Kathleen Bollerud (1995) reveals that:

1. 75 percent of women in treatment have a history of sexual abuse;
2. 50 percent of dissociative disorders have a history of chemical dependency;
3. 35 percent of women who are hospitalized for addiction have dissociative symptomatology.

Bollerud acknowledges that these findings are limited to women, but there is also evidence–though no accurate figures–that untreated sexual abuse is also an important factor with addicted men. She writes,

> Treatment failures for chemically dependent patients and sexually abused patients may well be due to the untreated secondary disorder. The impact of active chemical dependency or substance abuse is a crucial variable in both the prognoses and the rate of recovery in sexually abused patients. Untreated sexual abuse is most likely a common cause of treatment failure or relapse among substance abusers.

While Bollerud recognizes that the accurate diagnosis is difficult for both addictive and trauma-related disorders, she cautions that there is a potential to underestimate the impact of substance use on the emotional and/or cognitive functioning of patients dealing with trauma. Consequently, she recommends that the addictive disorder be dealt with aggressively and recommends a twelve-step abstinence-based intervention. She concludes that trauma patients–even patients suffering from multiple personality disorders–who are able to use AA have better recovery rates.

In a similar fashion, Minkoff (1995), working with patients who have both mental illness and addiction, recommends that these two disorders be approached as independent and primary, but interactive, illnesses. He draws parallels between the addiction disease model of recovery and the mental illness disease model of recovery. He suggests that the "steps" of the twelve-step program of recovery be applied to both addiction and mental illness.

In all four of the categories presented, it imay be concluded that only those individuals who fall into the first category are candidates for alternative methods of addiction treatment other than abstinence-based treatment approaches. In making this differential treatment recommendation, it is suggested that a false positive diagnosis (individuals diagnosed as addicted, but who really fall into the first category) is unlikely to have any far-reaching effects on the individual. As a treating physician on an inpatient unit once told his staff, "You know alcohol is not an essential nutrient for survival, so why all the fuss over whether this person can drink or not?" Conversely, false negatives (those identified as not truly addicted, but who are in actuality addicted) will increase the likelihood of the person eventually having to experience all of the inevitable consequences outlined in categories 3 and 4. It is more prudent to overdiagnose this condition than it is to underdiagnose it.

Gelormino (1995), in a reply to Marlatt's Moderation Management (MM) approach to addiction treatment, expressed very similar sentiments when he questioned the harm reduction hypothesis for addiction treatment:

> The second problem that I see with the harm reduction model is that any concept (such as the controlled drinking view), which al-

> lows for the notion of a timely reduction of use/abuse does not consider the workings of the addict mind. Self deception runs rampant in the addict mind. "I will use 'x' today and I will only 'x minus 1' tomorrow" makes perfect sense, but alcoholism and addiction are not disorders which cause the individual greater clarity of mind. On the contrary, for most addicts or alcoholics, after one beer "anything goes." To allow an addict to reduce his or her abuse over time, given the nature of the beast, is an error. Witness how although the formal MM treatment allows for a gradual reduction of dosage, leading to an abstinence state, this approach has almost entirely been abandoned. It is not a slow suicide. It often comes swiftly, without warning: the overdose, the interpersonal conflict leading to deadly weapons, the fatal automobile accident. Addicts/alcoholics do not have a cushion of time. The needle you supply could be the one that delivers the deadly dose. The reality is, for the serious addict, the only safe reduction is the COMPLETE ELIMINATION. Granted, oftentimes several attempts at treatment are required before lasting change occurs, but we need not develop such a compromise as such. We must go for the gusto, so to speak. (p. 9)

Another important and often ignored variable in this diagnosis and treatment recommendation process is the effect that drugs and alcohol have on the brain. This has important implications for a number of reasons. Most simply put, all forms of psychotherapy (individual, group, family, cognitive, psychodynamic, etc.) rest on the assumption that people will be rational enough to make decisions based on accurate insight and understanding of themselves and their situation. It is impossible to conduct traditional forms of therapy with addicted patients who are actively using drugs or alcohol or are in the early stages of recovery. While most therapists would agree with such a position, few fail to understand the significance of alcoholics' or addicts' cognitive impairment three, six, or even nine months into their recovery because these symptoms are often very subtle and specific. Because most alcoholics and addicts do not demonstrate significant difficulties in their verbal intelligence, they often "sound better" than they really are. For group leaders to be aware of the subtle differences in someone two, six, or twelve months sober, they must have some awareness and understanding of these cognitive deficits so they can adapt their treatment within group to match the needs and capabilities of the patient. Understanding these cognitive deficits will help the group leader realize why the confrontational techniques (i.e., coercion, leverage, intervention, etc.) described in Chapter 9 are so necessary for addicted patients during the early stage of their treatment.

Heyman, writing from a neuroscience perspective, emphasized that it must be remembered that addiction is a disease of the brain. "At the core of a disease model of addiction based on modern neurosciences is the concept that in a vulnerable individual, adequate drug use produces long-lived adaptions in brain functioning" (1995). Heyman goes on to say that adaptions in brain functioning that result from excessive chemical use produce somatic and psychological dependence, which in turn induces long-term changes in brain functioning that underlie drug craving in response to conditioned cues. An essential component of this adaption and change in brain functioning is the "commandeering of motivational systems of the brain" by the drug, and this results in denial or the loss of the capacity for awareness that this has happened. Heyman cautions treatment personnel not to confuse denial with lying and that denial does not mean that the alcoholic or addict is not telling the truth. Rather, it is the result of motivational systems of the brain becoming controlled by the reward circuitry of the brain. Brain adaptions, as the result of repeated drug use, are hypothesized to be absolutely central to the production of addictive behavior and behavioral priorities. Implications for treatment are profound. Much of addicts' or alcoholics' behavior is not under their volitional control or choice. Interventions that take into careful consideration the lack of motivation and the degree of denial on the part of the addicted individual are more likely to be effective than those approaches that assume the person has the emotional and mental capacity to choose and behave as someone who is in control of his or her brain functioning.

NEUROPSYCHOLOGICAL IMPAIRMENT

Within the last ten years there has been a vast accumulation of evidence related to the neurological functioning and neuropsychological deficits associated with alcoholism. Recent surveys and reviews of the literature (Wells, 1982; Parsons and Farr, 1981; Grant, Reed, and Adams, 1980; Wilkinson and Carlen, 1981; Ryan and Butters, 1980) reveal that the pattern of impairment associated with chronic alcohol abuse is identifiable and even predictable. Most important, the pattern of deficits noted in cortical compromise and cognitive deficiencies have important implications for treatment. Unfortunately, the significant contributions neurology and neuropsychology have to offer in the treatment of alcoholism often go unnoticed or are not utilized. Even when useful information about treatment is forthcoming, it either remains entirely academic and devoid of clinical application or is obscured in vague, nondescriptive terminology such as "organicity." Neurological consequences must be articulated and conveyed so that the implications these identified deficits may have in their clinical applications are practical. It is important to determine how certain patterns of neurological impairment may affect the motivation, abstinence, and recovery of the alcoholic patient. Do alcoholics who score in the impaired range of neuropsychological testing and who show morphological abnormalities as revealed by neuroradiological studies (CAT scan) and neuropsychological testing respond differently to treatment? In short, is there a relationship between neurological impairment and treatment outcome? Finally, what special strategies should be adapted and applied to an identified pattern of neurological impairment?

These questions have not been answered unequivocally, and replicated research addressing this problem is nonexistent with a few exceptions (i.e., Wells, 1982, Parsons and Farr, 1981). One purpose of this chapter is to present the available evidence and draw inferences about its application for treatment. Hopefully, such an exercise will help bridge the gap between pure research and clinical applicability of such research findings. Specifically, this chapter will attempt to delineate the relationship between Wernicke-Korsakoff syndrome, alcoholic encephalopathy, and alcohol-induced dementia. Each of these conditions will be briefly explored in relation to the continuum and premature aging theories of alcoholism. What is the pattern of impairment for each of these conditions and how might these patterns relate to treatment and recovery? Considering the evidence to be presented here, it is suggested that a highly structured recovery program like Alcoholics Anonymous owes much of its success to the very structure and directive strategies inherent in its intuitive design, which serves as a paradigm for recovery.

Gallant (1983) supports the importance of assessing cognitive functioning when planning treatment strategies for alcoholics and drug addicts. He writes,

> It is essential to evaluate neuropsychological impairment of every alcoholic before initiating any treatment plan. Even mild impairment of judgment or cognition can seriously interfere with both psychotherapy and the administration of medication such as Antabuse, particularly if the impairment is not evident to the therapist or the patient. Efforts to correlate impairment on simple neuropsychological tests and presence of brain atrophy may offer information on the future course or prognosis of the alcohol-induced damage. Such efforts may also show that inexpensive and readily available neuropsychological evaluation measures may be just as helpful as more costly computer-

> ized tomography (CT) for the evaluation and formulation of a treatment plan for the alcoholic patient. (Gallant, 1983, p. 448)

Most alcoholics and addicts hospitalized in an acute state of intoxication will stabilize after two to seven days of detoxification. A competent and experienced physician should be able to safely manage the detoxification period and accurately assess when the possibility of life-threatening seizures or delirium tremors is diminished enough to allow the patient to safely participate in group therapy and the rest of the treatment program. Many patients will not suffer the severe symptoms of withdrawal and will be able to benefit from group therapy much more quickly. Table 8.1 outlines the possible neurological complications that result from the chronic use of alcohol.

Alcohol and drugs usually produce striking central nervous system dysfunction. Researchers, until recently, have largely ignored the subtle effects that these chemicals have on the brain other than assessing the acute consequences of delirium tremors or long-term chronic effects as manifested in a Korsakoff's syndrome. Wells (1982) sums up this situation when he writes,

> . . . psychiatrists who are interested in organic brain disorders have centered most of their attention either on the consequences of its withdrawal (delirium tremens) or on the thiamine deficiency that so often accompanies its use and gives rise to the Wernicke-Korsakoff syndrome. Only recently have the long-term effects of chronic ethanol abuse per se on central nervous system function and structure begun to attract much attention.
>
> While deterioration of brain function has always been acknowledged in alcoholics, it usually has been attributed to malnourishment, hepatic failure, head trauma–in fact to just about everything but the effects of the alcohol itself. Even though a few doubts persist about whether functional and structural cerebral deterioration can be caused by alcohol abuse alone, there is no question that such deterioration can be demonstrated in many chronic alcoholics for whom malnourishment, hepatic failure, and head trauma have been reasonably eliminated as possible causes. (p. 111)

There had never been any doubt that neuropsychological testing would reveal abnormalities in alcoholics or addicts who were in acute withdrawal or suffering from a Korsakoff's syndrome. However, the application of neuropsychological assessment procedures to individuals without these conditions has revealed consistent findings that often agree with comput-

TABLE 8.1 Neurological Diseases Associated with Alcohol

1. Acute intoxication

2. Alcohol withdrawal syndrome (time of appearance after cessation of drinking)
   - Tremulousness (7-24 Hours)
   - Hallucinosis - visual or auditory (12-48 Hours)
   - Delirium tremens (36-96 Hours)
   - Withdrawal seizures (7-48 Hours)

3. Nutritional diseases of the nervous system
   - Polyneuropathy
   - Wernicke-Korsakoff Syndrome
   - Amblyopia

4. Possible nutritional or toxic effects of alcohol or metabolites
   - Alcoholic myopathy
   - Cerebellar degeneration

5. Secondary to cirrhosis - Hepatocentral degeneration

erized cranial tomography (CAT Scan). Wells summarizes these findings when he writes,

> The results of these investigations have been remarkably consistent. Tests of over-all intelligence often reveal no significant differences between groups of chronic alcoholics and matched controls, but tests designed to evaluate more discrete neuropsychological functions frequently show abnormalities among alcoholics. Many alcoholics demonstrate defects in short-term memory, performance on complex memory tasks, visual-motor coordination, performance on visual-spatial tasks, abstract reasoning, and psychomotor dexterity. Relative sparing of verbal skills is often observed and long-term memory is preserved. (1982, pp. 111-112)

Most of the results from these neuropsychological studies have been derived from data obtained by the Wechsler's Adult Intelligence Scale (WAIS) and the Halstead-Reitan Neuropsychological Battery (HRB). Tables 8.2, 8.3, and 8.4 show the differences in scores on the HRB for alcoholics, psychiatric control patients, and brain-damaged patients. As demonstrated by these scores, alcoholics generally score worse than control subjects and better than brain-damaged subjects. Alcoholics have the most difficulty with tasks sensitive to abstract reasoning, short-term memory, and motor speed (i.e., Category and Trails B). Table 8.5 demonstrates the number of studies that substantiate consistent difficulties in these areas for both alcoholics and addicts. Table 8.6 lists the percentages for a number of studies conducted with the HRB that substantiate the consistency of these findings. Table 8.7 provides a similar list of results from studies using the WAIS to demonstrate a clear disparity between performance IQ (new learning) scores and verbal IQ (old learning) scores.

The tables (8.2 through 8.7) presented reflect the results of studies conducted with alcoholics or addicts who were not suffering from Wernicke-Korsakoff syndrome. This is important to remember because it suggests that alcoholics or addicts need not be so severely and obviously impaired as a Korsakoff's patient before their cognitive deficits can be assessed. It also suggests that many, if not all, alcoholics and addicts suffer from subtle deficits in cognitive functioning that may interfere with their ability to process, retain, understand, and recall vital information necessary for their recovery. Considering that two of the leading theorists in the area of cognitive impairment in alcoholics suggest that chronic alcohol use may produce premature aging of the brain (Cermak and Peck, 1982) or that the Korsakoff's syndrome may just be a part of the continuity of this alcohol-induced process (Ryan and Butters, 1980), it is important to

TABLE 8.2. Mean Scores of Alcoholics (A), and Psychiatric (P) and Brain-Damaged (BD) Patients on Subtests of Halstead-Reitan Neuropsychological Battery

	A	P	B D
Trails, Part A	61.3	39.0	65.0
Trails, Part B	150.0	80.1	183.1
Aphasia Errors	4.7	2.2	6.5
Spatial Relations	2.7	2.0	3.4
Perceptual Errors	8.2	2.8	10.2
Seashore Rhythm Test	6.5	3.6	7.8
Speech Perception Test	9.4	6.1	12.3
Halstead Impairment Index	0.69	0.31	0.83
Average Impairment Index	2.18	1.06	2.47

Source: Parsons and Farr (1981)

TABLE 8.3

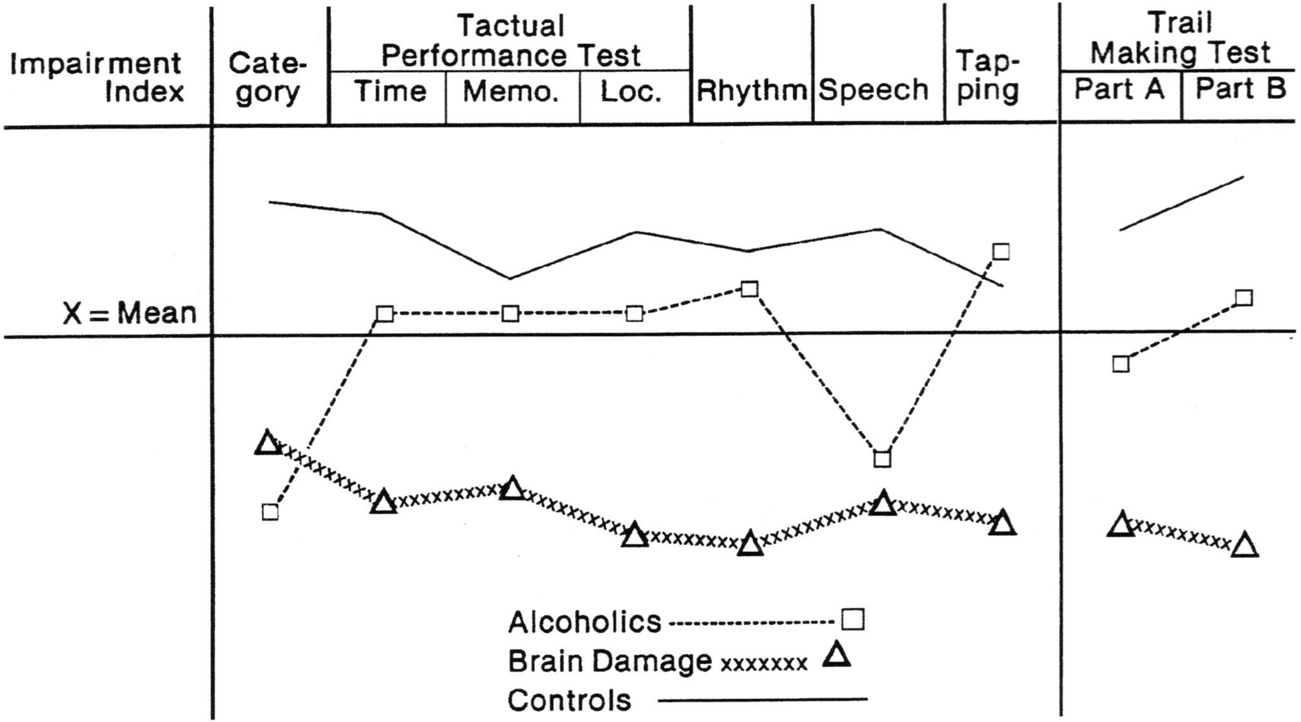

Impairment Index

Cate-gory

Tactual Performance Test

Time

Memo.

Loc.

Rhythm

Speech

Tap-ping

Trail Making Test

Part A

Part B

X = Mean

Alcoholics ----------------- □

Brain Damage xxxxxxx △

Controls ———

Source: Fitzhugh, Fitzhugh, and Reitan (1960)

TABLE 8.4. Mean Scores of Alcoholics (A), and Psychiatric (P) and Brain-Damaged (BD) Patients on Subtests of Halstead-Reitan Neuropsychological Battery

	A	P	B D
Category Test	90.0	51.5	93.7
Tactual Performance Test			
Right Hand	8.96	5.95	9.14
Left Hand	7.64	5.25	8.68
Both Hands	6.33	3.00	7.33
Total Time	22.9	14.2	24.3
Memory	6.75	8.14	4.93
Localization	2.44	4.18	1.70
Finger Oscillation			
Right Hand	38.1	50.0	37.8
Left Hand	36.7	46.2	32.6

Source: Parsons and Farr (1981)

TABLE 8.5. Pattern of Impaired HRB Subtests According to Halstead's Cutoff Points

	Alcohol		**Other Drugs**		**Other Drugs Excluding Marijuana**	
	Ratio of Impaired to Total Studies	%	Ratio of Impaired to Total Studies	%	Ratio of Impaired to Total Studies	%
Category	10-13	77	7-17	41	7-13	54
TPT-Time	9-13	69	4-12	17	2-7	29
TPT-Memory	0-13	0	0-12	0	0-7	0
TPT-Location	9-13	69	2-13	15	2-8	25
Rhythm	2-10	20	4-13	31	4-10	40
Speech Perception	5-9	56	1-9	11	1-7	14
Finger Tapping	6-10	60	5-12	42	5-9	56
Trails B	5-8	63	4-13	31	4-9	44

Source: Parsons and Farr (1981)

TABLE 8.6. Impairment Patterns on HRB for Alcoholics

HRB	No. of Studies	Impaired	Percent
Category Test	15	13	87
TPT-Time	15	12	80
TPT-Memory	15	3	20
TPT-Location	13	8	62
Rhythm	12	3	25
Speech Perception	10	5	50
Finger Tapping	12	3	25
Trails B	11	8	73

Source: Parsons and Farr (1981)

TABLE 8.7. Impairment Patterns on Wechsler Scales HRB for Alcoholics

Wechsler Scale	No. of Studies	Impaired	Percent
Information	7	2	29
Comprehension	8	2	25
Arithmetic	7	3	43
Similarities	8	1	25
Digit Span	8	1	25
Vocabulary	7	1	14
Digit Symbol	8	6	75
Picture Completion	8	4	50
Block Design	8	8	100
Picture Arrangement	7	5	71
Object Assembly	7	6	86

Source: Parsons and Farr (1981)

understand the degree of impairment in these patients because it will help the group leader understand the types of deficits commonly seen in less compromised alcoholics.

THE WERNICKE-KORSAKOFF SYNDROME

Tables 8.8 and 8.9 list the symptoms commonly seen in the Wernicke-Korsakoff syndrome. This is a two-stage illness, with Wernicke's encephalopathy being the early acute phase, and Korsakoff's psychosis usually the later, permanent, residual condition. Wernicke's encephalopathy usually responds quickly to proper medical treatment of which thiamine administration during the acute phase of withdrawal is crucial in preventing the structural alteration of portions of the brain that occurs in Korsakoff's psychosis. The Wernicke syndrome is reversible because the symptoms (i.e., ocular abnormalities, confusion, hallucinations, disorientation, etc.) are due to biochemical abnormalities that have stopped short of significant structural damage to the brain. Korsakoff's, on the other hand, is an irreversible condition due to the presence of permanent physical change to brain structure, usually involving the frontal-limbic-diencephalic system. Wernicke's is usually associated with thiamine deficiency, and this is why its symptoms are usually alleviated with vitamin B-1 injections. None of

TABLE 8.8. Korsakoff's Syndrome: Four Symptoms

1. Memory Difficulties
   a) Short-Term vs. Long-Term Memory
   b) Retrograde vs. Antegrade Amnesia
2. Intact IQ Functions
   a) Verbal vs. Performance
   b) Abstracting Poor
3. Confabulation

   Early Experiences Being Reported Out of Context
4. Personality

   Passive, Malleable, Emotionally Flat

TABLE 8.9. Amnesic Defect in Wernicke-Korsakoff's

1. Immediate and remote memory intact—verbal and nonverbal
2. Recent memory impaired—cognitive deficit, decreased attention
   a) Impaired use of semantic encoding—use associative and acoustic cues normally
   b) More sensitive to proactive interference
   c) Perseveration, inappropriate strategy

the animal studies conducted to date show that thiamine deficiency alone leads to irreversible memory problems, a condition limited to Karsakoff's patients. Although most textbooks on neurology accept avitaminosis as a primary cause of Wernicke-Korsakoff syndrome, impressive data exists showing that prolonged alcohol ingestion without malnutrition still results in permanent learning difficulties.

The most severe and noticeable condition in a Wernicke-Korsakoff patient is memory impairment. Patients' long-term memory, as well as their language and IQ functions, are usually relatively intact. The true Korsakoff patients suffer from the inability to retain and recall new information (antegrade amnesia) learned after the onset of their illness. These patients' old learning and long-term memory are usually unaffected, so they often appear "more together" than they actually are. Their personality becomes more passive and malleable. Because the medial dorsal nucleus of the thalamus, the mamillary bodies in the limbic system, and the hippocampus area are all structurally altered, these patients demonstrate a marked tendency to perseverate (i.e., keep repeating mistakes) and lack motivation (amotivation syndrome) to change. Since the limbic system alters their affective responses, they fail to care or be upset by situations that would normally alarm others. Consequently, they can be very accepting of their physical condition and continued old behavior (i.e., perseveration) despite its continual negative repercussions. Their capacity for foresight and planning is extremely poor because their abstract reasoning is compromised. Since they lack the ability to store new information into memory and their retrieval of old stored memories is impaired, they usually confuse old information with new information. This is a condition described as confabulation and is frequently confused with lying. Their damaged hippocampus does not allow them to recall new memories and it is this damaged hippocampus that is judged to be the reason for their increasing experience of blackouts. The normal acquisition and retrieval of information is continually compromised until attempts at recall produce early experiences being reported out of context. Confabulation is usually most pronounced during the acute early stages of Korsakoff's as the patients struggle to hide their difficulties from others. This condition is also exacerbated by personality characteristics that have been learned through the years as they attempt to cover over memory problems. Personality variables, along with the patient's lack of motivation, are inaccurately hypothesized as the reasons for their memory difficulties. It is rare to find confabulaton in patients who have had Korsakoff's for a period of five years or longer (Butters and Cermak, 1980). Their condition eventually deteriorates into one of apathy.

Table 8.8 illustrates the four most common symptoms in Korsakoff's patients. Table 8.10 lists evidence gathered from post-mortem autopsies on

TABLE 8.10. Evidence for Anatomical Localization

1. Post–mortem Autopsy
2. Symptoms similar to patients with lesions in this area
   a) Withdrawal symptoms (D.T.'s) parallel patients with acute lesions
   b) Inability to persist with cognitive set (Amotivation)
   c) Spatial perseveration responses
   d) Poor capability for insight and planning
   e) Personality typically malleable, carefree
   f) Field dependency problems

alcoholics and the symptoms experienced by patients with lesions in the same areas of the brain that are similar to those typically experienced by chronic alcoholics. All this evidence suggests a patient who will be extremely difficult to treat because of difficulties in these five areas:

1. Motivation (Lack of understanding and desire to initiate change)
2. New Learning (Perseveration–repeating of old mistakes)
3. Memory (Inability to learn and retain new information)
4. Affective (Inappropriate display of emotions)
5. Abstraction (Lack of insight and foreplanning)

Add to this the fact that the verbal IQ skills of most alcoholics remain intact, and the therapist is faced with an individual who can talk a "good game," but who does not have the ability to plan alternatives or the motivation and the capabilities to carry through with those plans. During a time of crisis, he or she can only fall back on old ways of coping and this is why the alcoholic continues, as AA says, "to repeat old behaviors and expect different results."

Many of the symptoms seen in a Korsakoff's patient will manifest in an alcoholic, although to a lesser degree. In fact, this is a hypothesis proposed by Butters and Cermak (1980). Certainly, the evidence presented in Tables 8.2 through 8.8 supports their contention. There is a unanimous rejection of the notion that alcoholics suffer from a generalized or global intellectual deterioration. Alcoholics, however, have a marked inability to learn new material as demonstrated by their relatively poorer performance on performance IQ tasks (Table 8.7). Their intact verbal skills leave them adept at hiding these deficits from both themselves and others. Their abstract reasoning difficulties as demonstrated by their poor Category and Trails B performance (Table 8.6) suggest they do not possess the ability to think abstractly or creatively and they will have a tendency to perseverate (keep repeating old mistakes).

However, there are some very important variables to this condition that the therapist and treatment team must take into consideration when assessing the degree of impairment in an alcoholic. Grant, Reed, and Adams, (1980) list four criteria that must be carefully evaluated.

1. Pre-Morbid Level of Functioning

A. IQ level prior to their alcoholism.
B. Age.
C. Social economic status (SES).
D. Education.

Each of these factors has an effect on WAIS and HRB measures of cognitive functioning. Higher IQ's, lower age, higher SES, and higher education are usually related to better scores on these measures. Higher scores can also indicate that these individuals may have had higher intellectual functioning prior to the onset of their condition and consequently could afford to "lose more" without it effecting them as dramatically.

2. The Duration of Alcohol Consumption

The duration of alcohol consumption has a direct effect on the degree of cortical compromise. The longer the duration of drinking, the more severe the damage.

A. Ten to twelve years usually does little damage to the cortex.
B. Twelve to twenty-five years is the pre-clinical period. Damage during this period is usually reversible if abstinence is maintained.
C. Twenty-five years and over is the clinical period. The chances of permanent impairment to the cortex are maximally increased, even if the person were to remain abstinent.

Table 8.11 summarizes Grant, Reed, and Adams's findings of the relation between poor performance on Category tests (abstraction, etc.) and age. The older alcoholics are and the longer they drink, the greater their risk for cortical compromise. Their level of cortical impairment is also dramatically affected by the age at which they started their alcohol consumption. A fifty-year-old alcoholic who started drinking at age thirty is likely to be less impaired than a fifty-year-old alcoholic who started drinking at age fifteen if the amount of their daily consumption is equal.

3. Level of Alcohol Consumption

The amount of alcohol consumption is directly related to the level of the alcoholic's impairment. Table 8.12 outlines an important distinction that must be made in assessing the severity of impairment in the alcoholic. A thirty-year-old alcoholic who has been drinking two-fifths of hundred-proof whiskey a day for ten years is going to be much more impaired than a fifty-year-old alcoholic who drinks two bottles of twenty-proof wine a week for twenty years.

4. The Length of Abstinence Since the Time of the Neuropsychological Testing

An alcoholic tested three days into his or her recovery is going to be much more severely impaired than an alcoholic tested three months or

TABLE 8.11

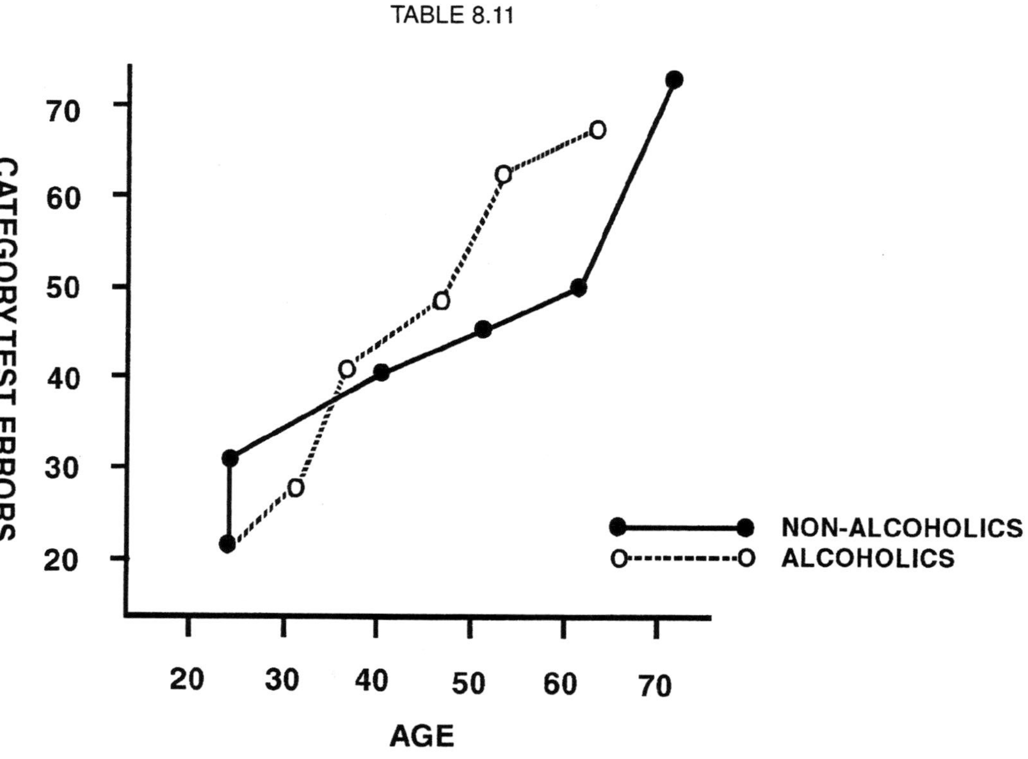

Adapted from Grant, Reed, and Adams (1980)

TABLE 8.12

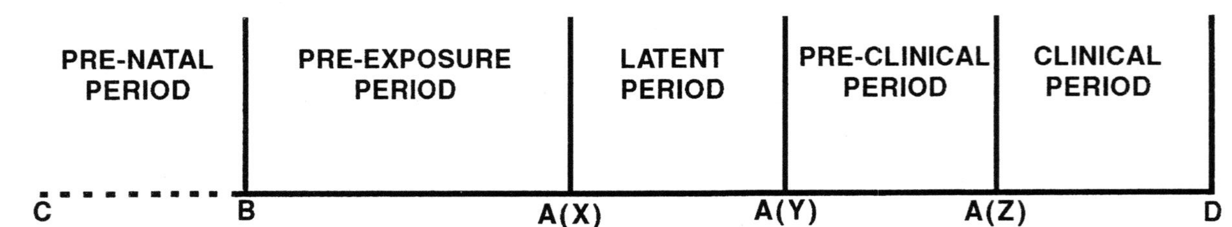

C = Conception
B = Birth
A(X) = Age of first exposure to drug
A(Y) = Age of first neurological changes due to drug
A(Z) = Age of first signs of dementia
D = Death

Adapted from Grant, Reed, and Adams

even three weeks into recovery. In fact, the length of time between the alcoholic's last drink and the date of neuropsychological testing is the most significant contributing factor to his or her assessed level of dysfunction.

If neuropsychological testing is to have any practical implications for alcoholics' treatment and recovery, it will be important to carefully evaluate the length of patients' abstinence at the time they were tested. Wells (1982) writes, "The level of impairment on neuropsychological tests, is to some extent, a function of when the subject is tested after he stops drinking; the defects found are generally greater immediately after" (p. 112). Most alcoholics do indeed show more impairment early in their recovery. Most studies demonstrate a continual improvement in cortical recovery up to and including one to two years after abstinence is maintained. The level of impairment in alcoholics, other than those alcoholics who suffer from a Korsakoff's syndrome, has been found to be reversible. Alcoholics experience spontaneous recovery from their deficits if abstinence is maintained. They only have to abstain from alcohol consumption to achieve this reversibility. The degree of the recovery in cognitive functioning is greatest during the first few weeks of abstinence. However, the degree of improvement continues on a positive gradient for many more months (Table 8.13). Such findings in neuropsychological research lend credibility to a very important AA maxim about recovery. Alcoholics are told by AA and their sponsors not to make any major decisions or changes in their life and to "keep it simple" during the first year of their recovery. The neuropsychological research evidence presented here substantiates the wisdom of AA's intuitive understanding and knowledge about alcoholism and its effect on a person's thinking process. As alcoholics' performance scores on the Category test and other neuropsychological measures suggest, they require at least a year before their abstract reasoning capacities return to normal levels of functioning. Consequently, it is best if they refrain from making major life decisions until they have had more time to stabilize cognitively.

This is where the pure research and neuropsychological testing has practical applications for clinical practice. A model of group therapy and treatment patterned after the AA philosophy has important implications for treatment because it is substantiated by recent neuropsychological findings. AA's insistence on abstinence parallels important cortical recovery changes that must be attained and considered before alcohol-induced dementia or encephalopathy can be properly treated. AA's insistence on keeping it simple and outlining concrete, distinct steps to recovery provides the alcoholic with a clear strategy and an achievable plan with

TABLE 8.13

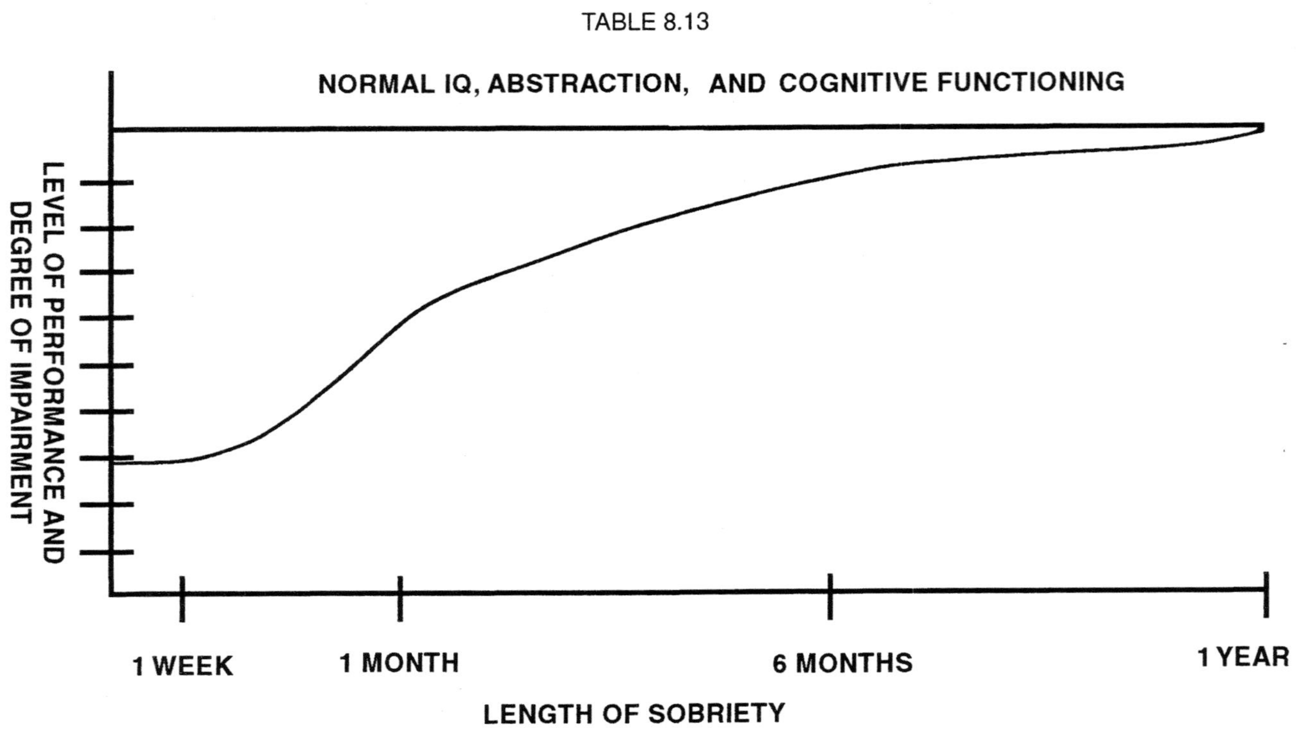
NORMAL IQ, ABSTRACTION, AND COGNITIVE FUNCTIONING
LEVEL OF PERFORMANCE AND
DEGREE OF IMPAIRMENT
1 WEEK
1 MONTH
6 MONTHS
1 YEAR
LENGTH OF SOBRIETY

measurable goals. This is crucial for individuals suffering from an impaired ability to think abstractly. It gives them what they desperately need at the beginning of treatment–direction, structure, and guidance. As alcoholics gradually recover their lost cognitive functioning, alternative treatment strategies can be implemented once their capacity for new learning, consolidation of information, abstract thought, creative thinking, and motivation have all returned to their pre-morbid level of functioning. At that point, alcoholics can utilize insight, self-understanding, and autonomous decision-making. Group leaders can then start to employ alternative modes of treatment in their therapy groups. Until alcoholics reach this stage, however, group leaders must conduct the psychotherapy groups in a more structured and directive manner.

Matching group interventions to stages of neurological readiness has important implications for treatment. Complicating the degree of neurological impairment is the motivation level and degree of readiness for behavioral change that will vary from individual to individual. While there is a strong correlation between psychological readiness and neurological readiness, not all individuals will present with the same levels of motivation or denial. Personality variables interact with the specific properties of specific drugs. Some addictions have a much more powerful impact on the brain than other addictive behaviors do. While many cognitive and behaviorally oriented researchers tend to classify all addictions under the general heading of addictive behaviors, they run the risk of overgeneralizing the addictive process. Addiction to nicotine, for instance, even though it is life-threatening and bears many similarities to the addictive process with alcohol and drugs, poses none of the immediate impairment and behavioral consequences that the abuse of substances does. Few would argue that nicotine abuse needs to be addressed with the same aggressiveness or immediacy that addiction to alcohol or drugs does. In a similar view, substance addictions are often compared to the addictions that involve compulsive activities such as gambling, sex, and spending. Outcome studies that generalize the results of smoking cessation or reduced caffeine intake to that of drug or alcohol treatment are guilty of seriously misleading the usefulness of such approaches. Despite these shortcomings, there is much to be gained from examining how motivational levels and stages of readiness to change can have important implications for treating the alcoholic or addict.

Within the last few years, behaviorally oriented researchers have attempted to quantify how it is that individuals change. Much of their work has been adapted to addiction and the identification of variables that influence a person's decision to stop alcohol or drug use. One popular conceptual model identifies five stages of the change process that have significant relationships with motivational levels of the individual and require intervention strategies of the therapist. Applying this conceptual framework to addictive disorders, it is suggested that motivation enhancement, or what some call "motivational interviewing," is of primary importance only in the very early stages of addiction treatment when individuals are ambivalent or have no interest in stopping their chemical use. Motivating individuals for treatment essentially consists of getting them to believe strongly in both the desirability and likelihood of change. Someone already convinced of this needs little help in this area, but needs more guidance in the latter stages of change where activities like preparation, action relapse prevention, and maintenance of recovery become the necessary priorities. In contrast to this position, others believe that early stage motivational interventions are all the assistance that some individuals will require in addressing their addiction. Once individuals are able to get past the precontemplative and contemplative stages, they will take the actions necessary to remain abstinent.

The stages of change model for addiction has been outlined by Prochaska, DiClemente, and colleagues (Prochaska and DiClemente, 1992; Prochaska, DiClemente, and Norcross, 1992; DiClemente, Carbonairi, and Velasquez, 1992) who have identified five stages of change that occur in both self-initiated and professionally facilitated interventions for addiction.

Horvath (1993) describes this model:

> The stages of change model suggests that precontemplation, contemplation, preparation, action, and maintenance are the five stages that the individual cycles and recycles through on the way to lasting resolution of a problem behavior. The model also identifies ten processes of change (e.g., consciousness raising, self-reevaluation, reinforcement management) which are viewed as specifying how change occurs. These processes of change are linked to specific stages. For instance, during the action stage the patient is focused in part on how to manage reinforcement (increase positives, decrease negatives of the new behavior). During the precontemplation stage the patient is focused in part on consciousness raising. Focusing on a process of change that does not coincide with the stage of change appears to be largely unproductive (e.g., attempting to teach reinforcement management to a patient still in the precontemplation stage). (p. 474)

Within this perspective, denial and resistance are viewed as the results of mismatched strategies on the part of the therapist with the addicts' or alcoholics' stage of readiness to change. Prochaska and DiClemente are suggesting that therapists can increase or induce resistance and denial if they do not carefully meet individuals with therapeutic interventions that are matched to their particular stage of readiness to stop their chemical use.

The stages of change within this model are:

1. *Precontemplation.* This is reflective of an individual having no intention to change because they either do not see they have a problem, or they believe it is not a serious enough problem to warrant change. Sometimes they hold the position that change is either too difficult or impossible. Usually, the individual in this stage is seeking therapy under some form of coercion because others (i.e., spouse, employer, judicial system, etc.) are of the opinion that there is a substance abuse problem. The task of the therapist at this stage is to engage individuals and establish some form of an alliance that will permit the therapist to raise doubts in the individuals' minds about the position they hold. They must be helped to see that they do have a problem and that the problem is directly affected or caused by chemicals. They must come to realize that change is not only beneficial, but achievable.
2. *Contemplation.* Awareness that change may be necessary, but ambivalence about initiating change dominates this stage. While individuals have some awareness of the consequences of their continual substance use, they either believe that they cannot change or that alternative and less drastic methods (i.e., controlled drinking) might work. The task of the therapist is to help tip the balance either by instilling hope (change is possible) or by presenting consequences of not changing (i.e., telling heroin addicts they will either end up dead or in prison if they do not stop using opiates).
3. *Preparation.* Awareness that change is necessary, but uncertainty as to how change is to be initiated is the crucial factor during this stage. Procrastination and avoidance can complicate this stage if the therapist does not help the individual determine the best course of action quickly. Imparting of information about treatment options and encouragement to the point of leading the person to take action is often necessary at this time.
4. *Action.* This is the stage of the shortest duration, a peak level of energy that can only be maintained for a limited period of time. Alternative behavioral options are tried and frustration is easily experienced if results are not rewarded or attempts are encumbered by excessive complications (i.e., hospital admission procedures or insurance documentation requirements). The therapist must remain sensitive to the fragility of this stage of the change process and

remove all possible impediments, helping individuals help themselves to take the necessary steps toward change.

5. *Maintenance.* There is a big difference between getting sober or clean and staying sober or clean. Strategies for staying sober and clean during the first few weeks of recovery will be far different than strategies necessary for staying sober or clean three, six, or twelve months into recovery. The learning of new behaviors, values, and attitudes that are incompatible with the old drinking and drug-taking behaviors, values, and attitudes is essential if maintenance of the change is to be obtained. Integration and assimilation into the twelve-step program and philosophy is one crucial component of this process. Learning how to use psychotherapy and the group will become another crucial component if recovery is to be maintained.

Relapse Prevention

While relapse will be a crucial part of the maintenance stage of change, it will be a continual focus after action is initiated to stop using alcohol and drugs. Relapses are inevitable for most, if not all alcoholics and addicts. They can be invaluable learning experiences if properly examined and integrated. Staying closely connected to other recovering addicts and alcoholics in the twelve-step recovery programs will ensure that the learning from relapses does not always have to come at the individuals' own personal expense since they have the opportunity to learn from each other by witnessing each others' relapses. They soon learn that relapses follow a predictable and recognizable pattern. This is vitally important since relapses can often be fatal. The therapist can provide information and direction and explain the typical warning signs of relapse that can help prevent and minimize its impact and occurrence. As important as this information is, it does not carry anything close to the impact and emotional learning that is provided by witnessing a fellow addict or alcoholic in the early throes of a relapse.

Prochaska and DiClemente's model for assessing readiness to change can provide some useful guidance for determining the strategies that need to be employed when initially treating chemically dependent individuals. Their work complements a growing consensus that traditional methods of psychotherapy cannot be applied to a practicing alcoholic or addict. While some controversy exists about when a chemically dependent individual can benefit from psychotherapy, there is a growing consensus that a person early in recovery is less likely than a person late in recovery to respond or benefit fully from more traditional methods of psychotherapy, whether it be individual, family, or group. A recent review article (Kaufman and

Reoux, 1988) recommended that treatment strategies be adapted to fit three distinct phases of treatment: (1) achieving sobriety; (2) early recovery or abstinence; and (3) advanced or late stage recovery. In a similar fashion, Washton (1992) recommended that addicts or alcoholics be moved through different sequential groups that focus on issues relevant to their particular stage of recovery: (1) early recovery; (2) relapse prevention or maintenance; and (3) long-term recovery.

Group therapy, especially during the earlier stages of recovery, is rarely a stand-alone treatment modality. It is usually part of a comprehensive treatment program that simultaneously provides individual therapy, drug screening or testing, family counseling, education sessions, detoxification, and integration into twelve-step programs. The question of how group treatment will be utilized depends on numerous factors and often conflicting variables. There is a confusing array of different theories of change, applications, approaches, and definitions of addiction. Which type of group, for which type of individual, in what type of treatment setting, with what level of addiction, to what kind of drug, with which level of motivation, in which stage of recovery, for what aim or purpose, must be evaluated and carefully discerned. The answer to each of these questions has to be carefully evaluated because it helps determine what role group treatment will have in addicts' and alcoholics' recovery. To help sift through this confusion, the next three chapters will be aimed at addressing how group therapy can best be adapted and applied to early, middle, and late stage recover issues.

Chapter 9

Early Stage Treatment Issues

Early stage treatment issues deal primarily with precontemplation, contemplation, and preparation stages of change that have been outlined by Prochaska and DiClemente (1992). Most of the therapist's energy will be directed toward getting alcoholics and addicts to recognize, admit, and move past their high levels of ambivalence and denial. Beginning group leaders soon discover that few alcoholics and addicts enter treatment of their own free will. Consequently, when these patients are initially introduced to treatment and group, usually they are either under extreme external pressure from their family, their employer, or a judge, or they are compelled by serious physical health problems related to their chemical use. Group leaders find that many of their group members are in a severe emotional state characterized by guilt, shame, and depression or are extremely obstinate and angry because others have forced them to comply with demands that seem to them to be unjust, unfair, and punitive. Even if chemically dependent individuals agree that they need treatment, they usually harbor wishes to be able to drink and use drugs in a safe and normal way. Their compliance to treatment is motivated more by their remorse and wish to avoid further condemnation than it is by their desire to actively learn ways to ensure that their treatment will be successful. Thus, the group leader is faced with the difficult task of dealing with resistant patients on two different levels. If the group members are not actively rebellious and resistant to treatment, they usually are working very hard to give the staff and group leader the impression that they are actively engaged in their recovery and treatment. This presents the group leader with a delicate problem because those group members who are actively resistant are usually easier to treat than those who are passively compliant.

Their facade of voluntary compliance must be exposed as a manipulation of the treatment process or their recovery will be motivated only by their desire to be free from external distress and pressure. In either case, the patient's postures need to be confronted and altered quickly, usually within twenty-eight days, the length of a normal inpatient program. Unless this is accomplished, the AA program will not be internalized and they will never be able to make the shift to personal responsibility for their recovery and abstinence. Although group psychotherapy can be a significant adjunct to alcoholics' and addicts' treatment, group leaders also discover that few patients are completely willing to do everything necessary to ensure the successful treatment of their addiction. Most alcoholics and addicts possess varying levels of motivation to abstain from alcohol and drug use. This is especially true during the early initial stages of treatment when their level of alcohol- and drug-induced cognitive impairment is most severe and they are more rigid and limited in their ability to explore alternative solutions to old problems. Even when addicts and alcoholics enter treatment completely of their own free will and possess a strong innate desire to stop their use of chemicals, many of these patients will have difficulty doing the things necessary to ensure their recovery because of the various degrees of character pathology they possess. This condition is also made more severe by the recency of their chemical use, which usually leaves them more rebellious, suspicious, and manipulative.

The art of treating addiction is to overcome the enormous denial and resistance–whether it be passive or active–that most alcoholics and addicts possess. Such a stance in treatment raises many important ethical and therapeutic issues. Confrontation, if done too punitively or if motivated by a group leader's countertransference issues, can severely damage the therapeutic alliance. However, the group leader cannot afford to stand back and take a stance of therapeutic neutrality, because time, the severity of the chemically dependent patient's condition, and his or her lack of motivation interferes with the normal evolution of psychotherapy that usually takes place with most non-addicted patients. Treating the chemically dependent patient requires group leaders to make a dramatic shift in focus and utilize techniques with which they usually have had little training or experience. Confrontation, intervention, coercion, and the use of therapeutic leverage are techniques that can have damaging effects on an individual or a group if they are applied inappropriately and indiscriminately. Such an approach to treatment is often completely contrary to most contemporary forms of psychotherapy, and many group leaders are either uncomfortable with its use or do not understand its proper application. Consequently, these methods are frequently misused, ignored, or overzealously applied. In some cases, group leaders who are unfamiliar with the proper utilization of these methods apply them indiscriminately to all group members with equal intensity all of the time. They fail to realize that some alcoholics and addicts require a little less and some require a little more. They fail to treat their group members as individuals, and these techniques become ends unto themselves. What would be an appropriate confrontation for an alcoholic at the beginning of treatment would be completely destructive for that same alcoholic later in treatment.

It is important to remember that defensive operations organize the self not only for effective normal functioning, but also to avoid anxiety. Therefore, confrontational techniques used solely as tools to hammer away at the rigid defenses of alcoholics and addicts are likely to increase anxiety and thereby precipitate avoidance responses and denial. Withdrawal, avoidance, or placating responses can be triggered by such techniques and will, in turn, reinforce rigid patterns of thought and behavior, thereby increasing resistance to change. In many cases, treatment can be enhanced with a more indirect use of confrontation. Also, any tendencies toward passive compliance (agreement with the staff and group leader to avoid the anxiety of confrontation) are amplified by direct attacks. Thus, indirect confrontation also decreases the likelihood of passive compliant forms of resistance.

This brings us to the purpose of this chapter. Each of these techniques—coercion, the use of therapeutic leverage, confrontation, and intervention—will be explored in an attempt to define the limits of its usefulness and applicability. Usually, if not always, these techniques are much more appropriate during the early part of treatment. They should be utilized either to get chemically dependent individuals to realize the extent of their difficulty in the hope that they will enter treatment or once they are in treatment help them to truly understand the severe disparity between their actions and feelings. In short, these techniques can help individuals take a more honest look at themselves and hopefully recognize that their self-deceptions are a significant contributing factor to the severity of their condition.

SPECIAL PROBLEMS OF THE ADDICTED PATIENT

The basic thrust of treatment for addicted patients is to get them to perceive and understand the relationship between their present difficulties in life and their alcohol and drug use. When this is accomplished, patients must be made to see the advantage of not drinking or doing drugs compared to the problems resulting from the continual use of chemicals. This choice must be weighed by each patient and a personal decision must be made. However, left to rely on their own resources, most addicts and alcoholics will cling to the belief that one day they can attain normal and healthy use of drugs and alcohol. While most therapists have been taught that it is important not to make decisions for patients and that a therapeutic alliance must never be compromised at any cost, the group leader must carefully evaluate such a stance when leading a group composed of members who are currently struggling with these decisions in the early stages of their recovery. As Shore states, "Therapists who remain inflexibly supportive while alcoholics continue to kill themselves by drinking need to reconsider the moral repercussions of their position" (1981, p. 13).

Alcoholics and addicts consequently present group leaders with new and unique problems in group. Working with this population requires group leaders to evaluate many of their conventional and unquestioned assumptions about treatment. An approach that is very effective with a non-addicted patient might be totally inappropriate for someone who is currently addicted or is in the early stages of recovery. The group leader must also be aware that many alcoholics and addicts have rather sophisticated defenses and are usually adept at applying these defenses in an effort to defeat the therapist. Unlike neurotics or non-addictive patients, who come to treatment of their own free will and are actively seeking help in the relief of their symptoms, most addicted patients want to convince the group leader and the treatment staff that there has either been a horrible mistake made in their referral for treatment or that they need the staff and group leader to focus on their real problem. This problem is often formulated in the patients' minds as the root cause of their pathological use of chemicals. Secretly, the patient hopes that once this root cause is discovered, he or she will be able to return to the normal use of chemicals. Chemically dependent individuals will emphasize this issue because drinking or drug use is frequently the only pleasure they feel they derive out of life–a pleasure that must be protected at all costs.

DEFENSE MECHANISMS

Alcoholics' and addicts' common misconceptions about alcohol and drugs are often the result of an elaborate set of defense mechanisms. Neo-Freudians were the first to make the distinction between healthy ego-defenses, such as sublimation and intellectualization, and unhealthy ego-defenses, such as denial and suppression. Group leaders should understand that repression and ego-defenses are a normal, healthy process that reflects an individual's tendency to selectively forget negative experiences that may be too painful or uncomfortable. Repression and ego-defenses are utilized by all of us in our attempts to cope with day-to-day problems. It is only when the degree of repression reaches such proportions as to deny reality that symptoms of illness are manifested. When ego-defenses are utilized with such frequency and intensity that reality-testing becomes compromised, individuals must be encouraged to face the inappropriateness of their defensive position. Confronting these misconceptions is crucial in treating the alcoholic and addict because inappropriate ego-defenses and repression are the key misconceptions that the group leader must recognize and deal with before any progress in treatment can be made. Borowitz (1964) hypothesized that the basic psychological effect of alcohol is to modify ego function, which involves a decrease in perceptual activity. In fact, alcoholics and addicts are generally thought to possess poorly developed egos with inadequate defenses. Vernon Johnson (1973) agrees, and he believes alcoholics are unable to perceive what exactly is happening to them because the dynamics of the illness are so complicated. Addiction is an intricate process that involves an interplay of repression, cortical deterioration, and impaired judgment. While it is not important that the group leader know why individuals are alcoholics or addicts in order to counsel and help them, it is important to have an understanding of the dynamics involved in the addiction process.

Alcoholics or addicts are individuals with a chronic disease that becomes progressively worse. This is important to remember because as their condition deteriorates, their ego strength weakens and their self-image deteriorates. Guilt, shame, and remorse are factors that frequently cause them to set up elaborate defenses to control these uncomfortable emotions. As the emotional pain becomes greater, their defenses become more rigid. Eventually, they become victims of their own psychological defense mechanisms.

Marty Mann (1973), among others, stressed the importance of straightening out the patient's misconceptions and fallacies about the disease of alcoholism. Alcoholics, Mann felt, share the view of society that alcoholism is a moral deficiency. Alcoholics and addicts generally do not view themselves as physically dependent, and this is one of the reasons why they make every effort to deny that addiction is their problem. The guilt and remorse they feel because of their drinking and drug use leads them to refuse to acknowledge or accept help. The disease concept convinces them that they are not bad, but rather, ill. This relieves their guilt. Any modality of treatment that helps addicts and alcoholics to accept themselves as individuals with some worth will help their recovery. Increased self-esteem and self-worth are important factors in treatment.

Ruth Fox sums up this position when she writes,

> The alcoholic needs to be reassured that alcoholism is truly viewed by the medical profession and other health authorities as an illness, not a moral falling or a wicked self-indulging weakness. The

> usual immediate result of this assurance is a draining off of the emotions which constrict and distort the alcoholic's self-image and view of the problem, and a release from the enormous guilt feelings which paralyze the patient's ability to take steps toward recovery. (1967, p. 54)

Fox's position is consistent with the psychoanalytic belief that when the cause of repression is discovered, the repressed material rapidly emerges into the patient's consciousness. In other words, if the threat is eliminated, it becomes safe for the repressed material to return to awareness. It is at this stage of recovery that alcoholics and addicts can look at their illness realistically.

The return to consciousness of repressed feelings is a crucial step in the recovery process for a number of reasons. Alcoholics and addicts can now become reacquainted with themselves at a more meaningful level. Admittance of one's illness and addiction is a significant first step in AA's twelve steps. Johnson suggests,

> The effect of this new degree of self-awareness has been to create the need for a reduction of the burden of moral anxiety and guilt which it has brought into conscious focus . . . . In some fashion, the alcoholic begins now to see the truth that these defects of character are the signs of his sickness, and that upon their removal, his recovery depends. (1973, p. 116)

Psychoanalytic theory generally supports Johnson's contention that an emotional component to this awareness is a prerequisite for recovery. In a similar fashion, Nemiah (1961) concludes,

> The pain is further heightened to an unbearable intensity by the anger that stems from their ambivalence. To protect themselves from pain, they employ abnormal mechanisms of defense: denial of loss leads to a blocking of the process of grief . . . resulting in a variety of somatic complaints, violent self-castigation, and suicide. (p. 63)

It is through the process of pain and grief that alcoholics' and addicts' awareness of their condition is realistically faced and accepted. Only through an emotional catharsis and crisis will alcoholics and addicts finally admit to God and to others that their life is hopeless in the face of their chemical use. This is the stage AA recognizes as the surrender to the acknowledgement that the alcoholic is ill. This process cannot be an intellectual awareness alone. It also requires understanding at an emotional and spiritual level.

For treatment to continue on at this point, it is important that the group leader not be manipulated into trying to perform insight psychotherapy with a patient who continues to drink or use drugs. The group leader must make it clear to the patient that abstinence will have to come first. Even when addiction is accompanied by an underlying psychopathology, the pathological drinking can kill long before its cause is found. Very often, abstinence brings about amelioration of most of the conditions previously blamed by alcoholics and addicts as the reasons for their drinking and drug use.

Johnson (1973) sees the removal and alleviation of guilt and remorse as an important factor in treatment. This only occurs after abstinence is attained. "Our most startling observation has been that alcoholism cannot exist unless there is a conflict between the values and the behavior of the drinker" (p. 75). Johnson goes on to conclude, "Very simply, the treatment involves a therapy designed to bring the patient back to reality" (p. 75). It is through the group leader's confrontation of repression and denial that the establishment of reality-testing takes place with an associated emotional catharsis.

Albrecht (1969) summed up this position when he concluded, "During this phase of heavy drinking, the individual becomes very skillful at using denial, rationalization, and projection to avoid full confrontation with his drinking problem. He denies that he has a problem; he finds a multitude of reasons for his drinking and he blames others for his drinking" (p. 15). Not only are alcoholics and addicts unaware of their highly developed defense system, they are also unaware of the powerful feelings of self-hate buried behind it. Their defense systems continue to grow, so that they can survive in the face of their problems. The greater the pain they suffer, the higher and more rigid the defenses become. Alcoholics and addicts therefore become more rigid in their defensive processes as time goes by. Consequently, this adds to the group leader's difficulty as he or she struggles to get alcoholics and addicts to see their situation more realistically. As alcoholics and addicts succumb more to their rigid defense systems, they become more and more out of touch with their feelings. Given these circumstances, the group leader's task during the early stages of treatment becomes clearly defined. He or she must help alcoholics and addicts to (1) discover themselves and others as feeling persons, and (2) identify the defenses that prevent this discovery.

Getting alcoholics and addicts to recognize their feelings is important for two reasons. First, feelings and spontaneous expressions tend to be much more honest. It is more helpful to be revealing than to be right. A spontaneous expression may release both positive and negative emotions that must be recognized and dealt with. This is the only way the alcoholics' and addicts' rigid defenses and repressions can be altered and reality-testing can be restored. Second, it is essential to know one's own feelings at a given moment, for it is necessary to sense with equal accuracy the feelings of another person. If alcoholics and addicts are to return to the world of the "living," they must be able to deal with other people accurately and empathetically.

Because of chemically dependent individuals' addiction, confrontation is often the only way to alter their self-destructive and rigid defenses. However, the way confrontation is utilized is crucial. There are constructive and destructive forms of confrontation. Alcoholics need someone who will call a spade a spade in a realistic fashion without adopting a punitive, moralistic, or superior attitude. As Vernon Johnson illustrates, attacking the individual is often mistaken for confrontation. Attacking serves only to raise defenses. Confrontation, on the other hand, can be defined as describing individuals in a way that is most likely to be received by them. Johnson states that, "We are most useful as confronters when we are not so much trying to change another person as we are trying to help him see himself more accurately."

COERCION

However, before confrontive techniques can be applied in group, alcoholics or addicts must seek treatment. In many, if not most, cases, this is the single largest obstacle to treatment. Pre-treatment strategies must be established and managed to ensure that reluctant patients are adequately coerced to seek treatment, especially when they are unable or unwilling to see the reality of their condition. Coercion to seek therapy, however, is a controversial issue having many ethical, legal, and practical implications. Questions concerning individuals' rights and freedom to refuse treatment even though their behavior may prove to be a menace to themselves and society are not easily resolved or answered (Wald, 1974). Aside from the crucial and currently popular issues of infringement of rights and invasion of privacy is the problem of the efficacy of forcing someone to seek treatment when cooperation and motivation to be treated are absent. An axiom in the field of psychotherapy and counseling is that clients must invest a large part of themselves in the treatment process if therapy is to be successful (Perls, 1969; Schultz, 1969; Rogers, 1942; Carkhuff, 1969). However, evidence is now mounting that perhaps this is not necessarily true, especially for alcoholics (Bourne and Fox, 1973; Johnson, 1973).

Ruth Fox (1967) announced that it is not necessary to wait for alcoholics to hit bottom or motivate themselves into treatment before taking therapeutic measures. Sterne and Pittman (1965) demonstrated plainly that it is often the psychotherapist or group leader, rather than the addict or alcoholic, who needs the motivating. Chaftez, Blane, and Hill (1970) showed that helping professionals can motivate reluctant patients to undergo treatment by promptly meeting patients' obvious dependency needs, by communicating through action, concern for the patient's low self-esteem, and by continuity of care. As Alcoholics Anonymous and Al-Anon have consistently illustrated, a new or changed attitude surrounding the problem drinker frequently motivates such a patient to seek help of his or her own volition (Bailey and Leach, 1965).

Denial

There is now a general consensus among theorists and practitioners in the field of addiction that alcoholics and addicts generally possess especially poor ego defenses (Johnson, 1973; Bourne and Fox, 1973; Jellinek, 1960; Weinberg, 1976).

Rationalization and denial are such frequent components of an alcoholic's and addict's illness that these ego defenses have become synonymous with the addiction process. Most theorists recognize the necessity of identifying and breaking through this denial system before successful recovery can be initiated (Hazelden Foundation, Johnson Institute, etc.). Denial is frequently a progressive part of the alcoholic's and addict's illness. It becomes overdeveloped, more rigid, and increasingly difficult to penetrate in its later stages until the alcoholic is almost completely out of touch with reality (Jellinek, 1960). Late stage alcoholics and addicts minimize, rationalize, and deny any problem with alcohol or drugs, usually projecting the cause of their problems onto others. Guilt, remorse, and deteriorating judgment perpetuate the drinking cycle until alcoholics and addicts totally reject any responsibility for their plight (Johnson, 1973). Weinberg (1976) saw the tendency on the part of family, friends, and helping professionals to avoid this issue when dealing with alcoholics and addicts in the earlier stage of their illness as providing a social environment that encourages denial. Until changes in cultural attitudes occur, Weinberg contended, professionals will continue to be frustrated by a stubborn resistance to change.

Other theorists disagree and suggest strategies for effectively dealing with this problem. It is understandable how alcoholics' and addicts' elaborate ego defenses and strong denial systems often lead many counselors, judges, and other helping professionals to erroneously assume that alcoholics or addicts must hit bottom before they can be helped. Evidence suggests that this is not the case (Bourne and Fox, 1973; Johnson, 1973). Fox (1967) contended that alcoholics will not consider giving up alcohol until the suffering it causes them is greater than the pleasure it gives them. The general consensus is that alcoholics and addicts must lose something important to them or at least be threatened with such a loss (Bourne and Fox, 1973; Johnson, 1973).

Vernon Johnson (1973) maintained that it is dangerous to wait for an alcoholic or addict to hit bottom. He sees the need to train counselors to recognize an alcoholic's and addict's "cry for help" and "defiant dependence" as components of the treatment process that the counselors can use to their advantage once they are identified. Evidence from industrial programs indicates that a crisis induced by individuals with the authority to confront and back up their accusations can be an effective alternative to previous modes of treatment.

Employee Assistance Programs

Substantial opinion and research evidence support a strategy of "constructive coercion" (Minovitz, 1973) or "forceful coercion" (Murray, 1973) as a viable alternative for inducing a crisis in an alcoholic's life. Lew (1973), in research conducted on industrial treatment programs, believed that alcoholics are motivated to change when they are in crisis, and that if they do not have to accept the consequences of their behaviors, they are not likely to be motivated toward recovery. Other research (Lemere, 1958; Gerard, 1962; Tiebout, 1961) indicated that the importance of employee assistance programs lies in the employer's right to bring about a job-related crisis in the alcoholic's or addict's life while he or she is still on the job. Because of the deteriorating effects of addiction, a written company policy confronting the individual's poor job performance and attendance, while directly avoiding accusations of his or her alcoholism or addiction, is generally successful in inducing treatment. Often, job security is the individual's chief vehicle for denial. Once that job security is challenged, his or her denial begins to crumble.

The strength of the employer and supervisor in confrontation centers in the intrinsic makeup of a supervisory role. Supervisors are trained to be more ready to act and have more power at their disposal than the alcoholic's spouse, friends, clergyman, or physician. Previous attempts to use the family as the locus for identifying the developing problem drinker have been unfruitful because of the diffused emotional relationships that characterize family structure and process (Department of Health, Education, and Welfare, 1974).

Independent research by the National Institute on Alcohol Abuse and Alcoholism (1962) indicates that the 70 percent success rate in industrial programs is often unparalleled, even by Alcoholics Anonymous. Most other treatment facilities report success rates that rarely reach above the 20 percent level. This suggests that the highly confrontational nature of industrial programs and AA produces an atmosphere that facilitates successful treatment for alcoholics. The court, too, has the power to bring about a crisis through confrontation.

The constructive confrontation strategy makes specific assumptions. Coercion, in some form, is necessary in human behavior (Simmel, 1950). Because society provides few clear norms about alcohol and drug use, developing alcoholics and addicts rarely face consistent sanctions; thus, they have few internal controls for managing this behavior (Inkeles, 1968). Enforced cooperation relieves alcoholics or addicts of the burden of developing motivation for themselves. The strategy activates and uses existing social controls within the system rather than moving the deviant from the system into a specialized control setting.

Coercion, Attitudes, and Motivation in Treatment

It appears that one of the problems in motivation of the alcoholic or addict to accept treatment is that reluctance on the part of the patient to seek or accept help is psychological in nature. This is particularly true if the procedure is unknown and possibly threatening. Canter (1969) tested this hypothesis and concluded that it is important to inform alcoholics and addicts about various treatment approaches to enhance their receptivity to treatment. Rossi (1972) reached a similar conclusion and suggested that the motivation of the alcoholic and addict to accept treatment is not only internal, but is related to the characteristics of the social environment and the personality of the helping professional. Rossi further suggested that the patient's motivation to recovery be seen as a multidimensional interaction of the patient, the setting, and the psychotherapist. Devito's research (1969) results were similarly encouraging and lend credence to the hypothesis of the value of firm external controls in the successful treatment of alcoholics and addicts.

Zax (1961) demonstrated that significant relationships in the counseling process enhance the tendency to remain in treatment longer. Wedel (1965), in a similar study, concluded that the efforts of social workers had great personal significance to some individuals. Wedel found that few alcoholics and addicts in his study had sufficient ego strength to stop drinking; the motivation had to come from other sources, such as religious faith, group involvement, or family considerations. Sterne and Pittman (1965) examined the concept of motivation to determine to what extent it was crucial to recovery. They concluded that the majority of individuals in the helping professions excessively rely on the belief that client motivation is essential for success in treatment. Failure to accept an alcoholic or addict as a client and the lack of success in treatment are often conveniently explained by the lack of motivation on the client's part. Their findings suggest a need for improvement of professional training. They also concluded that systematic research is needed to isolate factors that contribute to alcoholics' and addicts' acceptance of treatment.

While it sometimes is crucial for the legal system or employer to initiate the treatment process through coercion, there is research to indicate that addicts and alcoholics do not need pressures to keep them actively involved in the recovery process (Heitler, 1976). Other research, however, cites the importance of force as an essential part of treatment (Sexias, 1976). Other evidence suggests that individuals coerced into treatment do as well—no better, no worse—as those who presumably enter treatment on their own. Bibb's (1970) research concluded with the findings that outpatient treatment as a contingency of probation can yield results comparable to those of voluntary patients, as long as someone other than the therapist polices the terms of the probation.

Typically, these studies show that negative expectancies and attitudes on the part of the psychotherapists and group leaders frequently have an adverse effect on the success rate of the treatment. Effectively dealing with reluctant patients may be the most important overall competency that group leaders and psychotherapists can develop. Involuntary clients may account for the majority of a group leader's or psychotherapist's caseload and failure to learn how to deal adequately with hostility and reluctance on a patient's part may be the single largest contributing factor to failure in treatment. It is true that many professionals have simply not had sufficient training to deal skillfully and easily with reluctant patients.

It is important to point out that coercion takes many subtle forms and does not necessarily have to be so obvious as when practiced by the employer or court. Unhappy spouses, worried friends, concerned doctors, and disgruntled bosses all make up a contingency that often uses subtle pressure to force individuals with many different types of problems into counseling when those individuals do not agree that they have a problem. It is suggested here that individuals who seek psychotherapy completely of their own free will may be more the exception than the rule. Dealing with such patients requires that group leaders know how to utilize their therapeutic leverage to ensure maximum benefit from treatment.

THE USE OF THERAPEUTIC LEVERAGE

Group leaders must be aware that alcoholics and addicts will not give up their alcohol or drugs until the pain and dysphoria they experience outweighs the pleasure and euphoria they derive from its use. Consequently, alcoholics and addicts must be made to see the way alcohol and drugs affect important areas of their lives. Group leaders must also learn early in individuals' treatment what is significantly important to the addicts or alcoholics that continued drinking and drug use might threaten. For some individuals, it is their job. For others, it is their spouse, health, family, or self-respect. In some cases, it might even be the threat of incarceration. Such knowledge is important since it can be used to encourage and even coerce individuals to utilize the tools of treatment, group, or AA. Since alcohol and drug use affects judgment and in most cases of chronic use causes temporary but severe levels of cognitive impairment, many patients are unable to accurately understand, interpret, and perceive the true nature of their condition, much less make clear, rational decisions that will have profound effects on their life, family, health, and job. It is important for the group leader to understand the necessity of utilizing therapeutic leverage to guide alcoholics and addicts through the early stages of their treatment. This is required until patients are more capable of making rational choices for themselves. Convincing patients to try it the group leader's way under threat of loss of spouse, job, health, or incarceration can be tempered by telling group members that if they do not like this way after one year they can then try it their own way.

Group members who are concerned about their physical condition should have frequent laboratory testing and have ready access to a physician. Liver functioning tests and neurological examinations are particularly important. CAT scan evidence of cerebral atrophy, though costly and difficult, can be a very important source of therapeutic leverage, particularly with the abundance of recent research evidence demonstrating reversability of this condition if sobriety is maintained. Psychological testing, especially with an emphasis on neuropsychological assessment, can provide similar evidence to the patient at a much-reduced cost. Evidence presented from psychological and neuropsychological testing can be even more powerful, since it is concrete and concerns specific demonstrable behavior. Showing alcoholics or addicts that their IQ and abstract reasoning scores are markedly low can have a powerful influence on their motivation to abstain from further chemical use, especially if they are cautioned that further chronic use might produce permanent and irreversible brain damage.

If the alcoholic or addict is married, or involved in a significant relationship, the group leader will discover that there are usually multiple difficulties in the marriage or the relationship. In many cases, the spouse has either threatened divorce, is in the process of divorce, or is separated from the patient. If the marriage or relationship is important to the patient, and especially if the spouse is not also addicted, this can be a source of important therapeutic leverage. The alcoholic's or addict's spouse or significant other should be involved in the treatment process. This is especially true if the patient is hospitalized and being treated at a twenty-eight day inpatient program. Involvement in Al-Anon and conjoint therapy sessions will ensure that the spouse or significant other does not engage in self-defeating behavior that might threaten the therapeutic leverage. The input from this individual can be helpful to treatment if utilized properly. He or she can be supportive of the alcoholic and addict and can contribute information and observations that can help strengthen the therapeutic leverage. However, spouses or significant others must be taught not to make idle threats. They must be encouraged only to threaten separation or divorce if they intend to follow through with such threats. Such a stance by the spouse or significant other can often serve as a powerful motivating force in the chemically dependent person's recovery.

Patients who are suffering job-related difficulties because of their drinking or drug use can be under extreme pressure to remain abstinent. This is especially true if the referral comes from the employer. Under these circumstances, contact with the employer, the EAP (employee assistance program) representative, or the medical department of the company should be maintained. This, of course, will require that the group leader have a signed consent of release of information. This ensures that the group leader is protected legally, but, just as important, it is a clear therapeutic contract that defines the goals, motives, and intentions of the group leader. The purpose of this contract should be explained to patients not just as a threat to their job but as a clear message that the treatment program is serious about their recovery and expects them to face the consequences of their behavior. Patients should be told that the specifics of their personal sharing in treatment or group will not be discussed, but only their progress related to their drinking or drug use. This assures the group members that their confidentiality concerning matters unrelated to their progress with abstinence from drugs and alcohol will be maintained. For many alcoholics and addicts, the therapeutic leverage related to their job security and work performance is the most powerful motivating force in their recovery.

A very similar position can be taken with alcoholics or addicts if they are referred by a court. This is especially true if they have two or more convictions for public intoxication or driving while intoxicated (DWI) or driving under the influence (DUI). A therapeutic contract established through the court or a probation officer can serve as a powerful incentive in an individual's recovery. Utilizing a group therapy format for these referrals requires special adaptations of the group format. However, if this adaptation is accomplished successfully, group is the treatment of choice for court referrals. Later in this chapter, such a format will be presented and described in detail because such a format will contain the utilization of all the techniques (i.e., confrontation, intervention, coercion, therapeutic leverage) to be described in this chapter.

Certainly, the use of therapeutic leverage as outlined here raises many important considerations concerning the therapeutic contract. Trust is a crucial factor in all forms of psychotherapy and treatment. In many cases, trust and the therapeutic alliance will be severely compromised because of the nature of the disease of addiction and the circumstances leading the patient to enter group or treatment. There are a couple of ways that group leaders might avoid the pitfalls associated with the use of leverage in treatment. If the patient is in group under the auspices of a treatment facility or hospital, it would be beneficial to have someone other than the patient's primary therapist or group leader serve as the enforcer of this policy. This will allow group leaders to avoid compromising the therapeutic alliance too severely. However, group leaders should be definite in outlining the limits of the therapeutic contract. They should tell the group members explicitly that they must convey information concerning the members' progress to the rest of the staff at the hospital. After patients have completed the initial part of their treatment, group leaders could then establish a new contract with the group and its members. This will be especially important if the group is to be an ongoing, long-term, after-care group. However, it may be difficult, if not impossible, for some individuals to trust their group leader once they have felt coerced or manipulated into treatment–no matter how much it may have helped them. Trust and a therapeutic alliance may be impossible to establish or reestablish in such cases. Referral of the group or individual group members to other group leaders might be in order in these circumstances.

While the utilization of therapeutic leverage may create some difficulties for the group leader, the gains from its application usually outweigh its costs in terms of treatment effectiveness. Zimberg (1980) outlines the advantages of such an approach if it is carried out in a well-planned and therapeutic manner:

> When used judiciously, appropriately, nonpunitively and nonjudgmentally, therapeutic leverage can be very effective in directing the alcoholic into a more responsive therapeutic status. If used, however, by a therapist with serious countertransference problems, including anger and frustration at the patient, it can destroy the therapeutic relationship. One must be constantly self observing when

> treating an alcoholic to ensure that the therapeutic leverages are designed to facilitate the alcoholic's recovery and not to satisfy one's need for successful treatment or as retaliation and punishment for the alcoholic's provocative behavior. (pp. 112-113)

CONFRONTATION

Before group leaders can effectively apply the use of therapeutic leverage in group, they must understand the intricate interplay between the purpose of an alcoholic's and addict's defenses and the confrontive techniques necessary to alter them. Defenses are always there for a reason. They must not be stripped away too quickly and confronted too severely just for the sake of confrontation. It is a general axiom in psychotherapy that defenses should not be altered until patients completely understand their purpose and have developed enough ego strength and alternative resources to allow them to substitute more constructive ways of defending themselves from painful affective states. However, alcoholics or addicts can kill themselves or completely destroy their support system while the group leader allows them the necessary time it may require for them to figure this out by themselves. This is one instance where the group leader has to alter his or her normal stance of support and unconditional acceptance. Confrontation is one method that the group leader can utilize in dealing with the alcoholic's or addict's rigid, self-destructive defensive process. However, the parameters and limits of confrontation must be understood and appreciated first.

In contrast to empathic clarifications and interpretations, both of which are directed at what patients say and present to the group leader, confrontations address something that patients are unaware of or denying. Confrontations are more effective when they are directed toward something that patients could or should be addressing, but are not because they are either consciously or unconsciously avoiding it. Patients who describe incidents while omitting feelings, or whose description of an incident is notably similar to previous episodes in their lives, or who present a discrepancy between their thoughts, feelings, and actions are prime candidates for a confrontation, which might help them progress past their stuck position.

If, as the group leader, you only empathize with alcoholics' or addicts' pain and suffering, you run the risk of reinforcing their denial or delusional system. You must also be able to empathize with their denial that their suffering and pain is determined in a large part because of their refusal to give up their use of chemicals. The group leader must remember that empathy is not compliance and doing or saying what the patient wants or hopes to hear. Inevitably, there are critical moments in the group process when, in order to facilitate a significant step in the change process, responsible group leaders will take a well-timed risk by confronting a member with a painful truth, sensitively monitoring their own countertransferential feelings. In truth, the risk is a calculated one insofar as the group leader is implicitly saying with conviction, "In my judgment you are ready to face this issue, this truth about yourself at this time. I accept my responsibility as a group leader by confronting you and have confidence in the strength of our relationship and in your ability to face it." If the confrontation is delivered in the context of this attitude and not motivated by the group leader's frustration or anger, it is likely to be effective. As Louis Ormont (1985) said, "If you love your patients and they feel it, you can say anything to them."

Applied from this perspective, confrontations differ significantly from the way they have been used historically in addiction treatment. Historically, the use of confrontation in group therapy evolved out of the work of drug-free therapeutic communities such as Day-Top and Synanon and was in large part directed by ex-addicts. The original intent was to convey the message that if we did not care or if we were not concerned about you, we would not bother to point out something that might save your life. However, like any therapeutic technique applied overzealously, confrontation can have antitherapeutic consequences, especially when it becomes attack therapy (Rachman and Heller, 1974).

As Rachman and Heller caution, confrontation becomes "attack therapy" when:

1. In a confrontational atmosphere, individuals are often psychologically assaulted. Individuals who are rehabilitated from substance abuse can pay the price of losing their dignity, their freedom to disagree, or their sense of independence and opportunity to think, feel, or behave in a unique manner.
2. The mandate is to conform to a strict, inflexible code of behavior and philosophy known as the "concept."
3. Confrontation is often used before a working alliance is developed.
4. There is a lack of therapeutic flexibility, so that a variety of helpful interventions are not integrated along with confrontation.
5. A ritualistic interaction develops in which individuals confront each other over and over again without genuine internal change occurring.

As Rachman and Heller (1974) warn, members learn to "cop-to- the-game" in response to attack. They adapt by admitting to transgression in behavior in order to get the staff and group leaders off their backs. The use of confrontation exclusively promotes an increase of tension, anger, hostility, and resentment to the exclusion of empathy, concern, and caring.

In contrast to this position, Raubolt (1974) recommends that an atmosphere of "caring confrontation" be established under the following guidelines:

1. Confrontation and limit-setting are necessary when an individual's impulsiveness is out of control. Confrontation is used to peel away layers of defenses against the awareness of destructive effect of substance abuse.
2. The use of peers as agents of change rather than traditional authority figures.
3. The realization that addiction often involves a lifestyle and an identity that frequently consumes the individual.
4. Insistence that before personality change can occur, abstinence and a focus on alcohol- and substance-taking behaviors must occur.
5. Insistence that individuals take responsibility for their self-destructive and chemical-oriented behavior.
6. The use of nontechnical language in discussing psychological issues and personality functioning.

Confrontations are not usually delivered exclusively by the group leader. Peers and other members of the group are likely to be confrontational to each other, especially when the atmosphere established by the group leader permits and even fosters confrontation. This can have either beneficial or damaging consequences depending on whether the climate is one of "attack therapy" or "caring confrontation." Washton (1992) suggests presenting group members with the following guidelines to help them both understand the purpose of confrontation and become more receptive to its delivery.

Guidelines For Effective Confrontation

1. Confrontation is defined as giving someone realistic feedback about their behavior as you see it–it is a process by which you attempt to "hold up a mirror" to let a person know how he/she appears to others–it is not an attempt at "character assassination."
2. Confrontation is most useful when spoken with empathy, concern, and caring in a respectful tone of voice.

3. Confrontation is descriptive of what you have observed, giving examples of the behavior in question; it excludes guesses, explanations, interpretations, advice, and criticisms about the person's behavior.
4. Confrontation includes a statement of your concern about the person's dangerous, self-defeating behavior and, if possible, an example of similar self-defeating behavior from your own experience. (p. 514)

If these guidelines are followed, they can help the group leader avoid some of the difficulties that can be experienced with overly hostile group members who hold the mistaken idea that humiliation and aggression are acceptable ways to force resistant members to face reality. Washton, writing about the possible abuses of excessive confrontation, cautions the group leader to monitor its application in group:

> Group members typically have less tolerance for negative attitudes and "b.s." than do group leaders, especially when these attitudes are reminiscent of their own. Likely targets for attack are members who relapse repeatedly, who remain defiant, superficial, or insincere, and who minimize their problems and fail to affiliate genuinely with other members of the group.
>
> Sometimes group leaders feel ambivalent about stopping attacks on group members who have thorny problems that have been overlooked and are long overdue for being addressed. The group leader must never allow unpopular, frustrating, resistant, or severely troubled group members to be scapegoated and bludgeoned by their peers, even when the content of what is being said is entirely accurate. Harsh excessive confrontation must not be used as a means to push selected members out of the group and to discourage them from coming back. (1992, p. 514)

If confrontations are done properly, they will bring new understanding to the patient's awareness. However, if they are punitive or attacking, they will only raise defenses and increase resistance. In some cases, as with the passive compliant patient, there is some benefit to this tactic because it makes overt what would otherwise be kept covert by the patient, making it clear that what is hidden is an essential ingredient and component of effective confrontation. Consequently, group leaders are more effective when they limit their confrontations to observable events that will be obvious to the patient once they are pointed out. If group leaders do not keep their facts straight or misjudge the accuracy of their observations, their confrontations will lose their potency and impact. Confrontations are much more powerful as factual statements and should never be confused with a hypothesis about a patient's motives or behavior.

For instance, a confrontation by a group leader who tells an alcoholic, "I think you are an alcoholic because you drink too much" is offering a subjective opinion that at best suggests a plausible hypothesis about a person's behavior. It is a relative statement open to debate since what may be heavy drinking for one person may be moderate consumption for another. Such a statement is not based on observable facts and is likely to cause the confronted individual to counter with his or her own subjective opinion. However, group leaders can make a much more credible confrontation if they focus their observations on demonstrable facts. For instance, the group leader in this same instance could have said,

> It might be helpful for you to carefully and realistically assess the consequences of your drinking. Your wife is divorcing you because she finds you intolerable when you drink. You have two DUI arrests that have cost you a tremendous amount of money because of lawyers' fees and raised insurance premiums. Your boss is threatening to fire you because your work efficiency and attendance have been severely compromised by your weekend binges. This is certainly not normal drinking. Such a pattern of difficulties does suggest that you may be an alcoholic, or if you are uncomfortable with that word, someone who has a severe problem with his drinking.

The difference between the two confrontations is obvious. The first can be interpreted as subjectively biased and opinionated. The second deals with observable and undeniable facts. Even though the second statement is highly confrontational, it does not transmit an attitude of anger or disrespect. Confrontations should never come at the expense of a patient's integrity or respect. If done properly, they will not injure the person although the confrontation may trigger a painful awareness. Group leaders who "blast away" at patients "for their own good" need to carefully explore alternatives to such a stance. In most instances, they will discover that there are more effective ways to convey the same information without taking anything away from the impact of the message. An example will help clarify this point.

> John, a thirty-one-year-old, poly-drug abuser, had entered treatment because of mounting difficulties and concerns related to his escalating drug and alcohol use. His second wife had just filed for divorce and he was beginning to experience severe physical complications (i.e., memory loss, shakes, D.T.s and convulsions) relating

to his drug and alcohol use. Two weeks into a therapy group that met daily, he began to become more and more verbal after sitting quietly and passively while his thinking cleared and physical condition stabilized. As he gained strength and sobriety, his typical defensive maneuvers returned. He began to dominate the group meetings with his excessive rambling about extraneous events and circumstances in his life. The group leader carefully determined that this issue needed to be dealt with and corrected because, not only was it damaging to the group, it was a defensive maneuver that alienated others from John and was a significant complaint of his wife. Left to his own resources, John might have taken months to come to this awareness. At the start of the next session, John started into an elaborate explanation of his sister, describing her as a "big bullshitter," and appeared on the way to repeat his performances in the last two meetings. In the middle of his explanation, the group leader interrupted John briefly to say, "John, excuse me a second, but before you go on any further, I would like to ask you a question." John promptly stopped, his curiosity raised by the group leader's inquisitiveness. At this point the group leader gently confronted John with, "I ask this question in all respect John, and hope not to offend you, but does bullshitting run in the family?" John stopped and thought for a second, laughed out loud, and with a smile triggered by the awareness of his behavior said, "Yeah, now that you mention it, I guess that it does." The rest of the group laughed along with John and began to share that they, too, had noticed his tendency to ramble on in a nonproductive manner, but they had not wanted to say anything because he had been so quiet for the two previous weeks, and they feared that if they said anything, it might lead him to retreat once again into his shell. Further exchanges among other group members led to the awareness of the manner in which he and others often used words to cover over their real feelings. A productive exploration of fears and defenses by the group members accrued during the remainder of the session as a consequence of this confrontation.

In this example, the group leader could have easily confronted John earlier or more directly. A statement such as, "That's bullshit," would have certainly been more provocative and to the point. However, such a statement would have likely offended John, angered him, and led to his retreat from the group. It would have also set a tone for the group that might have had far-reaching, dire consequences concerning openness, trust, and safety. Also, as this example clearly demonstrates, confrontations need not be made punitively or in anger. A judiciously applied intervention mixed with a touch of humor and irony can be as, if not more, productive as one presented in an overly firm, provocative, or dogmatic manner.

The targeted intent of a confrontation needs to be cautiously assessed before it is delivered in a group composed of alcoholics and addicts. Since alcoholics or addicts usually utilize their defenses as a means of protecting themselves against painful affective states related to deep feelings of shame, low self-esteem, and overly intro-punitive self-loathing and hate, confronting these defenses prematurely or inappropriately can be counter-productive to their recovery. Group leaders will avoid the dangers associated with a "shotgun type, hit-everything-that-moves" approach if they limit their confrontations to the alcoholic's drinking or drinking-related behavior during the early or beginning stages of that individual's treatment. Group leaders will keep their feet on more solid theoretical ground if they follow the axiom of treating newly recovering or actively using addicts' and alcoholics' defenses differently from non-addicted individuals. While it is necessary to vigorously confront drug and alcohol use and all defensive operations related to their use, it will prove more beneficial not to confront other defenses while demonstrating empathic understanding and supportive soothing of feelings separate from patients' drinking or drug-using behavior. Many obvious inconsistencies and rigid defenses in newly recovering or actively using alcoholics and addicts may have to be tolerated by the group leader until these individuals are ready to look at these issues more realistically and honestly. This requires that group leaders temper many of their confrontations until they feel more confident that the addicts or alcoholics are able to tolerate the confrontation without relapsing and retreating into further alcohol or drug use.

Group leaders must maintain a delicate balance between confrontation and support when working with this population. Too much support for some individuals will only reinforce continued alcohol and drug use. Premature and inappropriate confrontation, on the other hand, may trigger a relapse or increased defiant resistance for other patients. Unfortunately, inappropriate and poorly timed confrontations do not always come from the group leader. Therefore, it is important that the group leader be adept at handling and managing confrontations between group members. Sometimes an accurate and empathic confrontation from someone else in the group can have a much more dramatic effect on the patient. However, a confrontation from another group member usually has a greater chance of being destructive because it is frequently triggered by anger at the individual. If the group leader can respond quickly when such a confrontation occurs, he or she can guide the interaction so it is not completely devoid of caring and support. An example will help illustrate this point.

> Fred, an immature and arrogantly defiant nineteen-year-old veteran had been required by the U.S. Army to enter an inpatient drug rehabilitation program in the VA hospital. A few months earlier, he had been given an early discharge on honorable conditions because of repeated disciplinary problems related to his drug use. In the three weeks he had been on the hospital unit, he had remained consistently oppositional, defiant, and angry. During the tenth meeting of a daily inpatient group, the group leader noticed Dave, another group member, shaking his head and glaring as Fred continued one of his frequent harangues about the innate badness and unfairness of the staff, the doctors, and the entire U.S. Army. At the end of Fred's daily tirade, the group leader quietly asked Dave, who was a rather large, burly, well-respected but feared, thirty-eight-year-old Vietnam veteran, what he was feeling as Fred talked. Dave, never one to mince words, replied, "Man, I see a bunch of self-pitying bullshit!" Since Dave, an IV heroin addict, was widely respected and feared by all of the other veterans on the unit, Fred was somewhat taken aback by his comment. Rather than leave the confrontation set at this point, the group leader asked Dave whom Fred reminded him of. Although initially startled by the question, Dave quickly responded, "You sound like me nineteen years ago and, man, if you do not change your attitude, you're going to end up like me–a junkie–or dead, or in jail." As the group leader explored Dave's exchange with Fred, it became more apparent that there was a great deal of concern underneath Dave's angry confrontation. Although it was somewhat uncharacteristic for Dave, he proceeded to demonstrate a soft, caring side of himself to Fred and the group. This softened the initial harshness of his confrontation and made it much more palatable to Fred. Such a confrontation would have lost much of its effectiveness if it had come from the group leader or if the confrontation had just been left with Dave's opening statement. Explorations of the reasons behind the confrontation led Fred to an awareness of himself that he had not previously possessed.

Confrontations conducted in this manner can be effective. But the group leader must remember that a confrontation is not an end in itself. It should be applied strategically, and when used in conjunction with other clinical skills and knowledge, it can enhance working with the alcoholic's and addict's denial and resistance to treatment. Confrontation need not always be direct or lacking in warmth and caring. Paradoxical interventions which take advantage of metaphors, humor, irony, and the use of counterforce, allow the group leader to assume a warm, empathic stance while placing the responsibility for change squarely on the shoulders of the alcoholic and addict–where it belongs–thus lessening the group leader's frustration and making treatment more effective. Sobriety and abstinence are impossible unless the alcoholic and addict are prepared to assume responsibility for that change. Confrontations only work if they are motivational and facilitative in nature. The group leader cannot and should not force or attempt to force the alcoholic or addict to change. In such a power struggle, no one wins. The addict or alcoholic has another excuse to continue his or her use of chemicals, and the group leader only becomes increasingly discouraged and frustrated.

The discussion of confrontation in this chapter has hopefully made clear criticisms and misunderstanding about the nature and appropriate use of confrontation in group psychotherapy. Confrontations, like good interpretations and clarifications, are attempts to make patients aware of behavior of which they had not previously been aware. As they develop more of an accurate and realistic understanding of themselves, the defenses they use and the reasons for these defenses can be examined. When working with alcoholics or addicts, the shift from an accurate awareness of their drinking and drug use to an understanding of their defenses and the reasons underlying the use of these defenses may take months, and in many cases, even years. With many alcoholics and addicts, the unconscious motives for their behavior should not be explored until they have enough sobriety and emotional stability in their life to handle this awareness. This is the most significant and important difference that must be learned by the group leader who is working with addicted patients.

The shift from confrontations, which are limited to behavior, attitudes, and actions that have a direct influence and connection with maintaining sobriety, to a more explorative examination of the unconscious motives behind all defensive operations, is a strategic decision that must be carefully assessed for each individual patient. Some will be ready for such a shift in treatment rather quickly; others will require much more time. Once the group leader feels that the recovering addict or alcoholic is capable of managing a more explorative form of psychotherapy, the leader can then transfer the addict or alcoholic to a more advanced group or shift the focus of the group.

The principle of making the unconscious conscious was originally conceived by Freud. "Where id was, there shall ego be" (Freud, 1936, p. 80) clearly summarizes Freud's position regarding psychotherapy. The psychotherapist or group leader is to bring to the patient's awareness (ego) what was previously unconscious (id). Yet, in no way did Freud intend the making of the unconscious conscious as the ultimate aim of psychotherapy. In other words, confrontation should never be done for confrontation's sake. Once more, in Freud's words, the intention of psychoanalysis is "to strengthen the ego, to make it more independent of the super-ego, to widen its field of perception and enlarge its organization, so that it can appropriate fresh portions of the id" (1936, p. 80). In many ways, Freud is suggesting that helping patients become aware of their unconscious is dependent on the strengthening of their capacity (ego-strength) to tolerate this awareness.

This is an accurate description of the strategic position that a group leader must take in working with an alcoholic or addict in group. It must also be kept in mind that increased awareness of unconscious motives should not be expected in itself to result in behavior change. The explicit purpose of confrontation, and eventually interpretation, is to bring thoughts and feelings of which individuals are not aware, and over which they have no control, into their awareness, where they can examine them, consider their relationship to other thoughts and feelings, and exert some conscious control over the extent to which they influence their behavior. To accomplish this task, group leaders must learn how to shift their tactics in group from a position of confrontation to interpretation and support.

Another ingredient absolutely vital to group leaders who want to help alcoholics and addicts work on a more accurate awareness of their unconscious motives is a healthy, informed, unambiguous, and relaxed attitude toward alcohol, drinking, drunkenness, alcoholism, and drugs. The group leaders who work most effectively with alcoholics and addicts are those who have the capacity to share deeply with others and who can relate to them with hope. Certain people seem to have a natural ability to feel deeply with those who hurt emotionally and physically. This capacity for empathy may be cultivated through self-awareness, but it cannot be learned as a technique or a skill.

Still, there are good, sound, basic communication skills that group leaders must be familiar with before they can hope to communicate realistically with the chemically dependent patient. First, certain assumptions must be made before any attempt is made to explain the individual's psychological state at the time of an emotional crisis and physical illness. Emotional disturbances and bodily disorders are often spoken of in terms of cause and effect. This erroneously presumes that humans are composed of two fundamentally different substances, mind and body, and that the two in some way reciprocally affect one another. It is the fashion in current thought to sidestep this vexing problem of the dualism of the mind and matter. The assumption psychoanalysis makes is that the basic unit that reacts to stimuli is neither the mind nor the body, but the organism. Neither takes precedence over the other. An emotionally distressing event may precipitate a physical disorder and a physiological disturbance will result in an emotional reaction.

The nature of the communication with the alcoholic and addict must take into consideration the nature of their addiction and should incorporate fundamental principles of interviewing techniques. The group leader should pay attention to the affect and style of what the patient says, rather than just the content. Knowing how to listen is an art. R.D. Laing (1972) suggests using the concept of paralinguistics when consulting with a patient. Pay attention not only to what is said, but to the way it is said, what is left out, bodily mannerisms, facial expressions, and the like. Communication with patients, whether they are addicted or not, should involve more than just language. The alcoholic or addict in a highly aroused emotional state may become quite receptive to the group leader's hidden agenda. If patients believe that the outcome of their rehabilitation is of concern to the group leader more as a reflection of his or her ability as a group leader, rather than as a real, genuine concern for the patient, treatment and recovery may be impaired.

Psychoanalysis operates on two basic principles, repression and suppression. Indirect methods of interviewing reveal not only an individual's significant fantasies, but also his or her train of thought. It therefore allows a patient to free associate, that is, to observe and to communicate, all the ideas that flow through his or her consciousness. If the group leader interrupts too frequently, or interjects too many of his or her own ideas into the flow of associations, that flow may be contaminated and distorted and may not reveal the underlying motivating factor. In fact, owing to the normal reluctance of all of us to freely disclose all of our thoughts and fantasies, true free association is an ideal rarely achieved. Moreover, the observation of where a patient seems to be holding back ideas and resisting the unfettered flow of thoughts, provides important information about his or her whole personality structure.

Group leaders must restrain themselves from impatient interrupting, premature interpretations, or personal reminiscence. They must know when to keep quiet even when patients are silent–to allow the patients to say what they have to say in their own way, at their own pace. At the same time leaders must observe the patients' behavior–their movements, their gestures, their tone of voice, the bodily show of their affects–for clues to the regions of emotional conflicts. Group leaders must know what to say and when. The content of questions depends on knowing what topics the patients are ready to discuss, and the timing depends on knowing when the moment is appropriate for discussing them.

Group leaders must also know what not to say. They must know when to give advice and when silence is wisdom. They must sense when patients are ready for communications. They must also know when to reassure and support patients to diminish intolerable anxiety and when to provoke it in order to keep the communication process moving. Too often, it seems that group leaders are too concerned with the rationale of the messages they send patients and they often miss underlying clues that indicate the possible reactions and fears of the individuals.

Reports and research findings indicate that treatment programs which stress insight therapy with the alcoholic or addict are not as successful or effective as AA-based therapy. Regardless of the treatment modality chosen, communication and psychotherapy should still remain an intricate part of an alcoholic's and addict's rehabilitation process. Successful treatment of addiction requires cooperation of persons from many disciplines. Although a cure is never possible, addiction can be arrested, and group therapy remains one of the proven approaches to its treatment. Under the proper management, group therapy can enhance the alcoholic's and addict's recovery process.

INTERVENTION

Conducting group with alcoholics or addicts who remain ambivalent about their abstinence and are reluctant to admit their illness is a problem somewhat unique to alcohol and drug treatment. The recognition that alcoholics or addicts must hit bottom, that they must face that existential crisis in their life before rehabilitation can actually begin is a popular maxim in alcohol and drug treatment. The problem of crisis, its recognition, its ramifications, and the methods of intervention that must be employed in the treatment approach are all important factors group leaders must take into consideration. But before group leaders charge into the treatment process, they should be aware of the games and tactics often involved in that treatment process. Steiner acknowledges that the games of alcoholics are an intricate part of their illness. Steiner postulates that people choose roles for themselves at an early age and those roles may turn them into alcoholics. He also warns that some forms of treatment may do more harm than good. He writes:

> The therapist's job is, first and foremost, not to play the "alcoholic game." That is to say, he should not play any of its roles–Persecutor,

> Rescuer, Patsy, Connection–in order to avoid providing the patient with a payoff from the therapist himself. This is the bare-bones necessity of alcoholism therapy . . . as soon as the therapist can see that self-destructive drinking is not the result of a defective ego but a deliberate strategic maneuver to accomplish certain ends, he will be much better able to treat alcoholics. (Steiner, 1971; p. 38)

Although Steiner himself does not recognize the disease model of alcoholism, he nevertheless has good therapeutic advice for group leaders. Foremost among his recommendations is that group leaders take precautions that will prevent them from being conned by alcoholics or addicts. While alcoholics or addicts may indeed be physiologically addicted to their drug or ethanol, social learning forces do come into play and life scripts do indeed play an intricate part in the illness itself. If, as Steiner says, alcoholics or addicts are playing out a life script, getting them to identify their problem and admit that their script is destructive and inappropriate is still a key ingredient to successful treatment. Once addicts and alcoholics have faced the conclusion that they are unable to control their drug use and drinking and that it is the cause of their problems, they can choose a new life script.

Choosing remains the crucial point. Alcoholics or addicts must take responsibility for their actions and at a gut level choose to change their lives. "Every time you try to rescue an alcoholic," Johnson warns, "you are delaying useful treatment" (1973, p. 59). The alcoholics' and addicts' decision to choose is usually made as a result of a crisis in their life. Johnson goes on to say, "When you examine the lives of those who claim to have had it, you discover that a buildup of crisis has forced them to look at the reality of their condition. The only way back to reality is through crisis" (p. 59). But Johnson warns that it is pointless and dangerous to wait until alcoholics or addicts hit bottom. The crisis everybody was trying to help the alcoholics or addicts avoid could actually be employed to break through their defenses. Frequently, it requires an act of intervention in order to stop the downward spiral toward death. Vernon Johnson has experimented with alternative useful methods of employing crisis at earlier stages of the disease. The group leader, Johnson says, must be tuned in and aware of the cry for help. "Crises do not have to be invented or created. . . . the problem is to get counselors knowledgeable enough to use them creatively" (p. 59).

Recent evidence generally supports the use of interventions that emphasize the importance of the job and court instead of the family. Vernon Johnson agrees: "Under the first principle of intervention, we said that an executive of the next rank up, or the boss, is likely to be the most fundamental person. So the boss instead of a member of the immediate family may set up the confrontation" (1973, p. 98).

The importance of intervening with alcoholics or addicts in treatment has been a long-recognized requirement for those who are familiar with the early history of Alcoholics Anonymous. Henry Tiebout (1961), a Life Fellow of the American Psychiatric Association and former president of the American Council on Alcoholism, has written extensively about the importance of intervention in an alcoholic's life. Because addiction tends to both isolate individuals and lead them to fall back on rigid, grandiose, narcissistic defenses, an intervention carries with it an important message from the real world. Tiebout says it informs individuals that their actions and behavior have consequences. The alcoholics' behavior is placed in its proper perspective, and the message is firmly delivered that they can no longer exist in blissful egocentricity. An intervention, if properly done, forces objectivity upon their denial. The therapist who is willing to intervene conveys an important message. The therapist is someone who not only cares enough to confront a painful truth and is forceful enough to intervene, the therapist is also delivering the message that he or she is a force, an objective representation of reality that must be reckoned with.

Interventions are a way of getting alcoholics and addicts to seek treatment before their alcohol and drug use has had irreversible psychological, physiological, and social ramifications as well as overwhelming marital, employment, and legal consequences. While evidence has been presented concerning the effectiveness of employee assistance programs, the criminal justice system is another source of early identification and intervention. This is particularly true for those individuals who are introduced to the court system as a result of DUI (Driving Under the Influence) or DWI (Driving While Intoxicated) convictions. The use of intervention with this population requires special considerations of the dynamics involved in this approach. Since there are general principles of intervention governing its application, a model for its use with DWI offenders will be presented and carefully outlined. First the reasons for this approach with DUI offenders will be presented since it will help explain the theoretical foundation upon which all models of effective intervention stand.

DWI and Intervention

Over the years of working with alcoholics and addicts, experienced professionals began to realize there were many factors that combined to contribute to the negative expectancies and poor attitudes concerning rehabilitation of alcoholics or addicts when these individuals were left to their own resources in deciding whether to seek treatment for their chemical use.

Building on evidence gathered from job- and family-based intervention programs, there were indications that DWI programs could provide an ideal opportunity by which effective treatment and early identification could be initiated. Perhaps most significantly, it was discovered that the great majority of drinking drivers arrested had not been treated previously for an alcohol problem (Scott, 1970). Highway safety programs were seen as another highly effective method of identifying individuals with alcohol and drug problems earlier in the course of their problem drinking and drug use when there is greater opportunity for effective treatment and intervention. The proceedings of the National DWI Conference (1976) concluded with the following recommendations to Congress.

1. Treatment is a supplement to an alcoholic's legal responsibility.
2. Evidence indicates that pressures are needed to keep alcoholics actively involved in their recovery process.
3. Three segments are required for effective treatment: early detection, creation of a crisis, and continual long-term counseling or care.

It has been recognized that the early identification of addiction plays an important part in the chances of successfully treating an identified patient. Due to the nature of the sample of the population that characteristically makes up each DWI class, these classes provide an optimal opportunity for both early identification and intervention in the addiction process. Therefore, it is important to make sure that this identification process is being carried out with optimum effectiveness.

The process of early intervention and treatment is only partially completed once an addict or an alcoholic is identified. Getting identified patients into treatment, when those individuals feel they have no problem, remains an area of controversy. The ethical consequences of intervention, when it is documented and obvious that individuals' excessive drinking or drug use will cause further harm both to them and to society, must be weighed cautiously by both the agency doing the evaluation and the criminal justice system doing the sentencing.

If the use of intervention is to be effective in getting identified alcoholics and addicts into treatment, it must be judiciously applied and followed up by a responsible representative from the court. Allowing this responsibility to fall entirely on the shoulders of the group leader or the agency providing the services only complicates and confuses the issue in a labyrinth of bureaucratic red tape and buck-passing. The authority to enforce recommendations lies within the realm of the criminal justice system, and it is within this system that the pressure should be applied.

The DWI intervention program should be adapted to take advantage of these circumstances. It is obvious that the DWI program provides an ideal opportunity for early identification and intervention in the alcoholism process. However, a program patterned after the solid principles of intervention and group psychotherapy would allow more individual time with each DWI offender. This would provide the group leader with a better opportunity to deal with the alcoholic's and addict's denial system and would also encourage more personal confrontation with group interaction if the group were conducted in a weekend marathon setting.

Principles of Intervention

Early intervention in the treatment of addiction, through the use of confrontational techniques, is designed to help the individual recognize the need for treatment. Intervention is most effective when it consists of a collective, guided effort by the significant others (i.e., spouse, employer, friends, children) in the person's environment so that a crisis is induced through confrontation that will remove or reduce the individual's defensive obstructions to recovery. Twerski (1983) sums up the principles of intervention when he writes:

> To be effective in the intervention, the participants must understand the disease of alcoholism and know its generally inexorable course if untreated. They must also act out of sincere concern for the welfare of the patient; be aware of the risks in confrontation; be adequately prepared to participate in the intervention as a well-orchestrated team if required; and be ready to endure the discomfort of confrontation and of describing sordid behavior to a patient or loved one, and to implement significant changes in their own lives if the subject rejects treatment. (p. 1030)

Twerski draws a distinction between two types of intervention. The first is conducted through conventional medical or psychiatric settings and involves the professional confronting the patient with the gravity of the alcohol or drug problem. The second consists of a collective, guided effort that is a more intense mode of intervention that requires the participation of as many people as possible who are significantly involved with the patient. Twerski (1983) meticulously outlines the strategy for both of these approaches and the interested reader should consult this cited article for more information on this procedure. At this point, a description of a third approach that combines elements of the two different processes as outlined by Twerski will be presented. This third approach emphasizes the use of a conventional psychotherapy group format and allows group leaders to adapt to a situation requiring that they deal with a number of reluctant patients who are coerced into treatment by the criminal justice system.

There are six principles of intervention that group leaders must be familiar with if they are to conduct a psychotherapy group with reluctant patients who are coerced into treatment for their alcohol or drug abuse.

1. Do not do interventions alone. They must be done in a small group with a supportive co-therapist and treatment team. If the group is conducted under the principles to be described, the group leader will be able to use the force of group peer pressure as a powerful mode of intervention. Since an actively using alcoholic or addict has little investment in the group leader, the professional has little if any credibility in the intervention process. The group leader's effectiveness is determined by his or her ability to mobilize the other group members as a source of support in the intervention process.
2. Establish and maintain specific goals for each group session. If the group leader does not structure the group so that each session is gradually more confrontive and addresses a deeper level of the individual's denial, the group process will deteriorate into an aimless exchange limited to war stories, acting out, and argumentative complaining. The group leader must remember that group intervention is not therapy. The goals of these sessions are training, identification, and intervention. Conventional approaches to conducting the group must be discarded or used more sparingly.
3. Focus on specific data that is obvious, concrete, and nondebatable. This is the most important component of the intervention process. The group leader must use the beginning group sessions to gather concrete information about alcoholics' and addicts' chemical use and determine how their use of drugs and alcohol has adversely affected their lives. This data must be gathered in a non-obtrusive manner and delivered back to the individuals in a way that will be palatable, undeniable, and non-debatable.
4. Create an atmosphere of care and concern. This must be the first task of the group leader. Confrontations must be used very sparingly until therapeutic atmosphere is created. If this atmosphere is not established, the group will remain argumentative, resistant, and defensive. Often, the only thing that will catch an alcoholic or addict off guard is the feeling that the group leader, the treatment team, and the group members care. Most alcoholics and addicts are afraid of highly confrontative behavior. They have their defenses up and ready. They

have usually been in control of similar situations for a long time and know that they can handle one group leader or counselor.

5. Operate from a well-established treatment structure. Allow no loopholes. Determine the agreed-upon treatment modality (i.e., inpatient, outpatient, AA, etc.) they and the other group members will accept if it is established that they are addicted. Once this is agreed upon, minimize the time between the intervention and their entering the chosen treatment program.
6. Consequences must be established if they refuse to go. In the situations where the intervention is conducted by the employer, it may be a loss of a job. If the intervention is done with the family, it may be a divorce. Interventions conducted with court-referred patients usually must rely on the support of the court system to enforce such consequences. In some cases, it may be probation, jail sentences, or fines.

A Group Intervention Format for Court-Referred Offenders

Many group leaders find themselves struggling with the difficult task of trying to conduct psychotherapy groups with reluctant patients who do not want to be in a group, but who are forced to attend because of an alcohol- or drug-related arrest. A format for dealing with DWI offenders who are coerced into group therapy and treatment by the court system will be described. While the specifics of this format will be somewhat limited to DWI offenders, there will be enough generalizability in this format to allow creative group leaders to adapt its principles to fit their particular situation. For instance, in many cases, the court will refer for treatment an individual who is suspected of having an alcohol or drug problem. Often, these individuals only commit crimes while intoxicated or to pay for their drugs. Treatment is often an alternative to a jail sentence since it is reasoned that their crime will stop if their alcohol and drug use stops. Conventional therapy, especially supportive individual therapy, is doomed to fail with these individuals. A psychotherapy group conducted in the prescribed manner should be the treatment of choice.

After an individual has been arrested and convicted for a crime (in this case, a DWI), the offender should be offered the option of jail or treatment. Most will choose treatment. This is important because this element of choice, albeit a somewhat compromised one, enhances their receptability to treatment. It is also important that this choice be given after the offender has been convicted because this allows the court leverage for ensuring compliance through its use of the probation sentence or plea bargain. If convicted offenders do not follow through with their agreed-upon commitment, they must be aware and assured that the court will enforce the alternative consequences to this choice. Such a contract should be clearly stated and defined by the court. Offenders must also be made aware of the limitations this contract imposes on the typical restrictions of therapeutic confidentiality. A signed consent should be obtained and the offenders told in no uncertain terms that the treatment staff is bound by this contract to let the court or the probation officer know if this contract is violated. Since such a stance will undoubtedly compromise the therapist-patient alliance, the treatment staff can salvage this alliance by assuring the offenders that personal information will not be shared with the court. In fact, it is often helpful to agree to show the offenders a copy of the correspondence that will be sent to the court and obtain their signature on the letter. This assures the offenders that they will be well informed about the information given to the court and re-establishes much of the compromised trust and safety that was lost in the original treatment contract.

The DWI offender is given the option of spending a weekend in jail or a weekend at a DWI school. Most offenders choose the school and arrive at the program on a Friday evening. Most do not know they are about to enter an intensive weekend marathon experience with time being split between large group lectures and small psychotherapy groups. The small groups are limited to ten members and the marathon setting ensures complete abstinence from drugs and separation from typical outside support systems.

The DWI program should not be geared toward treatment, and the group leaders should not intend to do psychotherapy during the weekend. Rather, the focus of the program and therapy groups should be on intervention, and emphasis should be placed on pre-treatment, identification, assessment, and diagnosis. The three-day marathon setting can be a very powerful, one-time situational experience in the individual's life if it is properly directed. Because of its structure, it will allow group leaders the time and intensity necessary to determine the extent of each offender's involvement with alcohol or drugs. Since it is often impossible for many group leaders to have such an intense treatment program or the support of an entire treatment team behind them, goals, objectives, and even the expectations of such an approach will have to be modified to fit their particular situation.

To reach the objectives of identification, group intervention, and treatment recommendation (if any), three goals must be established:

1. Assessment and data collection. One-third to one-half of DWI offenders typically have no significant alcohol or drug problems. Those who do need to be assessed, and this assessment must be supported by specific, concrete data gathered during the group sessions.

2. Utilize the group dynamics to break through the denial so that individuals can make a connection between their chemical use and the difficulties they experience.
3. Motivate the identified patients to seek treatment.

Group Intervention Format

Group conducted in this prescribed manner should not be confused with group psychotherapy as it is practiced with individuals who seek group therapy of their own volition. While many general principles of group process and group dynamics are utilized during the group intervention, the aim of each group session is distinctly different from most other conventional types of psychotherapy, both individual and group. The limitation of time, the dynamics involved in the addiction process, and the general resistance of the group members require the group leader to take a very active position in directing the focus of the intervention process. Each group member must be given information about the disease concept and this should be done in a lecture format in a large group setting separate from the small group meetings. The aim of the small group process is to incorporate the presented educational material so that it is relevant to each group member's life. Within this context, the group leader should direct his or her energies toward getting the group members to interact with each other. It is through the interaction of the group members that the group leader will gain the data necessary to confirm each member's possible addiction to alcohol and drugs.

Since most group members do not know what to expect at the start of the first group session, their anxiety and defenses are extremely high. The first session, or in some cases the first few sessions, should be directed toward alleviating this anxiety and reducing each member's defensive posture. This is accomplished best by asking group members to introduce themselves, explain the circumstances behind their arrest, and give their reasons for attending the weekend group meeting. The least guarded members should be encouraged to speak first and the group leader should respond supportively to any display of anger or agitation in the group. Anger must be diffused before the group can move to a freely engaging group interaction. Many members will be outraged (some justly, most unjustly) at either the court, their attorney, the judge, or the police who arrested them. If their anger is supported in a constructive and caring fashion during the first session or sessions, their hostility will begin to give way to reason and occasional displays of humor. Exploring these exchanges with good-natured laughter, which is not laced with hostility, can do a great deal to relieve the tension during the initial stages of a beginning group. When the group has begun to feel more comfortable, the group leader should give the group something to work with by taking away what they think will be the focus on the session. Most alcoholics and addicts will come ready to defend their drinking or drug use. State clearly that you, as the group leader, are not concerned with: (a) how they drink or use drugs; (b) what they drink or what drugs they use; (c) when they drink or use drugs; (d) with whom they drink or use drugs; or (e) where they drink or do drugs. Such a stance will diffuse their defensiveness and engage them in the evaluation process. Once they have discharged their anger and anxiety, many, if not all, group members can be persuaded to "make the most out of the situation now that you are here. You can either remain angry and make this a horrible weekend or you can use it to learn about yourself." At this time, if the intervention is conducted convincingly, the group leader will be surprised at the number of people, addicted as well as non-addicted, who want to understand how alcohol and drugs play a part in their lives. The appeal is most effective when presented in the following manner:

> People who drink and do drugs fit into two general categories. There are those who can do so without any problems and there are those who have a physiological or genetic propensity to become addicted or dependent. A hundred million people in this country drink. Ninety million of them are social drinkers. A small percentage, ten percent or ten million, cannot drink socially. If you are part of that minority, we want you to get involved in the group this weekend so you'll have a chance to understand your degree of involvement and how it is affecting your life. We want to encourage you to look at the consequences of your drinking and drug use. We would also like you to look at your life history and your involvement with chemicals and decide whether it is in your best interest to continue to drink or do drugs. There are eight critical major life areas we would like you to examine:
>
> 1. Self-Esteem (Self-Image)
> 2. Family relationships
> 3. Peer relationships
> 4. Job performance
> 5. Finances
> 6. Legal situation
> 7. Sexual activities
> 8. Health

> Explore each of these areas in relation to your drug or alcohol use. Have any of these areas been adversely affected by your drinking and drug use? If any of these areas have been affected, are you willing to continue to jeopardize them in order to continue to drink or use drugs? It is your decision. Until you decide, however, we would like to encourage you to explore these questions with other members in the group. We are not here to argue with you or try to convince you otherwise. It is your choice. But you have a unique opportunity here in group to get feedback from other group members who may be struggling with the same decisions or issues. We just want to hold up a mirror for you. Prove to us and yourself which category of people you fit in with–those who can or those who can't drink or use drugs socially.

If group leaders take this stance and avoid using the labels of alcoholic or addict, they can often engage and challenge most reluctant group members. Since most alcoholics and addicts suffer from various degrees of grandiosity or narcissism, and feel that they can convince anyone that they do not have an alcohol or drug problem, they will often readily take on such a challenge. They are usually unable to resist the opportunity to point out the ways alcohol or drugs are affecting others. Because of their own identification with other alcoholics and addicts, this is a skill at which they are acutely adept. With these two principles operating, group leaders will find that in a very short time they have an actively engaged group on their hands.

Usually at the beginning of the group, group leaders, and their co-therapists can expect to be questioned about their drug use. Such questions are inevitable and self-disclosure is essential. If group leaders do not volunteer this information, they can expect to be openly questioned about their own use of alcohol and drugs. Guardedness about this subject or an attempt to retreat into the safety of therapeutic neutrality will not work. Because of the short time duration of the group, its involuntary nature, and the fact that group leaders are asking everyone else to self-disclose about a specific topic, guardedness or evasiveness on their part will only increase the defensiveness of the other group members. On this subject, group leaders must model what they ask others to do. Freely volunteering personal information about drugs and alcohol early in group will enhance the group process. However, group leaders must be totally honest. If they happen to be recovering alcoholics or addicts, this should indeed be shared with the group. If group leaders have in the past abused drugs and do not use drugs now, this information, framed in the proper perspective, can lead members to increase their own self- disclosure about their own drug and alcohol use. If group leaders drink alcohol and do it in a non-alcoholic fashion, this should not be hidden from the group. Presented in the proper context, it will often enhance self-disclosure. However, if group leaders or their co-therapists use any drugs, even so-called recreational use of marijuana, this must not be shared. In fact, if therapists are using drugs of any kind, their effectiveness in working with this population is going to be severely compromised. One must not forget that drug use is illegal. Admitting one's own recreational use of drugs to the group conveys a subtle message that laws are for you and not for me. Not only is this position hypocritical, it is dishonest. It would be better for all concerned if a therapist who uses drugs refrains from working with all addicted patients. Addicted patients should be referred to another therapist, and the therapist should avoid work of any type that is associated with the addiction treatment field.

As the group members become more engaged with each other, cohesiveness will begin to develop. Confrontation up to this point should have been kept to a minimum. Self-disclosures, especially as the different group members begin to share the way alcohol or drugs have affected their lives, usually lead to a rapid deepening of feelings. As the group members begin to identify with others regarding concerns about alcohol and drug use, they can be easily encouraged to gently confront each other. With the proper timing and encouragement, the group leader can usually have the group very responsive to confrontations. It usually takes only a little encouragement to get some group members responding to others in an honest and open fashion. Openness and honesty can be enhanced by first focusing on the least guarded members. The more anxious and guarded members will have to be brought in more slowly. Caution should be used with those members who are reluctant to be open and honest. Allowing them to go first only establishes a norm of defensiveness in the group. As the group interaction increases, the group leader can use the more open group members to engage the more guarded ones in the group process. A statement such as, "Hey, Joe, do you think that Bill really wants any feedback?" can be a very effective way of engaging even the most reluctant member.

By the end of the third day, group members have usually become intensely honest and open with each other. Before the group ends, ask each member to assess themselves as either being harmfully involved or not harmfully involved with alcohol and drugs. Encourage them to go through the major life areas and determine how the drinking- and drug-using circumstances in their life relate to the information they have gathered this weekend from the personal issues they have heard shared in group, the lectures, and the feedback that they have received from others. Ask them to describe to the group what they feel would be examples of appropriate action for them to take, based on what they heard and discovered about themselves. Then, request that they state why they believe this is true. Upon completing this task, ask that each remaining group member indicate concurrence or disagreement with the stated assessment and plan. Consensus in the group is usually high, and this often leads to compliance. In some cases, individuals who have shared very little during the weekend will announce that the group has confirmed what they had long suspected, but feared examining, namely that they are alcoholic. Treatment recommendations are to be delivered at the end of group and individual sessions scheduled to discuss consequences of failures to follow through with agreed-upon treatment goals.

The main goal of the intervention is to help patients make a choice about their drinking and drug use. They must be able to determine by the end of the weekend the advantages of not drinking and doing drugs compared to the problems in their lives resulting from their drinking and drug use. This choice must be ultimately made by each member of the group. Despite an abundance of evidence to the contrary, some individuals will refuse to see their situation accurately or will fail to take adequate measures to change their self-destructive behavior. Group leaders must be aware that they cannot control the behavior of the chemically dependent person, nor can they dictate what that person must do. They can confront, coerce, intervene, and use all the therapeutic leverage at their disposal, but the choice of action is determined by the subject. Alcoholics or addicts have the choice of keeping or losing their job, going to jail, and preserving or dissolving their family. They also have the option of entering treatment. Hopefully, the techniques described in this chapter will increase the chances of a positive outcome.

Chapter 10

Middle Stage Treatment Issues

Once group leaders have helped to lead, guide, or even push the alcoholics and addicts past their precontemplation, contemplation, and preparation stages of change, the action components of recovery will become the dominant theme in treatment. Now, the group leaders' task will be to keep members actively engaged in the treatment and recovery process. This requires a series of special considerations concerning techniques on the part of the group leaders. Not only must they be keenly sensitive to the stages of an individual's recovery, they must also be acutely aware of the developmental stages of the group because it determines the functions that they will have to emphasize at each particular stage of recovery.

Allen Surkis (1989) has emphasized the distinction that must be made between leadership functions and therapy functions when conducting a group. Surkis maintains that leadership functions should take precedence over therapy functions because the former are necessary prerequisites for the latter. Leadership functions, if properly applied and managed, help dilute the anxiety and tension in the group, allowing the necessary atmosphere to be established so that the therapy functions can dominate the later stage of group. This stage parallels very closely that of Yalom, who recommends that the first of the three basic tasks of the group leader is to ensure the physical survival of group. Like Surkis's position, such a stance requires that the leader put his or her energy toward the establishment of a safe holding environment where time boundaries, therapeutic norms, and structure are clearly defined.

Surkis suggests that the differences between leadership functions and therapy functions be differentiated along a continuum. (See Table 10.1.)

There are other important differentiations that the group leader must be aware of when determining what approach to treatment will best match the addicted individual's particular stage of change. Early, middle, and late stage recovery issues will demand a different emphasis in both goals and activity requirements of the group leader. Table 10.2 outlines some of these differences.

TABLE 10.1

Leadership Functions: Early/Middle Stage	*Therapy Functions: Later Stages*
1. Reduce anxiety and manage tension. 2. Help group get past resistance and build cohesion. 3. Boundary issues are maintained (starting and ending on time, integrating new members, etc.). 4. Modulate the release of emotions and anger.	1. Promote a sense of discover and curiosity. 2. Provide opportunity for corrective emotional experience or relationship. 3. Help members discover or reclaim disowned shameful parts of self.

Minkoff (1995) recommends a four-phase approach to recovery that has some parallels to Prochaska and DiClemente's (1992) five stages of change model. Minkoff suggests:

1. acute stabilization,
2 engagement,
3. prolonged stabilization and
4. recovery with a focus on:
   a. continual stability
   b. continual sobriety.

Once stabilization has been obtained in the early portion of treatment, engagement and prolonged stabilization dominates the middle stage of the recovery process. From a disease concept and abstinence model perspective, this requires using the therapy group as a vehicle that will complement and encourage the addict's or alcoholic's engagement in the twelve-step recovery program and its support groups.

Recent recommendations by a number of authors suggest that an important part of the engagement process is getting the patient "acculturated" to the treatment milieu and the AA "culture of recovery." (Kemker, Kibel, and Mahler, 1993). Not only is this a necessary requirement for the patient, it is also necessary for many professionals unfamiliar with the language, culture, and treatment philosophy of twelve-step groups. Group therapy as an integral part of this acculturation process serves a unique function according to Kemker and associates. Because of its internal structure, the

TABLE 10.2. Goals and Activity Requirements of Group Leader

GOAL	*EARLY/MIDDLE STAGE*	*LATE STAGE*
1. Affect/Emotions	Minimal. Emphasis should be on cognition and containment	Optimal level of anxiety
2. Regression	Decrease	Increase
3. Here and Now	Decrease—More emphasis on there and then drinking behavior	Increase (immediacy principle)
4. Confrontation	Focus on drinking- or drug-related behavior	Less–With more emphasis on intimacy
5. Leader Activity	More active and transparent	Less active and opaque and transparent
6. Individual-Intrapsychic	More	Less
7. Interpersonal	Less	More
8. Group-as-a-Whole	Less	More
9. Support-Gratification	More	Less
10. Content vs. Process	Content	Process

small group experience has the most potential to establish the kinds of emotional bonds necessary during the middle stage or the engagement phase of recovery. Two essential elements of this process are: (1) acceptance of the need for abstinence, and (2) induction into the culture of recovery. Kemker, Kibel, and Mahler (1993) emphasize the unique properties of working with addicts and alcoholics within a structured treatment milieu. They state, "An addiction unit is the product of two very powerful institutions: psychiatry and AA" (p. 300). Successful addiction treatment requires some special adaptation by the therapist and "involves turning to the recovery movement for support and a sense of higher purpose" (p. 300). Therapists must learn that treatment of addicted individuals requires the recognition that they cannot treat these patients alone–"that addiction is too deeply entrenched, the patient too alienated." Unlike traditional forms of psychotherapy Kemker, Kibel, and Mahler point out, addiction treatment requires an "emphasis on groups and the self-help movement" (p. 299).

In a more recent publication, Matano and Yalom (1991) put forth recommendations that are very similar to those of Kemker, Kibel, and Mahler when they suggest that special considerations be given to integrating AA and twelve-step recovery principles into the group therapy format. Matano and Yalom warn that more traditional approaches to addiction treatment are doomed to fail unless the following guidelines are observed:

1. recovery and abstinence must always be accorded priority,
2. the patient needs to accept the identification as either an alcoholic or addict,
3. anxiety in group must be carefully modulated,
4. the proper distinction must be made between what the alcoholic or addict is and is not responsible for, and
5. the group leader must be thoroughly familiar with the language, steps, and traditions of AA and other twelve-step recovery programs.

Matano and Yalom emphasize two important issues in their recommendations that are often overlooked by therapists who are unfamiliar with working with the addicted patient in group. First, they caution that the group leader who is unfamiliar with the language and principles of twelve-step recovery programs is vulnerable to the misuse of AA concepts by group members who will distort them and use them as resistance to therapy. Thorough familiarity with the AA program not only helps integrate these principles into the therapy process, it also helps reduce the resistance that can be manifested through their manipulation by the addicted individual.

Second, Matano and Yalom help clarify an important distinction that must be made about responsibility. As they correctly point out, addicted individuals are not responsible for their disease or their inability to control their chemical use once they take the first drink or swallow that first pill. However, they are responsible for that first drink or the first use of the substances. Alcoholics, for instance, are notorious for avoiding responsibility for the first drink that triggers an alcoholic binge. They will often try to excuse their relapse as a "slip," implying it was something that just happened to them unsuspectingly. Seasoned AA members and addiction specialists are likely to confront such avoidance of responsibility by insisting that alcoholics own their decision to drink for what it truly is: "a premeditated drunk." They will be told, "It didn't happen to you; you did it! More important, if you deny responsibility for it, you won't learn anything from it." Consequently, addicted individuals must accept responsibility for all of their actions and behavior. In the short term, they must accept responsibility for working or not working the steps of the twelve-step program and applying for themselves what has worked for other addicted individuals to ensure their own recovery. In the long term, they must accept responsibility for how they choose to relate to others in the immediacy of the here and now of the group experience. In the later stages of recovery and treatment, responsibility for interpersonal relatedness will become the salient issue in treatment.

Matano and Yalom also address some of the sources of potential conflict between AA and psychotherapy. They present helpful suggestions on how these differences can be resolved or how these differences are sometimes induced by others' misperceptions. They conclude that these differences need not interfere with the establishment of a healthy, working alliance between twelve-step programs and the professional community:

> It is important to resolve these perceived areas of incompatibility between AA and psychotherapy. We believe that AA and psychotherapy are not competing forces that threaten the survival or efficacy of the other, but are mutually augmentative. Their goals are similar, and they share more common methods than generally thought. It must be remembered, however, that both psychotherapy and AA are diverse entities, containing a wide range of practices and interpretations of theory and traditions; there will, unfortunately, always be AA "hard liners," openly antagonistic to the idea of therapy, as well as psychotherapists who scorn AA (1991, pp. 284-285)

Integrating twelve-step recovery principles into more traditional forms of group psychotherapy is clearly one of the dominant themes and tasks confronting the group leader during the early and middle stages of recovery. Dies and Dies (1993) have outlined recommendations for a short-term group therapy approach that can provide some direction and framework for the group leader attempting to accomplish this task. The Directive Facilitation Model for short-term group treatment that Dies and Dies advocate is highly compatible with Yalom's recommendations because their approach is developmentally based and interpersonally focused. They outline twenty-one principles in their recommendations, the first ten of which will be presented here because these principles have the most relevance to the early/middle stages of group treatment.

1. Develop a Realistic Contract

Dies and Dies recommend much of the pre-group preparation that is outlined in Chapter 3 of this book. Adapting Kemker, Kibel, and Mahler's and Matano and Yalom's recommendations, Dies and Dies suggest that abstinence and identification of self as an addict or alcoholic must the primary components of any realistic contract with an alcoholic or addict.

2. Instill a Positive Climate

Recommendations are put forth that the group leader provide as much structure as possible, which promotes supportive norms and accents favorable interaction among group members. Many of Yalom's recommendations for the establishment of therapeutic norms and the leader as model-setting participant are relevant here.

3. React with a Process Rather than Content Focus

Much like Yalom, Dies and Dies emphasize that meaningful interpersonal contact between group members should be promoted at all times in group. They warn against excessive individual work or content focus in group. Twelve-step groups and individual sessions provide more than adequate time for members to tell their stories or explore the nuances of their individual experiences. Group therapy is best used when priority is given to a process focus that emphasizes individual interactions within the immediacy of the group.

4. Employ a Proactive Leadership Style

Dies and Dies, like Yalom, strongly recommend an active leadership style. A number of reasons for why this is important were discussed in Chapter 5. Primary among these reasons is that addicts and alcoholics do not generally respond well to passive or distant leadership styles that prevail in more traditional approaches to psychotherapy.

5. Confront Group Obstacles

The group will inevitably have to address the issues of safety, honesty, openness, and authenticity. Group members need to learn how real they can be with each other in group. It is crucial that the group leader be acutely tuned into these common obstacles in group and actively guide the group through the obstacles and resistance that are sure to present themselves.

6. Translate Group Conflict and Resistance

In Dies and Dies's opinion, clinicians have over-interpreted group resistance as representing unconscious collusions of group members to avoid doing the group work. While such a defensive process is certainly manifested in group, Dies and Dies have learned through their experience that personal reluctance to engage in meaningful therapeutic work in group usually derives from two primary sources: (1) the threat of personal vulnerability, and (2) the ambiguity about how to effectively use the group because of the lack of clarity about the group task. As they write, "As we persist in our efforts to foster interpersonal support and cohesion, and to clarify the framework for change, we find that personal guardedness dissolves rather naturally" (p. 180)

7. Illustrate the Theory of Change

New group members are generally naive about how group therapy functions most productively. Like Yalom, Dies and Dies believe that the power of the group to provide therapeutic assistance "is in the process of mutual exploration and sharing, not turn taking, advising, and staccato-style question-and-answering" (p. 181). Yalom, Ormont, and most other experienced group leaders are acutely aware of this important principle and encourage group leaders to help their group members learn this valuable lesson, not by giving them didactic information, but through the experience of it happening in the group.

8. Verbalize Frequently But Briefly

Group leaders' required activity is dictated more by the group leaders making their presence known by frequent, but brief interventions. This is not to be construed as Dies and Dies endorsing an autocratic perspective on group leadership. The best interventions in the group are always the ones that are short and simple. The art of good group leadership is the ability to say difficult and important things simply and briefly.

9. Encourage Members to Assume Responsibility

The best interventions are those designed to shift the responsibility to the group and its members. As Yalom recommends, a self-monitoring group is a highly effective group.

10. Facilitate a Here and Now Focus

Dies and Dies encourage the group leader to keep the group in the immediacy of the moment. As Yalom and Ormont suggest, the group is operating at maximum effectiveness when the members stay in the immediacy of the here and now.

The recommendations presented here by Dies and Dies supplement the model outlined by Yalom and elaborated upon by Ormont. While both Yalom and Ormont deal more exclusively with long-term outpatient groups, these ten principles can help the beginning group therapist determine which strategies will best match the requirements that are usually imposed upon them by a structured group therapy format that is part of a larger, more comprehensive treatment program.

Group therapists will quickly learn that many of the principles that dictate successful, long-term, outpatient group psychotherapy must be modified when doing short-term work in an inpatient unit or within an institutional setting. Within these settings, group therapy is not a free-standing therapy experience; it is but one component of a larger and more comprehensive treatment approach. Consequently, how it works and what the group leader can or cannot do is determined by the dynamics and restraints of the treatment atmosphere dominating the treatment program.

RELAPSE AND RECOVERY

It has long been a well-known axiom in the addiction treatment community that addicts or alcoholics will usually not give up their chemical use until the pain and dysphoria they experience from its continual use exceeds the pleasure or euphoria they derive from its present use. Conversely, addicts or alcoholics are likely to relapse or return to their drug of choice when the dysphoria and pain they experience with abstinence exceeds the pleasure or serenity they are experiencing in their recovery. Consequently, a great deal of addiction treatment is aimed toward monitoring this delicate balance between pleasure and dysphoria. Since most addicts and alcoholics are exceedingly intolerant of delaying gratification and will usually choose any certain source of immediate gratification (i.e., drugs and alcohol) over a possible source of probable satisfaction in the distant future, they will always opt for the quick, sure thing. In order to alter this ingrained attitudinal and habitual characterological pattern of behavior, they must first come to realize and accept the premise that their solution is the problem. They must be helped to realize that chemicals are not the answer; they only prolong the agony by delaying the reality of the situation. As AA members are told, "Nothing is ever so bad that a few drinks couldn't make it worse." Second, if treatment is to be effective, recovering addicts and alcoholics must be given hope and a new way of behaving with a different set of attitudes that will allow them to desire more long-term pleasure from their abstinence than they ever were able to get from the immediate euphoria of their alcohol and drug use.

Keeping alcoholics sober and addicts clean requires an entirely different set of strategies than getting them to initially stop their chemical use. The expectation that addicts or alcoholics will stay off of drugs and alcohol requires that they come to realize, accept, and experience the benefits of abstinence. Since the benefits of abstinence are not always immediately experienced, patients must come to accept on faith and hope that the benefits will come. Yalom (1975), expressing similar sentiments about an individual's capacity to derive benefit from psychotherapy, stresses the importance of belief and will in all forms of treatment. The expectation that patients will change is simply an extension of the moral philosophical belief that if humans know the good (i.e., what, in the deepest sense, is in their best interest), they will act accordingly. In the words of Aquinas: "Man, insofar as he acts willfully, acts according to some imagined good." (Yalom, 1975, p. 157). Therefore, addicted individuals must be persuaded that it is advantageous for them to stay abstinent and sober. An important aspect of relapse prevention is finding effective and influential ways to persuade addicted individuals that it is in their best interest not to return to drugs and alcohol. Logic and reason alone will not accomplish this task. Schopenhauer, a German philosopher, knew the limits of reason when he wrote over one hundred years ago: "Hence the uselessness of logic; no one ever convinced anybody by logic; and even logicians use logic only as a source of income. To convince a man, you must appeal to his self interest, his desires, his will" (Durant, 1926). Spinoza, another noted philosopher, addressed this issue nearly two hundred years prior to Schopenhauer when he wrote of the importance of substituting one strong emotion for another in bringing about change. "Passion always wins over reason. Unless we use reason to help steer our passions to a less destructive action. An emotion can only be mediated by another contrary or stronger emotion" (Durant, 1926).

One remedy for this dilemma requires that some desirable alternative be provided for alcoholics and addicts. This requires more than just appealing to the addicts and alcoholics to give up alcohol and drugs; it demands that they relinquish old sets of attitudes, behavior, and even friends associated with the addictive lifestyle. As AA members tell the new entry into the twelve-step program, "If you want to avoid a slip, don't go where it's slippery"; and "If you're serious about your recovery, you have to change your playmates and your playgrounds." In each case, the addict or alcoholic is being encouraged to substitute the fellowship of the program for the excitement or escape from reality that drugs and alcohol had previously provided. Epicurus, the early Greek philosopher, captured this realization over two thousand years ago when he wrote, "We must not avoid pleasures, but we must select them. Exalt the joys of intellect rather than those of sense. Be careful against pleasures that excite and disturb the soul which they should rather quiet and appease" (Durant, 1926).

Relapse prevention works on two levels. On a primary level, if addicts or alcoholics experience an immediate benefit from abstinence and recovery, this in itself will be all the motivation required to keep them from returning to alcohol and drugs. For many individuals entering treatment for the first time, this will be their experience. They will feel so relieved to have identified the source of their confusion, emotional pain, and despair that they will feel immediate relief, hope, and direction. Little else needs to be done except to stay out of their way and allow them to do what they will be pulled to do by their own intuitive knowledge. An example will help clarify this point:

> Ralph, a thirty-six-year-old poly-drug abuser and alcoholic had gained a notorious reputation in the small midwestern town he had lived in his entire life as a "hell-raiser and somebody not right in the head." Well-known and well-liked (when sober) by everyone who knew him, he had failed to respond to all efforts to help and rehabilitate him. His family was well-known and respected. Efforts were made by his family and other concerned citizens to get him the best possible professional help for his erratic behavior and "crazy thinking." Visits to two different and prominent psychiatrists in the large metropolitan city close by failed to produce any help or benefit. Finally, after a third DUI arrest, Ralph was forced for the first time to complete a state-mandated driver education program that emphasized the dangers of drinking and driving. A chance conversation with an alcohol counselor who was presenting one of the lectures that night resulted in Ralph attending an AA meeting at the counselor's suggestion. Following that meeting, Ralph initiated setting up some counseling sessions with the addiction counselor at the local mental health center because, as he said, "There was something about those people at that meeting. They were telling my story." Ralph agreed not to drink and put off any decision to identify himself as an alcoholic until he felt ready. He continued counseling and attendance at AA The immediate change in Ralph did not go unnoticed by the small community. Townspeople were talking about the "miraculous cure" that had come about at the hands of the counselor. No one in the town had noticed or even made the connection

> between the remarkable change in Ralph and the fact that he was no longer drinking. As far as they were concerned, he had gotten his "crazy thinking" straightened out. About four months into counseling, Ralph, after deciding he was an alcoholic, confided to the counselor, "You know the best thing that ever happened to me was finding out that I was an alcoholic. I didn't know what was wrong with me, but I knew something wasn't right. I was afraid that I was just plain crazy and there was no hope for me. Discovering I am an alcoholic is not near as frightening as believing that I was nuts."

Not all addicts and alcoholics will embrace sobriety and abstinence this strongly. For those who do not experience the kind of relief that Ralph did, their recovery will be marked by increased emotional pain and discomfort. This is the other level of relapse prevention. From this standpoint, relapse prevention strategies are geared to help addicts and alcoholics hold on to their abstinence until more stable emotional relief is achieved by furnishing them with a set of tools, practices, and recommendations that have proved beneficial and helpful to other recovering addicts and alcoholics. To understand how relapse can be prevented and how these strategies are beneficial, it is helpful to distinguish between two variables: (1) early stage versus later stage relapse contributors, and (2) the patient's contributions to relapse versus the therapist's contributions to relapse.

EARLY VERSUS LATER STAGE RELAPSE

Relapse is an observable symptom and concrete event that suggests one of the following problems: (1) an old pattern of thinking has returned (self-centeredness, narcissistic defenses suggesting unresolved feelings of shame, etc.); (2) the individual has failed to do what the program recommends; or (3) the therapist has neglected to address a crucial issue in the individual's treatment. A relapse, if properly examined, can provide an opportunity to learn what has not been done or addressed that should have been. Examining a relapse is not a search for an excuse. It should be motivated by a desire to come to a better understanding of what happened and why. Its aim is to help individuals who relapse gain some mastery and control over their inability to remain abstinent. Eventually, it leads them to take responsibility for the event to ensure that they do things differently in the future to prevent it from happening again. As Santayana said, "He who remains ignorant of the mistakes of history is doomed to repeat them."

Early stage relapses are usually marked by a number of common variables. Some of the typical patient contributions to relapse are:

1. Denial. The alcoholics or addicts still have not taken the first step of admitting they are powerless over alcohol and drugs. Sometimes newly recovering patients will have to test the first step to erase once and for all the possibility that they can drink "normally" or do drugs recreationally. Picking up another white chip will symbolize that they are willing to start over again in the program, and this is often all that they need to do in order to get themselves back in recovery.

2. Failure to Work the Steps of the Program. Many alcoholics and addicts hold onto the illusion that all they have to do in recovery is stay off of chemicals. Those who hold onto this belief will soon learn that recovery requires far more than staying abstinent. The first step of the twelve steps of recovery is the only one that mentions drugs and alcohol. The remaining eleven steps have to do with shame, guilt, honesty, altruism, removal of character defects, and a fearless moral inventory. While all of these efforts are required by the program, they also lend themselves nicely to the kind of therapeutic work that can be accomplished in group.

3. Honesty Is Too Difficult. The cornerstone of the twelve-step recovery process is honesty. This requires honesty not only with others, but most importantly with self. Because most alcoholics and addicts suffer from intense feelings of shame, admitting to even the smallest fault or failing can be an excruciating event. They cannot tolerate any more negativity about themselves and will go to great lengths to avoid, minimize, and deny the reality of a situation if it is even a little threatening to their fragile self-esteem. This leads to extraordinary measures of self-deception that at times can border on the delusional. They literally cannot see or admit to what everyone else around them knows to be true. This is why the group format and twelve-step meetings are so crucial to their treatment. Through the identification and acceptance of others who are like them, they can honestly face together what would be impossible to face alone.

4. Fantasy of Specialness. Because of the need for the excessive use of narcissistic and grandiose defenses to keep feelings of shame and worthlessness in check, most alcoholics and addicts will succumb to the belief that they cannot be like those other unfortunates because they are special. Humility is the antidote to this tendency to distance themselves from what they refuse to admit because to do so is too deflating of self-worth. The introduction of oneself in the AA manner, i.e., "Hello, my name is Joe and I'm an alcoholic," is so important to the program of AA. Contrary to the common misperception of those outside of the program who view this practice as harmful labeling, this is a constant reminder of the humility that is needed for recovery.

5. Haven't Bottomed Out Yet. Active members in AA and other twelve-step programs soon learn that there are those who need to lose everything (i.e., job, family, finances, self-respect, health, etc.) before they are willing to admit they are alcoholics. Such a stubborn refusal to face the reality of their situation is typically present in individuals who are referred to in the program as "low-bottom" alcoholics. In contrast, there are the "high-bottom" addicts and alcoholics. For many reasons, they are the individuals who are more able to address the consequences of drinking or drug use without having to experience the total devastation that befalls many others in the program. "Raising an alcoholic's or addict's bottom" is the intent of a well-conducted intervention where the facts and reality of the consequences and results of their drinking and drug use cannot be denied. This avenue of learning by seeing oneself in another is an additional unique benefit of group and twelve-step meetings that cannot be derived from individual treatment alone. Addicts or alcoholics need not make every mistake themselves before they know what to do or avoid in their recovery. They will be witness to it by learning from others.

6. Cognitive Impairment. Research evidence clearly demonstrates that, especially earlier in recovery, addicts and alcoholics often do not have the mental capabilities required to fully respond favorably to treatment efforts made on their behalf. AA's maxims of "keep it simple" and "one day at a time" provide the kind of structure and direction that many people early in recovery need. Insight-oriented psychotherapy is practically useless at these times. Inspiration, motivation, direction, and concrete suggestions are most likely to produce the best results with someone who has just attained sobriety or recently relapsed. As newly recovering AA members are told, "When you're up to your ass in alligators, it's difficult to remember that the purpose of your task was to drain the swamp." Survival takes precedence over understanding during a time of crisis.

THERAPIST VERSUS PATIENT CONTRIBUTIONS TO RELAPSE

1. Treatment Is Inadequate

Inadequate treatment is generally the result of too much or too little of some vital element necessary for recovery. In most cases, it will mean that there was too much affect too quickly in treatment. For some individuals, it may mean too little affect too late in treatment. It can also indicate too little motivation on the patient's part or too much apathy on the therapist's part, resulting in too little involvement in the treatment process. At other times, it might reflect too much confrontation and too little support. In other situations, it might mean too much support with too little confrontation. Knowing how to reach and maintain the delicate balance required for each patient is often the art of good effective treatment.

Sometimes, the addict's or alcoholic's refusal to participate or connect with the fellowship of the twelve-step program can be in part due to the patient's resistance and in part due to the therapist's resistance. While many primary care physicians, therapists, and other health care providers will pay lip service to the importance of abstinence and twelve-step recovery programs, it is rarely their referral or recommendation that gets the alcoholic or addict into recovery. A recent survey by Miller and Hoffman (1995) revealed that "Physicians do not generally identify or refer patients needing treatment to abstinence-based programs for alcohol or drug addiction. . . . Given the fact that addicted individuals are disproportionately represented in health care populations, such a statistic is problematic. The estimated prevalence rate of alcoholics and drug addicts in medical and psychiatric practices ranges from 25% to 80%" (p. 41). These findings are consistent with earlier statistics which had shown that a survey of state hospitals in 1964 revealed that only 3.3 percent of the daily census were recognized alcoholics, even though the surveyors estimated that alcoholics constituted closer to 30 percent of admissions (Moore and Buchanan, 1966). A later survey revealed that 23 percent of a random sample of psychotherapy patients seen in a large metropolitan mental health center who identified themselves as suffering either from addictive problems or excessive substance abuse were only identified 3.5 percent of the time by their own therapists (Cummings, 1979).

If alcoholics or addicts relapse and their lack of involvement in a twelve-step program is the primary contributing factor, there is an excellent chance they will get an inadequate referral to the right twelve-step program–if they get any encouragement to attend the twelve-step meetings at all. Uninformed or inadequately trained therapists can either be ignorant of how the fellowship works or hold an enormously negative bias about the program. Even though AA meetings are conducted along very similar and sometimes rigid adherences to the principles of the twelve-step program, different meetings will vary significantly in many important ways. The recently relapsed addict or alcoholic needs to "shop around" until the right meeting with the right mix of people is found. Failure to confront this as what it is, namely resistance, will only enhance the likelihood of more relapses in the future. An illustration might help clarify this point.

An alcohol counselor, strongly influenced by Bob Goulding's model of Redecision Therapy, was giving a lecture at an inpatient Alcohol and Drug (A&D) unit to a group of recently admitted alcoholics and addicts. Earlier in the day, the alcohol counselor had stressed the importance of dealing with resistance in treatment and had spoken about Bob Goulding's emphasis on the use of words such as *try*, *can't*, and *need* as indicators of a person's resistance and refusal to take responsibility for his or her own actions. Goulding, coming from a strong Transactional Analysis (TA) theoretical orientation, believed individuals often revealed their passive reluctance to change in the type of language they used. One key word for Goulding was *try*, which for Bob meant that they weren't really going to do it with all of their personal conviction, but were going to give an illusion of an attempt by *trying*. There was no real intent to succeed and when the inevitable failure came, they would justify it by crying "See, I *tried* and it didn't work." For Bob Goulding and TA, you either were going to do it or not, none of this *trying* business. Other key words within Bob Goulding's formula were *can't*, which meant *won't*, and *need*, which meant *want*. In this afternoon's lecture, the alcohol counselor was in the middle of a talk on the necessity and importance of AA in the alcoholic's recovery, when one of the patients interrupted the alcohol counselor to object to a point he had just made about AA. The patient (Bill) was a thirty-six-year-old alcoholic who had recently relapsed for the second time and had been unable to stay sober for more than six months following each treatment. Bill complained that AA wasn't for him and hadn't worked. He went on into a three-minute harangue about the failures and limitations of the twelve-step philosophy and its insistence on abstinence. Finally interrupted by the alcohol counselor with the suggestion that maybe Bill needed to search for the right meeting for himself, Bill quickly objected, saying, "I've been *trying* to find the right meeting, but I *can't* and I'm not sure I *need* one." Everyone at the lecture quickly recognized the key words in his statement because the morning lecture on Redecision and TA was still fresh in their minds. Quickly confronted by the entire group, Bill could not avoid the humor in his statement as he and the other patients good-naturedly laughed and they encouraged him to own his resistance by stating, "I *won't* find an AA meeting because I don't *want* one." This statement more accurately represented his position on abstinence and recovery, and helped him understand in a refreshing way how his resistance was contributing to his relapses.

Later Stage Relapses

While there are a myriad of factors that contribute to the early stage relapses, later stage relapses are dominated by two related variables. Alcoholics' or addicts' chances of relapse are heightened anytime they start to feel too good or too bad. Feeling too good is often an indicator that the old narcissistic defenses have returned. Grandiosity and a sense of specialness have the corrosive capacity to erode the humility that keeps the alcoholics' and addicts' defenses in check. As sobriety provides them with the opportunity to marshall the creative forces and energies that were practically sedated into submission, they rediscover the capacity for achievement and success. It is as easy for alcoholics and addicts to attribute all their success to their own special uniqueness as it is for them to harshly attack and blame themselves completely for any failure or mistake. As their achievements mount, they become just as vulnerable to the intoxication of success as they were to the intoxication of drugs and alcohol. It is a short step from being too busy with "important things," to skipping meetings, to "I can't be one of them" or "I have this thing licked." A few successful trials at controlled drinking and substance use only help solidify their new assessment of their own selves as unique and different. The inevitable relapse is set in motion.

At the other end of the spectrum is the recovering addict or alcoholic who continues to stay sober and clean without experiencing any relief from dysphoria or the benefit of increased serenity and contentment. It is important to carefully assess whether these individuals are doing more for their recovery than just abstaining from drugs and alcohol. All bets are off unless the individuals are really into recovery; specifically, they are working the steps, they are attending meetings, they have a sponsor, they are practicing honest self-exploration, and they are actively participating in a group. Despite making all the efforts required of them, many faithful twelve-step members continue to feel worse. Sobriety and the twelve-step program do not bring them any long-standing benefit. In many cases, they are deprived of the relief provided by self-medication (drugs and alcohol), however unpredictable and brief such relief may be. Slowly, but steadily, the steadfast resolve that they would never drink or do drugs again is gradually eroded by the dysphoria and gnawing unhappiness that dominates their existence. Eventually, they cease to care about their sobriety because their life ceases to have any meaningful purpose. Apathy in the form of "I don't give a damn" is a dangerous position for a recovering addict or alcoholic to reach. It is a short distance from "I don't give a damn" to "I might as well be drunk; it can't be any worse than this."

It is crucial that the group leader watch for such telltale signs in the person who is doing all that he or she should be doing in recovery and continues to feel worse. Often, antidepressants and other nonaddictive medications may be required if there is assurance that the prescribing physician is an addictionologist or well acquainted with the principles of addiction and its treatment. Dual diagnosis patients suffering from other mental health disorders often fall into this category. Because of the tendency of addiction to run in families, many addicts and alcoholics grew up with alcoholic or addicted parents. Unresolved ACOA issues can also contribute to their situation. More intensive, frequent, and adjunctive types of psychotherapy may be needed. With the increased recognition of the high percentage of substance and alcohol abuse by women and men who are sexual abuse survivors, a careful exploration of dissociative defenses and possible repressed memories is warranted in many cases. Recovering addicts or alcoholics in the above-mentioned situations may indeed have many contributing factors that will explain their unhappiness despite their efforts at recovery. To be told to "make a gratitude list," "stop feeling sorry for self," 'You're on the pity-pot," and "If you were working the program right, you wouldn't be feeling this way" is not only not helpful, it is also destructive.

RELAPSE PREVENTION

Within the last ten years, the large percentage of addicts and alcoholics who relapse after leaving the restricted confines, safety, and firm controls of an inpatient setting has led to the development of a number of models for relapse prevention. While concern about a potential relapse quickly becomes a consistent and dominant focus of treatment, almost from the very moment the addicts or alcoholics cease their chemical use, this concern becomes even more pronounced once individuals are discharged from a structured treatment unit and are faced with the pressures and demands of the street or the real world.

One serendipitous result of the relapse prevention models is that they have been structured in such a way that they provide an easy and useful conceptual framework for the delivery of outpatient abstinence-based substance abuse treatment. Relapse prevention was originally adapted to minimize the negative consequences of relapses and teach skills that would either help addicts and alcoholics avoid further setbacks or provide clues that would help them avoid emotional and situational factors that contribute to a relapse. Most approaches to relapse prevention are behaviorally oriented and structured in a way that helps the individuals identify specific situations or circumstances that will likely trigger a conditioned response that contributes to alcohol or drug use. These strategies can be extremely helpful and can easily be incorporated into a more psychodynamic group therapy approach such as the models that Yalom, Ormont, or Kohut advocate.

Rawson et al. (1993) provide an excellent overview of the relapse prevention approach. They cite a series of authors and researchers who have produced a number of different models of treatment utilizing relapse prevention as the central philosophy and methodology of their approach. Several other methods are described that outline clinical recommendations on the uses of relapse prevention for all forms of substance abuse (i.e., alcohol, marijuana, cocaine, crack, opiates). Rawson et al. also describes the work of a number of researchers who have created drug-specific protocols that allow for the evaluation of this approach with specific drug-abusing populations. The Rawson et al. article also provides an overview of techniques that are easily integrated into outpatient models of treatment, providing an easily replicated framework for delivering outpatient substance abuse treatment.

Structured Group Therapy

Rawson et al.'s (1993) review of recommendations for relapse prevention models is especially helpful because within the last few years, financial constraints, rising costs of medical care, and attempts by third-party insurance providers to reduce costs have had a profound influence on how addiction is treated. No longer are four- to six-week inpatient hospital stays the standard treatment regimen. More and more treatment is offered in day treatment programs and outpatient settings. Comprehensive treatment programs that were typically applied within an inpatient unit at a hospital have now been adapted to outpatient settings. Group therapy remains a crucial component of this adaptation, and much of what was utilized in an inpatient setting is applied in a very similar fashion in the structured outpatient programs.

Despite this rapidly changed treatment climate, it is still crucial to understand the special demands that an inpatient setting has for the group therapy process. Whether the group is conducted within a hospital on a closed or locked unit, or it is part of a day program outside of a hospital, the institutional setting will have a profound influence and impact on what the group leader has to contend with when doing group therapy.

Many of the difficulties and obstacles that a group leader will have to overcome when leading a group that is part of a structured treatment program will be similar to the difficulties that have historically presented themselves in hospital settings where group therapy has been part of an inpatient treatment program. Yalom has written an excellent book on inpatient group therapy in which he examines the special adaptations that must be applied to his model of group therapy when the group leader is required to lead a group within an institutional setting. Unlike inpatient psychiatric units, which Yalom perceives as being less receptive and appreciative of the proven impact that group therapy can provide in a patient's treatment, Alcohol and Drug (A&D) inpatient units historically have warmly embraced and enthusiastically applied group therapy as a crucial and integral part of an addict's or alcoholic's treatment. Despite this enthusiastic receptivity to group therapy, the application of it within a structured treatment program poses some unique considerations for the group leader. Yalom's recommendations for inpatient treatment have some important implications when considered and generalized to all forms of institutional settings.

As Yalom indicates, the goals, structure, and methods for the utilization of group therapy on inpatient units are not always consistent or clearly defined. This is true for both A&D and psychiatric inpatient groups. The confusion surrounding the application of group therapy is one reason many medical directors fail to appreciate its effectiveness. Contemporary forms of group psychotherapy, adapted from theoretical models derived from work with nonpsychotic patients treated in an outpatient setting, do not usually apply to inpatient populations. Inpatient group psychotherapy, with both psychiatric and chemically dependent populations, requires that the special circumstances surrounding inpatient treatment be appreciated and taken into consideration before the group leader embarks on the delicate task of treatment. Yalom outlines some necessary considerations that must be taken into account for effective inpatient group psychotherapy. These will be reviewed later in the chapter. First, it will be necessary to assess the special characteristics and circumstances surrounding the newly hospitalized alcoholic or drug addict because this defines the limits of the applicability of group psychotherapy for these patients.

Even as controversies concerning the validity and meaning of the disease concept remain heated outside the field of addiction treatment, group leaders within the field have attempted to define the disease and structure its treatment to fit a group therapy format. A stage-specific framework identifying the predominant problems and the complementary therapeutic techniques through the different phases of inpatient treatment is required in the development of an efficient inpatient group therapy model. While not all alcoholic and drug-dependent patients entering treatment require medical detoxification, it is generally the appropriate initial step in hospitalization. A discussion of the criteria utilized in evaluating the need for medical detoxification is beyond the scope of this book. However, it should suffice to say that these patients need to be excluded from group therapy until they are stabilized medically. A familiarity with, and understanding of, the symptoms of progressive withdrawal is essential for the group leader in all phases of alcoholism and drug-dependence treatment.

YALOM'S RECOMMENDATIONS FOR INPATIENT GROUPS

There are numerous difficulties confronting inpatient group leaders. They not only must contend with the resistant patient and the cognitively impaired patient, but they must also contend with difficulties that are specific to the special circumstances involved in all inpatient treatment. As Yalom writes, ". . . specialized skills are required for effective leadership. Neither individual nor outpatient group therapy training constitute sufficient clinical preparation for the inpatient group therapist. The acute inpatient ward constitutes a radically different clinical setting and requires a radical modification of group therapy technique" (1983, p. 36). The techniques and tasks of the group therapist outlined in Chapters 4 and 5 of this text must be modified to meet the demands of the inpatient setting.

Yalom (1983) lists the different factors that will impinge on the leader's attempt to conduct an effective inpatient group:

1. There is considerable patient turnover. The average length of stay is four to six weeks. There are some patients who only stay a few days. There is generally a new patient in the group almost every meeting.
2. Some patients attend the group meeting just for a single meeting or two. There is not time to work on termination. Some member terminates almost every meeting, and a focus on termination would consume all the group time.
3. There is a great heterogeneity of psychopathology: patients with neurosis, characterological disturbance, substance abuse, adolescent problems, major affective disorders, anorexia nervosa, and sometimes even psychosis are all present in the same group.
4. All the patients are acutely uncomfortable; they strive toward resolution of withdrawal or acute despair rather than toward personal growth or self-understanding. As soon as a patient is out of an acute crisis, he or she often desires to be discharged.

5. There are many unmotivated patients in the group: they may be psychologically unsophisticated; they do not want to be there; they may not agree that they need therapy; they often are not paying for therapy; they may have little curiosity about themselves.
6. The therapist has no time to prepare or screen patients.
7. The therapist often has no control over group composition.
8. There is little therapist stability. Many of the therapists have rotating schedules and generally cannot attend all of the meetings of the group.
9. Patients see their therapist in other roles throughout the day on the ward.
10. Group therapy is only one of many therapies in which the patient participates; some of these other therapies are with some of the same patients in the group and often with the same therapist.
11. There is often little sense of cohesion in the group; not enough time exists for members to learn to care for or trust one another.
12. There is not time for gradual recognition of subtle interpersonal patterns, or for "working through," and no opportunity to focus on transfer of learning to the situation at home (pp. 50-51).

Considering the difficulties a group leader will have to adapt to in running an inpatient group, the single most important task of the leader is to establish appropriate and realistic goals that can be attained within the confines of the situation, time, and patient population on an inpatient unit. Not establishing goals will lead the therapist, the group members, and the group to drift aimlessly. However, if the goals are unrealistic or overly ambitious, group leaders will become increasingly disappointed and stamp themselves, or group therapy, as hopelessly ineffective. Goal setting often involves two different but parallel processes. Explicit goals must be established with individual members regarding their sobriety and the attainment of the interpersonal tools necessary to ensure recovery. Implied goals, based on the group leader's assessment of the needs of the particular individual in relation to the group process, must also be monitored by the group leader. He or she must carefully determine which particular group member needs to be supported, confronted, encouraged, or left alone during group.

This situation is complicated by the fact that the goals of the therapy group are not always identical to the goals of the hospital or treatment facility. Unfortunately, some medical and program directors are not supportive of group psychotherapy. They fail to appreciate group therapy's potential as a powerful adjunct to a patient's recovery. In some cases, an inpatient unit can be so rigidly invested in AA and the disease concept that they view all forms of psychotherapy as counter-therapeutic to the alcoholic's or addict's recovery. Certainly, group therapy conducted by either overzealous group leaders who are too provocative and promote too much regression too soon, or group leaders who fail to adequately understand the disease concept, thereby neglecting the importance of appreciating the level of cognitive impairment and the need for abstinence before any type of introspective self-understanding can be achieved, can have detrimental effects on a newly hospitalized patient. This is why the goals of the group leader must be realistic and in tune with the goals of the treatment facility. If group is conducted in a prescribed manner that takes careful consideration of the special circumstances of the newly hospitalized patient, the therapy group will not be in conflict with AA and the disease concept. Group can be used to address those areas of the patient's recovery that the disease concept and AA neglect.

The disease concept and AA will be far more effective in helping a patient achieve and maintain sobriety. Since this is the essential first step of a patient's recovery, this goal must be given priority. Group therapy, if it promotes too much anxiety or introspection, or if it encourages the belief that controlled alcohol or drug use is possible, will only interfere with the recovery process. Group psychotherapy is most effective if it achieves two goals. First, by helping group members avoid and manage stress, it can play a vital role in reducing their propensity toward relapse. Second, and most important, according to Yalom, the primary goal of the inpatient therapy group is to engage the patient in the therapy process. This is a twofold therapeutic process that Yalom refers to as horizontal (the multifaceted therapy program in the hospital, which includes therapy groups, lectures, AA meetings, etc.) and longitudinal (post-hospital course of treatment, which includes aftercare groups, AA meetings, etc.).

The Horizontal Process

Group therapy is most effective during the initial stages of treatment because of its ability to help ameliorate the alcoholics' and addicts' isolation, shame, and self-loathing. Through identification with others in the group, alcoholics and addicts learn they are not alone in their wretchedness. They also learn they are not unique in their tendency to become intoxicated and engage in behavior that is offensive and disrespectful to themselves and others. Universality, as a curative process, allows alcoholics and addicts to learn they share a common bond with others with whom they come to identify with and care for deeply. Cohesiveness and trust with others in the group who are understanding and accepting of their defects of character lead to a loss of isolation and alienation–two profound circumstances that contribute greatly to their continual drinking and drug use. The disease concept places their difficulties within a concise, manageable framework, alleviates their guilt, and improves their self-esteem. One to two months of structured abstinence allows them to cleanse cognitively, emotionally, and physically. Often for the first time in years, alcoholics and addicts will feel some hope and have some understanding of their condition and a direction in which to guide their efforts.

The Longitudinal Process

As important as the horizontal process is in alcoholics' and addicts' recovery, their hospitalization and inpatient treatment will be effective only if it is coupled with continual aftercare therapy. Outpatient group therapy and continual attendance at AA meetings are two important components to this longitudinal process. Consequently, an important goal of inpatient group psychotherapy is to provide an introduction to group therapy that is relevant, comfortable, and effective. Such an experience will increase the likelihood that the hospitalized patient will participate in continual treatment in an aftercare group. If alcoholics and addicts learn that talking helps and that group can be used to identify major problem areas, continual involvement in an ongoing aftercare or outpatient group will be far more attractive to them.

COMPOSITION OF THE INPATIENT GROUPS

Yalom distinguishes between two basic strategies in composing an inpatient therapy group–the team approach and the level approach. The team approach has patients randomly assigned to different groups, usually according to the order of their admission to the hospital. The level approach requires patients to be assigned to a group according to the level of their functioning. More severely ill patients will be placed in one group, and higher functioning patients will be placed in another group. Both approaches have positive and negative consequences. To get the benefit of both approaches, Yalom advises having a team group every day and a level group every other day. Because Yalom is making these suggestions specifically for psychiatric patients, his recommendations must be altered before they are generalizable to chemically dependent patients. Since most alcoholics and addicts present with similar levels of ego functioning, Yalom's recommendations are not as germane for this population. On rare occasions, there are patients who present with far more serious psychiatric difficulties, and their symptoms, which were somewhat muted by their use of alcohol or drugs, become even more severe with abstinence. Transfer to the psychiatric unit may be required for these patients. Most chemically dependent patients will be able to enter group at the same level, and there is usually little need for a lower level and higher level group.

However, Brix (1983) suggests a variation of this two-stage format for chemically dependent inpatients that has some parallels with Yalom's suggestions. His recommendations call for a format involving a two-stage experience for the patients. The first stage is a leader-active group. The second stage emphasizes what Brix calls a "group-centered approach." Brix writes,

> As soon as gross effects of toxicity have abated to the point where the patient is lucid and reasonably attentive, he or she enters our so-called "A" group, which meets five days weekly in 45-minute sessions. My goal in this group is to orient the patient to the overall treatment program and especially to help the patient to begin to experience what it is to be a member of a therapy group without relying on a topic or exercise-centered format. Because of the wide variability in cognitive functioning among patients at this state of treatment, I remain very flexible in my approach–sometimes serious, sometimes more whimsical, but typically quite active. Following 7-10 days in the "A-group," most of our patients are transferred to our more group-centered "B-group." This transfer is viewed by practically all patients as a status symbol, and a sign of their progress by the staff. (1983, pp. 254-255)

In order for the hospitalized patient to participate successfully in a group-centered group, Brix feels they must first be able to tolerate the frustration and anxiety generated by such a format. He writes,

> The format of the psychotherapy groups grows out a belief that (1) a group-centered group experience, even if only of a few sessions duration, is at least equally valuable, perhaps more valuable, than any other group experience many alcoholic patients can have, but (2) patients profit more from the group if they are prepared for entry by participating first in a more leader-active group. (p. 254)

Following seven to ten days in "A" group, Brix transfers these patients to his group-centered "B" group. They are notified a day ahead of their entry with the following written message:

> For the remainder of your treatment you will be participating in the "B" psychotherapy group. The format of the "B" group as-

sumes one thing about you and that is that you want to better understand yourself and your emotions. It is not unusual for group members at times to be anxious and perplexed as they find they have been momentarily overcome with strong feelings. This is all a part of being a patient in group therapy. To make the most of this for yourself you really have to do only one thing and that is express openly and honestly what you are thinking and feeling about the group and your fellow group members. You are requested to be prepared to remain in the 1-1/2 hour session without interruptions. (Brix, 1983, p. 255)

Such a format with its emphasis on prepared instructions for entry into a therapy group accomplishes two important tasks for group leaders. It allows them to prepare the individual for the psychotherapy groups, and it provides the needed structure for conducting such a group. While Brix's suggestions for the "B" group format are questionable because they may provide too little structure for the newly recovering alcoholic or addict, his reasons for the shift from an "A" group to a "B" group approach merit careful consideration because they possess several advantages for treatment. Brix suggests the following advantages of a "B" group format:

As I see it, there are at least four compelling reasons to include a group-centered therapy group in an alcoholism treatment program: (1) this format tends to guard against the therapist's relying excessively on the use of confrontation, (2) the danger of the therapist's interventions being counter-transference based is reduced, (3) there is somewhat greater likelihood that therapeutic use of transference phenomena can occur, and (4) there is greater probability that patients will become therapeutic for one another. (1983, p. 256)

Because of the short duration of time, the rapid turnover of patients, and the other difficulties that Yalom listed, there are too many forces acting against Brix's "group-centered" format, at least the way he describes it (1983). However, his suggestions for the two-level approach and the way he implements the shift from "A" to "B" group is highly effective. If a group leader were to follow his recommendation, the "B" group format would be more beneficial if Yalom's strategies were incorporated into it.

YALOM'S STRATEGIES AND TECHNIQUES OF LEADERSHIP

Conducting an effective inpatient therapy group according to Yalom's recommendations requires the group leader to be very active and to provide structure for the group. As Yalom says, "There is no place in inpatient group therapy for the passive, inactive therapist. Nor is there a place in inpatient group psychotherapy for the non-directive leader!" (1983, p. 107). The rapid turnover of the patient population and their short duration of stay in the hospital prevents the group leader from operating from the perspective of a more passive, less structured leadership style. The group leader must therefore think of the life of the group as lasting a single session. This translates to a position where the leader must do as much effective group work as possible for as many patients as possible within the group framework. To accomplish this, the group requires an active and directive leader.

There are four essential tasks of the group leader on the inpatient unit:

1. The group leader must be active and efficient and should not allow the group to waste time.
2. The group leader must establish safety as a priority in group.
3. Supportive group leaders are necessary for inpatient groups.
4. The group leader must be directive and provide structure for the group.

1. The Group Leader Must Be Active and Efficient

Internal chaos within the individual requires that the group leader impose externally oriented structure as the first step in helping individuals develop a sense of internal control. Inpatients prefer and respond best to a leader who:

A. Ensures equal distribution of time within the group. Nothing is more destructive to group than to allow the rest of the group members to repeatedly suffer through a hyperverbal patient's repetitious and constant complaints.
B. Actively solicits group members, inviting different individuals to contribute and interact.
C. Actively focuses group attention on topics that are meaningful and relevant.
D. Prevents rambling patients from derailing the group work.
E. Provides a clear direction for the group sessions.

2. Safety As a Priority for Inpatient Groups

The group leader must create an atmosphere that is constructive, warm, safe, and trusting. Group members must experience the group as a place where they will be heard, accepted, and understood. Inpatient group therapy is not the place for destructive confrontation, criticism, or the escalation of anger. This does not mean that the group leader should pretend that anger does not exist. However, rather than escalate or encourage its expression, the group leader should move in for rapid conflict resolution. Most chemically dependent patients have little experience with the resolution of conflict or the nondestructive expression of anger. Learning that conflict can be resolved constructively without physical injury and harm can be extremely therapeutic for many patients. Often, encouraging discussion of little annoyances before they have a chance to build into a rage or tirade can be important to this learning process. If anger is ignited between two members, rather than have them express their anger directly, encourage them to direct it at an issue, policy, or even the group leader.

3. Supportive Strategies for the Inpatient Group Leader

Support in group is more than being nice or friendly. The group leader must balance his or her support with firmness and predictability. Explain explicitly what is expected of the group and its members. In turn, explain to them the reasons for your actions. A consistent, coherent group procedure will do wonders for providing the support that group members require before they will venture to share honestly with the group and its members. To encourage this type of interaction, the group leader must accomplish these tasks:

A. Acknowledge each group member's contribution to group. Members respond positively to a therapist's liking them, valuing them, and noticing and reinforcing their positive characteristics.
B. Take each member seriously. Do not discount or minimize their efforts.
C. Discourage self-defeating behavior. Although many group members are very sensitive to the behavior of others, they can be insensitive to their own behavior. They will keep alienating others in group without understanding how or why they are doing this. At times, it requires an extreme effort on the group leader's part to pick out the positive aspects of many patients' behavior.
D. Help the other group members to understand the reasons for another's behavior. As Yaloms states, "To understand all is to forgive all." The group will often accept another's irritating behavior if they understand the reasons why the person behaves as he or she does.
E. Identify and emphasize the group members' value to one another. Since most alcoholics and addicts have such strong feelings of self-

condemnation, the realization that they are of value to other group members can be extremely therapeutic for them. This is, in fact, one of the important aspects of the twelve steps in the AA program (see Chapter 8).

F. Do not attack a patient or support one group member at the expense of another. Each member must learn that group is a safe place for them. If confrontation does occur, either from another group member or the group leader, it must be nondestructive and follow along the guidelines outlined in Chapter 9.

G. Give the group member control of the depth of the sharing and openness they may show in group. One reason many group members are reluctant to open up in group is that they fear they may go too far and express or show more of themselves than they had intended. Members must know they can set their own limits in group in discussing their feelings. Drinking and drug-taking behavior should be excluded from these precautions (see Chapter 8). It is extremely important that alcoholics and addicts openly discuss their feelings related to their use of alcohol and drugs. Consequently, any techniques that interfere with this requirement should be used sparingly.

H. Treat each group member with respect and dignity. Do not interpret or expose their nonverbal behavior or their conflicts for their own sake. Only if this behavior is directly related to their alcohol or drug use should it be openly confronted against their wishes.

Provide Direction and Structure in Group

A clear, structured setting, preferably in a circle without a table in a closed private room with few chances for outside interruptions, is crucial. Starting promptly and ending on time provides the group members with clear boundaries. A unit policy that group not be interrupted and that attendance is mandatory instills an added sense of importance to the therapeutic setting.

Yalom suggests a basic blueprint for providing the optimal amount of structure for an inpatient group. (See Table 10.3.) It is Yalom's opinion that the gaining and accepting of a working contract with each group member is vitally important to the effectiveness of an inpatient group. If this is not obtained, the session can degenerate into a rambling, confused discourse.

Agenda Rounds

Yalom's description of agenda rounds is not without precedent. Robert and Mary Goulding operate from a Transactional Analysis (TA) frame-

TABLE 10.3. Yalom's Basic Blueprint for an Inpatient Group

1.	*Orientation and preparation* (The group leader introduces him- or herself and reminds the members of the purpose, length, and time of the meeting. If there are observers, new members, or a new co-therapist, he or she introduce them to the group.)	2 to 3 minutes
2.	*Agenda go-round* (Each member formulates a personal agenda for the group session.)	10 to 20 minutes
3.	*Work on agendas* (The group leader attempts to fill as many agendas as possible within the group time.)	60 to 80 minutes
4.	*Summary, comment, and close of the group.*	2 to 3 minutes

work in their use of Redecision Therapy in therapy groups (Goulding and Goulding, 1979). The Gouldings require a contract from each group member before they do any work in group. In their one-, two-, and four-week training groups, they spend the first part of the training period doing contract work. Members are required to decide what it is they wish to change about themselves in group that day. You do not enter a Gouldings's group without a "contract" for your work in group. Group members soon learn that these contracts must be explicit. If a person says they want to "try" to change, Bob Goulding reaches under his chair and begins ringing his famous "try bell." The Gouldings believe you either want to change or you do not. Such a stance prevents what Yalom refers to as the "moviegoers" turning up in group. Individuals do not come to the Gouldings's group to see what show is playing today.

While Yalom's recommendations are not as stringent as the Gouldings's, he accomplishes the same goals. First, the agenda rounds will provide structure, but not too much structure. After all, the group leader does not want a leader-centered group. The aim is to establish a freely interacting group. Too much structure will prevent free interaction between the group members and will encourage the group members to become dependent on the leader for direction and guidance. Too little structure promotes regression and wastes important group time as the members stumble around aimlessly trying to establish some direction for the group.

Second, the agenda rounds provide some contact with each member, although it may be brief and nondirected. This at least gives the group leader a "reading" of each member's emotional state at the beginning of group. Third, the leader's use of a structured opening to group gives the clear message that activity and participation are expected of each individual. A group member who repeatedly fails to come up with an agenda meeting after meeting needs to be assessed carefully by the group leader.

Group members need to be taught how to utilize the agenda rounds. A basic task of the group leader is to help each member formulate realistic agendas. The structure of the agenda can be very loose or it can be very specific. Yalom suggests the agenda be stated in a way that individuals identify some personal aspect of themselves that can be realistically attained within a single group setting. Yalom also feels that agendas are much more effective when they are channeled into interpersonal themes so they can be worked on in the here and now of the group process. It is not necessary for the group leader to hold to such a rigid format, and Yalom's recommendation reflects his bias toward his belief that the group work be kept in the "here and now." When working with alcoholics and addicts, the "there and then" can be as important and have as much significance for their recovery as the "here and now." Consequently, it is recommended that the group leader structure his or her agenda rounds in a style that Yalom recommends; the group leader must remain aware, however, that recently detoxified alcoholics or addicts may be capable of little more than following instructions. It may be best not to require them to come up with too elaborate a scheme or plan. In the wisdom of AA, "keeping it simple" may be best for them until they have had more time to stabilize.

For instance, the group leader might start his or her group off by stating,

> It's time to start group today. I'd like to start with an agenda round. Would each of you introduce yourself, say a little about how you are feeling and if there is anything you would like to talk about in group today. Who wants to go first?

At this point, rather than call on someone to speak first or direct the order of responses from the group members, the group leader should sit quietly. With this opening statement, the group leader has provided enough structure to get the group started and would be over-controlling if he or she proceeded to pick members to respond in turn. Usually the members will take up the direction at this point. It is rare for a group to sit in silence for very long with such a structured opening. If the silence goes on for more than five minutes, the group leader should avoid "picking" someone to start. Rather, it would be best to comment on the group's difficulty and wonder aloud why no one wants to start.

The example illustrates that the group leader's opening statement can be short and simple. If there are brand new members in the group on that day or it is the very first meeting of the group, the group leader may want to explain the purpose of the agenda rounds in more detail. For instance, the group leader could add to the opening instructions by saying,

> There are no restrictions on your topics in group. You may want to specifically work on some behavior you want to change or you just may want to take some time to report to the group how you are feeling. Sometimes, some group members want feedback from other members. At other times, people may have something left over from the previous group that they want to discuss further.

Formulating agendas can be difficult for many patients. One danger inherent in leaving the agenda vague is that the psychotherapy group can itself become vague or turn into a quasi-AA meeting. This is not to imply that AA meetings are bad, just that psychotherapy groups serve a different purpose and that it is the group leader's task to ensure that the purpose of the group is fulfilled. This requires that the group leader help the group members formulate their agendas. In one sense, it is the group leader's job to teach the group members how to think in specific and clear terms when it comes to utilizing the therapy group. The group members must come to realize the group is a unique form of treatment that serves a distinctly different purpose from that of AA, educational lectures, and discussion groups. This is especially important as patients begin to stabilize and their thinking clears to the point that they can meet Yalom's criteria for establishing realistic and "doable" agendas.

Yalom addresses this issue when he writes,

> The formulation of an agenda is not an effortless, automatic task. Patients do not do it easily, and the therapist must devote considerable effort to help them in this task.
>
> For one thing, the great majority of patients have considerable difficulty understanding precisely *what* the therapist wants and *why*. The task must be explained to patients simply and lucidly. The therapist may give examples of possible agendas and painstakingly help each member shape his or her own. The therapist must also explain to patients *why* he or she wants an agenda by stating the advantages of the agenda format.

> Agenda formation requires three steps, and the therapist must escort most patients, especially in their first meeting, through each of the three steps:
>
> 1. The patient must identify some important personal aspect that he or she wishes to change. Moreover, the task must be realistic; that is, the aspect must be amenable to change and appropriate for a group therapy approach.
>
> 2. The patient must attempt to shape his or her complaint into interpersonal terms.
>
> 3. The patient must transform that interpersonal complaint into one that has here-and-now ramifications. (1983, pp. 216-217)

Usually, most problems with agenda rounds concern the group members' tendency to state their agendas in a vague and overly generalized manner. For instance, a group member may give his agenda in the following way: "I'm depressed and I want to stop being depressed." As Yalom states, this is a useless agenda because it is a task that cannot be accomplished in one single meeting. The Gouldings suggest in their contract work that the group member start with small specific behavior changes that can be reasonably and successfully attained. They recommend building slowly on small successes and eventually graduating to more difficult tasks after members have begun to restore their confidence in their ability to change. Accepting a contract such as, "I want to be happy forever" is doomed to failure and is a set-up for both the group leader and the group member. In response to the group member who wants to stop being depressed, the group leader could say the following:

> Listen, Jim, I understand that this is a very important agenda for you because your depression has been very painful and incapacitating in the past. However, I wonder how realistic this is for you. You've been depressed for years and I doubt if you could change that in one session. As you've stated before, you can be very impatient and I'm concerned that this may be an example of you wanting too much too soon. One reason for your depression is your isolation. You've complained of not having friends and how this sense of loneliness leads both to your drinking and depression. Would you be willing to look at how you isolate yourself here in group? What is it about yourself that shuts off contact with others, even here in group? I would like to suggest you explore this issue in group as a means to understanding how this may contribute to your depression.

In this example, the group leader has moved the group member from the global to the specific. He has been gentle, but persistent in his efforts to get the group member to make a commitment to focus his agenda so it applies to interpersonal terms in the "here and now."

Examples of good clear agendas include:

1. I'm lonely. I want to change that.
2. I want to communicate with others.
3. I want feedback on how others perceive me.
4. I don't trust easily. I want to change that.

DIFFICULTIES WITH AGENDA ROUNDS

Each of the above examples of good, clear agendas can be easily turned into interpersonal here and now work. Unfortunately, not all group members are so concise and quick to formulate their agendas in such nice and neat packages. The biggest difficulty novice group leaders have with agenda rounds is their inability to contain their agenda round to ten or fifteen minutes. Each agenda, if properly conducted, should only take each member one to two minutes to relate. Before they are aware of it, group leaders often discover their entire group session has been consumed by the agenda round, or worse, they have only gotten around to half the group. Frequently, if a group member starts to demonstrate strong affect during his or her opening agenda statement, the group leader will find it difficult to move beyond that person for fear that this will disrupt or disturb the individual's sharing and openness. Group leaders should never allow themselves to be tied down to any technique, but most group members will respond to a gentle disruption. For example, the group leader might say,

> It's obvious, Mary, that this is a very important and painful topic for you. I'd like to stop you here for a minute and ask that you take some time in group today to talk about this further. I'm going to finish the agenda round first. Would you agree to make a commitment to talk about this when the agenda round is completed?

With this response, the group leader has maintained the integrity of the structure of the group without compromising a particular group member. Further, the group leader has acknowledged the importance of this issue and has gotten a firm commitment from the group member that she will pursue the topic after the agenda round is completed.

THE SPECIAL CIRCUMSTANCES OF INPATIENT THERAPY GROUPS WITHIN THE HOSPITAL

Inpatient treatment involves much more than the proper clinical management of the group, its members, and the group dynamics. Because inpatient therapy groups are conducted in a treatment facility that has many different components to its treatment program and these different components have a vast array of objectives and multiple associated personnel, it is necessary for the therapy group to adapt to fit within the total treatment picture. In outpatient groups, the boundary between the group and the outside world is typically distinct and clearly drawn. With inpatient groups, however, these boundaries are not as clear and are more diffuse. The inpatient group is a subsystem within the larger system of the hospital unit and the team approach to treatment. The blurring of boundaries between the group and many other hospital activities can be a source of added difficulty for the group leader. Management of these boundary issues is therefore of extreme importance to successful inpatient group treatment. If this were not the case, this chapter could end here and the group leader would only have to concern himself with the direct clinical issues presented so far. However, the hospital setting and the team approach require the group leader and the rest of the staff to work in concert with each other. If this is not successfully accomplished, the results could be disastrous for the patient. An extreme example of this would be a case where part of the staff requires total abstinence as the goal of treatment while a few others secretly advocate controlled drinking.

Vannicelli (1982) responds to these issues in describing the special difficulties alcoholics present in group therapy. In order for these difficulties to be managed on the inpatient unit, she recommends that six key issues be addressed:

> Our leaders are encouraged, however, to remain mindful throughout of some subtle differences between the defensive styles of alcoholics and neurotics and how these differences influence their relationship to the group. More specifically, we remain sensitive to the fact that alcoholics have well-developed skills for evading limits and for shifting or diffusing the focus. In contrast to working with neurotic patients, whose more focused anxieties provide motivation and direction for therapeutic work, the intense but diffuse discomfort of alcoholics does not perform these functions. In fact, quite often their diffuse defenses make working in therapy groups quite difficult. Thus, it falls to the leader to provide limits and focus in the group. To do this he needs to be able to intervene without generating more

> anxiety than necessary–a task which is considerably facilitated when the leader has knowledge of, and feels prepared to handle, the frequent trouble spots in alcoholic groups.
>
> There are six key issues which need advance thought so that the leaders will be prepared to respond in an unchallenging but firm manner. (pp. 19-20)

Vannicelli's six key issues are:

1. Group leaders must be prepared to respond to challenges to disclose information about their own drinking and drug abuse.
2. The patient's contract with the group and the group's contract with the hospital.
3. Confusion may occur regarding group expectations when members belong to other kinds of groups (AA, education groups, etc.).
4. Special problems arise concerning confidentiality because of the frequency of communication between the group leader and outsiders (other than staff, other patients, employers, family, etc.)
5. Active outreach by the group leader to provide intervention if needed.
6. Group defensive maneuvers regarding the drinking time and (for aftercare groups) abstinence and its consequences on the group when a member relapses.

LEADER'S TRANSPARENCY ABOUT ALCOHOL AND DRUG USE

Vannicelli warns that group leaders can expect questions about their own alcohol and drug use. Rather than avoid the question or answer it simply without questioning the underlying reasons for it being asked, group leaders need to explore the motives behind the patients' curiosity. For Vannicelli, this curiosity always translates into the implied concern of, "Will you be able to understand or help me?" The answer, of course, is a double-edged sword. If the group leader does not drink or do drugs, the members may wonder how the therapist could possibly understand their condition. If the group leader drinks at times (I will not repeat my stance regarding therapists who use drugs and work with alcoholics or addicts other than to refer to my sentiments in Chapter 9 and advise that they not work with such patients) and admits this to the members they are also likely to wonder if a person who can drink controllably will be able to be of help to them. A group leader who is recovering him- or herself may be a source of comfort for some members and suspect to others since the therapist is "not a professional, but just another recovering addict like myself."

A satisfactory response to such a question might be as follows:

> My guess is that you ask because you wonder if I'll be able to help and understand since I have (or don't have) the same problem. Could you say more about your concerns and has there been anyone else in your past who didn't understand?

Transparency about drinking and drug use has important implications for treatment. But, the issue is not limited to this subject. Yalom feels that a group leader should do more self-disclosure in an inpatient group. Many of the restrictions of the therapist's transparency that were outlined in Chapter 4 on outpatient group therapy also apply to inpatient groups. Self-disclosure on the leader's part is most appropriate when it helps facilitate the attainment of therapy goals. Transparency should be used in the service of providing support, acceptance, and encouragement. It is not the task of the group leader to manufacture positive feelings, but to locate and identify such reactions to patients through selective self-disclosure. A patient in need of support and help does not benefit from a group leader who manufactures false feelings or expresses distrust or anger toward the patient.

THE GROUP CONTRACT

In working with inpatient A&D groups, it is helpful to think of the group contract as having three major components. The first concerns the issue of abstinence. Certainly, this is a goal that is clearly advocated by AA and is a theme that runs continuously through this book. The second and third components of the contract concern the special circumstances involved in inpatient groups and are derived from recommendations made by Rice and Rutan (1981).

Vannicelli sums up the importance of the group norm of abstinence when she writes,

> The group norm regarding drinking should be made explicit as part of the initial group contract and should indicate that all members will be working toward abstinence and that any difficulties encountered in working toward this goal (in the form of either fears about drinking or actual drinking) will be discussed with the group. The

> importance of a set of shared norms about what it means to be working on one's drinking problem should not be underestimated. Although there is some disagreement about whether abstinence is the only appropriate goal for alcoholics, mixing patients with divergent goals in the same group poses an almost insurmountable challenge to the integrity of the group. Since the group members do not share a notion of what it means to get better, they find themselves at an impasse in terms of either helping one another to get there or assessing how they are doing. Furthermore, since the wish of nearly every recovering alcoholic is that he may some day be able to drink again, the presence of a member in the group who is acting on this wish may well arouse anxiety that is dealt with by means of unproductive and extreme proselytizing (in support of AA, abstinence, etc.). (1982, p. 29)

Inside and Outside Group Contracts

Rice and Rutan (1981) view the contract as a container for the group boundaries. Having clear and specific boundaries will ensure that the members of the inpatient group will profit more from their treatment. The contract will determine who will be in the group and for how long. It also determines how this material is used both inside and outside of the group.

Inside Contract

This is the contract made between the group leader and its members.

1. All group members will attend each session, be on time, and stay for the entire group.
2. Confidentiality between patients will be honored. Information shared within the group will not be given to patients outside the group by the other group members.
3. Group members will not subgroup. Information shared outside of group among group members in between group sessions most be brought back into group and talked about.

Outside Contract

The outside contract is the contract made between the group leader and the hospital or unit director. Specifically, it has to do with the relationship of the hospital treatment program to the treatment provided by the group. The agreement should include:

1. Group therapy will be congruent with the overall treatment program of the unit or hospital.
2. Group therapy will be recognized as a primary mode of treatment and not given a secondary status to other types of therapies.
3. The group boundaries will be respected by all staff members and patients. Group sessions and time will not be violated either by staff members entering uninvited or patients being called out indiscriminately for other appointments.

SIMULTANEOUS MEMBERSHIP IN OTHER GROUPS

Recovering alcoholics and addicts are likely to be members in a number of different groups simultaneously. Not only will they attend or interact in AA meetings that are held outside of the hospital, either before, during, or after their inpatient treatment, they will attend a vast number of different task-oriented and education groups while in the hospital, which will put them in repeated contact with group members in group formats having distinctly different orientations and objectives from that of the therapy group. This creates two distinctly different, yet very important obstacles that the group leader must overcome. First, the group leader will discover it will be impossible to prevent group members from having out-of-group contact. Most contemporary forms of outpatient group therapy recommend that out-of-group socializing between group members be discouraged. However, this rule will be difficult to enforce because recovering alcoholics and addicts frequently have a simultaneous dual membership in both AA and the therapy group. Beyond the uncontrollable reality of the situation, it may not be as damaging as many clinicians believe. Certainly, it should not be actively encouraged, and the possible hazards resulting from the mixing of therapeutic and social relationships should be carefully discussed and understood. Sexual contact between group members should be explicitly forbidden, of course. However, making all forms of socializing taboo often promotes acting out or forces the members either to hide their planned encounters or keep chance meetings secret from the group. Rather than set up questionable objections to out-of-group socializing, it would be better if the group leader encouraged the group members to agree to always talk with the group about any out-of-group exchange that may have taken place between group members. Whatever happens between two or more members outside of group should always be shared within the group. Vannicelli sums up this position when she writes,

> It is also common that members of the therapy group may belong to the same AA group. Thus, it is impractical (and not desirable) to try to limit group members' activities with one another outside of the group. However, since in a group of alcoholics, as in any group, it is desirable to keep as much of the group energy as possible within the group, patients should be encouraged to discuss with the group any "relevant" content that comes up outside. Although the word "relevant" is somewhat vague, and different patients will surely interpret it in different ways, there should be a shared understanding that if the outside-of-group contact exceeds the usual socializing at AA meetings, it should be discussed with the group. It is sometimes helpful to give patients concrete examples. (For instance, if two group members find themselves talking to one another about another member or about what happened in the group; if two or more group members find themselves socializing extensively; or if two patients find themselves having a "special" liaison.) Discussion with patients around these examples should help clarify that important business or relationships that go on outside and are not discussed with the group rob the group as a whole of the opportunity to explore these matters and rob the patients involved of the opportunity to get valuable feedback from other members. Equally important, the outside-of-group business that does not get talked about in group takes on the character of "special secrets," the existence of which runs counter to the group's shared goal of mutual openness and trust. (1982, p. 24)

Simultaneous participation in multiple groups that have prescribed expectations, goals, and ground rules that differ from those of a therapy group can create special problems for the group leader on an inpatient unit. Participation in groups that have either a substantially didactic component to them, such as education groups, or a more structural and supportive component, such as AA groups, is likely to create some confusion for individuals when they enter a more unstructured group therapy setting that offers little didactic information. It will be important for the group leader to clarify the difference between the therapy group and other types of groups patients may have to attend while in the hospital. The recommendations of Brix on the use of "A" and "B" level groups, which were cited early in the chapter, and the pre-group preparation conducted along the guidelines recommended in Chapter 3, are some excellent ways this difficulty can be avoided or corrected.

Specifically, the group members should be told about the complementary nature of AA and group. AA is to be used primarily to help them stop drinking. Group therapy is to help them learn new ways of coping and responding in their interpersonal relationships. While these two modalities are not mutually exclusive, patients must realize that what is required of them in group is far different than what is required of them in AA. For instance, they can go to AA meetings whenever they want to. In fact, they are often encouraged by "senior" AA members to sit passively and just listen at the beginning of their involvement in AA. Group therapy, on the other hand, requires that group members be there every session and be on time. They must be willing to be actively involved in the group process and realize there will be less structured guidance. Unlike education groups, they must be made aware that the information will not be given to them in a structured format. If group members do not fully understand that they are required to take a more active and responsible role in the therapy group, they may become confused or irritated, leading them to fail to appreciate the full benefits that can be derived from the group therapy experience.

THE SPECIAL PROBLEMS OF CONFIDENTIALITY ON AN INPATIENT UNIT

The rules governing confidentiality and information exchange are more complicated in a therapy group on an inpatient unit. In most contemporary forms of therapy, the patient can be assured that all information shared by the patient will be kept confidential. This is not the case with inpatient therapy groups. Many, if not all, chemically dependent patients are referred for treatment either by their employer, family, or court. Consequently, this often requires that the group leader share information with the referral source, since divorce, continual employment, or incarceration is often contingent upon or mitigated by the patient's participation in treatment and group therapy. In addition, the team approach to inpatient treatment requires that all pertinent information about the patient must be shared with the rest of the treatment staff. In order to avoid feelings of betrayal or deception, the group leader must have a clear contract outlining the limits of confidentiality. The group members must be told in advance that an exchange of information will occur. A signed release should also be obtained.

Of course, a signed release is not needed for the exchange of information that occurs between the group leader and the rest of the inpatient treatment staff. However, group members must explicitly understand that what they share in group will be shared with other members of the treatment team. For instance, they might be instructed in the following manner:

> If the co-leader or I feel that something we learn about you in group is important to your treatment and recovery, we will share this information with the rest of the staff. It is important to understand we are all equally involved in your treatment here at the hospital, and it has been our experience that a team approach is the most successful way to treat addiction. Occasionally, we may have to speak to others outside the hospital, such as your employer, spouse, attorney, or representative from the court. If we do, we will get a signed written release from you and we will avoid, as much as possible, giving them any personal information other than that you are or are not participating and progressing in treatment. After we have spoken with any of these individuals, we will let you know with whom we spoke, why, and what we told them.

Information given to outsiders is not the only source of difficulty plaguing group leaders on an inpatient unit. They must also be prepared to deal with the sticky problem of dealing with information that comes from sources outside of group about the members in group. There are two basic rules for dealing with outside information:

1. Make it a policy that group leaders will keep no secrets and that they will determine how the information will be used based on its clinical relevance. They should also make no promises to family members, friends, or employers that will bind them to some potentially damaging collusion with the informant. Group leaders may indicate that they may decide not to reveal the source of the information unless it is absolutely necessary. However, group leaders should retain the freedom to make this decision without pre-established restrictions.
2. Group leaders should never assume the information is more valid, truthful, or reliable than that supplied by the patient.

When given information about a group member, the group leader should first encourage the patient to talk about this issue on his or her own. Confrontation should only be used as a last resort. For instance, the following vignette illustrates how one group leader dealt with this dilemma:

> Arnold, a thirty-four-year-old alcoholic, had entered treatment after physically attacking his wife while he was in the midst of an

> alcoholic blackout. Since he was much too ashamed to talk about this with the treatment staff or the group, the group leader had to decide how to use the information of physical abuse he had gotten from Arnold's wife during her family assessment interview. As another member in group began to talk about his own difficulties containing his anger while intoxicated, the group leader noticed Arnold's discomfort and said, "It's obvious this brings up some strong and uncomfortable feelings for you, Arnold. I wonder if you share similar feelings of guilt and embarrassment about your anger when you have been intoxicated." This was a mild invitation for Arnold to speak, and it was presented to him in a nonthreatening or nonjudgmental manner. This was enough to help Arnold get through a very difficult issue. If this subject had not been addressed, it would have likely led Arnold to withdraw and hide more from himself and the rest of the group during the next four weeks. Since guilt and denial are such strong contributing factors to relapse, and since the group leader did not have the luxury of waiting weeks, or even months before Arnold felt trusting or safe enough to share this information, it was important to encourage him to open up about this topic. However, the group leader did it in a manner that was not too intrusive and allowed Arnold to maintain his integrity by giving him the opportunity to introduce it himself.

Sometimes, the exchange of information that occurs between a therapist and a patient during a private conversation can be another source of conflict for the group leader. Since most inpatient group leaders see some of their group members individually or in other capacities while they are in the hospital, they may find themselves privileged to information that has not been shared with others on the treatment team. Such a situation can put group leaders in a very compromising situation, especially if they have agreed beforehand to the patient's request to "please keep this information just between the two of us." If group leaders are part of an inpatient treatment team, they must realize that this is one important instance where inpatient treatment differs radically from outpatient treatment. The rules of confidentiality are altered in a team approach to inpatient treatment. Group leaders must never allow themselves to make a personal commitment of confidentiality to a patient on an inpatient unit. For instance, it may be very flattering to hear your favorite group member say to you in private, "I trust you more than anyone here at the hospital. There is something I just wouldn't tell anyone else because I don't think they would understand. But promise that you'll keep what I'm about to say between the two of us." At this point, group leaders should resist the temptation to succumb to such a flattering remark. Instead, it would be better for the group member and the group leader if the leader were to respond to this request in the following manner:

> Wait just a second before you share that with me. I am flattered that you've grown to trust me so much in such a short time and I want to encourage you to share what you're about to talk about. However, I can't promise I won't share this with other members of the treatment team. Now, I may not. But if I think it's important to your recovery and treatment at the hospital, I may have to let others know for your own good. Understand my concern is what is going to be best for you in the long run.

Patients will rarely object to such a stipulation on the therapist's part. If they were to refuse to share their "secret" after the therapist responded in this manner, it is likely that they were either trying to manipulate the therapist or caught up in their own destructive transference distortion. Such a stance by the group leader will keep him or her from contributing to a patient's primitive projections. Since many alcoholics and addicts suffer from primitive character pathology, they will be prone to split the treatment staff into all good or all bad segments. If group leaders carefully monitor their tendency to agree quickly to such requests, it will prevent them from placing themselves in a compromising situation. For instance, what if a patient were to share that he or she had plans to commit suicide this evening, or that he or she knew another patient had smuggled drugs or alcohol onto the unit? How could the group leader not break his or her promise of confidentiality in such a situation?

ACTIVE OUTREACH

Inpatient Alcohol and Drug (A&D) treatment has been made more complicated for the group leader because of two co-existing changes in addiction treatment over the last few years. First, many hospitals require that their inpatient group leaders conduct aftercare groups for those patients who have successfully completed their four- to six-week inpatient programs. Second, because of financial restrictions, more hospitals are now conducting day treatment programs that provide a treatment format very similar to the inpatient program except the patient is allowed to stay at home in the evening or continue to work during the day. In either case, group leaders must adapt and respond to situations that are somewhat unique to an alcohol and drug addiction population. Specifically, they will be required to do a considerable amount of active outreach work because most of their group members will either have a very short, unstable period of sobriety or they will be without the protective confines of a closed hospital unit. Consequently, the group members' sobriety will be much more tentative, and to compensate for this situation, group leaders will be required to do a considerable amount of active intervention, particularly in telephoning and reaching out to delinquent group members. While group leaders of a non-addictive group can afford to slowly explore the reasons why a group member's attendance is irregular or erratic, they cannot take such a leisurely approach with newly recovering addicts and alcoholics. Most contemporary forms of group therapy do not advocate that the group leader actively telephone or question group members if they have missed a therapy group. With a newly recovering alcoholic or addict, such an occurrence or unannounced absence should be interpreted as a warning signal or cry for help. For this reason, instead of waiting for the next session to explore the reasons for the group member's unannounced absence, the group leader must either telephone immediately after group meeting or within the next day. At other times, if a group member has been going through a particularly difficult time and the group member calls to say he or she is not going to be able to make it to group this evening, the group leader should carefully investigate any possible reasons the person might have for avoiding group. Often, with a little prompting or careful questioning, the group member might come to understand his or her reasons for resisting group and respond to the group leader's concern.

Although such an active stance by the group leader has advantages, in that it may prevent a relapse or bring forth unknown resistances to the patient's consciousness, it does place the group leader in a position that may be perceived as too controlling or parental. To minimize this, utilize the other group members to monitor attendance as much as possible. Focus more on the group member's behavior and conduct all interventions in a nonjudgmental style. Outreach delivered in a concerned manner can do much to help group members see the possible destructive overtones to their resistance and avoidance of group.

GROUP MEMBERS WHO RELAPSE AND COME TO GROUP

Because aftercare group and day treatment therapy groups operate outside of the protective confines of a closed hospital unit, the group leader is more likely to be faced with the difficult task of dealing with an active group member who relapses. Relapses, as addressed earlier in this chapter, can be an important learning experience for the alcoholic or addict if they are properly integrated and understood. The only bad relapse is an unexamined one. Not only would it be beneficial to examine the reasons for an individual group member's relapse, but it would also be a valuable learning experience for the other members of the group. It would help them all identify the different stages of relapse. First, it would be important for the group leader to take a position that most veteran AA members take when dealing with an alcoholic's relapse: Do not let individuals who relapse describe their experience as a "slip." This implies their return to drinking was due to something that happened to them. As AA says, "If you don't want to have a slip, don't go where it is slippery." AA members prefer to speak of "slips" as "premeditated drunks." Explore with alcoholics the reasons that lead them to return to their old "slippery ways" and how these patterns can be identified and avoided in the future.

DRINKING AND RELAPSE

The futility of attempting to apply psychotherapy to someone drugged or intoxicated was clearly illustrated in Brown and Yalom's classic study (1977). Although they never clearly resolved or fully addressed this issue, it was apparent that it caused them extreme difficulty. Beyond the detrimental effects of the drop-out rate, the intoxicated patients proved to be most damaging to the group process. In each case (fifteen times during the two-and-a-half year study), the intoxicated member stayed for the entire meeting and dominated the session. The individual captured and held the group's attention in ways that were impossible to ignore. "Members were especially frustrated by the knowledge that the meeting would rapidly vaporize, since the drinking member rarely retained much of the meeting afterward. Members felt the power of the alcohol and an overwhelming feeling of futility about the session" (p. 438).

Part of this difficulty can be explained by a failure of the therapists to recognize that the primary issue which must be dealt with in any treatment of addiction is the issue of drug and alcohol consumption itself. All too frequently, psychotherapists continue to hold the archaic notion that alcoholism is a symptom of some underlying pathology. It is difficult to understand why otherwise intelligent psychotherapists will continue to try to apply a mode of treatment (psychotherapy) built upon a rational foundation to an individual who is drugged into an altered state of consciousness.

Research has shown rather conclusively that learning which takes place during a drug-induced state of consciousness will not generalize to undrugged states (Fischer, 1976). A substantial part of all psychotherapy is the unlearning of old, self-defeating behaviors and the learning of more adaptive behaviors. This process is seriously impaired if a member is intoxicated because change often requires insight, cognitive realignment, and an emotional catharsis. Central to any therapy with alcoholics is the requirement of abstinence from alcohol.

Yalom acknowledged the fact that active drinking generally brought normal positive working forces in the group to a halt. Occasionally, he was able to process and integrate the incident into a form of therapeutic benefit through the use of videotape replay. Sometimes, by utilizing this medium, he was able to dramatically illustrate afterwards, when the group member was sober, how repulsive and self-defeating his or her intoxicated behavior actually appeared to the rest of the group. In each case, Yalom illustrated ways in which therapeutic gain could be derived from what may have seemed at the time the most discouraging therapeutic mishap. This should be the case with any instance of alcoholic relapse. Brown and Yalom (1977) mistakenly claim that AA "nonetheless considers a slip to be an unmitigated catastrophe: a slip is written in indelible ink in the AA member's personal story, differentiating him from those members who have maintained continuous abstinence" (p. 433). On the contrary, AA recognizes a slip as an inevitable process in some alcoholics' recovery. Rather than looking upon it as a catastrophe, relapse should be approached as a learning experience that indicates that the alcoholic is obviously doing something wrong. The task of the group and the therapist at this point is to explore circumstances that may have led to the drinking. Overconfidence, passivity, or old patterns of resentment and anger are common themes that may help other members realize that they too may be committing these same mistakes. Often such a relapse in group can be an extremely beneficial experience for the rest of the members as a whole.

In addressing this problem, Vannicelli lists four common drinking landmarks that can occur within the context of a therapy group:

1. Group members who come to group visibly intoxicated.
2. Group members drinking between sessions and refusing to acknowledge it even when confronted directly.
3. Group members drinking and admitting it, but not wanting to stop.
4. The group member who periodically drinks and continues to endorse the policy of abstinence while the behavior indicates otherwise.

Each situation requires a different strategy for appropriately responding to its unique set of circumstances.

1. Coming to Group Intoxicated

Ask the group member firmly, but politely, to leave the group and return next week. Explain quickly that group members are not allowed in group intoxicated, but that it would be important for them to return to the group. With a more obstinate and difficult individual, ask him politely if he would mind waiting outside. Suggest he have a cup of coffee and cigarette. This might give him a way out; then would allow him to save face in front of the other group members. Send the individual to a nearby AA meeting or call a sober member of AA to come in to speak with him. After the intoxicated member leaves, explore in detail the group's reaction to the incident.

2. Suspected Drug or Alcohol Use Without Acknowledgement

If it is not obvious that the group member is intoxicated, but the group leader has information from an outside informant that he is drinking or doing drugs (i.e., wife, etc.), it would be best to gently confront the group member. Often, invitations to speak about such issues are enough to get the individual started. However, if the group member is insistent that he is sober or clean, it is best not to push the issue. It is rare to have an alcoholic or addict who is using drugs or drinking who will continue to attend a therapy group that has a contract of abstinence. If the aftercare group or day hospital has a contractual agreement for periodic random drug screens, this will often eliminate such difficulties.

3. Continual Admitted Drug and Alcohol Use

After a repeated series of relapses, the group member needs to be evaluated for further supplemental treatment. If alcohol is the problem, Antabuse (disulfiram) should be prescribed. Inpatient hospitalization also needs to be considered. Supplemental individual therapy or increased AA meetings are other ways of adjusting the patient's treatment. If the member decides he does not want to agree to these requirements or openly acknowledges he wants to continue to drink or do drugs, it should be politely, but firmly, explained to him that group is only for those individuals who want to stop using drugs or alcohol. Tell the member a referral can be made to someone who will be able to see him on an individual basis and that he can return to group at any time in the future if he should change his mind. Under no conditions should the group leader try to mix an actively using addict or alcoholic in a group with newly recovering members.

Vannicelli stresses the importance of a solid group contract in order to avoid the possible pitfall associated with each of these problem areas. She writes,

> Effective handling of the last four issues [simultaneous membership in other groups, communication with outsiders, patients who drink, and drinking as a group focus] all require the presence of an explicit treatment contract that clarifies what will be expected of group members (and what they, in turn, can expect). This explicit agreement with the patient ideally will be laid out in a pre-group interview in which each of the ground rules will be stated. The rules should include the following: (1) a statement regarding minimum tenure in the group (e.g., we expect members to make a commitment of at least 3 months); (2) expectations of regular and timely attendance and advance notice when a patient absolutely must be late or away (and an indication whether the patient will be charged or not for missed meetings); (3) need for advance notice to the group if the patient is considering leaving; (4) commitment to abstinence and willingness to talk about fears of drinking or actual slips should they occur; (5) commitment to talk about other important issues in the patient's life that cause difficulty in relating to others or in living life fully; (6) commitment to talk about what is going on in the group itself as a way of better understanding one's own interpersonal dynamics; (7) specifics of the limits regarding outside-of-group contacts between group members (or requirements for bringing back into the group relevant material that comes up outside, or both); and (8) the nature and extent of communications between group leaders and outsiders. (1982, pp. 36-37)

SUMMARY RECOMMENDATIONS FOR INPATIENT GROUP THERAPY

Unlike most other forms of contemporary group treatment, inpatient group therapy with alcohol- and drug-abusing patients involves the simultaneous management of three diverse influences on the patient's treatment process. First, there are the neurological deficits commonly seen with most newly recovering alcoholics and addicts. Second, there are the more typical clinical management issues that confront any group leader who is leading a group on an inpatient unit. As Yalom outlines, these clinical difficulties are made more problematic by the special circumstances surrounding inpatient treatment. Third, because group therapy is a subsystem within a larger hospital system, the group leader must be able to negotiate the common difficulties that arise any time a subsystem has to exist within a larger suprasystem. Specifically, this problem usually manifests itself with group leaders who find themselves part of a treatment team. The usual principles for a therapy group are compromised by the special dynamics of the team approach to treatment. All three of these diverse influences–neurological impairment, clinical management, and the treatment team approach–must be brought together in a united, complementary effort if group leaders are to provide a beneficial treatment experience for their group members. The goals of group and treatment on an inpatient unit need to be adapted to fit these circumstances. Specifically, the therapy group must be complementary to the patient's overall treatment experience. If the therapy group is at odds with the goals of the rest of the inpatient treatment program, the patient's chance of successful recovery will be greatly diminished. Mueller, Suffer, and Pregaman (1982) identify and summarize eight important goals that must be achieved by patients during their hospitalization.

1. Have the patient identify where alcohol and drugs are in his life in terms of losses suffered due to drinking–(i.e., family, job, monetary, health, self-respect, legal, spiritual).
2. Individually tailor each treatment plan in terms of aiding each patient to identify the individual goals for his treatment.
3. Have the patient realize that being an alcoholic or addict means never being able to drink or use drugs again.
4. Have patient recognize alternatives to drinking and identify what he needs to do to stay sober (i.e., attend AA, outpatient groups, etc.).
5. Whenever possible, involve the patient's social-emotional support system in treatment–family, friends, AA sponsor, employer.
6. Provide a treatment experience whereby the patient feels valued by both staff and other patients through interaction, acceptance, and "permission giving" to experience and express feelings.
7. Educate the alcoholic and addict about the disease of alcoholism and addiction.
8. Provide a sober environment in which he can obtain treatment. This will involve both AA and ongoing outpatient groups. Particularly the

> inpatient group therapy experience will make the patient more receptive to continual outpatient group therapy. (p. 940)

The group leader's task is to lead the group members through these goals. Berger (1983) outlines this sequence when he writes,

> First, the therapist should increase the patient's motivation for sobriety by exploring the deleterious effect alcohol has had on his life, using a here-and-now emphasis, and avoiding the trap of looking with the patient for underlying causes of his drinking. The therapist should gently confront the patient's defenses (such as denial, projection, and grandiosity), and help him take responsibility for his actions, including the alcoholism. Furthermore, the therapist may have to deal with the patient's fantasy that one day he will be able to return to social drinking.
>
> Second, the therapist must help the patient learn to readjust to life without alcohol. He must learn to fill his time constructively, with alcohol no longer a central part of his life. Simultaneously, the therapist may optimize the alcoholic's chances for sobriety by suggesting family education sessions, encouraging him to attend AA meetings, and judiciously using disulfiram to minimize impulsive drinking. (p. 1043)

Through this tailored treatment process, the support systems that have enabled the patient's drinking and drug use must be cut off. Unlike techniques of most contemporary and traditional forms of group therapy, addicts and alcoholics must not be encouraged during the initial stages of treatment to look introspectively within themselves for strength or self-understanding. Rather, they should be encouraged by confrontation and life review to look at their failures so that their initial pain is intensified. This requires that the group leader not be conned by tangential discussions of coexisting internal conflicts. Alcoholics and addicts must not be allowed to escape from the paradox that their drinking and drug use is the problem. They must instead take responsibility for this. However, they must learn that within themselves, there lies no defense against their desire to use or drink. In short, they must learn they cannot drink and use drugs, but that they alone cannot quit drinking and using drugs. This position pressures alcoholics or addicts into hopelessness in themselves and their old support systems. They are then asked to accept guidance, help, and control from a source outside of themselves. Paradoxically, they are given no alternative. This combats their grandiose self-centeredness and isolation. Eventually, through AA and the therapy group, they must learn that others with whom they can identify are the new source of hope and strength.

Chapter 11

Late Stage Treatment Issues

Late stage treatment concerns with the addicted individuals will be dominated by two distinct issues that are related and closely intertwined throughout all phases of the treatment process. Foremost is the need to ensure abstinence while simultaneously addressing the need to bring about characterological change in addicted patients. As treatment progresses and as the individuals are able to put more time between the present and their last use of a substance, more emphasis must be gradually shifted to addressing the characterological features that usually dominate addicts' and alcoholics' personality makeup. Within the twelve-step treatment community, these two issues are often categorized under the rubric of relapse prevention and the removal of character defects. AA and other twelve-step programs have long recognized and intuitively known that if healthy sobriety is to be achieved and maintained, it requires the alleviation, modification, or removal of personality characteristics that are incompatible with recovery. From AA's perspective, the removal of character defects is essential if addicts or alcoholics are ever to obtain the only true aim of recovery, which is serenity. Long-term recovery from addiction requires much more than just stopping the use of alcohol and drugs. It requires "working the steps of the program" or employing some other viable alternative so that individuals can alter their basic character. Unless this is accomplished, they will stay as miserable as they were when they were using drugs or drinking. In such cases, a relapse is inevitable; the alcoholic or addict is a time bomb waiting to go off. "White-knuckled sobriety" leaves the person angry, dissatisfied, and miserable. AA views such an individual as essentially unchanged, "a dry drunk" who has only given up the use of chemicals, but whose personality or character remains unaltered. AA is well aware of the paradoxical dilemma that abstinence and long-term recovery cannot be maintained without the "removal of character defects," and that character defects cannot be altered or modified until abstinence is first achieved.

Group psychotherapy at this stage of the alcoholic's or addict's treatment becomes a much less restricted or rigidly structured treatment application than it was during the early and middle stages of treatment. Previously, concerns about modulating anxiety, regression, and hostility dominated the group leader's approach because the addicted individual's recovery and emotional stability were so fragile. Every intervention and application of technique had to be constantly weighed by the consideration of whether the therapist's actions might provoke addicted patients to return to old patterns of coping if they were emotionally stimulated too quickly or with too much intensity. Emphasis had to be placed instead on the addicts' or alcoholics' acculturation into the twelve-step community of recovery and their acceptance of the identification as an alcoholic or addict. While concerns about relapse always dominate treatment strategies from the very beginning of treatment, the focus of these concerns shifts during the later stages of recovery when individuals begin to achieve more sobriety, stability, and abstinence. No longer are alcoholics or addicts cautioned not to feel too much or open their emotions up too quickly (i.e., turn it over, one day at a time, etc.); they are now confronted with the realization that if they do not eventually deal with these emotional issues and conflicts that dominate their life, they are putting themselves in danger of a relapse.

Long-term treatment of the addict or alcoholic ultimately requires the treatment of the individual's character. Whether this takes the form of a personality disorder or a more benign manifestation of a deeply ingrained habitual pattern of dysfunctional behavior shaped in large part by the assault of chemicals on the patient's mind and body, this area of his or her life must be treated aggressively. For this reason, group therapy becomes even more of a crucial component of the recovery process. As clinicians and researchers are finding out, not only is group therapy the treatment of choice for addiction, it is also the treatment of choice for character disorders (Alonso and Rutan, 1993; Klein et al., 1991, Leszcz, 1989). Adaptations of technique for long-term treatment dominate the group therapy approach at this stage of recovery. As any well-trained clinician knows, character disorders do not respond to quick fixes and short-term strategies. In a similar fashion, relapse prevention is recognized as a lifelong process and overconfidence is one of the warning signs that the old narcissistic patterns of arrogance and specialness are returning. AA members, for instance, have long recognized that it is a short step from "I have this problem licked" to "I can have a drink every now and then" to "I can't be an alcoholic because I am different" to "I am special and unique and not like them." Humility and acceptance of oneself as limited is the antidote to the addictive lifestyle beliefs and attitudes that dominate the active alcoholic and addict. Successful long-term addiction treatment requires maintaining a delicate balance between chemically dependent individuals' primary defensive character (grandiose, narcissistic, and obsessive-compulsive features) and the feelings of shame and worthlessness that dominate their internal emotional life. The group leader must stay acutely aware that a relapse is potentially near anytime addicts or alcoholics sway too far to either end of these two poles (grandiosity and shame). When addicted individuals feel *too good* or *too bad,* their relapse potential is at its most crucial fragility. The art of long-term treatment for addicted individuals is the therapist's ability to help them maintain a fluid and finely tuned balance between these two extreme positions.

PARADIGM SHIFT

The long-term treatment of the chemically dependent person in group requires a paradigm shift from the typical medical model and more traditional forms of individual and group psychotherapy that are often utilized when treating the non-addicted patient. The relationship between character pathology and addiction is becoming better understood and more frequently identified as the schism between psychiatry and addiction is being slowly resolved. It is now more universally accepted that traditional approaches to the treatment of both addiction and character pathology must be modified if these patients are to be treated successfully. Interpretation and resolving transference, long the two cornerstones of psychodynamic treatment, are now viewed as inadequate in themselves for resolving character pathology and addiction. More and more evidence is being uncovered that in order for character pathology to be altered, patients must internalize and introject new realities, including an internalization of current relationships in the present maturational environment. Since most individual transferences stir up strong feelings of object hunger, dependency, and hostility in these patients, a group format where these feelings can be diffused through part-object gratification and support provides the necessary holding environment for the resolution of transference distortions and the internalization of healthy and more mature, gratifying relationships.

Alonso and Rutan (1993) are two of the more recognized authorities on group psychotherapy who have put forth clearly defined reasons why group therapy is the treatment of choice for character pathology. Following Leo Stones' (1961) critique of the position of the "cadaver model" of the classic stereotype of the analyst, they point out how such a stance "fails to offer any real opportunity for internalization or introjections to follow the interpretation of transference" (p. 441). In a very similar view, Louis Ormont (1992), writing about the pre-oedipal patient, contends that these patients pose special problems because their difficulties are the result of developmental failures that occurred very early in their life before they were able to use words effectively. Ormont correctly points out that such individuals are controlled by their emotions and are prone to emote or act out rather than talk. Such developmentally arrested individuals are prone to use external sources of gratification (i.e., drugs, alcohol, sex, etc.) and do not respond well to words or interpretations. They must be approached and influenced through feelings and actions.

A therapeutic approach influenced by the traditional medical model requiring an identified patient who is expected to dependently trust an authority figure to fix or resolve his or her difficulties simply does not work with addiction or character disorders. Usually these individuals do not feel they have a problem; they see their difficulties as external to themselves; have limited capacities to abide by any rules, including those of the treatment contract; tend to dissipate anxiety by acting out or through abuse of substances; and have notorious difficulties with truly intimate, interpersonal relationships. This last issue makes it extremely difficult for them to tolerate and manage a therapeutic alliance with any single individual unless attunement is perfectly accomplished. The therapeutic paradox is that even if it would be possible for the therapist to be perfectly attuned, confrontation, frustration, and limit-setting are crucial elements needed in order for chemical use to be stopped and characterological change to be made. Consequently, a group therapy approach based on a paradigm emphasizing interpersonal relationships, mutuality, and a sense of community is the most efficient model that can adequately address all the diverse issues and needs these patients bring with them to treatment.

Reviewing the theory of pre-oedipal or character pathology, Alonso and Rutan (1993) identify five main areas of common difficulties with these patients. Character problems generally are:

1. outside of the patient's awareness,
2. perceived as "that's who I am" when brought into awareness,
3. resistant to change even when the patient wants to change,
4. repeated compulsively until worked through, and
5. difficult to change even with motivation.

Elaborating on these five issues, Alonso and Rutan suggest how group psychotherapy uniquely addresses each of these areas.

1. Helping the patient become aware. Because character traits manifest themselves most prominently in the interpersonal field, group provides a substantial advantage over individual psychotherapy. In group, individuals do not have to talk about their difficulties; they will manifest in the immediacy of the interaction with other group members. Because the group allows individuals to experience themselves as reflected in the mirror of the entire group, there is less reliance on intellect or insight and more awareness of self in relation to the felt, lived experience with others in the group.

2. That's who I am. As Alonso and Rutan point out, "Because character traits are by definition ego-syntonic–that is they generate no particular sense of 'this is not me' in the patient–the undeniability of their presence in the group is often difficult to hear and usually leads to massive mobilization of character defenses" (1993, p. 443). Alonso and Rutan correctly point out that this inevitably leads to intense feelings of exposure and shame. They conclude that this is the first and most crucial obstacle that must be overcome in treatment. As they have written elsewhere (Alonso and Rutan, 1988) and as emphasized in Chapter 7 of this book, AA works because it uniquely addresses this issue of shame. In a similar fashion, Alonso and Rutan see the mutuality of exposure and acceptance, which is only possible in a group format, as the crucial element in the resolution of shame.

3. *I want to change, but I can't.* Alonso and Rutan identify the presence of shame and the threat of exposure as the primary obstacles to character change. Since most patterns of characterological behavior are habitual and established early in a child's life as the result of shame, altering these patterns requires working through the shame. Giving up habits related to earliest object attachments means that individuals will also have to work through the abandonment depression that is closely intertwined with habitual ways of responding to others. Because the alteration of character is so difficult due to the intense shame, rage, and abandonment depression it evokes, the promise of acceptance by a group of peers who are also committed to exposing their own vulnerabilities mitigates the agony of uncovering deep-seated, secret compromises.

4. Here I go again. Since character is by definition habitual, group members will repeat in group the patterns of behavior that contributed to their difficulties and prompted them to need treatment in the first place. Regression and the repetition compulsion dominate the long-term treatment of these patients in group. As Alonso and Rutan point out, because of the diverse possibilities of multiple transference reactions, the group provides for both the amplification of regression and the necessary safety, acceptance, and holding that these individuals need as they work through the repetition compulsion that dominates their lives.

5. Why change? What is in it for me? To give up habitual ways of behaving is painful and difficult. For many individuals, it feels as though they are compromising themselves at the basic level of selling themselves out in order to be accepted by others, and so it is a threat that must be avoided at all costs because it feels like a loss of personal integrity. Once again, it is shame that provides the driving force that prevents the amelioration of envy and other destructive or self-defeating behaviors. As Alonso and Rutan write, "The cohesion that surrounds a therapy group and the need to be included in the cohesive group can override a tenacious resistance to change. The power of the self-help movement attests to the force of that cohesive need" (1993, p. 445).

A GROUP THERAPY PARADIGM FOR THE CONCURRENT TREATMENT OF ADDICTION AND CHARACTER PATHOLOGY

Alcoholics and substance abusers usually do not respond well to passive, emotionally withholding group leaders or to strategies that do not provide emotional gratification, support, and responsiveness. Generally, addicted patients do not handle well the regressive pull that can be experienced in group if the group leader utilizes techniques that are applicable to Tavistock or classic psychodynamic theory as outlined by Bion (1961), Ezriel (1973), or Rice (1965). This is not to imply that the group leader must ensure that the group and its members are gratified in an infantile manner. Not only is this unrealistic, antitherapeutic, and ultimately impossible, it feeds the group members' narcissism and omnipotent expectations of immediate gratification. Rather, establishing a climate of *optimal frustration* provides the delicate balance necessary to ensure that enough of the alcoholics' and substance abusers' dependency needs are met until they are able to gradually internalize control over their own destructive impulses and emotions.

The task of group leaders is to ensure that the group members maintain abstinence while providing them with the opportunity to experience enough anxiety and frustration to promote the emergence of their typical destructive and maladaptive characterological patterns and coping styles. At the same time, enough support and gratification is required to ensure that they will not act out either in group (minimizing destructive transference distortions and pathological projective identification) or outside of group (dropping out of group or returning to alcohol or drug use to help manage painful affect) until they learn how to cope with adversity and stress in a more productive manner.

To attain this end, group leaders must be more active and gratifying than they would be if they were treating non-addicted patients. Yalom's emphasis on cohesion as an important curative factor takes on added significance when working with this population. The creation of a group climate that fosters understanding of self and self in relation to others will help the group members understand the ways that their psychological vulnerabilities can lead to alcohol and drug use and dependence.

In more traditional psychodynamic group psychotherapy utilizing object-relations theory, the group leader's task is to help group members work through the defenses each of them uses as an attempt to manage the anxieties associated with unacceptable or threatening forms of object relations in group. These anxieties are often related to unconscious instinctual drives, and the leader's task is usually to interpret these defenses and anxieties. However, drawing on Kohut (1977b) and the theoretical perspective of self-psychology, it is best to not interpret these anxieties or behaviors as distorted or maladaptive, but to help the alcoholic and substance abuser understand that these reactions are related to and a consequence of unmet developmental needs for self-object responsiveness that are repeated in the here and now interactions of the group. This approach, heavily influenced by self-psychology therapy, is much more supportive and gratifying and less threatening or shameful than traditional approaches to treating vulnerabilities typically manifested by most alcoholics and addicts.

The group leader must remember that an intervention made for a newly recovering alcoholic may be totally inappropriate for an alcoholic with one, two, or even ten years of sobriety. Early interventions need to be directed toward lessening the alcoholic's or substance abuser's denial while avoiding inducing too much negative affect too quickly. Eventually a gradual shift must be initiated requiring chemically dependent individuals to take a cold hard look at their character pathology and the defenses that prevent them from accurately perceiving their self-defeating behavioral patterns (i.e., alcohol and drug use). Eventually they must learn how to cope with interpersonal conflicts without relying on chemicals to self-soothe or regulate affect. There are some unique features in the treatment of alcoholics and addicts in a therapy group that the group leader must be aware of if the possible curative forces available in group are to be harnessed successfully. All of the curative factors (Yalom, 1985) that exist in any well-conducted group will also be available to the competent and well-trained group leader. However, it is important that the group leader emphasize some of these factors more than others. Some of the following curative forces are especially important during the early phase of treatment with alcoholics and substance abusers:

1. Positive peer support and pressure for abstinence from alcohol and drugs;

2. Mutual identification and the opportunity for individuals to learn they are not alone or unique as they struggle with their compulsive obsession with chemicals;
3. The opportunity to better understand their own attitudes and denial of addiction by having the opportunity to confront similar attitudes and defenses in other alcoholics and addicts;
4. Experiential learning and exchange of factual information which conveys that abstinence is always accorded priority, enhancing the patients' acceptance of their identification as an alcoholic or addict;
5. Identification, cohesiveness, hope, and support are provided in a setting that is structured and disciplined, with clearly defined limits and appropriate consequences that help the substance abusers make the proper distinction between what they are responsible for (i.e., taking the first drink) and not responsible for (i.e., the disease of addiction);
6. Chemically dependent individuals are granted the opportunity to become more aware of how their interpersonal characterological style interferes with their ability to establish gratifying, healthy, and intimate relationships with others.

This last issue is especially crucial since it is rare to find substance abusers who do not have either a character disorder or enough character pathology to cause them consistent difficulties in their interpersonal relationships. Difficulties forming and maintaining healthy interpersonal relationships is especially important because the inability to establish healthy relationships is a major contributing factor to relapse and the return to chemical use. As Khantzian, Halliday, and McAuliffe (1990) write, "While it is the drug-taking that initially brings the person to treatment, it is the treatment of character that leads not only to giving up drugs but also to profound change in one's experience of self and the world. . . . Ultimately we view the treatment of character disorder as the road to recovery from addiction" (p. 3).

The treatment of character pathology or deficits in self and psychic structure (Kohut, 1977b) becomes the eventual long-term goal of group psychotherapy for a number of reasons. Kohut and other object-relations theorists view addiction as a condition that results from a person's misguided attempts at self-repair because of deficits in psychic structure. *Vulnerability of the self* is the consequence of developmental failures and early environmental deprivation. Substance abuse, as a reparation attempt, only exacerbates this condition because of physical dependence and further deterioration of existing physiological and psychological structure. Prolonged and chronic stress on existing internal structures leads to exaggerated difficulty in regulation of affect, behavior, and self-care and increased characterological pathology.

Consequently, the addict and alcoholic will always be vulnerable to compulsive, obsessive, and addictive behavior, constantly substituting one addiction (i.e., drugs, alcohol, sex, gambling, work, food, or perversions) for another until the vulnerabilities in self-structure are repaired and restored. Repair and restoration of the self can only be accomplished within a healing and healthy relationship. It is usually necessary to provide the individual with a consistent nurturing, mirroring, and holding environment that can contain and manage negative, destructive impulses while giving the person the opportunity to identify, internalize, and incorporate a healthier set of introjects and internal object representations.

However, once psychic structure is repaired and restored, it can only be maintained if, like any living organism, it is provided an environment where it is continually nurtured, fed, and allowed to flourish and grow. This can only be accomplished if the alcoholics and substance abusers can learn how to maintain and establish healthy intimate interpersonal relationships—outside of the therapeutic milieu. Since relationships can also become compulsive and addictive, the group members need to experience themselves in relationship to others in order to fully understand how they contribute to difficulties within the interpersonal sphere. Until this is accomplished, the continued absence of satisfying and fulfilling relationships in their lives will leave individuals with an internal vacuum, a susceptibility to search for destructive external sources of gratification and sensation (i.e., drugs, sex, food, etc.) to help ward off the painful affect that constantly threatens to overtake them.

LATER STAGE TREATMENT STRATEGIES

Once the group leader has been able to skillfully use the power and leverage of the group to help alcoholics and substance abusers gradually internalize their responsibility for abstinence from alcohol and drugs, he or she must gradually begin to get the group members to recognize the internal factors that have contributed to their propensity to use external factors (i.e., drugs alcohol, sex, food, etc.) as sources of affect regulation and gratification. This requires that group members begin to explore and understand the connection between drug use, their character pathology, and their inability to form healthy, satisfying, intimate relationships. This understanding requires members to take a cold, hard, honest look at their past and their early history of relationships with their family of origin.

Because most alcoholics and substance abusers came from dysfunctional and alcoholic families, unsatisfying and dysfunctional relationships are the norm for them. Much of this is due to their experiences of early childhood deprivation and is fueled by repetition compulsion that drives them to repeat their dysfunctional interpersonal styles over and over again in the present. Consequently, they usually choose poorly, or through the power of projective identification, unconsciously coerce others into behaving and treating them as they have been treated in the past.

It is within the realm of the interpersonal relationships experienced in the here and now of the therapy group that the group members began to get a glimpse of how they contribute to creating their past in the present. As Alonso (1985) says, "Group members don't have to talk about their problems in group, they don't have them!" Through the power of group feedback and support, the group members can begin to identify and become aware of their subtle and not so subtle destructive interpersonal styles.

Members in a mature group, who have been able to put some distance between the present and their last drink or use of chemical are more able to profit and learn from a strategy that focuses on the here and now exchanges between group members. Since increased sobriety and abstinence frees them from their preoccupation with withdrawal and physiological craving, they are able to tolerate an approach that is less gratifying and more demanding. The ultimate aim of group at this point is to help them develop healthy interpersonal skills within the group so that these skills can be generalized and applied outside of group in the "real world." They have to come to understand how to savor, nurture, and establish mutually satisfying relationships without succumbing to the destructive impulses that sabotage them. As Kohut and other object-relations theorists suggest, the group leader needs to help the group members understand that we are all object-seeking creatures from birth and that the drive to form satisfying relationships is innate. As Kohut (1984) suggests, no person ever outgrows his or her need for satisfying relationships, and cure in therapy is obtained when a person can establish healthy relationships outside of the therapeutic milieu.

YALOM'S MODEL AND SELF-PSYCHOLOGY

One of the implications of self-psychology in the treatment of addiction within a group therapy format is the notion that there are often two levels of interaction going on simultaneously in every group member's interpersonal exchange in group. There is an external interaction between members and the people they interact with in the external world. At the same time, there is an internal interaction that is also being experienced and played out in their internal world. Each level of interaction influences the other. The external interaction has an impact on the internal representations of self and object relations, while the internal world of an individual colors, distorts, and influences others in the external world to behave or act in ways that "fit" the individual's projected unconscious expectations. Each level of exchange must be appreciated if the group leader and the members are to fully understand the dynamics occurring for each individual in the group.

While Yalom's interactional model is the best systematic model for understanding and explaining the group members' external behavior, object-relations theory and self-psychology provide the best explanation for understanding the group members' unobservable internal experiences related to the external events occurring in the here and now of the group. The group format is better able to accomplish this task because it provides many key elements that individual therapy cannot provide. Group therapy can more readily do this because it gives substance abusers a far wider array of individuals upon whom they can either depend or direct their anger. By virtue of the number of group members, the group format dilutes the intensity of the feelings that are sure to be activated in any close interpersonal relationship and that have to be worked through if characterological change is to occur. While this process is likely to be too threatening in a one-to-one relationship, the group provides a safer holding environment that gives substance abusers more "space," while permitting them to deal with the intense hostility and ambivalence they are sure to experience as their needs for approval, dependence, and caring surface. Usually, most addicts and alcoholics cannot tolerate the stimulation of "object hunger" or their own dependent yearnings that are activated in individual therapy as well as any in intimate relationships. As Kosseff (1975) outlines, the group can become a kind of "transitional object that protects the patient from the intensity of the fear of dependency on the therapist because this dependency is transferred to the group. The group carries within it a degree of freedom or support which the dyadic relationship cannot provide while at the same time serving as a bulwark against too great feelings of frustration and fear of punishment if he should function autonomously" (p. 237).

A clinical vignette will help illustrate this point.

> Mary, a recovery addict with nearly two years of abstinence, had been progressing nicely in her therapy group, which she had entered shortly after her discharge from an inpatient A&D treatment pro-

> gram. Along with the immediate comfort she was able to establish with the group, she also quickly developed an idealizing transference with her female group leader. Hanging on intently to her every comment, she would revel in any show of attention and support given her by the group leader. Her admiration came to an abrupt end after nearly a year in group when the group leader supported another group member's observation that Mary was intolerant of anyone disagreeing with her. Mary exploded into a rage, screaming she was "sick and tired of people betraying and blaming her," directing most of her anger at the group leader. Attempts at containment and interpretation by the group leader proved futile. However, Mary was able to gain some solace from other group members who expressed their understanding of her feelings because they too had felt similar feelings with others in their lives. Following this emotional explosion, weeks went by where Mary refused to even look at the group leader, much less speak to her. Her only comments during the next two months were mumblings about leaving the group because she "no longer felt safe here." However, Mary had enough of an emotional connection with many of the other group members that she was able to respond to their urging that she stay because they cared for her and would miss her if she left. Consequently, Mary continued to attend the sessions regularly, eventually interacting more and more freely with the rest of the group members, while remaining somewhat cautious and distant from the group leader. Gradually, she was able to engage the group leader and even respond favorably to some of her interventions. Finally, one evening she was telling the group about an argument she had with her female supervisor at work. She looked directly at the group leader and openly confessed, "You know, I think I was distorting her comments and over-reacting just like I did with you a couple of months ago."

No interpretation was required. The group had provided her with a safe holding environment and its group members had given her enough "good objects" to connect with until she was able to work through the intensity of the transference feelings with the group leader who represented the internalized bad-object parental figure. If the group members had not been able to provide enough safety for Mary by their "holding" of her, she would have likely dropped out of therapy or sought previous sources of gratification (alcohol or drugs).

Usually, alcoholics or addicts cannot tolerate the hostility that eventually surfaces in any relationship and consequently leave it feeling threatened by their own anger, abandonment, or retaliation fears. Because the group provides a safer "transitional object" or holding environment, it allows addicts or alcoholics to achieve an appropriate mutually dependent relationship with the other group members without the crippling interference of their own anger, dependency, or fear of intimacy with the therapist. The group helps create a safe space between the substance abusers and the therapist. Eventually, due to their need to please and be with others, they can identify and internalize a more stable set of internal representations modeled after the group leaders and the other members of the group. The group provides an alternative to the destructive drug-using environment that has up to now dominated their lives. The constant availability of the group can also perform a soothing function for members whenever a crisis occurs. Group supplies members with a number of different objects upon whom they can depend or direct their anger and allows them to deal with the ambivalence that comes up for them in their relationships without feeling severely threatened by the loss or closeness of any single relationship.

TREATMENT OF INTERNAL STRUCTURAL DEFICITS

Krystal (1982) disagrees with Kohut's view that the alcoholic's inability to obtain self-soothing gratification can be cured by treatment through the process of "transmuting internalization." In many ways, the fellowship of AA allows this to occur. Krystal disagrees that the alcoholic's and addict's difficulty is related to a deficiency in the self-structure. Krystal feels this problem is due to "an inhibition resulting from a mistaken attribution of these functions to the object rather than the self-representation" (p. 611). He believes these individuals see themselves as victims of childhood deprivation and expect the therapist to supply them with the missing love in the belief that all will be good and well if this is done. Krystal sees the addicts' and alcoholics' stance as follows: "If you love me, you will make me feel good; therefore, as long as everything is not perfect and I do not feel blissful, you do not love me." He also adds that "these patients have terrible resentments about their past, and demand that the therapist roll back the reel of their lives and fix everything retroactively" (p. 611).

Krystal is correct in his assessment of their demands and expectations, but what he fails to appreciate is the reality of their experienced deprivation. Their needs have not been met by a supportive, empathic self-object. This is what drives them to search for what is unavailable and to constantly confirm their view that the world is rejecting and unfair. Krystal believes that this condition is an illusion, supposedly something that these individuals fabricate. Such a stance does not correlate with Mahler's developmental theory, which is essentially a deprivation model. Granted, alcoholics and addicts do distort objects in their world and perceive others as unempathic and ungratifying. This is precisely why therapists who take a nongratifying, nondirective stance provoke such anger and rage in chemically dependent individuals. Such an unempathic stance on the part of the therapist rekindles painful memories of archaic self-objects who have failed them in the past.

Krystal is also correct in pointing out that their expectations are unrealistic and can never be fulfilled or gratified. This is exactly the realization that chemically dependent individuals must come to accept. They must admit their search is futile, and then they must surrender to this realization. In AA terms, they hit bottom. They must then accept the fact that no one can give to them what they want and that they alone are responsible for accomplishing the arduous task of structure-building via internalization of the twelve steps of the AA program. This is why AA and group psychotherapy work while individual therapy frequently fails. AA and the group become substitute self-objects or transitional objects allowing recovering individuals to identify and internalize those aspects they are lacking structurally. Self-object distortions, triggered by too much identification and expectation of one individual, are minimized and the person is given enough time and distance to diffuse the transference distortions. In AA language, "We can do what I couldn't accomplish alone."

Krystal fails to understand all of the ramifications of a child's early experience. When the parents' behavior is rejecting, angry, or persecutory, children, because they are unable to give up the external objects since they need their parents for their survival, cannot change their outer reality because they are too helpless and dependent. They consequently handle the frustration and disappointment by internalizing the loved-hated parent. This is done in an attempt by children to master and control the object in their inner psychic world. This love-hate relationship is repressed and retained as an introjection, a psychological representation of the children's inner world. It is the emotional relationship between the self and the external object that is internalized, not the feelings as such. These introjections become part of the structure of the personality.

The earlier in life this splitting and introjection occurs, the more painful and frustrating the external world becomes. For instance, alcoholics are likely to see others as either all good or all bad. When the all-good objects inevitably disappoint them, they feel enraged at again being deprived. They are either forced to perceive them as all bad to preserve their all-good introjection or feel that they are all bad and undeserving of the good object. They may may have a strong yearning for merger with the good object only to feel trapped and engulfed when they get close, leading them to have to break away. Individuals are perceived only in terms of the alcoholic's introjections or denied split-off traits. Not only are relationships in the outer reality unconsciously interpreted in light of the alcoholic's inner world, resulting in distorted expectations, but the alcoholic engages in an unconscious attempt to force and change close relationships into fitting the internal role models.

If a parent was demeaning and critical, individuals will force others in their external world to change into a critical, demeaning object so that their external reality fits their internal world. The relationship takes on the form of a third entity and becomes introjected. Children grow up demeaned and criticized. As adults, they demean and criticize themselves. In their relationships, they perceive others as demeaning and critical, eventually forcing the others to fit their internal experience of them.

TREATMENT OF INTROJECTIONS

As Kohut has pointed out, the building of psychic structure occurs as infant and parent misunderstand one another's signals and try again to come to a better understanding of each other. The concepts of good-enough mothering and optimal frustration play an important part in the therapist's stance during treatment. It is when the therapist and patient struggle to overcome the obstacles to their relationship and their misunderstanding that maturation takes place and psychic structure is laid. While the most rapid and fundamental features of structuralization take place in the early years of life, development is a process that continues throughout life. The therapeutic task is to walk the line between optimal frustration on the one hand and optimal anxiety on the other hand, with just enough gratification provided to keep the chemically dependent individual from leaving treatment.

Because alcoholics and addicts cannot tolerate technical neutrality, they require a therapist who is active, alive, and who will gratify them on some level. They must be made aware that the therapist cares. However, complete support and gratification will not lead to internalization, correction of introjections and structure-building. It requires empathic understanding first and then conveyance of that understanding to the patient. This requires a therapist and group leader who will face misunderstandings and see that conflicts are resolved. As Basch writes, "It is only unexamined errors that have catastrophic consequences" (1980, p. 101).

Individual therapy usually has little success with alcoholics and addicts. The one-to-one traditional setting evokes too many transference distortions and frequently results in the therapist being frustrated and defeated. Individual therapy, at least during the beginning of recovery, is too threatening for addicts or alcoholics. They cannot tolerate the stimulation of their dependent yearnings, nor can they handle the hostility that will inevitably surface and threaten the continuity of the relationships. Nevertheless, alcoholics and addicts must establish a capacity to relate to others on a meaningful level. They must be helped to achieve an appropriate dependent relationship without the crippling interference of their own hostility and fear of closeness. Only under the sway of their wish to please others and be with others can they identify and achieve a more stable, internalized set of values patterned after the model set by those trying to help them.

How can this potential for healthy relationships be internalized? The group approach and Alcoholics Anonymous is effective for a number of reasons. First, by virtue of the number of group and AA members, it dilutes the intensity of feelings that otherwise inundates the patient in a one-to-one setting. Thus, alcoholics or addicts can spread their attachments to several people. The group offers alcoholics and addicts a way of dealing with the intense hostility and ambivalence in their relationships by supplying them with a number of figures upon whom they can depend or direct their anger. Their fear of closeness, hostility, and dependence is therefore not as severely threatened. Thus, the structure of the group and its relationship to AA permit maintenance of the splitting defense as long as needed. Of similar impact is the response of the group leader, who, by his or her firm yet nonhostile ability to absorb anger, can lay the foundation for later identifications.

The group and AA can also provide an alternative to the alcoholic's and addict's lifestyle in the bars and on the streets. This is an alternative that can supply the need for a transitional object and thereby pave the way for the development of a more stable and adequate sense of object constancy.

This is where the group and the AA program can become the opportune agent of change in the chemically dependent individual's life. Much as the scrap of blanket or teddy bear serves the infant, the group and AA program allows the individual to begin the strenuous business of movement toward autonomy and separation. The group can become the transitional object for addicts and alcoholics who are seeking to emancipate themselves from their symbiotic tie to their drugs and alcohol as well as their self-object.

Kosseff (1975) outlines the transitional qualities of the group in this process of internalization:

1. The group is a tangible representation of the relationship between the patient and the therapist. However, the patient is protected from the

intensity of the dependency on the therapist because it is transferred to the group.

2. The group carries a degree of separation from the therapist and allows the patient a combination of support and freedom that the dyadic relationship did not provide.
3. The group is a bulwark against too great feelings of frustration and fear of punishment if the patient should function autonomously. The group offers its support of other members as an alternative to dependence on one object.
4. The group provides a "space between" the therapist and patients and allows an area of freedom for patients to fill creatively. They can use the group as they choose, relaxing or tightening up their relationships with the therapist and splitting their transferential identification as they need.
5. The group serves as a convoy in the patient's efforts to deal with his or her internalized bad objects.
6. The group as a "good-enough, facilitating environment" substitutes for and also denies the possibility of being controlled by or controlling the therapist.
7. As the patient gives up his or her internal distortions of the therapist, with the help of the group, he or she becomes more able to differentiate reality from distortion. Boundaries between group leader and patient become firmer.
8. The group as transitional object promotes the emergence of the real self and facilitates the mastery of the self as the patient experiments with objects in a new way. Giving and receiving empathy, reassurance, understanding and self-assertion in group leads to freeing of impulses, and capacity for greater closeness emerges.

In summary, the group's value as a transitional object is in its facilitation of the identification process. It helps alcoholics and addicts "(1) shift from a set of internalized split-images of self to a more unitary representation of self by identification with other group members; (2) shift from the part object seen as if it were the whole object (the therapist seen solely as bad object); (3) shift the fears of being engulfed by the group leader to a gradual recognition through other group members that this cannot happen because the group leader is not so powerful and because they, by sharing the leader with the patient, interfere with the patient's longing for fusion" (Kosseff, p. 237). Kosseff (1975) sums up this process when he writes:

> The group helps the patient let go of primitive idealizations of the therapist and his omnipotence by pointing out both the reality and the shortcomings of the therapist. As the patient is able to face these

> less positive attitudes toward the therapist, he is able "to change places" with him and see himself in a more worthwhile light. Where the patient in individual treatment would tend to overlook differences between his view of the therapist and the reality of the therapist, the other group members jar the patient's efforts at continuing pathological identification with the therapist or themselves and force him to acknowledge, and ultimately accept, his differences from others. Where the therapist's relative silence in individual treatment may tend to foster such pathological identification, visible group behavior and interaction force objective recognition of differences. What had been a sealed-off, dead-end identification with the therapist, a giving up of the real object and a substitution of an internalized, possibly idealized object, along with a giving up of the real potentialities of the self in favor of a false compliant self, now gives way to a recognition of the self as good and different from others. As the danger of fusion and immolation with the therapist subsides, the patient develops the hope and possibility of separation and true individuation. (p. 237)

Often after alcoholics have completed treatment, they will want to return for visits, especially when anxious. This is where the lifelong availability of the AA program provides an even clearer illustration of this transitional function. Many individuals have difficulty weaning themselves from the AA program and are likely to seek continual contact with it. They gain continual confidence from the AA activities that win approval of the AA community. In this way, the unfolding of a sense of self-approval, defined as object constancy, can be discerned. What was not completed in childhood may take place later on as the program itself gradually acquires a maternal function, first as a transitional object and later, after individuals have internalized some of values of the program, as the source of object constancy.

The alcoholic's reliance on AA is often judged with concern and suspiciousness by professionals. Some critics of AA express fear that the addict and alcoholic may become too dependent on the program. A common suggestion is to get the individual prepared to "face the world as it really is." From the point of view of the addict's and alcoholic's inner life, the emergence of such dependent behavior signals an important change in a positive direction. It is unfortunate that so many professionals view it as a negative turn of events. It is fortunate that alcoholics become "hooked" on the people in the AA program. Such an occurrence is often the first evidence of the alcoholics' ability to engage in one-to-one relationships, which allows them to accept their need for help and to find new people with whom they can identify. This process takes time. Such individuals do ultimately develop a healthy independence.

Closely related to this principle of healthy dependence on others is the maturation of narcissism as Kohut defines it. Alcoholics and addicts are narcissistically oriented. Their reliance on their grandiose self is manifested within the fabric of values expressed by the drug and alcohol subculture. Thus, there is a need for a principle of treatment that will interfere with the narcissistic fixations of the alcoholic and addict, those that perpetuate lowered self-esteem. There is also a need for a principle of treatment that will facilitate the maturation of healthy narcissism. Thus, treatment should foster an idealized attachment to a program that allows an individual's narcissistic needs to be met in a healthy fashion. It is helpful if the alcoholics and addicts admire the values expressed in the philosophy of the program in which they participate. AA is a useful illustration since its values are so often enthusiastically held and so frequently represent a direct confrontation with the tenets held by the drug and alcohol subcultures. By idealizing the values of their group or AA program, alcoholics and addicts not only become less enamored of drinking and drug use, but they are tempted to allow some dependence upon those they idealize. Since these new objects of admiration are more dependable and far more empathic than their drinking or drug-using friends and earlier parental figures, alcoholics and addicts are more willing to risk relying on another human being. It is within this climate that a sense of hope can be generated, a beginning faith that personal change is possible and that with the help of new objects for identification, a more adaptive patterning of relationships can emerge.

GROUP THERAPY AND ACOA

As group therapists work more and more with alcoholics and substance abusers, they begin to realize that many of their group members have also grown up in homes where one or both of their parents were alcoholic. Eventually, group leaders will begin to discover that an equal quantity of their group members will have a disproportionately high number of spouses and significant others who have also grown up with alcoholic parents. Addiction seems to run in families. If individuals do not become addicted to chemicals themselves, they are likely to become drawn to people who are addicted. Because of the alcoholic's and the substance abuser's likelihood of being exposed to related twelve-step programs patterned after AA (i.e., Adult Children of Alcoholics, Al-Anon, Co-Dependency,) the group leaders will soon discover that much of the jargon and concepts will become intertwined during treatment and recovery. Consequently, it will be important for group leaders to familiarize themselves with the similarities and differences between those ACOA who are addicted and those that are not addicted to chemicals. Each will usually present with a somewhat different set of dynamics requiring different treatment strategies. While alcoholics or addicts who grew up in an alcoholic home will more likely act out their difficulties and manifest more overt character pathology, non-addicted individuals who grew up with alcoholic parents are more likely to act in, hiding their psychopathology from others. Consequently, as children, they are more likely to "look good" and go unnoticed by schoolteachers, counselors, and family therapists. As a result of their learned ability to hide their internal pain and conflicts, they will, as adults, frequently go unnoticed by others in the helping professions.

ADDICTION AND THE FAMILY

Alcoholism and substance abuse is now recognized as a condition or disease that impacts every member of the family (Gitlow, 1973, Jellinek, 1960, Johnson, 1973). Children growing up with an addicted parent are likely to be left with the aftereffects of this experience long after they grow into adults and leave their original family. There is a shared opinion (Brown and Beletsis, 1986; Cermak, 1984; Kristbergh, 1985) that individuals who grow up in an unsafe, chaotic, dysfunctional alcoholic home are prone to develop common symptoms and characteristics as a result of these common experiences. These shared symptoms and characteristics have become popularly known and identified under the general rubic of Adult Children of Alcoholics (ACOA).

Whether ACOA is an accurate diagnostic entity is an assertion currently open to debate. Cermak (1984), for one, feels strongly that it is a label, not a diagnosis, and has made attempts to clear up the overgeneralizations used by many authors who write on this subject. In fact, the literature on ACOA has been dominated by the anecdotal, clinical, impressionistic, and the personal experiences of its authors. Most good empirical research is either lacking or equivocal in its ability to clearly identify a set of traits or characteristics that clearly separates ACOA from other individuals who grow up in non-alcoholic dysfunctional families. However, despite the current lack of solid empirical evidence to support this label, an ever-increasing proportion of the population are identifying themselves as ACOA groups. While there is some disagreement as to whether all ACOA share a common etiology, there is evidence to support the possibility that many, if not most, individuals who have grown up in an alcoholic home will share a very similar chaotic experience that often leaves them with a similar distorted sense of self and others.

At times, it can appear that it is almost a tautology to describe an alcoholic home as dysfunctional. The two cannot be separate from each other when speaking of the impact of alcoholism. To grow up in an alcoholic family is equivalent to growing up in a dysfunctional family system. It is important to remember that it is not the alcohol or its consumption that disrupts the family system, it is the pathological behavior and erratic emotional displays of the alcoholic parents that lead to the development of characteristics within the child that are commonly referred to as ACOA traits.

There are many confounding variables (e.g., age of the child at the onset of parental alcoholism, number of other siblings in family, position of the child in the birth order, availability of surrogate parents, one or both parents having alcoholism, etc.) that must be carefully assessed before one can accurately state that all individuals who grew up in an alcoholic home will have the same characteristics. It is probably more accurate to say that growing up in a dysfunctional alcoholic family system is going to produce certain types of psychopathology in most people, and that as a result of this common psychopathological experience, many individuals are going to emerge with similar personality styles and traits.

Recent research by Jarmas and Kazak (1990) revealed some empirical evidence that supported previous clinical impressions of ACOA. Using Blatt's (1974) developmental model, ACOA were found to exhibit greater *introjective depression* than non-ACOA. In contrast to anaclitic depression, introjective depression involves more feelings of guilt, inferiority, worthlessness, and a sense of having failed to meet expectations. Jarmas and Kazak write,

> Blatt's developmental model hypothesized that introjective depression develops when a child internalizes parental images (i.e., object representations) that are fragmented and ambivalent and when the child cannot resolve contradictions among these disparate images. Apprehensive about losing parental love and acceptance, such a child may experience excessive self-criticism and guilt as a way of maintaining emotional contact with its internalized parent. (1990, p. 245)

COMMON IDENTIFIED CHARACTERISTICS OF ACOA

Understanding ACOA can be accomplished best if their most common identified characteristics are placed within an object-relations developmental framework (Bowlby, 1980; Mahler, 1979; Wood, 1987). The most common characteristics identified in reviewing the literature on this subject are the following:

1. ACOA are compulsive caretakers whose self-worth is disportionately reflected by their need to maintain control and their determination to be overly responsible for others.
2. ACOA are shame-dominated individuals who go to extreme lengths to look good, act right, and avoid drawing attention to themselves.
3. ACOA lack a stable sense of self and are likely to be compliant, adaptive, and chameleon-like in their relationships with others.

Compliance in Group

Leading a group composed entirely of ACOA will pose some unique difficulties for the group leader. Foremost among these will be the ACOA's propensity to feel, act, and behave in a manner that is reflective of how they perceive the group leader wants them to feel, act, or behave. Because they have had to develop a hypervigilance in determining the sobriety and mood of an alcoholic parent, they are extremely skilled in picking up subtle cues from others and using these cues to dictate their actions, behavior, and statements. Along with their compliant, adaptive, and chameleon-like qualities is their deep fear of shame at the thought of exposing their feelings. A lifetime of learning how to hide their feelings, behaving appropriately, and controlling their actions will leave the group leader with a very polite, dependent, frightened, and compliant group that will go to great lengths not to hurt or upset anyone, especially the group leader. Exacerbating this process will be the tendency of ACOA to diffuse any affect by overutilizing labels and slogans they have learned in twelve-step programs. Vannicelli (1991) encourages the group leader to help the ACOA explore their use of labels in defining themselves by requiring them to be specific when describing their behavior. For example, Vannicelli suggests that the therapists ask the following questions: "What do you mean when you say you're an ACOA?" or "When you describe this as your typical ACOA behavior, can you tell the group what this specifically means?"

Control in Group

Control is the most frequently identified character feature of ACOA (Ackerman, 1979; S. Brown, 1988; Whitfield, 1987). Cermak and Brown

(1982) identified control as the most compelling source of difficulty for their group members. Fears of being out of control and being controlled were paramount. Trusting others was difficult because this was viewed by most ACOA group members as giving control over to others, which "left them feeling more anxious and vulnerable." Responsibility for self and others was viewed as a way to stay in control, while maintaining self-worth. This excessive sense of responsibility contributes to what Bowlby (1958) describes as *compulsive caregiving.* Behaving in this manner allows the ACOA to remain in control while maintaining some essence of interpersonal contact. ACOA usually have great difficulty allowing themselves to be on the receiving end of any emotional support. Mutually satisfying and intimate relationships are as difficult for them as they are for alcoholics and substance abusers, although for diametrically opposite reasons. Alcoholics and substance abusers are usually takers who cannot give and ACOAs are givers who cannot take.

Treatment Strategies in Group

Most of the treatment strategies suggested for the long-term treatment of the alcoholic and substance abuser that have been outlined previously in this chapter will be applicable for ACOA. Both populations find it extremely difficult to establish satisfying intimate relationships. Until ACOA are able to accomplish this, they will be as vulnerable to their obsessive need to be responsible and in absolute control as alcoholics and substance abusers are vulnerable to their obsessive need for alcohol and drugs. However, there are some important differences in these two populations. Alcoholics and addicts are more likely to act out, and through their use of projective identification, are more likely to induce anger and hostility in the group leader. ACOAs are more likely to act in, berating, blaming, and condemning themselves for any shortcomings or failures. Their use of projective-identification is more likely to induce feelings of incompetence and failure in the group leaders, compelling the leader to try harder and be more available, only to fail and feel similar disappointment in his or her self and abilities.

Helping ACOA give up their absolute need for control and responsibility will be difficult because this is often the only source of self-worth and identity that they have ever had in their lives. Most ACOAs have tremendous ambivalence about the power bestowed upon them as either a surrogate spouse, confidant, or substitute parent when they were children. Because of the deteriorating competence of the alcoholic parent, they were often thrust into a unique form of role-reversal, where they parented their parents. This is especially true for the oldest child in the alcoholic family.

Consequently, giving this up will not only be difficult, it will also be painful and shameful.

ACOA AND SHAME

Alonso and Rutan's (1988) description of group therapy as the preferred mode of treatment for shame takes on added ramifications for this population for a number of reasons. Foremost among these is the intensity and the depth of the shame that children typically experience with the alcoholic parent. Not only do the children internalize their own shame, but they also feel contaminated and responsible for the contempt in the community and the embarrassment that was generalized to the entire family as a result of the alcoholic parent. As Hibbard (1987) writes: "While being reared by one or more alcoholics provides many opportunities for being shamed by them in the sense of irrational narcissistic traumatization, this is not unique to alcoholism. What is unique . . . is the deep sense of being ashamed for them and the fusion (or reciprocity) of these shameful self and object representations amalgamated at different development stages of psychic structuralization" (p. 784).

As Rice (1988) says "while the cure for guilt is forgiveness, the cure for shame is acceptance." However, acceptance can only be experienced if and when the feelings of shame, and the events that contributed to or caused its activation, are exposed to others and the "light of day." Shame, by definition, implies that something must remain hidden. Exposure, which provides the opportunity to experience acceptance from others, is therefore crucial. It is sometimes argued that this would be more easily accomplished in the pristine privacy of the individual therapist's office. But as Alonso and Rutan convincingly point out, this is precisely why it is important that it be done in a group setting. First, it removes the unspoken implication that this dirty little secret should never be shared with others but should be kept hidden—except from a select few who are "trained to understand." Second, and perhaps more important, the group provides ACOA with the opportunity to experience the hidden shameful aspect of themselves through their identification with another who shares the same shameful experience as them. Accepting in the other what they have been unable to accept in themselves provides them with a bridge, allowing them to experience that acceptance from others. The principle that before a person can be healed, that person must know that he or she can provide healing to another is what Searles (1973) identifies as the "therapeutic symbiosis." Such an experience and awareness is often only possible in group psychotherapy. This is the heart and soul of the healing process, not only for ACOA, but also for alcoholics and substance abusers.

Chapter 12

Characteristics of the Leader

There are many contributing variables that influence successful group therapy. Of all the multiple influences occurring within a group setting, none has more of an impact or importance than the intangible qualities of the group leader. Most important, the intangible, nonspecific qualities that influence successful group therapy have more to do with the type of person the therapist is rather than what the therapist does. This is not meant to imply that techniques, training, and experience have nothing to contribute to successful group therapy. To the contrary, all forms of successful psychotherapy, both individual and group, are impossible without these factors. However, these elements of psychotherapy can be acquired by the dedicated student through learning. The nonspecific contributing factors to successful therapy include such important intangibles such as caring, sensitivity, and empathy. Is it possible to teach another to be able to tap into a deep source of ultimate concern and authentic respect for another human being if that quality does not exist in the individual before he or she embarks on the vigorous course of training that is required of any competent professional?

In his book, *The Healer's Art,* Eric Cassell (1985) has raised this important question and exhorts the physician and the therapist to retain his or her role as a healer, that is, as someone who views the patient in a holistic sense without regulating disease as an entity. Cassell urges the group leader, therapist, and physician to be aware of the effect that all forms of disease have on the patient in terms of the feeling of disconnectedness, loss of sense of omniscience, and loss of control they produce. These complications are well known to most seasoned and competent group leaders, but they are often difficult to convey to the therapist in training. In fact, Cassell asks if it is possible to teach sensitivity. He suggests that it be attempted, despite the ever-increasing stress on techniques, theory, and technology.

Today, alcohol and drug treatment is falling prey to the same difficulties confronting all forms of medical care. More and more emphasis is placed on greater technology, large group practices, multimillion-dollar corporate hospital chains with revolving treatment personnel, bureaucratic state and federal treatment policies, and multiple specialties–all factors tending to discourage a close therapist-patient relationship. Cassell, like others before him (i.e., Yalom, Polster, Goulding, Ornstein, and Kohut), offers an important reminder of the need to restore or reestablish the necessary human connection between the patient and the person or persons providing the care and treatment if the individual is going to fully benefit from these advances in technology.

VALUES OF THE GROUP LEADER

The values of the group leader are an integral part of his or her individuality. While it has been well documented that the therapist's values and characteristics have an important impact on successful treatment, the research in this area has been limited to non-addictive populations. A brief review of this research will be presented later in the chapter even though the material does not pertain exclusively to group therapy with alcoholics or addicts. Much of this information is generalizable to all forms of treatment and should prove to be helpful for the group leader in working with addicted patients. However, the therapist's characteristics are made more significant to alcohol and drug abuse treatment by the special circumstances induced by the dual impact of group therapy and the common characteristics of the addicted patient. First, group therapy is a much more active and interactional mode of treatment than individual therapy. Consequently, the personality of the leader plays a much more significant part in successful treatment than it would in individual therapy. Second, the addicted patient requires a leader who is more alive, exciting, and active. Before venturing to give a plausible explanation for why this may be so, a brief example of this author's experience at a national alcoholism conference with Irvin Yalom and Father Martin will help clarify this point.

> Toward the end of the conference, after both Yalom and Father Martin had presented equally excellent but totally divergent all-day workshops, the participants and presenters were invited to an "informal" get-together one evening. Father Martin came early and shortly after his arrival had quickly attracted a rather large gathering of individuals who sat around him in an "informal" circle, laughing, joking, and exchanging stories with the lovable, leprechaun-like priest. Many of the participants at the conference were recovering alcoholics and addicts like Father Martin, and they were eager to be

> in the presence of the priest who had become famous for his charisma, charm, and excitement. Father Martin didn't disappoint them, as it was obvious that he sincerely enjoyed their company and loved exchanging small anecdotes about alcoholism, recovery, and spirituality. Yalom arrived a couple of hours later and quietly circled the reception hall, often unnoticed by many of the conference participants. Eventually, Yalom stopped and talked politely to a few individuals who asked him about some of his more obtuse, yet stimulating, comments about existential psychotherapy. Yalom remained kind and courteous in his responses, but it was apparent that the participants were somewhat uncomfortable in his presence, and at times, he was a little awkward in his social interaction with many of them. On numerous other occasions, a small gathering of individuals would point toward the direction of "Yalom's presence," speak softly to each other, look as if they wanted to approach, but would drift off or engage each other in conversation, giving the appearance that they thought better of the idea. It was apparent that Yalom was somewhat intimidating to them, and unaware of this, he did nothing to discourage their discomfort. After a half an hour or so, Yalom turned to leave. However, he stopped very briefly at the gathering in the corner of the room from which loud billows of laughter would sporadically emerge. He stared somewhat inquisitively at the Catholic priest who was entertaining the gathering with his stories and jokes. He hesitated ever so slightly then departed as quietly as he had entered the room. For one brief moment, I caught glimpses of both men and the different personality styles of each were placed in sharp contrast as they stood there in the same proximity. I wondered which man would be most effective in treating alcoholics and addicts. The kind, quiet, polite man with the piercing intellect or the charismatic, charming, lovable elf with the sparkling eyes and contagious wit. Certainly, each had something equally important to offer. Which would a recovering alcoholic or addict respond best to? At least based on this experience, it was apparent that the characteristics possessed by Father Martin were far more inviting to alcoholics than those possessed by Yalom.

The divergent personal characteristics displayed by Yalom and Father Martin represent an important variable in the treatment of the addicted patient. In many cases, those characteristics embodied by Yalom would be preferred by certain types of patients. Certainly, those individuals who have fears of intrusiveness and need a more insightful approach in their treatment would have difficulties with a Father Martin-type therapist. It is a well-documented fact that certain patients respond more favorably to certain types of therapists. The therapist-patient match is, in fact, one of the most significantly influential factors in successful treatment, and the research on this will be reviewed later in the chapter. However, one therapist cannot be everything to all patients, no matter how skillful and charismatic he or she may be. There are certain characteristics of a therapist that are more likely to evoke a favorable response in either an alcoholic or addict. Because of the nature of the characterological deficits commonly seen in addicted patients, it is suggested that those characteristics embodied by Father Martin are more likely to produce a positive effect than those characteristics embodied by Yalom.

Because so many addicts and alcoholics suffer from the characterological deficits commonly seen in narcissistic and borderline conditions (see Chapter 6), they must constantly battle the feelings of boredom, deadness, and emptiness that threaten to overtake them. One cocaine addict aptly described his need to capture some excitement or "rush" in his life because without it he felt dead or empty:

> You know, doc, how your foot feels when it falls asleep after it is kept in the same position too long so that it cuts off your circulation. You stand up suddenly and your foot feels like it's dead. You have to stomp it on the ground and smack it with your fist so you can start to feel it again. Well, this is how cocaine is for me. Without it I feel dead, like I've got no circulation. Cocaine gives me a smack, a stomp, to help me come alive.

Many therapists do not fully appreciate the impact of their personalities or values on addicts or alcoholics who are struggling to identify some viable alternative lifestyle that will allow them to fill up the emptiness or deadness within them. Addicts and alcoholics are suspicious of others whom they perceive as dead or empty trying to make them adhere to their values. Most of the dominant values shared by middle-class professionals (i.e., delay of gratification, control of impulses, rational thought, hard work, responsibility, etc.) are not the same values or characteristics shared by most alcoholics and addicts. While the professional therapist may look upon the use of alcohol and drugs as an escape, addicts or alcoholics view their alcohol or drug use in a far different light. Unlike the professional who holds the position that drugs and alcohol are for those who cannot cope with reality, addicts see that reality is for those who cannot cope with drugs. In many ways, addicts or alcoholics view many professionals as dull, dead, or timid people who cannot tolerate excitement within themselves because of their meekness and deadness.

Addicts and alcoholics frequently adhere to values and behavior that is foreign to many professionals who do not suffer from such character defects. Impulsiveness, spontaneity, action, and excitement are often judged by professionals to be forms of "acting out" that must be curbed or modified in treatment. To addicts and alcoholics, this is a compromise that must be avoided at all costs because they view it as trading one's soul for a condition that is lifeless, boring, and dead. Consequently, therapists are dealing with patients who frequently see them as dull and unspontaneous individuals who have sold their soul to "make it" in the world.

This situation can be exacerbated by a therapist who adopts a stance of technical neutrality. An unresponsive therapist stirs up unconscious fears of annihilation and nothingness that are associated with primitive identifications. Transference distortions are heightened and alcoholics or addicts are reminded of the dull, deadened, and distant parental figures who tried to shape them to fit their expectations. Resistance is consequently heightened as the alcoholics or addicts are forced to deal with the therapist in the same manner as they were forced to deal with their unresponsive parental figures. This is why they need a strong, exciting self-object to fill them up or stimulate them like drugs or alcohol does. A passive, unexciting therapist will be perceived as just another bad object who is withholding, dull, and lifeless. Addicts are searching for an idealized other who is a model or representation of what they wish they could be. If they can be stimulated interpersonally and can come to identify with those positive aspects of an exciting, alive therapist, they will react more positively to treatment. This is especially important during the initial stages of treatment because it will enhance the establishment of a working alliance. Addicts need someone exciting and alive who will serve as a model for them in their own attempts to combat the emptiness and deadness that threatens to overtake them.

Masterson (1981), writing about the borderline patient, expresses similar sentiments about the importance of the personality characteristics of the therapist. Therapist dynamics that Masterson thinks interfere with effective therapy are: passivity, compulsivity, submissiveness, and dependency. The passive therapist negates the patients' need to have an active, real person who can help them distinguish between reality and internal distortions. The submissive therapist will fail to confront patients, leading them to feel that the therapist does not care. The compulsive therapist will be more likely to react angrily at the alcoholics' or addicts' anger and acting out since in Masterson's view, the therapist's compulsivity is a defense against his or her own anger and need to control. Since it is rare to find an addict or alcoholic who will readily comply with the demands of treatment, a therapist who is easily angered or frustrated when the patient does not do as he or she wishes will have a difficult time when working with this population. The therapist who is dependent and needs patients' approval is in danger of repeating part of the patients' developmental problem. Patients need to achieve their separation, individuation, and autonomy in treatment. They must be free from disapproval, even when they do not comply exactly to the pre-established expectations of the therapist. All of these described therapist characteristics will also interfere with the therapist serving as an appropriate role model (external object) that the patient can internalize.

THE THERAPIST AS A PERSON

Erv Polster, Irvin Yalom, Carl Whitaker, and numerous other theorists have written extensively about the importance of the therapist as a person in effecting successful change in therapy. Yalom suggests the therapist's personal characteristics are why some interpretations click and why others do not. Change is produced by those interpretations that are made when the relationship is just right. If patients feel they are controlled, approached in a superior manner, or treated as an object by the therapist, they will not benefit from the interpretation. Any interpretation, even the most eloquent, has little benefit if the patient does not hear it. Genuineness, concern, acceptance and empathy take precedence over all technical considerations because it is the relationship that serves as fertile ground for the techniques to take root.

Erv and Miriam Polster feel that the personhood of the therapist is one of the key elements that helps facilitate change in psychotherapy. Most excellent therapists are exciting people. They have access to a wide range of human emotions. They can be tender or tough, serious or funny, courageous or respectfully cautious. If their patients spend enough time with them, the Polsters feel that these traits will rub off. Their patients will experience someone who knows how to accept, arouse, tolerate, and frustrate. They will eventually learn a respect for what it is like to be a human being who can meet surprise and adventure without hiding characteristics of themselves when they appear.

Carl Whitaker and Tom Malone (1953) differentiate between three different types of therapists. They identify the three types as the Non-Therapist, the Social Therapist and the Professional Depth Therapist. Each serves a very different function in therapy. Whitaker and Malone describe their different roles in detail when they write about their differences.

1. The Non-Therapist

> Included in this group would be the professional administrator and the psychiatrist whose relationship to patients is a business one. The

nontherapeutic psychiatrist seldom reacts to the child in his patients; he does not really accept them in terms of their potential capacity. His artificial role-playing contributes little to the patient's growth, though it may make significant contributions to their current adjustment. He denies his own patient needs, does not identify with patients in any but the most superficial sense, and has never had any adequate therapy himself. The non-therapist has access to his own fantasy life, but is unable to make that part of his life available to other people. One of the most conspicuous examples in this category is the psychiatrist who has had an incomplete psychotherapeutic experience, and is thereby categorically determined to keep himself from any entangling alliances. (Whitaker and Malone, 1953, pp. 135-136)

2. The Social Therapist

In contrast, the Social Therapist forces growth in persons around him. He accepts his own patient needs and his fantasy life. He thereby can identify with patients and their needs and can go with the patient into the symbolic experience of a therapeutic relationship. In the course of this, he accepts their projections upon him, reacts positively to the child in the other person, and carries the person into "therapy," although in ordinary circumstances, not through the *core* phase of therapy. Because he has satisfied his own patient needs, he knows his own limitations and will frequently refer patients who need deeper therapy to a professional therapist. (Whitaker and Malone, 1953, p. 136)

3. The Professional Depth Therapist

Like the social therapist, the Professional Depth Therapist has been a patient, and has resolved the major portion of his infantile transference needs. He can identify with his patients in the specific sense of seeing the patient as his child self while he is critically aware of his limitations in the therapeutic sense. As a professional, he learns to separate his therapeutic function from his real life. His motivations have to do with his own efforts at reconstructing his body image, and he thereby accepts the therapist-vector in the patient as a specific dynamic in the therapeutic process. He can take patients through the therapeutic experience, help them constructively with the symbolic relationship and also with their relationship to him as a person. By virtue of his personal motivations in the therapeutic relationship, he goes to sufficient depth with each patient to gain from the therapeutic potential of the patient. In thus being patient to his patient, he strengthens the patient's capacity to become a separate, growing person. (Whitaker and Malone, 1953, p. 136)

QUALITIES OF THE GROUP LEADER

Martin Grotjohn (1983) has described certain qualities of the group leader that he feels are essential to effective group treatment. The group leader is of central importance in group therapy because group therapy, more than individual therapy, is based on the dynamics of interaction. Grotjohn lists six important qualities of the group leader:

1. Reliability
2. Spontaneity and Responsiveness
3. Trust
4. Firm identity
5. Humor and creativity
6. Fallibility

Reliability

The group leader must be reliable. Group members require a consistent parental figure whose behavior is predictable and understandable.

Groups must start and end on time. Group members must learn that the leader will not support them for some behavior one moment and then attack that very same behavior in another moment. Only then will group leaders invite trust and confidence from the group members. This first requires that the leaders have trust and confidence in themselves. This can only be accomplished if they have experienced life to the fullest. They must know fear, anxiety, courage, and dependence. They must not be afraid to love and they do not need to be strangers to anger. Group leaders must possess the capacity for what Karl Jaspers (1975) calls "unlimited communication" or be what Erv Polster (1981) calls "a connoisseur of contact." They must also have the capacity for what Franz Alexander (1950) calls "dynamic reasoning"–the ability to see their patients not only in the here and now, but how they became as they are. Group leaders must listen with what Theodore Riek calls "the third ear" if they are to truly understand their patients (cited in Grotjohn, 1983, p. 294). However, while group leaders should always strive to understand, they must be able to tolerate the tension of not understanding rather than force their own explanations or interpretations. As Riek says, "It is better not to understand than to misunderstand."

Spontaneity and Responsiveness

While therapists in individual therapy have the time to wait, think, and speculate, like a slow-moving chess player, group leaders must rely more on spontaneous responses to the multiple situations and interactions in group. Grotjohn compares the group leader to a conductor of an orchestra. He or she leads, but he or she is also a central part of the presentation. The individual therapist is like a critic who sits in the audience and has the advantage of standing up, stopping the music, making a comment, and then sitting back down. The group leader on the other hand not only interprets, but does something that shows what or how it is done. This requires the group leader to split himself or herself and be both participant of and observer to the group.

Trust

This requires that group leaders not only possess the ability to trust others, but that they have basic trust in themselves. This means they must have the capacity to tolerate bad experiences and despair in themselves and others. However, as Erikson notes, people cannot develop basic trust by themselves. Group leaders must know how to develop and protect the trust of the group, for as they will discover, the group members will come to trust the group more than they trust the therapist. One aim of the group is to restore the members' belief and trust in their fellow members and themselves. Trust in others reduces narcissistic, self-centered preoccupation and teaches members to care about each other.

Trust does not imply simply being nice, kind, and accepting. It requires the willingness to risk pointing out painful truths and self-deceptions. It means knowing that one cannot help but have an influence on the patient. The question raised here is one of timing. It is the therapist of the Gouldings's, Ormont's, or Polsters's caliber who knows when to encourage, confront, and influence. The avoidance of these issues is impossible. Frank (1961) agrees that "psychotherapists must be aware of their influence on patients. This cannot be helped. The only question is whether the therapist uses his/her influence consciously or unconsciously" (p. 234). As Modell (1955) says, "It would be well to remember that in all therapy, trouble is apt to follow the ignorant application of important forces" (cited in Frank, p. 234).

Persuasion or influence does not mean that manipulation is sanctioned in order to satisfy the therapist's own interests and needs. As Kant wrote many years ago, "A man must never be treated as a means, but only as an end in himself" (cited in Durant, 1926). Once the patient or the group member becomes only a means of determining the therapist's worth as a skilled practitioner, the true aim of mutuality and help is compromised. If the patient's getting well or the alcoholic's or addict's stopping his or her chemical use becomes important only as a reflection of the therapist's ability as a group leader, treatment is compromised. As Buber (1964) wrote,

> Help without mutuality is presumptuousness; it is an attempt to practice magic. The psychotherapist who tries to dominate his patient stifles the growth of his blessing. As soon as the helper is touched by the desire, in however subtle a form, to dominate or to enjoy his patient other than a wrong condition needing to be cured, the danger of falsification arises, besides which all quackery appears peripheral. (p. 395)

Not only is this an illustration of trust in another being manipulated, it also demonstrates a violation of one of the canons of existential philosophy. Martin Buber (as well as Yalom and every existential-oriented therapist) supports existential therapy's goal of making patients more aware of their own potential for choice and growth because it parallels his early teachings of Hasidism concerning the uniqueness and potentiality that each individual possesses and is responsible to fulfill. The existential psychotherapist's insistence that patients take an active part in the healing process, rather than being passive recipients who have something done to them, is not only an intricate part of existentialism, but is also at the core of AA and its treatment philosophy.

As most individuals working with addictions will attest, getting alcoholics and addicts to change is difficult. Coercion, manipulation, confrontation, intervention, and persuasion are important and necessary techniques in the therapist's repertoire if he or she hopes to work successfully with addicted individuals. While many counselors working in the addictive disease field are familiar with the use of these techniques, those outside the field of addictions often shudder at the implications of such a treatment approach. However, as Jay Haley (1976) notes, manipulation is an integral part of human interaction and occurs whether or not therapists recognize or identify it as such. Haley and others therefore suggest openly identifying and understanding the implications of such an approach rather than applying such principles in ignorance.

All of these aspects of addictive treatment–coercion, manipulation, intervention, and confrontation–were explored at length in Chapter 9. Now, the relationship of persuasion to the trustworthiness of the therapist must be examined. This is a necessary endeavor, because the elements of persuasion play an important part in all forms of psychotherapy. Psychotherapy, in fact, is viewed by many as a subtle form of interpersonal persuasion (Frank, 1961). However, persuasion or the lack of it in a psychotherapeutic relationship is not always clearly definable. Most therapists agree that persuasion is influenced by a number of important factors, of which the personal characteristics of the therapist are generally recognized as the most significant. Experience, credibility, training, dedication, values, and enthusiasm are attributes usually agreed upon as being important contributors to the therapist's power to persuade. Understandably, psychotherapy conceptualized in this manner raises significant issues of values, ethics, and responsibility in treatment. While not all agree upon or recognize the existence of persuasive influences in psychotherapy, many suggest that persuasion is a salient feature of psychotherapy whether or not it is identified. Further, it is suggested that these persuasive influences cross doctrinal differences and can be augmented by applying them within a group therapy setting when treating alcoholics or addicts. In the hands of a skilled and ethical psychotherapist, these persuasive influences can be enhanced and the group can be a powerful tool in the addict's and alcoholic's recovery process.

More specifically, these issues need to be explored in relation to the notion that learning by doing (as in Alcoholics Anonymous) is preferred to learning by talking. This is why the Alcoholics Anonymous maxim of "Walk your talk" is so effective. It requires a recovering individual to "do" rather than just talk. Members of Alcoholics Anonymous, like most good therapists, are not fooled by what an alcoholic or addict says. Alcoholics and addicts are advised to go to ninety meetings in ninety days. "Take you body and your mind will follow," they are told. In essence, this is the principle William James proposed years ago: If you want to change your belief, act as if you believe and you will soon believe as you act.

Firm Identity

The central firmness of the group leader allows the group members to recognize the therapist for what the leader is–a real person and not just an imagination of transference. A firm identity will allow the therapist to have an openness to the group and its members so he or she can be a parent to one, a friend to another, or a disciplinarian to another. Group leaders will be able to be many things to different members, yet they will maintain a firm identity to all. At times, they may be a blank screen in order to invite transference distortions, but simultaneously, they will be able to be real and human enough to develop a working alliance with the group and its members. This requires them to be active, but not so active that they dominate the group or its members.

A firm identity will also help the leader with his or her own countertransference reactions while at the same time allowing the group to use the leader for three different transference resolutions:

1. Transference to the leader as a central figure, as in individual therapy.
2. Transference to peers in group, as among siblings in a family.
3. Transference to the group as a whole, as a symbolic mother.

In reflecting upon the way that gifted and well-trained group leaders such as Ormont, Rutan, and Alonso lead groups, it is important to remember Frank's suggestion that an important part of the effectiveness of these group leaders is determined by their own belief in their modus operandi. Research has in fact shown that this is frequently the case. Those therapists who are most involved and committed to their particular mode of treatment apparently instill their own enthusiasm in the treatment process in their patients. Consequently, accepting and believing in the therapist's approach to treatment requires taking some of their assumptions on faith and for those patients that do, the therapist's mode of therapy can be quite effective.

Both Transactional Analysis and Gestalt theory are sometimes criticized as being overly simplistic explanations of personality that do not share the sophistication of object-relations theory, self-psychology, or classical Freudian psychology in describing the intricacies of the dynamics of personality. It may be that Transactional Analysis, Gestalt, and even Alcoholics Anonymous are effective modes of treatment precisely because of their simplicity and the emotional involvement of the practitioner. This is not intended to imply that all therapy can be explained by the placebo effect, but that it can be an important part of the treatment process.

For instance, Wallace (1978b) recognizes that one value of AA as a treatment modality is that it places the alcoholic's behavior within an alcoholism paradigm and places the alcoholic's experience within some cognitive structure. Helping the alcoholic achieve a self-attribution of alcoholic and hence an explanatory system for his/her behavior is a central role of the therapist. Frank (1961) sees this cognitive component as a very vital part of therapy.

> First, they provide a cognitive structure that enables the patient to name his symptoms and fit them into a causal scheme. Since major sources of anxiety are ambiguity and fear of the unknown, this, in itself, can powerfully reduce the patient's anxiety and enhance his self-confidence.

Yalom (1985) agrees when he stresses that both catharsis and insight are very necessary components of change. If you do not obtain both, Yalom doubts whether any significant change can occur.

In truth, psychotherapy with the patient at this point is very much the teaching of what Wallace describes as an "exotic belief," wherein the true value of describing what has actually occurred in an alcoholic's life (in this case, alcoholism) is held irrelevant. Yalom addresses this issue extensively. Each of us holds constructs that are important for our survival. In other words, our defenses exist for a good reason and a sensitive therapist should not rip them away too rapidly. Yalom wrote about the issue of responsibility being salient to honesty. Honesty for honesty's sake is an overly rigid posture that does not guarantee therapeutic gains. "Vital lies," as Yalom describes them, are sometimes essential for survival, and it is the prudent therapist who knows when to remove and when to build up defenses.

Humor and Creativity

Often, the best therapists are the ones who can use humor creatively. For instance, both the Gouldings and the Polsters usually share an enthusiasm for the good-natured kidding of ourselves and our neurotic struggles. They repeatedly demonstrate this at their respective training programs, as their workshops are frequently spiced with humor. "Laughter does not obscure a point," the Polsters write. "Often it makes it even clearer and lubricates what might otherwise be a lugubrious passage. This is true of therapy itself as it is of teaching" (Polster and Polster, 1974, p. 40). The creative use of humor can also help correct transference distortions because, if used properly, it invites the group to look upon the group leader as a more complete and real person. However, humor must never be used to hide hostility or to wound. The group leader must not fight with members for dominance because of his or her own narcissism or display of brilliance. The best interventions or interpretations are never the ones the group leader makes, but rather those the individual or the other group members make. Humor is best used when it supports honesty, courage, and frankness.

Creativity can take on many forms. As Jerome Frank (1961) points out, the personal attitude of group leaders is often one of the most important qualities they can have in their repertoire. Likewise, Bergin (1971), among others, has presented convincing research evidence showing that the personal characteristics of the therapist are the most important contributing factors to treatment effectiveness. Frank's thesis of psychotherapy actually being a subtle form of persuasion takes on added significance when one looks at the relationship of the therapist's personal magnetism to the values change in therapy. Beutler (1979b) provides evidence for sufficient reason to believe that patients' values, attitudes, and beliefs change in psychotherapy and that to some degree, these changes are associated with the degree to which therapy is successful. However, these values change in a systematic fashion, and the successful patient usually takes on the values of his or her therapist.

Frank (1978) has identified two sources that invoke the patient's expectancy of help. One is the personal magnetism of the healer, which is often strengthened by his or her own belief in what he or she does. This was clearly evident with therapists of the caliber of the Gouldings, the Polsters, Ormont, Rutan, and Alonso. All are exciting people and enthusiastic about their modus operandi and truly believe that they can be of help to anyone. They all are also very charismatic individuals, and there is an abundance of clinical evidence that . . . "confirms the hypothesis that part of the healing power of all forms of psychotherapy lies in the therapist's ability to mobilize the patient's hope for relief" (Frank, 1961, p. 62). Consequently, part of the success of any therapist may be attributed to his or her ability to mobilize the patient's expectation of help. As Frank suggests, "The therapist's power is based on the patient's perception of him as a source of help and it tends to increase the greater the patient's distress." As Frank (1961) points out:

> Another source of the patient's faith is the ideology of the healer or sect, which offers the patient a rationale, however absurd, for making sense of his illness and the treatment procedure, and places the healer in the position of the transmitter or controller of impressive healing forces. In this he is analogous to the shaman. The healer may pose as a scientist who has discovered new and potent scientific principles of healing, thus surrounding himself with the aura that anything labeled scientific inspires in members of modern Western societies. (p. 60)

An example may help clarify this point. While being supervised by Mary Goulding, I was a therapist with one of the other trainees at her and Bob's training programs at Mount Madonna. I made an intervention and an interpretation concerning a dynamic or pattern I thought my trainee "patient" was manifesting. This was quickly denied and discounted by the trainee as not fitting for him. However, when Mary agreed it did fit for him, he quickly changed his resistant stance and the therapeutic work consequently had a profound effect on him during the rest of the month of training at Mount Madonna.

Fallibility

Group leaders must be expected to make mistakes. More important, they must be allowed to do so. They will learn that they do not lose their position by admitting a mistake. To the contrary, their central position will be confirmed even more by the humanness of their fallibility. The only unforgivable mistakes are pulling rank on group members or not being able to tolerate patients moving slowly in treatment. Treatment of alcoholics and addicts is not the kind of work for a person who demands immediate success and dramatic results. This was a point explicitly made in Janet Malcolm's book, *In the Freud Archives* (1984). Malcolm emphasizes that it is the psychotherapists who are able to plod along in a sometimes dreary, slow pace with their patients who are the most successful analysts. Those who only have the sharp, quick intellect, often do not possess the capacity to tolerate their patients' inability to keep pace with them and their discoveries about the patient. Such psychotherapists can become easily frustrated and dissatisfied with the lack of immediate success in treatment.

Demanding success and quick results can lead some therapists to avoid recognizing aspects of the individual that might indicate fallibility on the therapists' part. There is at least some research evidence that sheds light on this issue. Beutler (1980) has presented some preliminary findings indicating that those therapists who perceive more dysphoria in patients are more effective in achieving successful treatment outcome. Further, those therapists who perceive the patient as more resistant are also more successful in treatment than those therapists who identify resistance less. Both of these factors have important implications for training and treatment. It may be that those therapists who are more successful in therapy are more sensitive to resistance and the hiding of dysphoria.

While experienced group leaders such as Ormont and the Gouldings may work out of two distinctly different models, in actuality there may be more similarities in their approaches than differences. Research in this area (Frank, 1978) indicates that the type of relationship offered by therapists seems to be determined more by their levels of experience than by their theories. One experimental study found that therapists of different schools agreed highly as to the nature of the therapeutic relationship and that experienced practitioners of different schools agree more highly than did junior or senior members of the same persuasion. Further, studies of taped interviews showed that experienced experts of different schools created relationships more similar to each other than novices of the same school. Apparently, experience in actual practice overcomes doctrinal differences.

As suggested earlier, the differences between the Gouldings and Ormonts may be greater in theory than in actual clinical application. It is not so much what they each do as it is how they do it. All competent and well-trained group leaders are able to make interventions work because of their timing and their personalities. For instance, within the mystical Jewish tradition of Hasidism, the religious leader (Zaddick) was not an impersonal vessel or medium through which great powers operated, nor was he the great scholar and seat of religious reason (Buber, 1955a, Kopp, 1971). Rather, as the Zaddick, he first of all would be a person in his own right, one who helped those who trusted him and who was able to help only because they trusted him.

The relationship between the Zaddick and his disciple was the crucial factor in this attempt to give spiritual help, just as the relationship between the therapist and the patient is crucial. The personality of the teacher takes the place of doctrine. He or she is the teacher. As one student of the Zaddick said: "I did not go to my Zaddick to learn Torah from him, but to watch him tie his bootlaces." Likewise, there is much that group members learn from watching the way the group, its leader, and its members deal with their own individual anger, sadness, confusion, and fear in therapy.

GUIDELINES AND PRIORITIES FOR THE GROUP LEADER

Rutan and Stone (1993) make a valuable effort in identifying, organizing, and assigning priorities to the numerous roles and tasks confronting the group leader. In their attempt to make sense of the chaos that presents itself when the leader is determining how to intervene, they suggest separating the options into two categories. One is the leader's *role* and the other is the leader's *focus*. They present these options on a continua. (See Figures 12.1 and 12.2.)

ROLES OF LEADER

Activity versus Passivity

As Rutan and Stone suggest, the leader's activity level will be dictated by a number of factors. Developmental stages, target population, goals, theoretical orientation, composition of the group, and even the personality of the leader will all have some influence on how active or passive the group leader will be. As stated repeatedly in this book, addicts and alcoholics do not respond well to passive, withholding leaders. However, they also do not do very well with overcontrolling leaders whose style is apt to evoke competition, judgment, and dominance. The leader's activity level, especially in the earlier stages of recovery, needs to be directed toward providing firm boundaries, limits, and structure while avoiding power

FIGURE 12.1. Roles of Group Leader

1. Activity .... Passivity
2. Transparency .... Opaqueness
3. Gratification .... Frustration

FIGURE 12.2. Focus of the Group Leader

1. Past .... Here and Now .... Future
2. Group-As-a-Whole . . Interaction .... Individual
3. In Group .... Out of Group
4. Affect .... Cognition
5. Process .... Content
6. Understanding .... Experience

struggles with individual members. Passivity on the leader's part lends itself too easily to misinterpretation as disinterest, detachment, and weakness, all personal attributes that are likely to provoke strong transferential reactions that will impede the progress of the group.

Transparency versus Opaqueness

How open the therapist will be should always be dictated by the question of how helpful will this be to the patient? As Rutan and Stone recommend, "It is usually helpful to reveal only that which is in the service of the treatment process" (p. 130). It is usually best to avoid openness or transparency when the response arises from the group leader's own inner needs or from pressures from the group members. Requests by members for personal information should always be explored to understand their roots. Group leaders who are working with alcoholics and addicts will soon learn that this request for personal information will always center around their own history of drug and alcohol use, as well as their experience with addiction in their own family of origin. To avoid directly answering such questions runs the risk of disturbing the therapeutic alliance. Unlike patients who are seeking help for mental health difficulties, alcoholics and addicts will not grant therapists immediate credibility because of their educational degrees and professional training. Some of this mistrust may be the result of the influences from more experienced members of twelve-step programs who caution them to be careful of "ignorant professionals." However, most of their questions will be driven by fear and a need for assurance that they will be understood and helped. Since most addicts and alcoholics strongly identify with others in the program, they often feel immediately understood and accepted by others who are addicted. Group leaders must remember that this is usually at the root of patients' requests for information regarding the therapists' own personal history with alcohol and drugs. If group leaders are not from an alcoholic family or have no personal history of addiction, they need not apologize for this. Addicted patients are more interested in knowing that they will be understood, accepted, and helped than they are in knowing the facts about a therapist's own personal life. What is important though is that the therapist be able to speak to this in a straightforward way without flinching or showing discomfort with the topic. Such a stance demonstrates more to the group members than any piece of personal history.

As Rutan and Stone point out, no matter how strictly a therapist holds to the belief that it is best not to reveal personal information about yourself, it is impossible for the group members not to learn a great deal about the personal characteristics of the leader. While the therapists can avoid revealing facts about themselves, they cannot avoid revealing themselves as people. As Rutan and Stone write:

> No matter how *strictly a particular therapist holds to the opaque pole of this continuum,* after a time members come to know a great deal about the therapist. As an actively engaged participant in the group, albeit in a role different from that of a member, the therapist reveals a great deal in nonverbal ways. Patients learn to read body language and facial expression; they know when the therapist is pleased or displeased. It is not necessary or useful for group therapists to be bland screens. Groups are intensely human encounters, and it is often impossible (or inhuman) for a therapist to avoid laughing at funny moments or feeling tearful when a group is struggling with sadness. If therapists are empathically attuned to their groups, they are not immune to the affect that engulfs everyone. *It is through the therapist's steadfastness to the tasks, through the concern, caring and thoughtfulness and through the ability to be introspective, to tolerate affects, and to move forward in a therapeutic manner that the group members come to know a great deal about their therapist.* (pp. 130-131)

Gratification versus Frustration

The degree to which the group leader frustrates or gratifies the group is one of the most consistent dominating themes presenting itself in the treatment of addition. Alcoholics and addicts demand and require certain levels of gratification in group if they are going to be able to tolerate the relinquishing of their primary source of gratification—namely, alcohol and drugs. Self-psychology's perspective on this issue is most useful in helping the therapist determine when and how much gratification is necessary when treating the addicted patient. Addiction, as self-psychology defines it, is the result of deprivation of developmentally appropriate needs for gratification. Alcohol, drugs, food, sex, and other forms of potentially addictive behavior are attempts at self-repair. The addict and alcoholic tries to acquire externally what cannot be provided internally because of defects in psychic structure. This is not to imply that therapists should "love their addict or alcoholic into health." Not only is this impossible, it is counter-therapeutic since this is what the addict or alcoholic has been trying to do symbolically with chemicals. Rather, the addicted individual needs to learn how to tolerate frustration without immediate gratification since it is through managing tolerable levels of frustration that psychic structure is laid. It is here that the concept of *optimal frustration* captures the necessary stance of the group leader when working with alcoholics and addicts in group. As Anne Alonso has stated, "The group is working best when it is functioning at the most tolerable level of anxiety" (1985). If there is too little anxiety, the group does not promote the stimulating atmosphere needed to challenge the group members' capacity to cope and adapt. Too much anxiety interferes with the necessary trust, safety, and cohesion required for openness, exploration, and the revealing of one's self to occur. *Optimal gratification* means that the group leader will help the group provide enough nurturing or emotional responsiveness until the addicts or alcoholics are able to provide it to themselves without returning to old methods of gaining immediate gratification. A group composed of individuals early in recovery will require more gratification while a group composed of later stage recovering addicts and alcoholics will require less gratification.

FUNCTIONS OF THE LEADER

Past, Present, and Future

All well-trained and experienced group leaders know that a focus on the immediacy of the here and now is likeliest to produce the most therapeutic benefit in group. The past is only important to the extent that it is influencing what is happening in the present. While current events always take precedence in group, they can often seem confusing and unexplainable unless they are understood within the context of the past. However, it is almost always unproductive to examine the past in an attempt to discover the reasons that may have lead the person to become an addict or alcoholic. On the other hand, it can be extremely valuable to understand how past situations or affective states have lead to recent alcohol and drug use. Such methods are crucial elements in relapse prevention strategies. Trying to explain how events in one's past may have caused one to have originally started to use alcohol and drugs is usually futile, especially if this venture is motivated by the spoken belief or unspoken hope that this understanding will allow the addict or alcoholic to be able to use drugs and alcohol again–every alcoholic's or addict's secret wish.

In a similar fashion, focusing excessively on the future can become just another way of avoiding what needs to be done in the present. Too much emphasis on tomorrow can be deadly for the addict or alcoholic unless it takes the form of some structured, behavioral rehearsal to reduce anxiety and minimize surprises. Addicts' and alcoholics' preoccupation with the future can become a source of unmanageable anxiety and fear. This is especially true for those early in recovery. Drugs and alcohol are usually the methods that have been used to control these uncomfortable affective states. This is one reason why newly recovering addicts and alcoholics are reminded constantly by their fellow AA members to stay in the here and now by taking it "one day at a time."

Group-as-a-Whole, Interpersonal, Individual

The skill and art of leading a group is determined in large part by the leader's ability to discern which level of intervention (group-as-a-whole, interpersonal, individual) at a particular moment will benefit the group and its members the most. Generally, exclusive group-as-a-whole interventions, as strictly applied in the Tavistock model, promote too much regression and not enough gratification for the alcoholic and addict. However, the judicious application of group-as-a-whole interventions can be invaluable at those times when personal and group dynamics have collided in a way to create an impasse. While individual interventions are absolutely necessary at times, especially in the early stages of an alcoholic's or addict's recovery, they should not be used excessively, as this will not only make the group leader-dependent, it will rob the group of its most potent and useful force–other alcoholics and addicts helping each other. While the promotion of interpersonal interactions needs to dominate the group leader's efforts when working with an addicted population, the form that this promotion must take will vary depending on the stage of recovery and the stage of development of the group. Early on, interpersonal exchanges need to be encouraged to help establish a climate of support, cohesion, and responsiveness. Similarities between member's issues, circumstances, and experiences should dominate all early interventions. Later in the group and later in recovery, interpersonal interactions need to be emphasized as a means of uncovering the way internalized object relations get projected and played out in the external world with other individuals. Group therapy now becomes a vehicle for treating the character pathology that dominates much of an alcoholic's or addict's life. Differences between group members, rather than similarities, now need to be emphasized to help addicted individuals deal with the rigidity and the "black and white, all or nothing" thinking that dominates most of their relationships.

In-Group versus Out-of-Group

If a group leader values the importance of the here and now and believes that interaction between group members is crucial, it follows that the emphasis on in-group experiences will take precedence over out-of-group experiences. While it is always necessary to look for parallels for reported out-of-group events that might reflect avoided in-group happenings, it is imperative that important out-of-group events be treated with the concern and responsiveness they deserve. This is even more significant for a group composed of recovering addicts and alcoholics. The danger of a relapse, an out-of-group event, is always, without fail, the most salient concern when treating this population because treatment is essentially stopped if the addict or alcoholic returns to drugs and alcohol. However, just as a group composed of non-addicted individuals are apt to do, alcoholics and addicts can use out-of-group events as a resistance and a way to distance themselves from emotionally charged events in the group. This is especially true if the leader allows his or her addicted group members to escape into old drinking and drug using "war stories" under the guise that telling these stores will somehow enhance their sobriety and recovery. Louis Ormont offers one good suggestion for determining whether a reported out-of-group event is resistance or a genuine attempt to communicate something of emotional importance to the group. Ormont recommends that the group leader assess whether this outside event is being reported in a drab, detached manner or in an emotionally charged way that provokes strong feelings that enhance the responsiveness of others in the group. Any event that has occurred outside of the group can have important implications for the group as long as it is brought alive within the immediacy of the moment.

Affect versus Cognition

All experienced therapists know there is an important difference between a cognitive understanding and an emotional understanding. Exclusive attention to affect without cognition or cognition without affect is generally ineffective. The skilled practitioner knows how to balance these and discern which patients need more of one and less of the other at a particular time in their treatment. The evaluation of how much affect at this time for this individual takes on special considerations when working with alcoholics and addicts. Frequently, too much affect too soon can lead to a relapse. However, there are numerous exceptions to this position. Sometimes, the failure to release pent-up emotions can just as easily contribute to a relapse. Determining which addicts or alcoholics need to contain their emotions and which need to release them is not always easy. How much affect is too much for this individual at this particular time in recovery is a question that needs careful consideration. Clinical experience and recent research suggest that catharsis is especially important for some addicts and alcoholics early in their recovery. Orchestrating this within the confines and safety of an inpatient unit will ensure that the limits and containment will be in place to prevent addicts or alcoholics from having easy or ready access to their drug of choice. It is important to discriminate between the promotion of regression for regression's sake and the creation of a safe, therapeutic environment that will allow and invite the natural release of blocked emotions. Avoiding unnecessary invasive procedures, when less intrusive methods of effective treatment are available, is just as crucial in psychotherapy as it is in surgery.

Process versus Content

There is usually a strong pull in groups for individual members to respond to the content of a person's communication. Process commentary is usually the group leader's domain and responsibility. While process can occur intrapersonally (e.g., an individual's own free association), group process generally reflects the free exchange that needs to take place among and between group members. In order for this to occur so that the entire range of feelings will be available for the group, all of the group members must feel free to respond openly and spontaneously to whatever comes to their minds. While this is difficult for everyone, it is especially difficult for alcoholics and addicts. Alcoholics and addicts do not handle interpersonal conflicts or differences very well. Burdened by their own overwhelming feelings of shame and vulnerability to narcissistic injury, they will go to great lengths to avoid inflicting similar feelings on others. Consequently, their interactions are usually superficial, highly structured, and avoidant or combative if forced to deal with an emotionally threatening issue. Through the influence and misuse of AA and other twelve-step programs, they will keep their exchanges superficial, controlled, and highly supportive except when it comes to the area of chemical use. This is the one area where they have been granted complete freedom to speak as openly and honestly about their feelings as they can. AA and the twelve-step tradition discourages "cross-talk" at their meetings. Content, therefore, is the primary focus of a twelve-step meeting, and an exclusive focus on the content usually elicits responses that predominantly take the form of advice-giving. This is almost totally contrary to the tasks expected of patients in a psychotherapy group. Consequently, group leaders will have to direct a great deal of energy toward educating their group members on the ways they can use the therapy group most effectively. Distinguishing between what is helpful at AA and what is required in group will help members see that each format has something valuable to offer, and that neither format should be degraded or devalued.

Understanding versus Experience

Rutan and Stone (1993) emphasize that while insight and understanding are vitally important in all forms of treatment, they are usually insufficient by themselves to bring about any real change in an individual. The opportunity to experience life and others in a different and more satisfying way is at the bottom of any effective change or healing process. Just as AA and other twelve-step programs provide this for the recovering addict or alcoholic, the group can provide its members with a unique learning experience. Yalom's concept of cohesion in group captures the potential benefits of belonging to a healthy holding environment where the primary emotional experience is that of acceptance, empathy, support, nurturing, caring, predictability, and honesty. It is impossible for any individual, addicted or not, to have such an experience and not be profoundly changed. While there is some controversy regarding the definition and benefits of a corrective emotional experience, it is now recognized that it involves more than just loving an individual into health. It means giving him or her an authentic, real, and caring experience with an authentic, real, and caring individual. More appropriately called the corrective emotional relationship, such relationships are inherently built into a well-functioning group.

Alcoholics and addicts, perhaps more than those who are not addicted, have extreme difficulties establishing mutually satisfying relationships. Being able to do so requires the opportunity to learn by experiencing it, rather than being given a formula that explains how to do it. Rutan and Stone sum this up when they write:

> Groups provide uniquely therapeutic opportunities to acquire both understanding (emotional and cognitive insight) and corrective emotional experiences; they provide opportunities to build new psychic structures via better, more authentic, and more nourishing relationships and to try out and practice new behavior patterns. Group leaders need not choose between the ends of this continuum; they need to ensure that both ends are operative and that patients are receiving both information and experiences. (1993, p. 141)

PSYCHOTHERAPY OUTCOME RESEARCH

While many of the qualities of the therapist described by Grotjohn and others are certainly admirable, science has taught us that things are not always as they seem to be on the surface. Research has demonstrated that while many of the innate characteristics described by experienced clinicians such as Whitaker, Yalom, Polster, and others do indeed play a very significant part in successful treatment, the interplay between a therapist's characteristics and successful treatment is a subtle and delicate one. However, before the reader is left with the impression that the possession of these described innate human characteristics is all that is needed for successful treatment, it is important to understand what research has discovered about this factor. Strupp and Hadley (1979) concluded that while nonspecific factors such as therapist characteristics were crucial in setting up an initial alliance with a patient, they were not enough to produce successful treatment outcome if long-term treatment was required past the first two or three meetings. After the initial meeting, specific factors such as technique, training, and experience played a more significant part in treatment. Strupp and Hadley discovered that individuals who were not professional therapists, but who possessed important innate characteristics such as the capacity for caring and warmth, could provide immediate relief to many patients during the first couple of sessions if these individuals could demonstrate their ability to understand and empathize with the patient. However, after the initial relationship was established and more specific interventions were required of the nonprofessional therapists, they were at a loss as to how to respond. This is where the specific training and skills of the professional therapist are required to move the patient beyond the limits of their presenting condition.

In one of the most thorough and complete reviews of all treatment outcome studies, Bergin (1971) agreed with this position when he concluded that successful psychotherapy is determined in large part by the characteristics of the therapist. Bergin found that the three most significant contributing factors to successful treatment are (in order of importance):

1. The patient's characteristics
2. The therapist's characteristics
3. The therapist's technique or theoretical orientation

Bergin's findings suggest that two of the most important contributing factors in successful treatment outcome are beyond the control of universities, training institutes, and teaching facilities. In the words of Cassell from earlier in the chapter, "Is it possible to teach sensitivity?" Certainly, the capacity to care represents a crucial variable to successful treatment, but it appears that this is something therapists bring with them to the therapy situation. However, as Whitaker and Malone (1953) suggested, therapists may be far more effective if they have had a successful therapy experience themselves. This is one good argument for therapists in training to receive their own therapy before they are turned loose on their patients. Certainly, this suggestion would hold true for group leaders. It would be important for them to have a good group therapy experience before they could be expected to be effective group leaders themselves. Bergin's findings also stress the importance of the patient's contribution to successful treatment. The fact is that many patients are just not suitable for psychotherapy. They are either too disturbed or too resistant to benefit from treatment. The specifics of these patients' characteristics will be explored later in the chapter.

Psychotherapy Update

In recent years, research concerning psychotherapy process and outcome has increased greatly in sophistication and has generated interesting findings with important clinical relevance. The upsurge in treatment outcome research was, in large part, stimulated by earlier claims that psychotherapy was found to be no more beneficial than no treatment (Eysenck, 1952). Greatly improved methods of reviewing and aggregating the vast amount of literature on this subject have demonstrated that much of the early research methodology had been seriously flawed. The most powerful conclusion of this massive review was that psychotherapy works. The average treated patient was found to be as well off as the patient in the 80th percentile of the control groups.

Specific Effects

Another result emerging from this review was a failure to demonstrate that some therapies are better than others. One interpretation of this result is that different psychotherapies, however diverse they may seem in their specific techniques, are really effective by virtue of their shared, or nonspecific, ingredients, such as the healing ritual that provides hope, reverses demoralization, establishes a helping relationship, and provides patients with an increased sense of understanding and control over their present situation (Frank, 1961).

The quality of the therapeutic alliance, even when it is measured early in treatment, has been found to be the best and most consistent predictor of outcome. It appears that a good therapeutic relationship between patient and therapist is more important in predicting change than are factors that reside only in the patient or the therapist. Moreover, it appears that the patient is more powerful than the therapist in determining the nature of the therapeutic alliance. However, there is evidence suggesting that part of the success in all forms of psychotherapy may be attributed to the therapist's ability to mobilize the patient's expectation of help. Frank (1961) specifically suggests that the common effective factor in all forms of therapy is the patient's faith in treatment, and this factor should be deliberately mobilized in treatment.

Mobilizing a patient's faith in treatment and his or her expectancy of help is a crucial issue when working with alcoholics and addicts. Treatment approaches such as AA that encourage, engage, and promise relief may work better with these patients because they mobilize a patient's expectancy for help. Treatment approaches that are passive and unresponsive and rely on the alcoholic's or addict's own source of motivation frequently fail because they do not address this crucial issue in treatment.

Frank identifies two important sources that will evoke the patient's expectancy of help. First is the personal magnetism of the healer, which is often strengthened by the healer's faith in what he or she does. Another source of the patient's faith is the ideology of the healer or sect, which offers the patient a rationale, however absurd, for making sense of his or her illness and the treatment procedure. Anyone who has attended AA meetings on a regular basis knows that each of these forces are operating strongly in the AA program.

Frank sees any procedure that places the healer in the position of transmitter or controller of impressive healing forces as enhancing the patient's faith in the treatment process. Whether that position is defined as an enthusiastic recovering alcoholic with many years of happy sobriety or a professional psychotherapist is irrelevant for Frank. Healers in our present-day society characteristically back up their pretensions with an elaborate scientific-sounding pattern of theories and diagnostic labels.

Frank further posited that since the success of psychotherapy does not seem to be linked to any particular type of therapy and since the relief of discomfort was the same regardless of the types of treatment utilized, relief of the patient's suffering may have more to do with the therapist"s ability to mobilize the patient's trust, hope, and faith in the treatment process.

Patients' Characteristics and Contributions to Successful Therapy

Based on the abundance of research evidence gathered over time, the most powerful vehicle for producing significant therapeutic change seems to be an emotionally charged interpersonal relationship. This relationship need not be with a professional therapist, but it does need to be an emotionally charged one with a real person. The effectiveness of this relationship in producing desirable therapeutic change is determined in large part by the therapist's personality and his or her skill at managing interpersonal relationships, especially with individuals who have a history of difficulties in this area. Some patients, such as severely psychotic individuals, cannot tolerate the closeness of a real interpersonal relationship. Others, who are severely mentally retarded, brain-damaged, intoxicated, or suffering from a severe character disorder are incapable of forming a true working alliance with a therapist. What patients bring to psychotherapy, at least as far as their interpersonal skills are concerned, determines in a large part the potential success of a therapeutic encounter. The more the patients have to offer the therapy situation and the less severe their difficulties, the more likely treatment will be successful. Conversely, the more severe the patients' disorders, the less chance that they will benefit from treatment–no matter how skillful and "together" the therapist may be.

Initial Phase of Treatment

Patients' willingness to enter treatment is determined by a number of important factors, of which their level of experienced distress is the most influential. The effectiveness of the initial stages of treatment is enhanced by the therapist's ability to mobilize patients' expectancy for help, and this is influenced in large part by patients' ability to possess a favorable expectation from treatment. This requires the patient to be able to accept and respond to symbols of healing. Good responders to psychotherapy expect treatment to help them and are better integrated socially and less mistrustful than poor responders. The ability of a person to respond favorably is not so much a sign of excessive gullibility as it is of easy acceptance of others in their socially defined roles. However, the more suggestible the patient and the greater the experienced distress, the more likely he or she is to stay in treatment.

There are a number of important factors that will enhance the patient's willingness to perceive the therapist as a source of help. Certainly, the therapist's ability to inspire the patient's confidence in him or her as a credible psychotherapist or healer is essential. It should be understood, however, that there is not a close correspondence between these inferred attributes as rated by either the therapist him or herself, external observers, or the patient whom the therapist serves. The most consistent relationship found between therapeutic outcome and inferred therapist qualities is that derived from the patient's perception of the therapist rather than either from the therapist's perception of him or herself or the ratings of external observers.

The patient's willingness to continue treatment is, in turn, dependent to a large extent on the patient's personal liking of the therapist. It has also been found that if the patient perceives the therapist to be a credible person, there is more of a chance that he or she will find the therapist more attractive. The concepts of credibility and attractiveness are not mutually exclusive. Research has demonstrated that those who are perceived as experts and who engender trust wield greater influence over attitude and behavior change. Consequently, patients are more accepting of explanations or interpretations that conflict with their own perceptions of the world and belief systems when these interpretations and explanations are presented by therapists who are perceived as attractive and credible. The acceptance of advice-giving is thus dependent on the patient's perceived estimation of the therapist's competence, skill, anticipated thoroughness, and attractiveness. Like credibility, attractiveness interacts completely with issues of interpersonal similarity and compatibility.

The patient's perception of the therapist as an interpersonally attractive person facilitates the initial development of perceptions that in turn produces positive outcomes. Attractiveness is more important than credibility during the initial stages of therapy and results in the patient's remaining in treatment long enough to develop the therapeutic alliance necessary for real change. Credibility, which usually includes such qualities as trust, competence, and ability, is a more subtle feature of the therapist and has more influence on the patient's gains throughout therapy.

THE THERAPEUTIC PROCESS: THERAPISTS' AND PATIENTS' CONTRIBUTIONS

Therapists' Contribution

Therapists must have the capacity to be empathic. They must be able to experience what the other person is experiencing without losing themselves or becoming the other person. However, as Ornstein (1981) says, this empathic understanding is useless if therapists are unable to communicate to the patients what they understand. Therapists who just sit there with their empathic understanding do little good for their patients if they are unable to convey their understanding back to the patients.

Therapists must also be able to listen to what patients say. More important, they must also be able to listen to what patients do not say and leave out of their conversations. This requires listening with a third ear. Listening is not a passive process. It is an alert activity that is necessary if therapists are to be able to make understandable, for themselves and the patients, what the patients are experiencing. This in turn helps the patients make sense of their own experiences. This is where theory plays an important part in patients' treatment. The more sound the theory, the more it will give the patients cognitively. A solid framework for understanding will help patients master their situation more completely.

Therapists must also possess a nonjudgmental attitude. They must listen without judging. Freud referred to this as neutrality. However, many therapists have come to confuse neutrality with a nonresponsive, blank-screen-stance in therapy. Despite Freud's caution, therapists will be more effective if they realize it is impossible not to form a judgment of their patients. Therapists form constant opinions on what patients have to say. But they must not impose their opinions or judgments on the patients unless this opinion concerns alcoholic drinking or drug use. While it is generally a therapeutic maxim that therapists should not impose their standards on their patients, this stance can be destructive for an alcoholic or addict. In most cases, it is best if patients discover their own value system. Because of their shared characterological deficits and cognitive impairment, however, alcoholics and addicts may require an imposed value system such as AA until they have had enough time to restore their cognitive functioning to the point where they are able to think clearly and rationally for themselves.

Therapists should also avoid provocative behavior when their patients are hostile. It is important for therapists to tune into their own feelings and use their counter-transference as a barometer to help them understand their patients better. If this understanding leads to a calculated confrontation with an alcoholic or addict, there is less chance that it will be triggered by the therapist's own unconscious anger.

Patients' Contributions

There are three basic patient contributions that need to be assessed in treatment.

1. Patients usually come to treatment with anxiety, doubts, and fears. These feelings are often unexpressed. If patients are court referrals, they will also present with anger and hostility. Such feelings have to be expressed at the beginning of treatment, or the therapist will lose the patients. Repressed feelings increase the likelihood that these feelings will be acted out. Talking, on the other hand, diffuses their intensity.
2. Patients present with a certain level of psychological development that is the result of their previous experiences. The more troublesome these experiences were at an earlier age, the more difficulty the patients will have. The more difficulty the patients have, the more disturbed they will be and the more difficulty they will have understanding and relating to the therapist. The more disturbed patients will not be able to understand or handle passivity or interpretations. They will require support, calming, and soothing from the therapist.
3. Every patient comes to treatment with certain expectations. Many come with what is commonly referred to as the curative fantasy. Their hope is that the therapist will somehow magically remove their discomfort and ills. Many will have a silver-platter attitude. On an unconscious level, they still cling to magical thinking much like small children who believe that if their mother will only kiss their hurt, their pain will go away. For such individuals, their parents are frequently viewed in an unrealistic, omnipotent fashion. If children hurt themselves, for instance, they will often blame the mother. If they view the therapist like they did their mother, they will believe on some level that the therapist will be so powerful as to be able to magically cure them.

With alcoholics and addicts suffering from more severe characterological deficits, such as borderline patients, the therapist can expect to easily provoke their rage and anger. Because patients frequently view the therapist as magically powerful, they will expect him or her to remove their hurt and pain. Since the therapist does not, they reason that he or she must have the power but is withholding it. Their rage is, in one sense, saying, "Why do not you make me feel better? If you cared, you would give to me so I wouldn't hurt so badly. Since you aren't removing my pain, you must dislike me. Since I've done all you've asked and still hurt, you must be uncaring and awful because you have treated me so badly."

As distorted and unrealistic as the curative fantasy may be, it should not be interfered with too quickly. Often, this belief may be the most salient motivating factor in an individual's continual investment in treatment, abstinence, and recovery. This situation was dramatically demonstrated by a newly recovering alcoholic who had little more than one year's sobriety and decided to attend a national conference on alcoholism treatment. A nationally recognized alcoholism treatment expert, who also had nearly fifteen years of sobriety through AA, openly stated that AA does not have all the magical answers. He further added that if a person were to just stop drinking, this would not cure him of all his problems. Abstinence was just the first step in the long and difficult process of recovery. Upon hearing this, the newly recovering alcoholic admitted to the other group members the next week, "That scared the hell out of me. If I would have heard that just one week sooner, I don't think I could have handled it. Thank God, that information wasn't given to me sooner."

The curative fantasy and its proper utilization in treatment can have an important influence on recovery, as demonstrated by the following vignette:

> Angie, a thirty-two-year-old artist and photographer, had sought treatment because of an unhappy marriage. Her husband refused to respond to her requests that they seek conjoint therapy and he had a history of physically abusing her when he became intoxicated. After a few weeks of therapy, it became obvious that she, as well as her husband, was an alcoholic. She promptly responded to the therapist's request that she stop drinking and join AA. After nearly a year of individual therapy and regular AA attendance, she divorced her husband and eventually entered a psychotherapy group at her therapist's suggestion. Six months into the therapy group, in a moment of extreme frustration, she screamed at the other group members and the group leader, "Look, I've done everything you've told me to do and things still aren't perfect. I still get angry and people still hurt me!" The next few sessions following her outburst were marked by her sharing of deep feelings of sadness and hurt as she struggled with the

realization that things were not ever going to be perfect. This was a stance that she had taken early in her life as a child. Her parents, who were brutally critical of her, demanded that she live up to their expectations and only showed her love or affection when she performed perfectly. After more than two months of struggling with this realization, she finally stated to the group and its leader one evening, "I realize that even if things aren't perfect, they are a lot better than I imagined they would ever be. I guess I kind of like this reality thing. But, if I knew it was going to be this hard when I started out, I do not think I would have had the courage to put myself through all this pain. I thought a couple of months ago that I would just go back to my old ways of dealing with things, but I realized that wouldn't work for me either. I think that's why I got so angry. I didn't like where I was and I couldn't go back to where I've been. I felt stuck and cheated by you. Now I realize this place here isn't really so bad."

GROUP PSYCHOTHERAPY RESEARCH

The most extensive controlled research on the effectiveness of group therapy was conducted in part by Yalom (Lieberman, Yalom, and Miles, 1973). The research project was complex and, as Yalom states, expensive. The full description of the project will not be explored here. However, one major aim of the study was to investigate the effect of leader technique upon treatment outcome. Eighteen experienced and expert group leaders from ten different ideological schools (i.e., Gestalt, psychodrama, TA, psychodynamic, etc.) were each recruited to run a group that met for a total of thirty hours over a twelve-week period. An extensive battery of psychological and personality measures was administered to each member of each group three times: before the start of the first group, immediately after the twelfth group session was completed, and six months after termination from the group.

Yalom discovered some disturbing results. Two-thirds of all the subjects who participated in the study found it to be an unrewarding experience. In fact, some individuals actually became worse as a result of treatment and were judged by Yalom to be casualties. A casualty is one who, as a result of group experience, suffers considerable and persistent psychological distress. Since several types of groups had been studied, it was found that the key causative factor of casualties was not the type of group, but rather the individual, personal style of the group leader. Leaders with the highest casualty rate were described as "aggressive stimulators" by Yalom. They were intrusive, confrontive, and challenging. They also revealed a great deal of themselves and surprisingly were judged by most members to be the most charismatic. Groups that experienced low casualty rates had leaders who were described as "loving" and who created an "accepting, trusting climate."

Yalom further discovered that if he analyzed the research data for each group independently, he was left with an equally interesting conclusion. In some groups, almost every member underwent some positive change with no casualties among them. In other groups, there were cases where not a single member benefitted from treatment. All were either casualties or were fortunate to remain unchanged. Again, it was discovered that the leadership style was the most important contributing factor to successful treatment. In fact, the group that had the highest success rate was led by a leader who belonged to the same ideological school as the leader who had the lowest success rate and highest number of casualties. The ideological school to which the group leader belonged actually had little to do with the success rate of any of the therapy groups in this study.

Yalom, trying to answer the question of what determines successful group therapy writes,

> The next obvious question–and one very relevant to psychotherapy–is: Which type of leader had the best, and which the worst, results? The T-group leader, the gestalt, the T.A., the psychodrama leader, and so on? However, we soon learned that the question posed in this form was not meaningful. The behavior of the leaders when carefully rated by observers varied greatly and did not conform to our pre-group expectations. *The ideological school to which a leader belonged told us little about the actual behavior of that leader.* We found that the behavior of the leader of one school–for example, transactional analysis–resembled the behavior of the other T.A. leader no more closely than that of any of the other seventeen leaders. In other words, the behavior of a leader is not predictable from one's membership in a particular ideological school. Yet the effectiveness of a group was, in large part, a function of its leader's behavior. (1985, p. 501)

Yalom's discovery of the lack of congruence between what group leaders say they do in group and what they actually do in group was made clear in a statement Bob Goulding made about Fritz Perls. After having worked and trained with Perls for many years, Goulding confessed that the way Perls wrote about doing psychotherapy was often quite different from the ways Perls actually did psychotherapy. Certainly, Yalom's research findings support Goulding's personal observation of one universally recognized expert in group therapy. This observation is made more relevant by the fact that

Robert Goulding was one of the eighteen group leaders who participated in the original Lieberman, Yalom, and Miles study. Also, Goulding was the group leader who had the most improved group members with no group therapy casualties and was consequently rated the most effective group leader in this study.

Yalom and his cohorts attempted to determine exactly what it was about Robert Goulding and the other successful group leaders that influenced successful treatment outcome. Yalom (1995) derived a factor analysis of a large number of leadership variables and categorized them into four basic leadership functions.

1. *Emotional stimulation* (challenging, confronting activity; intrusive modeling by personal risk-taking and high self-disclosure).
2. *Caring* (offering support, affection, praise, protection, warmth, acceptance, genuineness, concern).
3. *Meaning attribution* (explaining, clarifying, interpreting, providing a cognitive framework for change; translating feelings and experiences into ideas).
4. *Executive function* (setting limits, rules, norms, goals; managing time; pacing, stopping, interceding, suggesting procedures).

These four leadership functions were found to have a powerful relationship to successful treatment outcome. (See Figure 12.3.) As Figure 12.3 illustrates, there was a direct linear relationship between caring, meaning attribution, and successful treatment outcome. In other words, group leaders cannot care too much for their group members and they cannot provide for them too much meaning for their confusion or suffering. On the other hand, group leaders who do too much or too little emotional stimulation and too much or too little executive functioning increase the likelihood of having an unsuccessful group. In any of these cases, leaders can either be too passive and not provide the group with enough direction or they can be too provocative or confrontive and the group will become leader-centered and too dependent upon the leader for direction and leadership.

THE IMPLICATIONS FOR CONDUCTING A SUCCESSFUL THERAPY GROUP

It was through the examination of the individual subjects' ratings of the different leaders that Yalom was given the first indication of any trend in positive success of group participation. The leaders studied ranged from

FIGURE 12.3

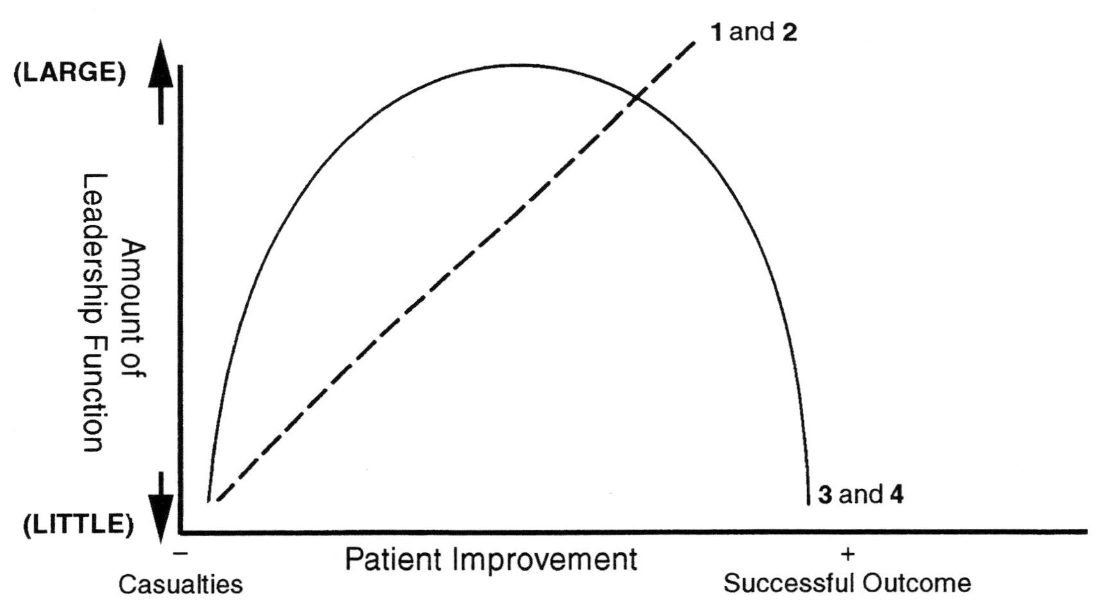

1. **Caring** (Support, Warmth, Concern, Loving, Protection)
2. **Meaning Attribution** (Explaining, Providing a Cognitive Framework)
3. **Executive Function** (Norms, Goals, Setting Limits, Direction)
4. **Emotional Stimulation** (Confronting, Risk Taking, Self-Disclosure)

those who were primarily analytic and interpretive, to those who saw the management of group forces as their distinctive function, and to still others who offered instructional, often nonverbal exercises almost exclusively. Some of the leaders believed passionately in love; others just as passionately in hatred. Some leaders depended solely on talk therapy; others used music, lights, and the touch of human bodies. The study found that the most effective leaders–the ideal type–were moderate in the amount of stimulation and executive behavior they showed and high in caring, and that they actively utilized meaning attribution. Meaning attribution showed the strongest association with positive outcome.

The nature of the group as a social system was judged by Yalom to be very important. Whether participants identify with the group, whether they like it, their role in the group, and whether the group likes them are all relevant to the outcome. The study further indicated that group members who liked their groups, who participated actively, and who were valued by other group members learned more. All these indications illustrated that the leaders who instilled norms favoring moderate emotional intensity and confrontation were the most popular.

Contrary to what many encounter group leaders and members seem to believe ("There is no group, only persons"), the study indicated very clear evidence that the nature of the group as a social system is important in affecting outcomes. Also contrary to the opinion expressed by some that "the group can comfort, but it can't cure" (Back, 1972), Yalom studies indicate that under the proper leadership, group therapy can have a significant effect on a person's life. Groups in which the leader instills a sense of cohesion functioned better, and individual members related their experience more favorably. The clear indication is that nonauthoritative leaders operating in a more democratic manner were viewed more favorably by members due primarily to the feeling of autonomy on their part when in the group. Many intangibles combine to make up what may be described as a good leader. Back sums it up best with his definition that "a good sensitivity trainer combines the religious healer's charisma with the scientist's language." Undoubtedly, the early criticism of psychotherapy groups was misdirected, in that all group therapy is not bad, but rather it is the poorly led group with a poorly trained or inadequately prepared leader that must be evaluated with a critical eye.

ALCOHOLISM TREATMENT OUTCOME STUDIES

Many reviews of alcoholism and substance abuse treatment studies have generally revealed mixed and conflicting findings. However, when older studies are excluded because of methodological flaws due primarily to the inconsistency of diagnostic criterion (alcoholism in one study did not fit the criterion for alcoholism in another) and because there is now more effective treatment for addiction, a consensus begins to emerge from the more recent research efforts. Studies generally support the conclusion that some treatment is better than no treatment (Emrick, 1974). Longer treatment enhances success more than shorter treatment. Psychotherapy, especially group psychotherapy, can positively affect treatment success unless it discourages abstinence and involvement in outside support groups, in which case those who do not receive therapy have more success than those who do (Miller, 1995). Few meaningful differences are likely to be found in outcome among opiate addicts in methadone maintenance, residential drug-free, and outpatient drug-free treatment that are either a function of client difference or of time in treatment. Most well-conducted studies with substance abusers are unanimous in showing substantial changes in clients who remain in treatment, with longer treatment generally being correlated with better outcome. Individuals who dropped out of treatment early generally showed much less improvement over time.

The changing third-party reimbursement climate is also having a potent impact on addiction treatment. Cost-containment concerns have resulted in dramatic shifts from residential to outpatient services and from individual to group treatment and also have resulted in considerable decreases in length of treatment (National Institute on Alcohol Abuse and Alcoholism, 1995). Cost-effectiveness concerns influence expectations about cure and total abstinence that are often unrealistic. A comprehensive review of comparative chronic diseases such as diabetes, hypertension, and asthma found that rates of re-treatment and compliance with treatment were not superior to those for substance abuse treatment and, in most cases, were less impressive (NIAAA, 1995).

Studies overall support the view that addicts and alcoholics are better off after treatment than they were before treatment. The type of treatment appears to make little effective difference, as some studies have found that all procedures have the same degree of success (Matakas, Koester, and Leidner, 1978; Emrick, 1974; and Miller, 1995). The success rates–including spontaneous remission–lie between 40 and 50 percent. There were some reported exceptions to these general findings. Some treatment programs treating skid row alcoholics had success rates as low as 5 percent while some private hospitals utilizing a select patient population reported success rates as high as 90 percent. The treatment effect may last two years or longer if continued treatment or support groups are included. If not, treatment is usually short-lived (Miller, 1995). Overall, the one-year recovery rate was found to be very close to the five-year rate because most of the recidivism occurs in the first year of treatment. Consequently, like most other psychotherapeutic treatment modalities, addiction treatment research has shown that most therapeutic procedures are more or less effective if certain variables, especially abstinence, are held constant.

In one of the most recent and extensive reviews of addiction treatment outcome studies, Miller (1995) has concluded that the treatment of addiction "as generally practiced has not been well recorded in the psychological and medical literature" (p. 4). He goes on to speculate that this may be due to the arbitrary exclusion of twelve-step forms of treatment because they do not always fit neatly into research paradigms and because "there is a striking dichotomy between actual clinical methods and experimental investigations" (p. 4). Miller concludes that the most compelling explanation for this set of circumstances is that "the contemporary treatment of alcohol/drug disorders with few notable exceptions has developed outside of mainstream medicine/psychiatry/psychology" (p. 4). Because the abstinence-based method of treatment has not, until recently, been studied extensively, its critics have been slow to acknowledge that this form of treatment is a highly effective form of addiction treatment.

One final criticism put forth by Miller concerns the lack of well-controlled studies (one notable exception is Vaillant's extensive work) that look at treatment beyond a few months. This is especially critical in light of the twelve-step community's assertion that addiction is a lifelong disease. Based on this understanding, treatment outcome research has thus far confirmed the existence of a large variety of treatment methods that appear to work in the short run (weeks or even months).

However, looking at treatment outcome over an extensive period of time reveals abstinence as the only viable treatment option. Millers writes:

> Treatment outcome research confirms that only one method of treatment appears to be effective and to consistently work in the long run (years to lifetimes), namely, abstinence based treatment when combined with regular, continuous and indefinite attendance at Alcoholics Anonymous meetings (Narcotics Anonymous is probably as effective, but sufficient data are not yet available). (1995, p. 18)

PATIENT CHARACTERISTICS RELATED TO TYPES OF THERAPY

Inpatient therapy was found to be basically no more successful that outpatient therapy. However, there were some identified characteristics indicating that one form of treatment may be preferable to another depending upon the patient's circumstances. Patients with more severe levels of addiction as well as more social and psychological instability were judged to be better candidates for inpatient treatment. On the other hand, patients who have a stable and permanent work relationship that might be compromised by long-term inpatient treatment were more likely to benefit from outpatient treatment. This is especially significant since those patients who respond best to treatment are those who have a permanent work situation, intact marriage, and continual family support (Matakas, Koester, and Leidner, 1978). Very similar findings were reported by Collins (1995), who wrote:

> Outcome differences were related more to patient factors, including motivation, chronicity, and severity of alcoholism, age and gender, and personal, interpersonal, familial, educational, and vocational resources rather than to treatment factors, including theoretical orientation, content, focus, and intensity of treatment, which generally predict treatment outcome poorly. The possibility that patient variables are a better predictor of outcome than program content does not mean that treatment per se is ineffective. Rather, in a way analogous to an educational model, those who bring more to the process, even if only in the form of greater motivation, seem to achieve greater success. (p. 35)

At the other end of the spectrum is research evidence clearly demonstrating that the lower-class, less-educated, and socially disadvantaged alcoholic and addict has the worse treatment prognosis. Detox is not enough, nor is impatient therapy by itself sufficient to bring any long-standing change. One recommendation is that treatment of an undetermined length of time–possibly lifelong–is the most realistic approach. Certainly, this suggests that involvement in twelve-step programs and their affiliated support groups is the most viable option for these individuals.

A voluntary model of treatment utilization was found to not work well for alcoholism and drug addiction. Research has deemed that entry into addiction treatment services usually involves some degree of coercion, including sanctions from the criminal justice system, the workplace, or welfare office or pressure from family and community (NIAAA, 1995). Self-help groups such as AA, NA, and CA dominate the treatment field. In fact, national survey data have shown that more individuals attend AA than formal treatment programs. The mainstream chemical dependency treatment model relies heavily on AA's approach. However, the addiction treatment field is marked by ideological controversy and differences. Besides the abstinence-based treatment modalities, there are controlled drinking, harm reduction, and Moderation Management techniques that are heavily influenced and advocated by behaviorally oriented researchers (NIAAA, 1995).

Psychotherapy

Research also demonstrated that group therapy was the treatment of choice, although it was noted that "there is a lack of adequately based clinical investigations regarding its effectiveness" (Matakas, Koester, and Leidner, 1978, p. 5). Bakeland, Lundwall, and Kissin (1975) cited some controlled studies that reported results ranging from total abstinence in 15 percent of the cases to significant improvement in 47 percent of the cases. Empirical research into the effectiveness of group psychotherapy in the treatment of substance abuse has been until recently either limited, anecdotal, or equivocal, despite its popularity (Cahn, 1970; Matakas, Koester, and Leider, 1978; Stein and Friedman, 1971). However, the little empirical research that was previously available was enthusiastically supported by anecdotal reports and clinical impressions (Kanas, 1982). Cahn (1970), for instance, found in a national survey that group psychotherapy is a widely preferred method in alcoholism treatment programs. Matakas, Koester, and Leidner (1978) agreed when they expressed similar sentiments that group psychotherapy is viewed as dogma in the treatment of alcoholism and drug abuse even though there is little empirical research to support its popularity. Pattison (1979) was of the opinion that there has not been enough empirical research to support the popularity of group psychotherapy as a method of choice for treatment of alcoholism and drug abuse. What is lacking, he suggested, is a clear differentiation of the types of group methods that can be selectively used for specific therapeutic goals with different types of patients. Pattison (1979) suggested that this was not to imply that group psychotherapy is not useful, but that there is a need to construct specific guidelines for group psychotherapy. Kanas (1982), on the other hand, cited clinical research, both anecdotal and empirical, that has generally been enthusiastic regarding the effectiveness of group psychotherapy with addicted patients. Furthermore, group psychotherapy has a long history as a significant, if not major, therapeutic modality in the treatment of alcoholism (Stein and Friedman, 1971). Many studies have shown that the treatment of choice for addiction, in most instances, is group psychotherapy. In some cases, the estimation is that the recovery rate for patients in group psychotherapy is two to three times higher than for patients who only receive individual psychotherapy (Kanas, 1982, Yalom, 1985). In a review of the treatment outcome literature on group psychotherapy and addiction, Kanas (1982) found most studies supported the claims made in the anecdotal literature regarding the effectiveness of group psychotherapy as a treatment modality.

Within the last few years, group therapy has become the preferred mode of treatment for substance dependent patients. Many types of group therapy have been used with this population, including behavioral, cognitive, psychodrama, Gestalt, and rational emotive, to name a few (Zimberg, 1980; Brandsma and Pattison, 1985). Some researchers have suggested that psychodynamic and insight-oriented therapy is not effective with this population (Holder et al., 1993; Miller and Hester, 1986). However, most of the extensive reports by group leaders who work exclusively with this population strongly recommend otherwise.

SPECIFIC GROUP STRATEGIES AND REQUIREMENTS

Within the last few years there has been an increasing body of research and clinical literature addressing the ways that group psychotherapy can be adapted to fit the specific needs of the addicted patient. Generally, there has been a growing consensus among those who regularly work with addicted patients in a group therapy format. Khantzian, Halliday, and McAuliffe (1990), Vannicelli (1988), S. Brown (1985), Matano and Yalom (1991), Flores and Mahon (1993), and the author of this book (Flores, 1988b) have provided extensive suggestions about the ways that proven group therapy strategies can be adapted and modified to address the unique problems and characteristics of the addicted patient. All of these authors agree that abstinence is a crucial, if not the most important, element in the substance abuser's recovery. All are supportive of the chemically dependent patient's involvement in twelve-step programs while he or she is also participating in a therapy group. All of these authors operate from a group therapy format that usually includes an interpersonal approach to group psychotherapy that relies heavily on Irvin Yalom's (1985) theoretical model of interactional group therapy or a modified form of psychodynamic group psychotherapy (Flores and Mahon 1993, Khantzian, Halliday, and McAuliffe, 1990). In combination with Yalom's theory, most have also adapted many of the principles of psychodynamic group therapy, with some modifications in technique that take into special consideration chemically dependent individuals' propensity to return to chemical use if their anxiety, shame, anger, and guilt is not carefully modulated. This is especially true during the early phase of treatment.

Because of the heavy influence of AA and other twelve-step programs, it is also important that group leaders become well-versed in the language and philosophy of these twelve-step programs. Matano and Yalom (1991) strongly recommend that group therapists become thoroughly familiar with Alcoholics Anonymous, its language, its twelve steps, and its twelve traditions. They recommend this for numerous reasons, foremost among them the addict's or alcoholic's propensity to use AA as a therapy resistance either because of deliberate avoidance or misperceptions about the twelve-step program. As Matano and Yalom suggest, "It is important that therapists not permit misconceptions of AA to be used as therapy resistance and that they be able to harness the wisdom of AA for psychotherapeutic ends" (1991, p. 269).

Most research into group psychotherapy has focused on outcome rather than process (Kassel and Wagner, 1993). A recent survey attempting to delineate the mechanisms of change that are most influential in group therapy with alcoholics suggested that different factors play more or less important roles at different times during the course of treatment. Utilizing Yalom's curative factors as an assessment tool, it was discovered that catharsis or the release of repressed emotions was much more important and influential for *inpatient groups.* In contrast, instillation of hope and altruism were more important for *outpatient treatment.* Group cohesiveness and interaction (interpersonal output and input) remained constant for both types of group treatment. Comparisons were made to a study by Emrick, Lassen, and Edwards (1977) in which the curative factors operating in AA were identified. Similarities were discovered between AA and outpatient groups, as altruism, cohesion, instillation of hope, and identification were the curative factors most frequently cited in the AA literature (Kassel and Wagner, 1993) .

Behavioral Therapy

Matakas, Koester, and Leidner (1978) reported varying success rates for both classical and aversive conditioning therapies. However, as Emrick (1989) and Wallace, Forbes, and Chalmers (1979) are correct in pointing out, there is much evidence to suggest that this research, such as most other research on alcoholism treatment success, is seriously flawed. Since it has been clear from the start that this author's bias leans heavily toward abstinence as the primary goal of treatment and since the effectiveness of "controlled drinking" has not yet been clearly established, the research findings in this area will be limited to those behavioral strategies that encourage abstinence from alcohol rather than continual alcohol consumption.

As Emrick (1974) demonstrated in an extensive review of 478 alcoholism treatment outcome studies, some treatment is better than no treatment.

However, Emrick (1979) later noted that some types of behavioral intervention may actually do more harm than good for some patients. Emrick further suggests that research should be directed toward identifying those patients who might be harmed by this type of treatment.

Along similar lines, Matakas, Koester, and Leidner (1978) stated that "the criteria for conditioning therapy mentioned in the literature are not entirely convincing" (p. 2). The usefulness of drug therapy with disulfiram was also reported to be doubtful, and it was suggested that it should be employed only supportively with other forms of treatment.

A review on the controlled drinking research conducted by Miller (1995) revealed that the groups that did the best most consistently in most of the studies surveyed were those that abstained the most or had the greatest days of abstinence. In general, alcoholics who have the greater number of days of abstinence do better than those who have fewer days of abstinence. Miller suggests that such data indicates "that abstinence rather than controlled drinking led to better outcomes early on" (p. 14). Miller also found that one- and two-year follow-ups often show a gradual deterioration into the familiar patterns of alcoholic drinking. In general, Miller concludes, "Among those who receive training for controlled drinking the abstainers do the best; actual controlled drinking is associated with poorer outcome" (1995, p. 14).

The use of behavioral and cognitive techniques appears to be most helpful when used in the service of maintaining abstinence. Wallace (1978a) has written an excellent review for using behavioral techniques in the treatment of the addicted patient. He deliberately avoids the controversial topics of behavioral methods for controlled drinking, aversion conditioning, and systematic contingency-management techniques for many reasons. Namely, his many years of clinical experience with alcoholics have taught him that these methods do not work. Wallace realizes that most relapses occur within the first year and that the skillful utilization of some behavioral factors can enhance recovery, especially during the first few crucial months of abstinence from alcohol. In fact, Wallace sees AA operating within a behavioral change format. He writes,

> Attendance at AA meetings is, in effect, a behavioral change in the life of the alcoholic of significant proportions. Going to such meetings alters his typical schedule of activities, enables him to make new friendships, exposes him to a host of social supports and reinforcements, and permits him to gather information about other alcoholics and the disease of alcoholism very directly. In many respects AA itself is a behavioral change. (1978a, p. 102)

Self-Help Groups

Emrick, Lassen, and Edwards (1977) noted that AA is more successful than other therapeutic approaches when the alcoholic's goal is total abstinence. In his earlier research (1974), he suggested that AA was only suited for certain alcoholics with certain shared characteristics. This was a position he later reversed in another survey when he concluded that no clear profile emerged of the alcoholic who was most likely to attend AA. He suggested that all alcohol-troubled patients could wisely be regarded as possible members of AA and that at the very least, they needed to be informed of the organization's potential benefits (1989). His reversal illustrates a common misconception that many researchers had and still have of AA membership. Typically, AA has been erroneously described by many as best suited for middle-aged, white males with middle-class values who possess religious beliefs and dependency traits.

A recent AA membership survey (Alcoholics Anonymous, 1992) destroys many of these myths and stereotypes. Thirty-five percent of AA members are women, and this number is increasing each year. Forty-three percent of women and 57 percent of men are under the age of 30, and this number is increasing each year. The average length of sobriety is five years with 35 percent having more than five years of abstinence. An increasing number of members (46 percent) are also addicted to other drugs. Attendance at AA is very stable, with the average number of meetings per week at three. Before coming to AA, 63 percent of its members had received some type of therapy or counseling such as medical, psychological, or spiritual. Eighty percent reported that this treatment had played an important part in directing them to AA. After coming to AA, 56 percent have gone on to receive some type of treatment and counseling. Eighty-seven percent of those members who did receive some form of professional treatment said it played an important part in their recovery from alcoholism.

Empirical research has supported the view that AA participation is correlated with good outcome and cost-effectiveness. Individuals who attend AA weekly have better treatment outcomes, and less frequent attendance correlates with lower rates of sustained sobriety. In a similar fashion, controlled studies generally find significant treatment outcome for abstinence-based programs, particularly when combined with referral to AA (Miller, 1995).

RECOMMENDATIONS

Definite conclusions can be drawn from the data available on over 8,000 patients who have entered treatment programs throughout the

United States. A conclusion that Miller and his associates draw is that abstinence-based treatment works more effectively than those treatments that do not emphasize abstinence. Despite the relative lack of this recognition by more behaviorally oriented researchers, abstinence-based treatments dominate the treatment field. Controlled drinking appears to have little significant impact outside of academically oriented research. Miller goes on to conclude that it is unrealistic to assume that the higher differential-reported success between abstinence-based treatment and other treatment approaches is due to patient selection (higher patient motivation variable, etc.). He recommends that more competent research be done to determine how and why it is that some will avoid abstinence-based treatment when it is clearly more beneficial. He also recommends finding ways to encourage patients' participation in AA and other self-help groups. In a similar fashion, other researchers (Kellogg, 1993) suggest that therapy for addiction should be centered on helping the individual make a connection to a twelve-step group. Patient resistance and therapist resistance to this needs to be explored and better understood.

CONVERGENCE OF PATIENT AND THERAPIST CHARACTERISTICS

While psychotherapy research has succeeded in demonstrating that treatment works for most patients, there is not a clear understanding of why some patients profit more from it than other patients. Indeed, the research cited in this chapter suggests that the techniques and the theories to which psychotherapy outcome are usually attributed account for relatively little of the patient's actual change. In contrast, there is an abundance of evidence suggesting that most of the treatment gain is determined by virtue of the patient's coming to perceive the therapist as a competent, trustworthy, accepting, and caring individual who is responsive to his or her presenting difficulties. These perceptions are not dependent upon the therapist's theoretical orientation, training, or technique. Nor are these perceptions consistently evident from one patient to another. While it is evident that the characteristics of the patient determine to a great extent whether they will be able to perceive the favorable qualities of the therapist, it is not clear why some patients click with some therapists and not others. Certainly, the convergence of patient and therapist values and personalities plays a large part in the establishment of the therapeutic relationship. There is evidence suggesting that success in both psychotherapy and alcoholism treatment is very much dependent upon the establishment of a good working alliance. It is therefore important to understand the nature of the therapeutic relationship and the working alliance if one is to be an effective group leader.

Hans Strupp (1978) has succinctly outlined the process of establishing a good working relationship in therapy. The matching of therapist and patient characteristics is determined to a large degree by the successful management of the early hours of therapy. Furthermore, a good human relationship is judged by Strupp to be a precondition for the therapist's technical interventions. Strupp writes,

> There is ample evidence that any "good" human relationship–i.e., an interaction characterized by understanding, acceptance, respect, trust, empathy, and warmth–is helpful and constructive. If such a relationship is provided by one person (therapist) for another (patient) who is unhappy, demoralized, defeated, and suffering from the kinds of problems which our society has diagnosed as requiring the services of a specialist in mental health, the outcome will generally be "therapeutic," provided the recipient is able to respond to, or take advantage of, what the therapist has to offer. Some therapists believe that psychotherapy begins precisely at the point where a patient cannot profit from a good human relationship, and the professional is needed specifically by those persons who are chronically unable to seek out and profit from a good human relationship. (1978, p. 9)

Strupp emphasizes repeatedly that it is not the utilization of techniques or the eludication of historical antecedents that produces change in a patient. It is the reliving and modification of historically meaningful patterns that come alive in the here and now of the therapist-to-patient relationship or group-to-member interaction that produces change. Understanding is determined by reason, and the weight of therapeutic change is not carried by reason but by the emotional relationship between the patient and the group and the group therapist.

Certainly, the therapist as a person plays a crucial part in determining how important and effective this relationship will be. A therapist who is just a nice person will fail to provide the entire range of stimuli that the patient will need in treatment. Therapists must be able to challenge, soothe, care, love, and fight with the patient if they are to provide the full range of emotional experiences that can potentially come alive in any authentic relationship. Therapists will hopefully have free access to all their passions and will discipline them to achieve their own goals. Whenever therapists are kind, altruistic, or generous, they should not be motivated by their desire to be nice or thought of as kindly. Rather, their ability to soothe another and be generous should emerge out of the depths of their own self-worth. Nietzsche (1968) captures these sentiments exactly when he writes,

> Gracefulness is part of the graciousness of the great-souled. When power becomes gracious and descends into the visible, such descent I call beauty. And there is nobody I want beauty from as much as from you who are powerful. Let your kindness be your final self-conquest. Of all evil I deem you capable: therefore I want the good from you. Verily, I have often laughed at the weaklings who thought themselves good because they had no claws. (1968)

In concluding this chapter, there is an important message for beginning group therapists. It is important, as stated previously, that they learn from the masters and make themselves familiar with the basic principles of group therapy before they embark on developing their own style. Yet, it is important that each group leader not try to be another Yalom, Polster, Goulding, or Whitaker. These individuals are all experts in their own right, and each is uniquely different in their approach to group therapy. It is important that beginning group leaders not try to completely emulate others or make themselves a carbon copy of a therapist they admire. It is best that each group leader develops and discovers his or her own style. This principle is clearly demonstrated in Sheldon Kopp's story of the Hassidic religious leader's (the Zaddick) advice to his young disciple:

> Thus, the relationship between the Zaddick and his disciple was the crucial factor in this attempt to give spiritual help, just as the relationship between therapist and patient is crucial in its secular equivalent. The personality of the teacher takes the place of doctrine. Even this must be guarded against turning into dogmas. As we read the stories of the many Zaddicks, we see that what best characterized them was their dissimilarity, their startling individuality. This was not always pleasing at first to those people who wanted not only help, but also a model, a way of behaving which they could emulate. And so in one story the followers of Rabbi Zusya asked him, "Rabbi, tell us, why do you teach in this way when Moses taught in another way?" "When I get to the coming world," answered Rabbi Zusya, "there they will not ask me, 'Why were you not more like Moses?' but instead they will ask me, 'Why were you not more like Zusya?' " (1971, p. 36)

Chapter 13

Transference in Groups

The concept of transference has long held a central position in psychotherapy. It was one of Freud's greatest discoveries, and nearly sixty years after his death, it continues to be of central importance in psychoanalysis and all psychodynamically oriented therapy. While every competent and well-trained therapist recognizes the importance of transference in psychotherapy, in the past some critics doubted whether transference could actually occur in group. Some believed that group therapy watered down transference reactions and neutralized transference phenomena. Many individually oriented theorists believed that transference could only occur within the context of free association. Since group was believed by some to interfere with free association, it followed that transference could not occur within the group. Of course, free association does occur within group, especially if the group is conducted within a psychodynamic perspective. Every experienced group therapist knows that transference not only occurs in group, but is actually expanded because of the wide array of available transferential objects. Transference not only occurs with the group leader, but is also manifested with each of the group members and the group as a whole. Yalom went so far as to state the obvious in his attempt to justify this view when he published the first edition of his text nearly thirty years ago. He outlined six principles of transference addressing the atmosphere of doubt that existed for some theorists at that time.

1. Transference does occur in therapy groups; indeed, it is omnipresent and radically influences the nature of the group discourse.
2. Without an appreciation of transference and its manifestations, the therapist will often not be able to understand the process of the group.
3. The therapist who ignores transference considerations may seriously misunderstand some transactions and confuse rather than guide the group members; but if you see only the transference aspects of your relationships with members, you fail to relate authentically with them.
4. There are patients whose therapy hinges on the resolution of transference distortion; there are others whose improvement will depend

upon interpersonal learning stemming from work not with the therapist, but with another member around such issues as competition, exploitation, or sexuality and intimacy conflicts; and there are many patients who choose alternate therapeutic pathways in the group and derive their primary benefit from other therapeutic factors.

5. Attitudes toward the therapist are not all transference based; many are reality based, and others are irrational but flow from other sources of irrationality inherent in the dynamics of the group (As Freud knows, not all group phenomena can be explained on the basis of individual psychology).
6. By maintaining flexibility, you may make good therapeutic use of these irrational attitudes toward you, without at the same time neglecting your many other functions in the group (1975, p. 194).

If Yalom's principles are followed, the group members will come to discover the extent to which they invest one another with early familial qualities. Under the group leader's guidance and leadership, the group members can have the opportunity to learn how they project parental and sibling images onto the group leader and the other group members. They will hopefully see how these distortions are determined by their own circumscribed experiences as children and that the investment of others with attributes they do not possess is a result of their own distorted character structure.

DEFINITION OF TRANSFERENCE

There are a number of elaborate definitions of transference. Simply defined, transference involves two separate characteristics:

1. It must be a repetition of the past.
2. It must be inappropriate to the present.

If both of these characteristics do not occur in conjunction, it is unlikely that the phenomena being observed are really transferences. For instance, if a group member perceives the group leader as controlling and demanding and the group leader is, in fact, controlling and demanding, this is not transference. In this example, the group member's perception of the therapist is totally appropriate to the present. Further, if the group member has not had a history where he or she has repeatedly perceived neutral people as controlling and demanding, it is unlikely that the person will do so in the present, unless he or she is given a valid reason for reacting that way currently.

However, if a group member has experienced someone important in the past (i.e., father, mother, sister, brother, etc.) as cold, indifferent, exploitative, or unfair, and there is an unrealistic imposing of these attitudes or characteristics on neutral people in the present, there is a high probability that the person is caught in a transference distortion. Transference makes other people appear to be what they are not.

For instance, if Mary perceives Burt as an angry, critical man who cares little for the other group members' feelings and the rest of the group members perceive Burt as kind, caring, and gentle, there is obviously some incongruence in Mary's perceptions. There are seven other individuals who perceive Burt in a totally different light. What is it about Mary that leads her to distort Burt in such a way that it defies the reality of the rest of the group members? Mary is an otherwise successful woman, wife, mother, and accountant. She makes her living by dealing with accurate perceptions. Mary, who grew up in a home with an overly punitive and critical alcoholic father, is reminded of his presence every time Burt speaks in his own characteristic style. Mary is transferring her own feelings of anger and resentment at her father onto Burt. These feelings are inappropriate to the present because Burt is actually nothing like her father except in his size and speech.

Levy (1984) writes about this process:

> Psychoanalytic theories of psychopathology are rooted in the idea that the past distorts the present, that past difficulties are continually repeated, and that recovery is based upon uncovering old conflicts and resolving them in such a way that their distorting influence is abolished. The patient can be expected to distort his important adult relationships significantly, in a way that conforms to the structure of his unconscious difficulties, which usually have to do with his conflict-ridden relationships to his parents during the formative years of development. (p. 94)

Transference, as it occurs within the therapeutic setting, allows the group leader to get a glimpse into the patient's past. Examining the group member's interaction in the group becomes a means of understanding the way the patient's past, recreated in the here and now of the group member transference reactions, interferes with the patient's present relationships. The transference is a means of knowing the past by re-experiencing it in the present. We all possess the tendency to repeat the past by distorting the present and until patients are aware of their own idiosyncratic distortions, they will be doomed to repeat them.

Levy stresses the importance of recognizing that these repetitions occur with all individuals:

> Such distortions need not be limited to people with significant psychopathology. All personal interactions are colored by past experiences that shape current expectations and responses. Especially conflictual and unsatisfying relationships with parents and other influential figures from the childhood years have a particularly lasting and distorting influence on people's adult relationships. How can one relate such ubiquitous distortions to the concept of transference in a manner that ensures that the latter term will keep its specific clinical meaning? Transference is the manifestation, within the psychotherapeutic relationship, of the ubiquitous distorting influence of past relationships on current ones, intensified by the regressive forces inherent in the treatment situation and clarified by the therapist's neutrality, relative anonymity, and objectivity in the face of the patient's distorted view of him. (1985, p. 94)

Transference as a means of interpreting a person's past can be a valuable tool in therapy. However, like any technique, it can be destructive if used as an end in itself, instead of a means for better understanding the patient. If they are not cautious in its application, therapists can hide behind transference interpretations because of their own difficulties in dealing with an emotionally arousing encounter. As Kernberg (1984) warns, transference usually crystallizes around some realistic aspect of the therapist's personality. Like paranoia, there is always an element of truth in it. However, it is a perception that is usually exaggerated and distorted by the observer. If therapists are not careful, they will fail to appreciate the part they are contributing to the transference distortion.

Scott Rutan (1983) tells a story that captures the essence of this type of predicament:

> During a case conference, a medical student was having particular difficulty managing his first psychiatric referral. From the student's description, it was apparent that his patient was a chronic drug abuser and a street-wise borderline character disorder. It was also obvious that she was well aware of this student's nervousness and incompetence. This only infuriated her more. As he proceeded to make one therapeutic blunder after another with this woman, week after week, her narcissistic rage continued to grow in proportion to every narcissistic injury she suffered. Finally, after more than three weeks of being subjected to repeated affective storms of this woman,

> one senior resident, noting that the medical student was beginning to show some wear and tear as a result of these encounters, kindly offered the suggestion of medication. As this possibility was discussed, the residents and medical students turned to Rutan and asked him what he thought of the idea of medication. Without blinking an eye, Rutan replied, "I think it's a great idea; but for the medical student, not the patient."

Therapists, unattuned to their own countertransference reactions, can attribute qualities to the patient that are inaccurate, distorted, or exaggerated. Or, as the previous case illustrates, they can act out against the patient because of their own internal discomfort or anger. Too often, the patient is on medication because the patient's affect is intolerable for the therapist.

Transference often takes time to develop. However, there are numerous instances where it will be immediately and powerfully demonstrated by the patient. In more cases than not, this will be the situation with many addicts and alcoholics. Resolving transference distortions often takes skill, patience, and time. Unfortunately, time is the one commodity that is often unavailable and is becoming more scarce to the group leader. This is especially true for inpatient treatment and the shrinking time constraints imposed by managed care and third-party insurance coverage. Group leaders often must respond quickly and directly to negative or destructive transference distortions. Positive transference reactions such as idealization need to be utilized in the service of the patient's benefit. Yalom recommends that the skillful and judicious use of transparency, gratification, and self-disclosure can help with many early negative transference reactions. At times, this can be invaluable because time constraints and treatment issues do not always provide the group leader with the luxury of slowly working through such transference distortions.

Yalom does not believe that transparency or self-disclosure, if carefully applied, will necessarily interfere with transference phenomena. However, the use of therapist transparency and self-disclosure must be dictated by the determination of whether it will impede or enhance the facilitation of therapeutic goals. Self-disclosure and transparency should be used to provide support, acceptance, and encouragement when necessary. This is especially true for addicts and alcoholics early in recovery when abstinence is still being held in a delicate balance. Transferences that might interfere with abstinence must be resolved quickly. Yalom reminds the group leader that it is not the task of the therapist to manufacture positive feelings, but to locate and identify them through selective self-disclosure. A patient in need of support, help, and guidance does not benefit from a therapist's feelings of dislike, distrust, or anger. Neither does the patient benefit from a therapist who has an unhealthy need to be liked, admired, and idealized.

Anonymity and its counterpart, transparency, are often misunderstood concepts even within the realm of psychoanalysis. The therapeutic stance of neutrality is often confused with the blank screen, or the non-obtrusive position of the analytic therapist. Therapists, even within the analytic tradition, need to be able to establish warm relationships while not allowing their prejudices, conflicts, and outside distractions to interfere with the therapy session. This does not mean therapists should be distant, aloof, cold, or uninvolved. Therapists must be emotionally involved in their patients' lives, just as group leaders must be emotionally involved participant observers within the group.

Transference occurs not only with the patient, but also with the therapist or the group leader. The early concept of countertransference was first used to differentiate therapist transference from patient transference—a distinction that unfairly implied one was uniquely different from the other. The view on countertransference has been going through some radical changes within the last few years. Initially, countertransference was applied rather narrowly. It had generally referred to something that the therapist should avoid and was limited to the therapist's reactions to the patient's transference. Many classic analysts used to believe that countertransference reactions were the result of unresolved or not fully analyzed conflicts within the analyst. Having such countertransference feelings toward the patient was unacceptable and usually meant the therapist needed to get back into his or her own psychoanalysis. Currently, the growing consensus is that such countertransference reactions not only cannot be avoided, but that they should not be avoided. They can be a rich source of powerful and useful information about the patient if properly understood and used by the therapist. To help understand how transference from both the patient and the therapist can interact and consequently reveal important information that will enhance treatment, these concepts will be explored at length.

TRANSFERENCE POSSIBILITIES IN GROUP

Harry Stack Sullivan's (1953) influence on Yalom has been outlined in Chapter 4. It is important to repeat briefly here the significance that Sullivan's concept of parataxic distortion has on Yalom's approach to resolving transference distortions in group. Parataxic distortion refers to our proclivity to distort our perceptions of others. These distortions are self-perpetuating and lead to self-fulfilled prophecies. A primary distortion of addicts and alcoholics is that people cannot be trusted. They continue to choose as friends and lovers other addicts and alcoholics who are notoriously untrustworthy. Consequently, their view of others and the world as untrustworthy is kept consistent. Therefore, they feel justified in keeping others at a distance and not trusting anyone. This is the game of addicted individuals. Their payoff is that they do not have to get too close to someone who is trustworthy, because their underlying fear is that they will not measure up and will be found to be inadequate and unacceptable by others.

Distortions like this can only be modified by what Sullivan refers to as "consensual validation." For children who are developing psychologically, this requires that they compare their perceptions with their peers'. It is the isolated individuals who keep their distortions self-perpetuating. They come to believe they are unique in their "badness" and that if others truly knew them as they really are, they would reject them. Perceiving others as untrustworthy is a defensive operation that protects alcoholics and addicts from exposing their true selves to others. Group psychotherapy requires members to address their unconscious fears and modify their distortions through consensual validation. As members in the group begin to understand their transference distortions, they will be forced to look at themselves more realistically and subsequently reveal more of their true selves to the group. Eventually, through corrective emotional experience, they will come to realize that they can be accepted for who they really are and need not continue to relate to others in a manner that is based on their early past experiences.

The group leader must remember that transference is an unconscious phenomenon. Group members do not realize that they are doing it. Only when they are acting in a way that does not make sense to other group members does the transference distortion have a chance to be exposed for what it is. Group members' reactions or overreactions are usually obvious to others in the group before it is obvious to the individuals. The reliving of their infantile reaction in the present is needed before this behavior can be changed. Change is subsequently impossible without the members being aware of their transference distortions. The therapy group allows its members to deal with these infantile distortions as adults now that they have the capacity to more fully understand them. They can be relived in the safety of the group and changed so that old unconscious patterns need not continue to plague the members. As one group member exclaimed after an enlightening awareness of her transference distortions, "The great thing about this group is that I can go back and experience what I had to struggle with alone as a child and have all these people here to help me."

While transference occurs in every form of psychotherapy, group therapy expands the transference possibilities. Not only does each group member trigger separate individual transference reactions, there are three distinct transference processes inherent in every group experience that must be differentiated. These are the vertical, the horizontal, and the symbolic. (See Figure 13.1.)

1. Leader transference (vertical)
2. Peer transference (horizontal)
3. Group-as-a-whole transference (symbolic mother)

Leader Transference

Leader transference usually refers to libidinal distortions related to unresolved oedipal issues. Consequently, power, dependency, success, and authority conflicts will manifest around the vertical pole. These are the

FIGURE 13.1

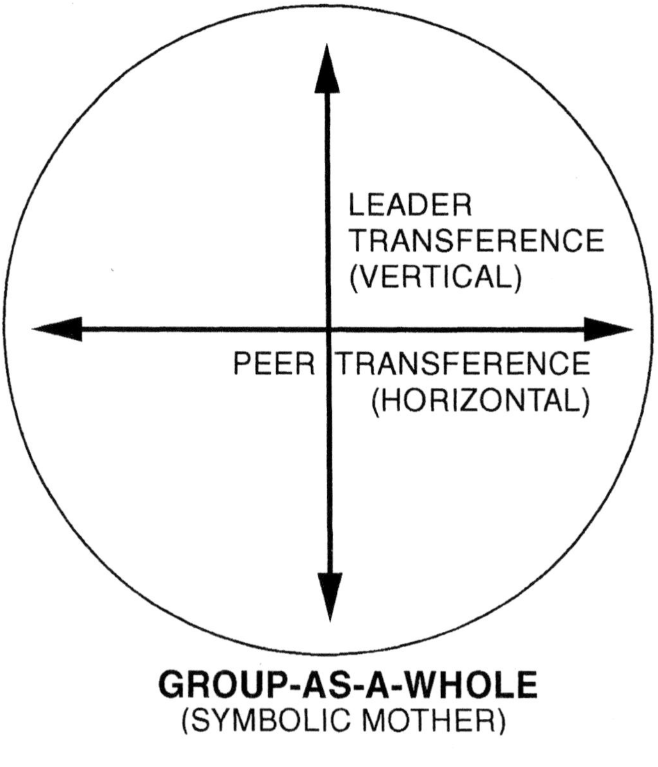

type of transference issues that most readily emerge in individual therapy. Depending upon the group members' individual early experiences, some will see the group leader as cold and distant; others will perceive the group leader as warm and supportive. Some will be fiercely protective or dependent on the group leader for guidance and direction while others will be defiantly independent and challenging of the group leader.

Peer Transference

Peer transference involves competition issues related to jealousy, envy, and cooperation. Group members will often rekindle sibling rivalry issues. Members may frequently remind each other of brothers, sisters, husbands, wives, or lovers. At other times, group members will evoke parental transference distortions. It is because the group offers such a diverse source of transference stimuli that it allows more distortions to be experienced and ultimately resolved.

Group-as-a-Whole Transference

The group as a symbolic mother helps steady the course of therapy. A great part of the group's therapeutic efficiency is based on a pre-oedipal maternal transference. If the group is a symbolically bad mother, it will stir up primitive feelings of anger and rage. Few alcoholics or addicts can tolerate such feelings and will find the group much too threatening. This is why cohesion, trust, and safety are so crucial to a beginning therapy group. The group's benevolent tolerance, acceptance and safety may amount to an experience of dissolution of the mother-infant symbiosis and rebirth. The intensity of the individual transference distortions, be they rebellious anger or fears of dependency and engulfment, are diluted by the presence of the other group members. A symbolic good mother will serve as a container for the group members' anxiety and will allow the necessary holding environment to be established so that the transference distortions can be addressed and modified.

MODIFICATION OF TRANSFERENCE DISTORTIONS IN GROUPS

Once a proper therapeutic climate has been established, group leaders can turn their energies toward exposing and modifying each group member's transference distortions. Group leaders have at their disposal three primary means for accomplishing this task:

1. Interpretation
2. Consensual validation
3. Transparency

Interpretation

Interpretation plays a very special and unique part in psychoanalysis and psychoanalytic group psychotherapy. While every form of psychotherapy has its own means for bringing about change in a person's life, interpretation is the cornerstone upon which information is conveyed in psychoanalytic group psychotherapy. Interpretation is a statement made by the group leader referring to something patients have said or done in such a way as to identify features of their behavior that they have not been fully aware of. Transference interpretations are intended to expand patients' awareness of their own personal idiosyncratic distortions of others that occur in group. The harnessing of transference is a key task for group leaders. But they must not confront or expose transference in an attacking, premature, or embarrassing manner. Timing is the key. A poorly timed interpretation can result in more repression or regression in group. Accuracy is another important factor. With an inaccurate interpretation, group members will often latch on to the statement as a way of defending themselves. An accurate interpretation will trigger deeper associations and deeper feelings. However, accurate interpretations can also evoke strong negative feelings in patients. Do not expect group members to respond appreciatively to accurate interpretations by saying, "Thank you so much, that was really helpful." Accurate interpretations expose individuals and are frequently experienced as narcissistic injuries. With an accurate interpretation, the group leader is essentially saying, "Your slip is showing and I know it." It is often embarrassing to members because the group leader has penetrated their defenses and the result is usually fear, anger, or shame.

Consensual Validation

Transference distortions are most readily corrected when members of the group start comparing their perceptions to those of the other group members. This is especially important for alcoholics, addicts, and character disorders. Interpretations rarely work with these patients because of their tendency to overutilize ego-syntonic defenses. Their characterological defensive posture protects them too well. They frequently do not experience the same degree of internal discomfort that neurotics experience, so they rarely seek therapy on their own. They are usually sent or brought to therapy by others who find their characterological features disturbing, offensive, and troublesome. These patients are convinced that it is "others out there" who are the problem. They would be fine if only they were left alone. Consensual agreement from the rest of the group members is needed to countervalidate their distortions before they are able to even entertain the idea that they might be the reason for their difficulties. Such validation from peers carries far more impact than validation from the group leader.

Transparency

Transference distortions can also be corrected if leaders are more transparent and reveal more of themselves. However, if leaders reveal themselves too soon, transference may be disturbed. Since transference, like free associations and dreams, is a way to reach a person's unconscious, the premature use of transparency can interfere with a valuable and important source of self-discovery and awareness. While it is important for group leaders to use transparency as a way to correct destructive transference distortions, they must carefully evaluate their reasons for revealing more of themselves to the group and its members. Transparency should not be used by leaders as an excuse to dominate the group or use the group to gratify their own needs. Group leaders should not fight with members of the group for dominance by narcissistically displaying their brilliance or by showing their superiority in other ways. Group leaders should use their transparency as a means of allowing peer relationships to effectively exercise therapeutic pressure. Leaders should be able to handle their relationships with the other group members not with envy or interference, but by carefully respecting the relationships. A jealous parent is not a good parent.

TYPES OF TRANSFERENCE IN GROUPS

Transference will reveal itself in many forms. While individual therapy will create a specific type of atmosphere that will lead to the likelihood of particular types of transferences being manifested, group therapy contributes to its own unique influences. The group leader can expect to witness three common types of transference in the therapy group:

1. Displaced transference
2. Acting out transference
3. Repetition compulsion

Displaced Transference

Some theorists believe displaced transference is the kind most likely to manifest itself in a therapy group (Alonso, 1985). Group members will use their history as a way of displacing their resistance. For instance, a group member may say that he is angry with his father, while in actuality, he is very angry at the group leader. His historical material may appear very rich and the group leader will be tempted to chase off in pursuit of his affect, failing to realize that he is the actual source of its manifestation. Group members may also displace their transference reactions onto each other, rather than risk demonstrating such feelings directly to the group leader. In extreme cases, this can result in scapegoating. The group will direct its aggression onto one group member rather than the group leader.

Acting Out Transference

Acting out is a term that is often confused by therapists in its application. Acting out is usually used to describe aggressive, antisocial behavior that is frequently directed against society. This is too narrow a definition. Acting out is really a transference phenomenon. Rather than talk about their feelings, individuals will discharge them directly instead of utilizing sublimation. If angry, they will miss a session or scream at the group leader. They may also idealize the group leader. When the inevitable disappointment occurs, they will then act on their anger, rather than talk about their feelings of disappointment or frustration.

Acting out is really a form of communication. While it has been viewed by some as a form of resistance, it is not so much resistance to transference as transference itself because it carries communicative significance. There has been unwarranted overemphasis on motoric action in defining acting out. Actually, acting out involves more than behavior. It involves thinking and the processing of information. In this context, acting out frequently results in the group members' either doing to the group leader what they wish would be done to them, or what they fear might happen to them. They treat the group leader affectionately because this is what they want from the leader, or they attack the leader because they fear that the leader will attack first.

Blanck and Blanck (1974) define acting out as "behavior motivated by unconscious, object-related fantasies repressed by the ego" (p. 101). Kernbergh (1975) sees acting out as closely tied to the relationship between the patient and therapist. He writes, "A patient may tend to act toward the therapist rather than reflect feelings about him" (p. 85). Acting out, in the classical sense, is a discharge of drive tension that is achieved by responding to a present situation as if it were the original situation that first gave rise to the drive. The term *transference* is employed if the attitude or behavior is in response to certain definite persons. It is called acting out (proper) if it is done indiscriminately.

The character structure of a person is an example of a chronic and habitual pattern of acting out that develops as a result of conflict between instinctual demands and a frustrating outer world. Alcoholics and addicts, because of their propensity to utilize characterological patterns in defending themselves, will overutilize acting out in therapy. Group therapy, due to the nature of its regressive pull, will elicit acting out from even those individuals who may not normally act out.

Consequently, there is a general agreement among group leaders that acting out is more likely to occur in a therapy group than in individual therapy. It is also more likely to occur with chemically dependent patients. It is futile to prohibit it. Rather, the group leader must use it as information. The amount or kind of acting out is dependent not only upon the composition of the group, but also upon the conscious and unconscious attitudes of the group leader.

COMMON TYPES OF ACTING OUT TRANSFERENCE

Three common types of characterological acting out transferences are captured in Kohut's description of the narcissistic transference (1977a). They are the idealizing, mirror hungry, and merger transferences (see Chapter 6).

Idealizing Transference

The origination of idealizing transference is established in the need for the small child to have a secure relationship with a strong parent in order to feel secure and safe. The parent is idealized and perceived as more powerful and stronger than he or she actually is–as a means for the child to ward off intruding fears of anxiety and environmental threat.

Idealizing can also take on the form of ideas or ideals. Ideals can be goals for the child to pursue and identify in a healthy fashion. A child's sense of self-worth is often guided by his or her ideas of achievement and recognition. As the child grows older, this culminates in a mature capacity for pride and self-esteem. Self-identity is established, and the ability to satisfy the self is internalized. If this process is successfully negotiated, the child will grow to an adult who does not need the constant presence of a strong other or ideological cause to feel secure.

Individuals who grow up in an environment that deprives them of the idealized other will constantly search for this throughout their adult life. They will seek strong leaders, just causes, or rigid belief systems in order to feel secure. In the more pathological cases, they may fall victim to the charismatic religious leader who provides them with a rigid, predictable belief system that will protect them as long as they abide by all the rules. In other cases, such deprived individuals will pursue political systems with authoritarian leaders, or, on a less dramatic level, choose a spouse who will be harsh and controlling. Since they will not allow themselves to see others as they truly are, they will distort their perceptions in order to only focus on the strengths or the admirable qualities of the other. These are the patients who idealize their therapists and see them as all-wonderful. They only feel secure in the therapist's presence. In order to defend themselves against their need to see their leaders as strong, they will not allow themselves to see faults in others upon whom they must depend.

Yalom (1985) gives an excellent example of such an idealizing transference in a passage from Tolstoy's classic novel, *War and Peace*. The protagonist, Rostov, finds himself overwhelmed emotionally when thrust into the presence of his idealized leader, the Tsar.

> He was entirely absorbed in the feeling of happiness at the Tsar's being near. His nearness alone made up to him by itself, he felt, for the loss of the whole day. He was happy, as a lover is happy when the moment of the longed-for meeting has come. Not daring to look around from the front line, by an ecstatic instance without looking around, he felt his approach. And he felt it not only from the sound of the tramping hoofs of the approaching cavalcade, he felt it because as the Tsar came nearer everything grew brighter, more joyful and significant and more festive. Nearer and nearer moved this sun, as he seemed to Rostov, shedding around him rays of mild and majestic light, and now he felt himself enfolded in that radiance, he heard his voice–that voice caressing, calm, majestic, and yet so simple . . . and Rostov got up and went out to wander about among the campfires, dreaming of what happiness it would be to die–not saving the Emperor's life–(of that he did not dare to dream), but simply to die before the Emperor's eyes. He really was in love with the Tsar and the glory of the Russian arms and the hope of coming

> victory. And he was not the only man who felt thus in those memorable days that preceded the battle of Austerlitz: nine-tenths of the men in the Russian army were at that moment in love, though less ecstatically, with their Tsar and the glory of the Russian arms. (cited in Yalom, 1995, pp. 195-196)

In some cases, idealizing patients will go to great lengths to maintain their perception of the therapist as one who does not make mistakes. It is often too threatening for idealizing patients to see the therapist as one who has faults. This is also manifested in the patients' relationships outside of group. For instance, this is why these patients frequently choose as a marriage partner someone who is entirely "wrong" for them. They have the propensity to only perceive the idealized good qualities of their partners, failing to see the more negative aspects of the partner's personality. Once the realization of what the person is really like begins to "sink in" over time, they feel disillusioned and betrayed. A case vignette will help illustrate the lengths that an idealizing patient will go to to keep their image of the "idealized other" intact.

> Fred, a thirty-six-year-old accountant, had an intense idealizing transference for his group leader and would fiercely defend him against criticism by the other group members. He would also inevitably look to the leader for approval whenever he spoke in group. During moments of confusion, Fred would actually ask the group leader, "What am I feeling now?" Finally, after a painful empathic failure by the group leader, Fred finally exploded angrily at him for failing to understand the nature of his discomfort. Unable to tolerate the realization that the group leader had faults or could err, Fred was overcome by his disappointment and responded in an uncharacteristic rage. After Fred's outburst had subsided, the other group members eventually congratulated him for his assertiveness, as this was the first time the other group members had witnessed him not readily complying to the demands of the group leader. Toward the end of the group, the leader also voiced his support of Fred's uncharacteristic challenge of him. In the next session, Fred announced to the leader that he had thought about the incident over the week and concluded that the leader had actually made the blunder on purpose. Fred said that he discovered, after "thinking about it carefully," that the group leader had actually done this in order to provoke him to react in an angry manner because the leader knew it would be good for him to do so. Fred promptly thanked the leader for his skill and foresight in utilizing such a creative strategy. So strong was Fred's need to keep

> his image of the leader as an idealized other, that he went through elaborate intellectual somersaults to ensure that the leader's mistake was perceived as a well-planned and calculated strategy. This was also Fred's dilemma outside of group. He had been repeatedly passed over for promotions at his job because of his tendency to turn over his good ideas to his boss, who was extremely exploitive of him. Fred could not tolerate seeing his boss as someone other than what he wanted him to be.

Mirror Hungry Transference

If children are not given the unconditional admiration and recognition of an uncritical mother or father while they are developing emotionally, they will seek this confirmation constantly in their adult lives. These individuals will require a relationship with another who will be an agreeing and reflecting mirror. They will demand that others constantly respond to them, admire them, and confirm them. They will be forced to seek externally in their adult life what they lacked internally as a child. Others become for them what Kohut calls self-objects. They will often be very successful people who will be obsessively driven to be recognized, acknowledged, and admired by others. They will thrive on recognition and will feel deprived, empty, and depleted if recognition and admiration is not forthcoming. If their sense of entitlement is challenged or not immediately gratified, they will be narcissistically injured and fly into a rage or become extremely depressed. A case vignette will illustrate this transference problem.

> Tom, a thirty-year-old cocaine addict was being seen simultaneously in both individual and group psychotherapy. He flourished in the individual sessions because all the time and energy was focused exclusively on him. He would literally start each individual session by asking the therapist how he looked today. He sought and needed confirmation from the therapist that he was all right. Much like someone standing in front of a mirror to make sure his tie was straight, Tom would pose in the same manner in front of the therapist. While he was able to get the mirroring he needed in individual therapy, he experienced much more difficulty with the group. The other group members began to tire of his insistence on talking about himself each week. Tom was reluctant to share the group spotlight and this eventually reached a crisis one week when it became blatantly obvious to the rest of the group that Tom was unwilling to give up "his time" in group, despite the acute emotional discomfort of

two of the group's most supportive members. Since it was uncharacteristic of these two women to be so visibly upset, or to ask for group time, the other group members were enraged at Tom's insensitivity. Tom's behavior was especially provocative to the group, since both of these women had been consistently supportive of him in the past. Tom was unable to tolerate the group's reaction and eventually refused to return to the group, stating, "I don't want to be part of any group that is not going to be supportive of me. I get too much of that in the real world."

Merger Transference

Another variant of the narcissistic transference is referred to as the twinship, alter ego, or merger transference. It is characterized by the patients' assumption that everyone in the group is either like them or similar to them. In some cases, the group members will expect the group leader's psychological makeup to be just like or very similar to their own. This phenomenon explains the uncomfortable feelings all of us experience in strange surroundings, such as when we visit a foreign city for the first time. In contrast, the merger transference explains the comfort we experience when we are in the presence of others whom we perceive to be like us.

In the most developmentally arrested group members, merger transference will manifest in their refusal to see others in the group as different. They will protest any attempts to differentiate between group members, insisting that "we are all just alike," or "I like everyone equally here in group." If this transference distortion is not challenged by the group leader, the members of the group will continue to hide their individual differences behind a facade of forced compliance and feigned similarity. They will never learn whether they can risk truly being themselves with others. Unless this is altered, the group will become a shared illusion, in which everyone will be squeezed into a mold of sameness and equality. The group leader's task is to contrast the individual group members' personal histories and repeatedly point out their differences. The aim is to get the group members to gradually move from the "we" to the "I." Each individual member must eventually come to realize that there is no threat in individuation and separation.

Repetition Compulsion

The repetition compulsion is the transference phenomenon most likely to occur first in group (Rutan, 1983), and it will manifest itself in the here and now of the group interaction. Through its manifestation, group members will attempt to undo what has been done and is left uncompleted from their past. It involves the repetition of an experience. There is a general tendency in all human behavior to repeat painful experiences and to be haunted by any experience that is unfinished or incomplete. The repetition act, in adult experience, is usually self-defeating, but the underlying motive is assumed to be that the individual seeks to redo the original trauma in the hopes that it will be mastered.

In an extreme case, this is what takes place with children who grow up in an alcoholic home. An example will help clarify this point.

> As a doctoral student completing my graduate work, I was employed part time as an intake counselor at a local alcoholism treatment center. Late one evening, around midnight, as I sat alone in my office catching up on my progress notes, the telephone rang. It was unusual for the phone to ring so late in the evening, as the agency had an answering service that took all incoming calls after midnight. As the telephone continued to ring repeatedly, some inquisitive impulse prompted me to answer the call. This was very uncharacteristic of me, but I felt compelled to discover what would lead a person on the other end to insistently pursue a call that went unanswered for such a long time. Since I expected to hear an intoxicated individual on the other end, I was somewhat startled by the gentle, soft, and meek voice of a troubled woman. There was a profound sadness to her as she spoke, the type of sadness that emerges after a person has struggled and discovered some unpleasant truth about herself. I politely informed her that the agency was closed for the evening, but that I would be happy to refer her to another number if it was an emergency. She kindly agreed that she could wait until morning and politely informed me that she would call back the next day. As I was about to hang up the receiver, she wondered if I would be so kind as to possibly answer one question that was presently plaguing her. Since her voice had the sound of a troubled soul who was struggling silently with a very personal and crucial issue, I quickly agreed that I would try. She paused, then asked in complete sincerity, "My present husband is an alcoholic, my first husband was an alcoholic, and my father was an alcoholic. Is there anything wrong with me?" I was deeply moved by the sincerity of her question. Unable to answer immediately, I sat silently with her as my mind conjured up the image of a troubled young woman sitting alone at her kitchen table after midnight, begging for an answer to a troubling question. No answer was necessary,

> as the full impact of her past had already come barreling down on her with the stark realization that the repetitive nature of her unconscious compulsions had already traced out a definable and painful pattern to her life.

This woman, like so many other adult children of alcoholics, is a perfect example of someone caught up in the throes of a repetition compulsion. This is why so many children who grew up with an alcoholic parent defy logic and continue as adults to marry or choose partners who are alcoholic. On an emotionally developmentally arrested level, they feel responsible for the family chaos. If only they had gotten Daddy to stop drinking, everything would be all right. Since they couldn't fix Daddy, maybe they can redo it differently this time with their spouse. The original traumatic experience (father's alcoholism) leads them to redo the experience in their adult life in the hope that this time it will be mastered. The awareness of this process remains buried, because the repetition compulsion, like most transference phenomena, is unconscious. Many adult children who "end up" married to alcoholics will protest that their spouses did not even start to drink until they had been married for years. It is the personal characteristics of the spouse that they are drawn to alter, rather than the drinking itself.

Since the repetition compulsion will manifest in the here and now of the group interaction, the group leader only has to observe the group members' interaction to decipher each member's personal history. Each member will manifest his or her particular idiosyncratic transference distortion in group. Those who have difficulties with anger in their life will have difficulties with anger in the group. Those who are taken advantage of by others in their life will be taken advantage of by members of the group. Group members will play out their uncompleted trauma of the past in the present. The group leader's task is to repeatedly point out the members' distortion as it occurs in the present and force them to examine in detail the many ways they keep repeating their past in the present.

ABUSE OF TRANSFERENCE

Group leaders must keep a careful watch on the way they deal with transference in group. Interpretations can often be used by group leaders as a means of defending and distancing themselves from the group. Transference interpretations are only helpful if they come from empathic ties to group. Freud wrote of the danger of hurling interpretations in the patient's face if interpretations are used by therapists to defend against their own feelings of discomfort. Interpretations should never be used by group leaders to give the impression of superiority. Once leaders try to position themselves in a one-up position, they have abandoned the group.

Group leaders must ensure that they are not hiding behind the safety of their therapeutic technique when they elect to demonstrate to the group their awareness of transference phenomena. Their own fear, anxiety, anger, or need for recognition can color their therapeutic objectivity. A case vignette will demonstrate this potential problem.

> During the tenth hour of a group psychotherapy training experience, a young woman angrily confronted the group leader, stating he was arbitrary, indifferent, and aloof. The group stopped in its tracks and the group members all sat poised on the edge of their chairs, for this was the first confrontation of the leader and the group was eager to see how he would respond. Finally, after a very agonizing few seconds, the group leader replied, "Do I remind you of your father?" The woman, relieved at the opportunity to move the exchange from the heat of the here and now encounter to the safety of the there and then, quickly agreed that this was indeed so and proceeded to explore the more familiar terrain of her relationship with her father. The initial crisis of the confrontation had been watered down, and the rest of the group sat back comfortably in their chairs, relieved on some level that this issue could be dealt with on less threatening ground. Although the group members were relieved to be allowed to move away from the overt expression of anger in the group, they had been cheated out of a valuable therapeutic experience. They were, in fact, given a demonstration on how to avoid direct confrontation. The issue between this woman and the group leader was unresolved. In fact, it remained unresolved for the rest of the group members during the remainder of the group experience, for her accusation was very true. The group leader was, indeed, arbitrary, indifferent, and aloof. His urgency to move into the woman's there and then relationship with her father was motivated by his own need to avoid facing the painful accuracy of this woman's accusations, more so than by his desire to understand her transference distortions. Remember, transference is only transference if it is inappropriate to the present.

COUNTERTRANSFERENCE

Group leaders, like all therapists, remain human and are more similar to their patients than they are different. Consequently, they suffer their own transference reactions. In addition, the patients' intense transference toward the therapist may evoke in the therapist many unconscious responses that can interfere with his or her ability to respond therapeutically. This was technically referred to as countertransference. As the term was classically used, it referred to the total emotional reaction of the therapist to the patient with full consideration of the entire range of conscious, preconscious, and unconscious attitudes, beliefs, and feelings in the therapist as a result of his or her contact with the patient.

However, as stated earlier, the more classical definition of countertransference is now judged to be too narrow and too limited. Countertransference indicates much more than just the therapist's inability to respond therapeutically because of the patient's own intense transference. Emotional and unconscious communication is occurring all the time in every intimate encounter. It is the skilled therapist who is able to distinguish his or her own feelings and reactions from the induced feelings that the patient may be communicating unconsciously. To fully understand all of the possible implications and ramifications involved in the process of therapists' utilizing their induced feelings in treatment, it is important to examine some of the key concepts related to this phenomena. As Louis Ormont (1992) wrote, "The worst therapists are those out of touch with their feelings or in bondage to them to the degree that their feelings dictate their performance" (p. 52). Not all feelings that a therapist feels are necessarily induced by the patient. To be able to discern which feelings the patient is evoking and which ones reflect the therapist's own emotionality is crucial to all forms of psychotherapy, not just addiction and group therapy.

Definitions of Countertransference

1. Freud's early definition of transference limited it to the unconscious response of the therapist to the patient's transference. The therapist's countertransference was viewed as unconscious reactions that interfered with the therapist's analysis of the patient. The two important elements in this definition were that it must be unconscious and that it must interfere.
2. Freud's definition was gradually expanded by classical psychoanalytic theory to include the entire repertoire of possible therapist's responses in reaction to what the patient triggered in the therapist. Countertransference came to be viewed as the therapist's transference to the patient.
3. Countertransference eventually came to be viewed as an indicator of neurotic difficulties in the therapist. Such a reaction was thought to be reflective of problems within the therapist that were not *patient specific* or necessarily evoked by the patient. In many cases, the difficulties

within the therapist were thought to be *topic specific* (i.e., sex, anger, jealousy, competition, etc.). Because of the therapist's own unresolved conflicts, certain neurotic reactions would be stirred up because of the subject matter presented by the patient.

4. Object-relations theory began to expand the definition even further. Countertransference came to be defined as any response that was the result of the psychological impact that the patient had on the therapist. Such responses or reactions were not necessarily problematic to therapy or necessarily unconscious. In its broadest definition, countertransference was meant to include all feelings (conscious and unconscious) and thoughts that a patient triggers in a therapist. Often referred to as unconscious perceptions or empathic process, the therapist is required to monitor and analyze his or her own unconscious feelings or associations that are triggered internally as the patient talks. It is recommended then that the inner stimulated thoughts and feelings induced by the patient be used by the therapist to formulate a hypothesis about the patient's feelings and unconscious.
5. Current views on countertransference take into account that it is impossible and in most cases unproductive to not be influenced emotionally by a patient's transference and emotional demands. Eventually, the therapist–any therapist–will be influenced in some way by the patient's demands for responsiveness. The way in which the therapist responds to a particular emotional demand made upon him or her, especially if the patient unconsciously evokes some action (withholding, gratifying, etc.) that the therapist would not normally do is called enactment. The process of enactment usually involves an intense, unconscious experience that includes projective identification and the therapist's reliving of aspects of his or her own unresolved past.

It is tempting at times, as Adler (1994) suggests, to view these difficulties as residing in "other therapists" who are either inadequately trained or who possess rare instances of psychopathology. Adler writes,

> It is important to remember that I am describing these difficulties as potentially present in all therapists. It would be easy and reassuring to believe that some therapists have these vulnerabilities and others do not. However, even though there is obviously a continuum of psychopathology between those who may never act upon these vulnerabilities and those who do, such issues are present to some degree in all therapists. (p. 156)

Adler goes on to explain that it is important to remember that some patients with certain painful backgrounds and experiences are more likely to tax individual emotional resources in certain therapists, placing them in a position where their own unresolved difficulties will be used destructively in relation to their patients. To help understand how the potential for induced countertransferential feelings can be use productively rather than destructively, it is important to become familiar with the concept of projective identification and its relation to objective and subjective countertransference and enactment in therapy.

Objective and Subjective Countertransference

Louis Ormont and others have attempted to explain the relation of projective identification to transference and countertransference by first making the distinction between *subjective* and *objective* countertransference. *Subjective* countertransference is just what the term implies–a subjective reaction on the part of the therapist to the patient that is tied into the therapist's own past and personal idiosyncrasies. *Objective* countertransference, on the other hand, refers to feelings or thoughts that the patient induces in the therapist. Rather than provoking a subjective reaction on the therapist's part, the patient communicates an objective piece of data that gives the therapist a glimpse into the patient's emotional life. Objective countertransference also implies that this induced feeling is objective in the sense that it is a feeling that this patient would likely evoke in most people. For instance, if a group member is managing to provoke you and everyone else in the group to be as angry with him as his wife and friends are outside of group, it is safe to assume you are dealing with objective countertransference. If as a group leader you find yourself overly solicitous and protective of a particular group member while none of the other group members respond in a similar manner, chances are good that this is a subjective countertransference reaction.

Subjective Countertransference

One simple, yet concise definition of subjective countertransference is as any feelings the therapist has for significant figures in his or her past that are reawakened by a patient's or a group's transference. While this can take on many different forms, three types are commonly experienced:

1. *Positive.* The therapist feels too much love, protectiveness, and responsiveness to the patient. In the most severe cases, loving can become eroticized or cause infantilizing of the patient. In group, the therapist's demonstration of favoritism or overprotectiveness can contribute to scapegoating or intense rivalry, competition, and envy.

2. *Negative.* The therapist feels too much hate or anger for the patient. In more severe circumstances, this can contribute to excessive confrontation, unresponsiveness, and nonprotectiveness. The group could act out the therapist's anger and the patient could easily be scapegoated or ignored.
3. *Narcissistic.* The therapist's feelings will be unrelated to the patient. Attunement, empathy, and responsiveness will be missing or inadequate. The patient will be used for the therapist's own gratification (financial or personal). The therapist will use the group as a vehicle to foster compliance and admiration from its members.

Objective Countertransference

Object countertransference can be divided further into two major categories. One category involves the therapist's feelings, thoughts, and actions that are evoked as a result of the patient's transferential feelings, thoughts, and actions. The other category consists of his or her own feelings that are reflective of his or her ability to resonate with feelings that the patient is experiencing at that moment.

In the first instance, patients may respond to the therapist or another member of the group as they have responded to parental or other important authority figures in their past. Being perceived as cold, aloof, and withholding is often difficult, especially if the therapist has made a lifelong commitment to be warm, available, and responsive to others. This situation can be compounded even more, if the therapist has an exorbitant need to be liked, admired, and respected. In many cases, this could result in therapists drastically altering their normal therapeutic stance. They could either become more gratifying in order to compensate for the transference distortions or become more withholding because of their anger at the patient for judging them unfairly and behaving in such an ungrateful manner.

As Adler (1994) points out, therapists never reach a state of development that leaves them immune to countertransference reactions. As he suggests, it is important to stay aware of them in order to minimize their impact on the patient. In an article that examines reasons why patients either drop out of therapy prematurely or fail to gain benefit from group therapy, Har Paz (1994) suggests that the therapist's personality, character, and countertransference reactions are important contributory factors. Citing Yalom's (1975) list of nine reasons for patients dropping out of treatment, Har Paz notes that the role of the therapist is not mentioned. Har Paz goes on to show that the unresolved, irrational fears of the therapist are major contributors to failure in group psychotherapy. Weiner (1983), exploring the causes of failure in group psychotherapy, suggested that, "the most subtle and most potentially destructive factor is the therapist's narcissistic vulnerability" (p. 320). Drawing on this countertransference variable, Har Paz goes on to caution group leaders to be keenly aware of their need to be treated in a certain way by their patients (i.e., liked, admired, needed, etc.), in order for the patients to receive effective psychotherapy from them.

To help prevent the therapist's countertransferential fears and narcissistic vulnerabilities from altering the effective delivery of treatment, Har Paz suggests that the following questions be answered:

1. Are the therapist's countertransference reactions unique to the group?
2. Is the therapist using the group to resolve or to act out his or her own conscious, preconscious, and unconscious feelings and wishes?
3. How is the therapist's therapeutic style or the therapist's activity level influenced by his or her fears?
4. Which irrational fears (anxiety) are activated and impact negatively on the therapist in the group setting. For example:
   a. Is he or she afraid of intimacy with men or women?
   b. Is he or she afraid of authority, power, or loss of control?
   c. Is he or she afraid of open, powerful expression of feelings?
5. What type of fear or anxiety dominates the therapist's own psychological organization, that is, the fear of abandonment or the fear of engulfment? (1994, p. 7)

In the second category of induced countertransference reactions, the therapist's ability to resonate with their patients' unconscious emotional communication will be an important source of information if properly utilized and applied. It is in this area of unconscious emotional communication that the concept of projective identification needs to be thoroughly understood.

PROJECTIVE IDENTIFICATION

Projective identification involves both interpersonal and intrapsychic components. Projective identification differs substantially from projection in that it exists only in the context of an interaction between two or more individuals, whereas projection can happen alone and does not necessarily take place in an authentic personal relationship. Projective identification requires both a projector and a receiver. The more the receiver's defenses are down, i.e., the more open, emotionally close, and vulnerable the receiver to the projector, the less able the receiver will be able to avoid "taking on" the projection from the projector. Ogden (1982) has suggested it is easier to understand this process if it is looked at as occurring in three phases. (See Table 13.1.)

As Ogden suggests, there is some emotional pressure exerted on the recipient to experience and take on the projection. Projectors need to rid themselves of an emotion or part of themselves because it is intolerable for them to own or contain it. So they will project it onto another and coerce that person to experience it and give it back to them as verification of their expectation. For example, because the projectors already feel so bad and worthless about themselves, they cannot tolerate having a feeling that might verify in their minds how bad they are (i.e., "Good people don't get angry. I'm a good person, so I can't be angry. You must be the one who is angry because I can feel it!"). The receiver is then forced to contain it and act it out with the projector, thus confirming the projector's expectation (i.e., "See I was right, you are angry, you do hate me and think I am a bad person!"). Ogden, writing from an object-relations perspective, elaborates on this process when he writes,

> In association with this unconscious projective fantasy, there is an interpersonal interaction by means of which the recipient is pursued to think, feel, and behave in a manner congruent with the ejected feeling and the self and object representation embodied in the projective fantasy. (1982, p. 2)

Projective identification, however, is much more than a defense. Ogden identifies three other important functions it serves: (1) communication, (2) object relatedness, and (3) pathway for psychological change. These last three functions provide the therapist with some valuable therapeutic information if they are properly understood and utilized. (See Table 13.2.)

Projective Identification as Communication

Projective identification, if properly understood and utilized can provide the therapist with valuable pieces of information about the patient.

TABLE 13.1. Ogden's Phases of Projective Identification

1. Expelling part of the self into someone else, where it takes hold.
2. Pressuring the other person to experience it.
3. Getting it back from the other person.

TABLE 13.2. Ogden's Four Functions of Projective Identification

1. Defense–to distance oneself from the unwanted part or to keep it alive in someone else.
2. Communication–to make oneself understood by pressing the recipient to experience a set of feelings like one's own.
3. Object-relatedness–to interact with a recipient separate enough to receive the projection yet undifferentiated enough to allow some misperception to occur and to foster the sense of oneness.
4. Pathway for psychological change–to be transformed by reintrojecting the projection after its modification by the recipient, as occurs in the mother-infant relationship, marriage, or the patient-therapist relationship.

There is much to be gained if the projective identification is examined as a source of emotional communication about the person's past experience and his or her inner emotional life, which is reflective of that experience. The patient will not only be communicating how it felt to be the child of abusive, neglectful parents, but will also provide a glimpse into how the abusive or neglectful parent may have felt toward the patient. Consequently, the therapist can be induced by the patient to identify either with the patient's self, which is termed a *concordant identification*, or with the patient's internalized object, which is termed a *complementary identification*. It is important to remember that the two forms of identification (concordant and complementary) available to the therapist provide an important source of emotional communication and understanding. Their ultimate value is that they can increase the therapist's capacity for empathy. Empathy is the optimally desired outcome resulting from the successful processing of a projective identification and leading to a better emotional understanding of the patient's experience.

Complementary Projective Identification

Not only does complementary projective identification provide the therapist with an opportunity for understanding how it feels to be the abuser (object-representation), it will also give a therapist a more complete empathic understanding of the patient's experience in the past. If, for instance, the therapist finds him or herself becoming impatient with patients' "whining" and has to fight the impulse to tell them to stop feeling sorry for themselves, chances are good that the concordant identification is revealing how the patients experienced their parents as children. A greater empathic understanding can help the therapist respond to how difficult it must have been to get one's parents to listen in a caring and understanding way. Instead of giving in to the pull for enactment, by criticizing the patients, the therapist will be able to resonate to the patients' experience.

Concordant Projective Identification

In its simplest and purest form, concordant projective identification represents the therapist's capacity to directly experience very similar feelings to those of the patient. Much in the way that self-psychology uses terms such as *vicarious introspection* and *empathy* to describe the therapist's ability to accurately resonate to another person's experience, concordant projective identification conveys the same sentiments. It is synonymous with empathy, at least the way self-psychology defines the term. Empathy is described as the inner experience of sharing with and comprehending the momentary emotions and psychological state of another person. The empathic experience is further characterized by feelings of harmony and closeness with the patient, as well as by the experience of positive regard. In its most concise definition, empathy is not exactly the same as concordant identification, but is the optimal outcome that is possible if the therapist is successful at processing the inner induced experience. It is knowing what it felt like to be the self in relating to the internalized object.

Object-Relatedness

Many alcoholics and addicts, especially those early in recovery and those with significant character pathology, will prove difficult to treat because of their excessive use of projective identification as a defensive process. The closer and more intimate the relationship, the more likely that internal self- and object-representations formed as a result of early relationships in past will become activated in the present. Transference and countertransference reactions, if properly managed, allow a bridge to be built between the past and the present. The intertwining of transference and the real relationship, past and present, and you and me is often unclear, even to the most skilled therapist. Hopefully, the therapist in such circumstances will be able to tolerate the ambiguity that is present in any real, authentic relationship, but that is more intense in a dependent relationship such as the one that the patient must form with the therapist. No matter how hard a therapist may try to form an equal and nonauthoritative relationship, it cannot be avoided. As long as the patient comes to the therapist's office or to the hospital where the therapist is employed and either pays for the service or the therapist gains financially for providing the service, it is not an equal relationship.

The ability to tolerate ambiguity in a relationship, especially a therapeutic one, is something that many patients do not possess. Individuals who do not have an adequate supply of good introjections or good internal self-representation will not be able to tolerate much ambiguity. Such individuals have usually not had a sufficiently responsive or protective relationship with reliable parents. Consequently, they will be prone to experience any ambiguity on the therapist's part (i.e., empathic failures, poor attunement, distraction, tardiness, etc.) as another failure to protect or evidence of disinterest.

PATHWAYS FOR PSYCHOLOGICAL CHANGE

It is with the fourth function of this process that the therapist's tasks become clear and crucial. The recipient must give projection back to the projector, but not in the original form it was delivered. Since the projectors' aim is to get rid of some part of themselves they cannot tolerate, the projection must be returned by the recipient in a digested manner that can be tolerated by the projector. The therapist must contain and detoxify the feeling before giving it back in a way that the patient can bear and integrate into his or her experience. This sometimes requires that the therapist not react too quickly to the affect, "hurling interpretations" at the projector. Containing the feelings and detoxifying and digesting them before helping the projector understand or make sense of what is happening requires some deliberation on the therapist's part. A three-step procedure may provide some clarity to this process:

1. First, the therapist must strive to suspend defensiveness and criticism of the patient while tolerating the experience of perceiving him or herself in a temporarily unfavorable light.
2. Second, the therapist must possess the ability to manage the current self-experience, however uncomfortable, without feeling it as an intolerable threat to self-esteem, which requires it to be experienced in relation to a predominance of positive self-representations that must be available internally for the therapist.
3. Third, the therapist must have the capacity to understand that the induced experience is temporary and an indication of projective identification.

To help illuminate this process, some examples may help clarify useful ways of responding to a patient's projective identification. For example, a woman in group, whose husband has just relapsed, attacks the group leader vehemently after he makes some ambiguous statement about blame and responsibility. Rather than respond too quickly, the therapist conveys to her a response that acknowledges a full understanding of her anger and how the statement could have sounded blaming to her. The therapist would then venture an interpretation from either a transference- or countertransference-based perspective.

1. Transference-based communication:

   "Despite the fact that to all appearances you are angry, I can't help but feel that somehow it might be more comfortable for you to be angry with me right now than to be left with how threatened and devastated you are about your husband's relapse."

2. Countertransference-based communication:

   "I feel as though I am being pulled into a fight here at a time when your husband's relapse seems too pressing. Do you suppose there is anything to that?

   "You seem to me to be looking for a fight today. Any ideas what that might be about?"

   "I feel as though there is a great deal of tension in the air here that I, for one, do not believe we understand."

In another related circumstance, the group leader might not be able to readily identify or understand the source of a group member's transferential anger, as was the case in the previous example when the group member's husband relapsed. In such circumstances, the group leader's task will be to contain the transferential feeling and acknowledge it in a way that the group members feel heard without conveying that they are justified to act as they are acting toward the therapist. Not only must they be assured that the therapist will not retaliate, but they must also know that the therapist will not be a patsy or a pushover who will be intimidated or frightened by their anger.

An example:

> "I am willing to be seen or perceived as a weak, ineffective, cold, cruel, etc., therapist until we work this through."

"I'm angry and unhappy with your treatment of me right now, but I'm not going to punish or attack you for it. . . . and will be willing to hang in there with you through this until we get it resolved."

ADDICTION AND COUNTERTRANSFERENCE

While countertransference is an important concern for all therapists, it is frequently more of an issue for those who work with alcoholics and addicts because of the intense hostility, anger, disrespect, and distrust these patients commonly provoke in others. While countertransference can manifest itself in therapists who use patients as a source of their own gratification or pleasure, it is likely to be the negative emotions that give group leaders the most difficulty. Imhof, Hirsch, and Terenzi (1984) agree and caution those who work with these patients to be careful of the intense feelings that alcoholics and addicts are likely to evoke in the course of treatment. They write:

> The drug-abusing patient, with his sense of worthlessness, self-hate, and destructive rage, now meets his obverse–the "good" therapist, a "paragon of virtue," and essentially everything the patient is not. The resultant good-bad dichotomy is a serious threat to the ego identity of the patient, and the first order of psychic business for the patient is to reverse the imbalance. More specifically, the patient (unconsciously) begins to employ any strategy available to provoke, cajole, humiliate, and deceive the therapist–in essence to make the therapist more like himself, or worse than himself. Without the concurrent presence of the therapist's skill and understanding of the dynamics at work, including his own countertransferential and attitudinal postures, the proposed treatment may be short-lived, and the probable negative results all too frequently ascribed to the patient alone. (1984, p. 26)

Without an accurate awareness of possible countertransferential responses, therapists will find the clinical management of the alcohol- or drug-dependent patient to be virtually impossible. In addition, negative countertransference attitudes can be acted out in derivative forms. Therapists who are chronically late, cut short their sessions, fantasize during the treatment hour, become drowsy, or refuse to return phone calls to patients within a reasonable amount of time may need to carefully assess their reasons for these actions, as chances are good that they are being influenced by unconscious feelings toward their patients.

Imhof, Hirsch, and Terenzi (1984) list six common countertransferential reactions stimulated by alcoholic or drug-dependent patients. They point out that these reactions may be overt or transparent, and at other times quite camouflaged.

1. Therapists can assume the role of the good parent who rescues the bad impulsive child. Therapists may become overinvolved, protective, maternal, permissive and overly nurturing, hoping that their outpouring of "love" and "goodness" will cure the patients of their drug and alcohol use. Much like the typical untreated Al-Anon member, therapists may believe that if they try hard enough and give their all to the alcoholic or addict, they will get the patients to stop their drug use and drinking because of their love for the therapist.
2. Physicians can inadvertently contribute to patients' addiction by overprescribing medication. Misdiagnosis or failure of physicians to appreciate the drug abuse potential of their prescriptions can contribute significantly to the addict's or alcoholic's problems. The addict's or alcoholic's own sense of futility may stir in the doctor his or her own countertransference need to do something for the patient. To not respond with something concrete that can help the patient immediately may be tied into the doctor's own need to be valued as one who brings relief to another's suffering. Such a countertransference need to be valued may result in the physician prescribing drugs even when his or her judgment tells him or her that it may not be best for the patient.
3. Therapists can be captured by the remarkable and quick recovery of the addicted patient. They can be led to believe in the illusion of the dramatic cure that has taken place due to the effectiveness of their therapeutic skill. In the extreme, the therapist can come to hold the belief that the patient is "well enough" to try controlled drinking. The inevitable relapse can lead the therapist to feel deceived, resentful, angry, or that he or she is a "bad therapist" who has failed the impulsive child.
4. The therapist can get vicarious satisfaction from the patient's acting out and establish an alliance built on "you and me against the world." Therapists who are struggling from their own unresolved unconscious impulse fantasies can overly identify with the patient. They can develop the attitude of "only I really understand you," which frequently leads the patient and the therapist to "play off" of each other.
5. Therapists can develop the commonly referred to syndrome of "burn out." They can become callous and indifferent to their patients. Instead of caring, the therapist employs different defense mechanisms

of which withdrawal, narcissistic distancing, boredom, or anger are the most common.

6. Stereotypical classification by the therapist of his or her alcohol and drug dependent patients can lead to an attitude that his or her patients are nothing more than "junkies," "drunks," or "addicts" who will never change.

Self-reflection and self-analysis by group leaders into their own participation and impact on the therapeutic relationship and treatment outcome is necessary if they are to enhance their effectiveness in group. The cause of the alcoholic's and addict's failure in treatment is too often attributed to the patient's own psychopathology rather than the negative derivatives of the patient-therapist interaction. If group leaders are going to be able to avoid their own destructive countertransference influences, they must be emotionally and cognitively receptive to receiving, recognizing, and analyzing the intense feelings generated by most chemically dependent patients.

Imhof, Hirsch, and Terenzi (1984) make five recommendations for the group leader to follow so that the potential for destructive countertransference derivatives is minimized.

1. The field of addiction treatment is unique in its use of former patients (i.e., recovering alcoholics and addicts) as treatment providers. In many cases, this has numerous advantages to treatment (i.e., identification, alliance, altruism, etc.). In other instances, it can have detrimental effects. Recovering alcoholics or addicts might be inclined to use the exact identical format for treatment that they themselves experienced. In such cases, a "what worked for me will work for you" attitude may result in unreasonable therapeutic expectations. In some cases, more emphasis can be placed on prior personal experience in relation to clinical training. It is important to realize that nothing can substitute for good, sound clinical skills, whether the therapist is recovering or has never suffered from an addiction problem. The recovering person who has become well-trained clinically has much more to offer than a therapist who is either just recovering or just well-trained clinically.

2. One's own personal therapy is a very important asset to providing quality therapy. This is especially important in the field of group therapy. The group leader who knows what it is like, from personal experience, to be on the other side of the therapy group encounter, will be more sensitive to the issues that are likely to manifest in group. Yalom (1985) writes about the importance of a group training experience:

> Such an experience may offer many types of learning not elsewhere available. The student is able to learn at an emotional level what he may previously have known only intellectually: he experiences the

> power of the group, its power to wound or heal; he learns how important it is to be accepted by the group; he learns what self-disclosure really entails, how difficult it is to reveal one's secret world, one's fantasies, one's feelings of vulnerability, hostility, and tenderness; he appreciates his own strengths as well as his weaknesses; he learns about his own preferred role in the group; and perhaps most striking of all, he learns about the role of the leader as he becomes aware of his own dependency and his own unrealistic appraisal of the leader's power and knowledge. (p. 523)

Imhof, Hirsch, and Terenzi share a similar opinion about personal therapy when they write:

> We maintain that only through an examination of one's own emotional development can the therapist most effectively recognize, tolerate, and begin to sort out the infinite range of countertransferential and attitudinal considerations inherent in the treatment of such patients. (1984, p. 29)

3. Clinical supervision, especially in the field of alcohol and drug abuse, is essential if therapists are to successfully manage all of their countertransferential considerations that are likely to be evoked by these patients.

4. Continual education is required. Group leaders must continue to familiarize themselves with an ever-greater understanding of the multifactor influences of alcoholism and drug dependence.

5. A constant evaluation of one's own personal values and attitudes toward individuals who abuse or are addicted to chemicals is required. This also means therapists must carefully monitor their own attitudes toward their own personal alcohol or drug use. Therapists who are "recreationally" using marijuana or cocaine are ill-suited to treat someone who has an alcohol or drug problem. This is made more problematic by the fact that cocaine and marijuana are illegal. The moral and ethical stance of such a position has important ramifications for treatment. At the other extreme, therapists who, for religious reasons, perceive drug or alcohol use as a moral issue need to carefully assess whether working with alcohol or drug dependent patients is in their best interest–not to mention the detrimental effects this attitude can have on their patients.

If group leaders can discipline themselves to follow these principles in the course of their work with addicted patients, their chances of having a successful therapy group will be increased. Awareness of one's own countertransferential influences and reactions is essential while working with alcoholics and addicts in a group setting. Group leaders who are finely tuned into themselves have a valuable diagnostic tool at their disposal. How is each patient affecting them? What are the feelings they are having at this moment in regard to the group and its members? Constantly monitoring questions like these can give group leaders much valuable information about their group and its members. Each group member reacts differently to the group leader. Studying members' individual reactions not only teaches group leaders about the individual members in the group, but it also gives the group leaders an opportunity to understand themselves better. Individual members often pick up on reactions, feelings, and attitudes of group leaders that the leaders may not be aware of in themselves. An openness to self-reflection and a willingness to critically examine one's contributions to the group and its individual members' reactions can give group leaders a valuable therapeutic tool if they have the courage to honestly monitor themselves. In the words of Socrates, group leaders must "Know thyself."

Chapter 14

Resistance in Group

One of the most difficult technical problems confronting group leaders is the recognition and resolution of group resistance. The extent to which group leaders are successful in helping the group members deal with their individual and colluded efforts at avoiding emotionally charged issues determines to a large degree the success or failure of the group therapy experience. Group leaders must not only manage the different individual resistances in group, but they must be able to identify the phenomenon of a unified group resistance and successfully resolve the simultaneous resistance of each and all of the members in group. Group leaders' handling of group resistance is crucial. Unless they successfully develops strategies for coping with it, the group may remain at an impasse indefinitely, become fragmented, or dissolve totally.

In working with a unified group resistance, group leaders' previous experiences dealing with individual resistances in individual therapy will be of little use to them in the group setting. It is essential that group leaders develop special skills for detecting its occurrence in group and for working resistance through on a group level. Group leaders must learn to gauge the group's characteristic operating efficiency by noting the extent to which the group and its members contribute or detract from the group goals. The success or failure of a therapy group is determined to large degree by how group resistance is managed by the group leader. Successfully negotiating its resolution requires that two important principles of group resistance be addressed before the group can be a true working group.

The first required principle that must be established for dealing with group resistance is to be able to recognize it when it occurs. It is impossible to cope with group resistance successfully if group leaders cannot see it or feel it. This requires that the group leaders understand the different forms resistance can take in group and how their reaction or inaction contributes to its duration, intensity, and resolution. Group leaders must help the group members come to recognize when they are being resistive. It is necessary to call their attention to the resistive pull of the group process. However, simply calling this to their attention will not be enough to resolve its occurrence. Resistance is always there for a reason, and the group members should not be expected to give it up until the emotional forces held in check by it are sufficiently discharged or converted, so that they are no longer a danger to the safety of the group or its members. Each group member has to be able to come to understand the meaning of resistance in terms of his or her own life history and experience.

The second principle for dealing with group resistance requires that group leaders clearly understand the part they play in the establishment and maintenance of resistance in the group. Resistance is always a product of the interaction between the patient and the therapist. In group, resistance can be induced by leaders who are passive, hostile, ineffective, guarded, weak, or in need of constant admiration and excessive friendliness. Group leaders must be able to differentiate between the part they play in this process and the part the individual group members play within the context of the group's regressive pull. If leaders do not establish a cohesive, safe atmosphere for their group members, resistance will be promoted by the very nature of the group's inherent threat to the safety of the group's individual members. Any group approach or technique that is applied without the careful evaluation of these principles is apt to decrease the chances of therapeutic success in group treatment.

RESISTANCE: A DEFINITION

There are a variety of definitions for resistance. Two simple definitions that best capture its essence are:

1. Resistance is a force that prevents the freeing of unconscious material.
2. Resistance is the avoidance of feelings and the denial of emotions.

The first definition reflects a more classical, psychodynamic definition of resistance. Psychodynamic-oriented group therapists define resistance as any force that opposes the patients' primary task of making conscious their repressed, unconscious feelings. Resistance prevents individuals from freely conveying to the group leader all of their thoughts and feelings. Until this is accomplished, the patients will remain unaware of the unconscious motives that continue to compel them to act in a self-defeating manner. The second definition is a more generalized one pertaining to an individual's tendency to avoid presenting any emotionally meaningful material to the therapist. Patients do this despite the fact that it is the emotionally charged conflicts in their relationships with meaningful others, both in their past and present, that have led them to enter therapy in the first place. The patients' affect and the content of their verbalizations will remain inappropriate to the material and consequently work against the primary goals of therapy.

Resistance can take many forms in groups. It can manifest as silence, anger, excessive intellectualization, compliance, indifference, or even boredom. Boredom is an especially troublesome form of resistance because many group leaders fail to identify it as resistance. It is a commonly accepted fact that groups promote regression. Every group member is forced to deal with emotionally arousing issues related to survival, acceptance, rejection, and closeness. Boredom is literally not feeling one's emotions. If someone feels bored in group or starts to doze off as other group members speak, the group leader can feel confident that the bored individual is keeping powerful emotions out of his or her awareness. It is the group leader's task to bring such repressed feelings to the surface, where they can be examined and altered.

Nowhere is the principle of boredom as resistance more dramatically applied than in a therapy group conducted by Erv Polster. The group member can count on attracting Erv Polster's attention by just appearing bored in his group. In fact, the surest way to attract Erv Polster's interest is for a group member to announce in group that he or she is, in fact, bored. Nothing stimulates Erv's interest as much as a group member who can be in a close intimate setting with six to eight other people and not feel some emotional stirrings within him or herself. Erv's eyes will light up in his own unique penetrating fashion, and he will lean forward and ask with sincere inquisitiveness, "Now, that is interesting! Would you please tell me and the rest of the group how you manage to keep yourself bored in such an intimate gathering as this?"

Erv Polster (1981) also has his own unique definition of resistance. He views resistance as that which occurs when the patient does not do what the therapist wants him or her to do. Resistance does not exist for Erv Polster. For Erv, resistance is "the stuff" that therapy is made of. Operating from a classical Gestalt perspective, Erv Polster "goes with" the patient's resistance. Utilizing a Zen-type, martial arts stance when exploring resistance, Erv Polster moves in to use the resistance to his advantage. He magnifies the resistance because this is where the patient's energy is frequently blocked. Exploring and expanding the resistance will usually lead to a release of the repressed material.

Heinz Kohut (1977a), coming from a more classical psychoanalytic point of view, expresses similar sentiments to those of Erv Polster when he writes about resistance. Kohut views resistance as being enhanced by the iatrogenic effects of an unempathic therapist. Resistance is lessened either by the group leader's empathic understanding or by another group member's sympathy and shared similar experience. If the group leader is vicariously introspective and remains empathically in tune with the patient, resistance will be greatly diminished.

Robert and Mary Goulding (1979) see resistance somewhat differently, yet they agree that its resolution is one of the most important ingredients to successful therapy. For the Gouldings, therapy with the patient is much like a chess match. A part of the patient wants to change and get better. This is the part that brings the patient to the therapy session. However, there is an equally strong part in the patient that wants things to remain as they are. This is the part that is resistant and tries to defeat the therapist. This is why the Gouldings caution the therapist to watch for the first con. The first con will usually manifest itself in the patient's initial statement (e.g., "I don't think this will help, but . . .") or in other key words such as *can't, need, should,* or *try.*

While Kohut, the Gouldings, and Polster each view resistance somewhat differently, they agree on the significance it plays in a person's psychological functioning. The group leader must never lose sight of the understanding that resistance is part of an individual's defensive system and that defenses are always there for good reason. As Scott Rutan (1983) said, "Patients come to us with solutions, not problems." By this, he meant that resistance must be recognized as a defensive maneuver constructed by patients to protect themselves against painful emotional experiences, usually of a longstanding nature. The only problem is that the defenses they have erected to protect themselves are often worse than the original emotional trauma that led to their establishment. Their defensive operations usually end up more disruptive than the feelings or thoughts they were originally intended to protect them from. In dealing with resistance of this nature, the group leader must remember a simple principle about resistance: The more guarded and defended the person, the more pain, hurt, and fear that is hidden behind the guardedness. Anger is almost always an emotion that is erected in direct proportion to the amount of hurt that a person has experienced in his or her life. The more angry group members appear, the greater the likelihood that they are protecting themselves from the exposure of powerful negative emotions such as shame, guilt, hurt, and self-loathing. Therefore, defenses must not be stripped away too quickly. Defenses must never be exposed just for the sake of their exposure. They must be slowly and carefully removed or altered as the individuals gradually develop new and healthier methods for protecting themselves.

GROUP RESISTANCE AND THE WORK OF WILFRED BION

Wilfred Bion is one of the most influential figures in psychoanalytic group psychotherapy. He earned his reputation and fame in group therapy without the benefit of working with therapy groups himself. This makes his contributions all the more remarkable, since his book *Experiences in Groups* (1961) continues to have a powerful effect on psychodynamic approaches to group therapy.

The most widely known aspect of Bion's work is his basic assumption theory. Bion drew a distinction between the basic assumption group and the work group. Within Bion's perspective, there were always two groups present in every group setting–the overt or work group and the covert or basic assumption group. While the work group is always established to accomplish an overt task, a covert group exists alongside the overt group and often operates out of its own unspoken rules. Bion asserted that the primitive states of mind operating covertly in the basic assumption group tended to dominate the work group and would come to interfere with the declared task of the group. The emotional attitudes organized in these basic assumption states were described as unconscious processes and were differentiated into three categories. These categories possessed an "as if" quality and were identified as dependency, fight-flight, and pairing.

I. *Work Group*	II. *Basic Assumption Group*
A. Overt	A. Covert
B. Task-Oriented Activity	B. Hatred of Learning by Experience
C. Readiness to Cooperate	C. Opposition to Development
D. Ego Activity, Reality Testing, and Responsibility	D. Preferring the Comfort of Magical Ideas Rather than Ego Ideas Which Require Work
E. Composed of Individuals	E. Group Mind
F. Real and Quantitative	F. "As If" Quality

Dependency

The group will behave "as if" satisfaction, safety, and the future of the group depends on a strong leader. The aim of the group is to obtain security by seeking the protection of a leader who can be seen as all-powerful and all-wonderful. The aim of the group is to find someone who will take care of them.

BASIC ASSUMPTION OF DEPENDENCY:

1. Leader Idealized as Omnipotent and Wonderful
2. Helpless Dependency on Leader
3. Attempts to Extract Power from the Leader

Fight-Flight

The group acts "as if" there is an internal or external threat that must be challenged or from which they must escape. Action is essential within the fight-flight basic assumption. The group can flee into the abstract dialogue of the there and then or the group members can fight with each other, often giving the illusion that their fighting is doing "real work" in group. In actuality, their fighting is a defense against the real overt task of the group. If the group leader cannot tolerate internal strife, the group will direct its anger outward and find a cause, ideology, or other group to hate.

BASIC ASSUMPTION OF FIGHT/FLIGHT:

1. Outfighting: Group Unites Against Foe
2. Infighting: Between Subgroups
3. Flight from Task

Pairing

The group acts "as if" assertive feelings of anger or depressive feelings of despair do not exist. Passive contemplation is maintained through idealization and a mood of hopefulness that prevents the emergence of destructive rage or persecutory anxiety and depression. The group lives in a state of hope that the intimacy of the group members may give birth to a new idea or a Messiah who will save them.

BASIC ASSUMPTION OF PAIRING
1. Intimacy of Pairing Subgroup 2. Tolerance of and Collusion with the Pair 3. Hopeful Expectation of Salvation through the Resolution of Conflict by the Pair

Fusion

A fourth common basic assumption that Bion did not identify is that of fusion. The group acts "as if" all the members of the group were the same. The group and its members retreat into "we-ness." This is represented by the group members who comment that they see everyone equally in the group. "I trust everyone here equally," and "I care equally for everyone in the group" are examples of how group members will go to great lengths to deny their individuality. It is a defensive reaction brought upon by the regressive pull of their need to be part of and included in a group, society, or family. Bion asserts that we are forever social animals. (See Figure 14.1.)

Bion uses the term *valency* to describe an individual's tendency to be attracted to others with similar underlying motives, values, and propensities. These valencies can exercise a powerful regressive pull and lead to the activation of basic assumptions when the group is faced with the frustration entailed in sustaining the requirements of the group work. Basic assumptions are primitive states of mind generated by the dilemma created by the dual pull of the group. Each member wants to be part of the group, yet they want to maintain their individuality. As Bion wrote, "The individual is a group animal at war, not simply with the group, but with himself for being a group animal and with those aspects of his personality that constitute his groupishness" (1961, p. 131).

While it is true that basic assumptions exist in group, it is important for the group leader to be aware that basic assumptions are stage-specific and can be induced by the behavior of the group leader.

Stage Specific Basic Assumptions

1. Early phase of group development is marked by the dependency group. The group expects magical solutions will be bestowed upon them by the group leader. The emotional state is one of dependency and awe.

2. Middle phase of group development is marked by flight from tasks or engagement of battles within or outside of the group. The emotional state is one of hostility and fear.
3. Late phase of group is marked by a state of hope. The group possesses the curative fantasy and hopes the intimacy of the group will given birth to ideas or a person who can bring about an ultimate answer to the group's dilemma. Pairing carries an emotional state of optimism and hopefulness. The group waits for the birth of a Messiah who must never be born because it would end hope.

THE LEADER'S INFLUENCE ON THE BASIC ASSUMPTIONS

Otto Kernberg (1984), writing about the leader's influence on group development, emphasizes the important effect that the leader's personality has on the group's development. He has correctly pointed out that a passive, inactive, and quiet group leader is more likely to provoke Bion's basic assumptions. Basic assumption states owe their existence, therefore, in large part, to the conditions imposed by the group leader him or herself upon the group. D. G. Brown (1985) takes a very similar stance and questions whether many followers of Bion have taken his basic assumption theory too literally and suggests that they have applied his ideas incorrectly to group therapy. Brown writes, "For some of his ideas are, I think, ultimately inadequate and misleading as a basis for therapy, particularly the unmodified concept of basic assumptions" (1985, p. 192). Brown further states that Bion ignores the more mature ego states in his work and is preoccupied with primitive processes. Bion's viewpoint, Brown feels, is "based on a Kleinian approach to mental functioning that is preoccupied with primitive processes to the neglect of more mature ego functions" (1985, p. 215). This is why Bion overemphasized the basic assumption group. The work group is not opposed to the more primitive functions; rather, it develops out of them and eventually supercedes them unless the group leader fails to guide the group through this process. Basic assumptions are, therefore, indications that the group is struggling unsuccessfully against resistance. Resolution of resistance, however, does not require that the basic assumption states be the focus of therapeutic interventions.

The group leader's attempt to resolve the basic assumption is a misdirected effort. This is where most psychodynamic group leaders fail to appreciate the impact that they have in inducing a basic assumption emotional state. Unmodified basic assumptions arise as a result of avoidances of genu-

FIGURE 14.1

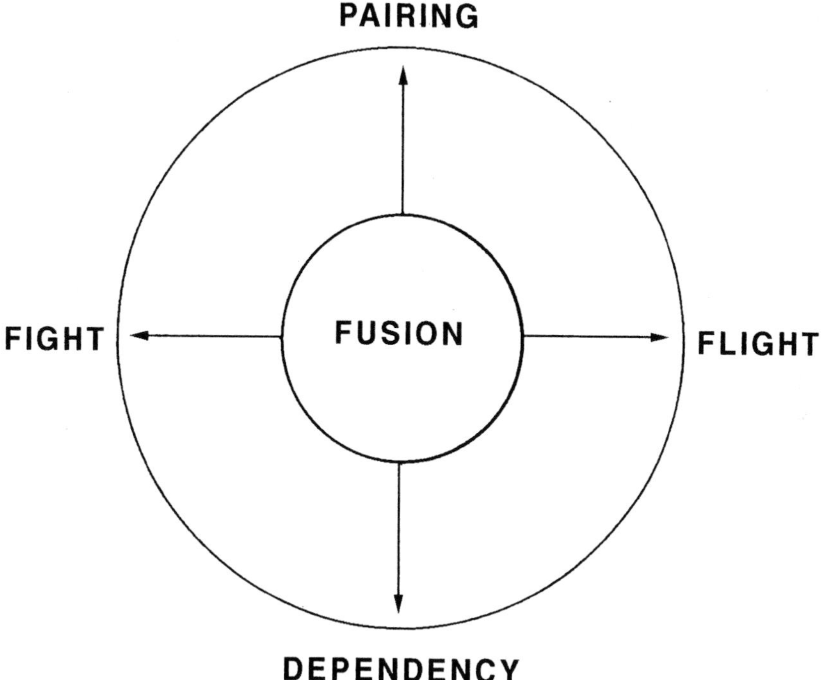

BASIC ASSUMPTIONS

GROUP RESISTANCE

1. **Dependency**
2. **Fight - Flight**
3. **Pairing**

ine personal encounters. Difficult feelings in relationships are thereby disavowed and repressed. Repression and denial lead to basic assumption states.

It is with the choice of the intervention that group leaders are most likely to misdirect their efforts. Unmodified basic assumptions arise as a result of a situation that prevents genuine personal encounters. Difficult feelings in relationships are disavowed either through dependency, fusion, fight-flight, or pairing. Any gathering of three or more people that does not permit true intimate contact is likely to induce a basic assumption emotional state. Group members must be encouraged to deal honestly with all feelings that emerge in the group climate. Negative as well as positive feelings must be expressed and acknowledged or the group will stay stuck in a basic assumption state. Basic assumption states reflect ways that group members try to cope with and rid themselves of dangerous feelings and impulses. Group members will attempt to engage the group leader on the basis of wishes and fantasies, which will protect them from their prohibited emotions. Ezriel (1973) states that group members will first try to establish three types of relationships with the group leader in their attempt to defend themselves:

1. Each group member will first try to establish the *required* relationship since he or she requires it in order to protect him or herself from the second relationship.
2. The second relationship is called the *avoided* relationship that the group member attempts to establish in order to avoid external reality because he or she is convinced that if he or she gave into his or her secret desire to enter into the avoided relationship, it would result in the third relationship.
3. The third relationship is not a relationship at all, but an expected result of the avoided relationship which is *calamity.*

Calamity is the feared result that must be avoided at all costs by each group member. Ezriel describes this process:

1. Required relationship: Idealization of therapist.
2. Avoided relationship: If established, it would result in the group member attacking the therapist.
3. Calamity: Based on the group member's fear that he or she would either harm the therapist or the therapist would retaliate and in turn destroy him or her.

During treatment, as the group leader induces more reality testing, the expected unconscious calamity does not occur. The need for the required relationship is removed, and the avoided relationship and its related behavior pattern emerges. Both negative and positive emotions are experienced and expressed. True intimacy is established in group. In the basic assumption group, the leader of the dependency group must be omnipotent; the fight-leader must be unbeatable and the flight-leader uncatchable; and the leader of the pairing group must be marvelous but unborn. As the expected calamity is corrected, the group members learn that they need not resist their true feelings toward the group leader. In the mature work group, which makes a more adaptive use of appropriate assumptions, the leader of the dependency group is dependable, the leader of the fight-flight group is courageous, and the leader of the pairing group is creative.

The group leader plays a very significant part in determining whether the group makes the transition from the basic assumption group to the work group. The group leader who needs to be idealized keeps the group dependent. Bad feelings are subsequently split off and projected onto other group members. The possibility of scapegoating is subsequently increased. The scapegoat serves an important function for the group. He or she is the container for the frustrations the group members have but cannot express toward the group leader. In every group, there will usually be one or two volunteers for the role of the group scapegoat. The group will eventually choose from the list of volunteers to determine who is to serve in the capacity of the container for their anger.

The group leader who requires that the group be highly cohesive so that negative feelings cannot be directed between group members contributes to the group directing their negative feelings to the there and then outside of group. The group leader who encourages pairing in group allows the group members to use their need for hope to prevent the emergence of negative feelings such as anger and despair.

However, pairing, like the other basic assumptions, can be viewed as a testing of the group leader. Pairing will continue if assertive feelings cannot be mobilized in a way that makes the defeat of rage and despair less dependent upon a leader who continues to foster a hopeful situation. If the group leader can help the group members accept his or her limitations and the rage or disappointment this realization produces, he or she will lead the group to become more autonomous. The negative forces of fight-flight will not be split off. In pairing, the group has the chance to accept and realize its fantasy wish. Pairing in group is really an experiment by the group in their effort to determine if it is safe to be intimate in group. Fantasy or illusion is not always defensive. It can be a creative adaptive response. It allows the group to perceive and imagine what does not exist and create it. The group will eventually learn that it can establish intimate relationships without sacrificing hope. More important, it can eventually learn to accept relationships, even if they are not perfect, without becoming depressed or enraged or losing hope.

This is where Bion's original concept of basic assumptions must be carefully evaluated and modified. Basic assumptions are not the result of the group's attempt to avoid intimacy as much as they are a reaction to a leader or a situation that prohibits intimacy. As Brown suggests, basic assumptions arise in group when there is an "avoidance of genuine personal encounter, so that difficult feelings in relationships are disavowed" (1985, p. 216). Basic assumption states are more likely, therefore, in settings where personal contact is forbidden, inappropriate, or best avoided (i.e., disturbed families, large groups, work situations, or therapy groups run on strict Bionian lines). In situations such as these, it is easy to understand how a strong leader, an enemy, or a utopian idea can appear as a viable and entertaining alternative to all the group's problems.

Brown suggests that settings which promote genuine contact, such as a well-functioning therapy group, will reduce the emergence of basic assumption states. A therapy group that faces up to its problems and differences and allows the full expression of all emotions–be they awkward, negative, or positive–will prevent the emergence and persistence of basic assumptions. The group leader's task is not to encourage basic assumptions in order to analyze or study their occurrence; rather the leader's task is to ensure that they do not manifest or persist in group.

In those group settings that are not intended to be therapeutic, basic assumptions serve important functions. The basic assumption states can be recognized in society through the institutions of the church, army, and aristocracy. The function of the church is to organize dependency on a deity; the function of the army is to defend the realm; and the function of the aristocracy is to ensure the next generation of superior leaders.

If Bion's and Ezriel's interpretations of the basic assumption phenomenon are correct, their analysis of this process has two important implications for group therapy. First, their work implies that the basic assumptions are the result, not the cause of a group setting, where true intimate dialogue is prohibited. Second, as Brown clearly states, the group leader's task is not to analyze or heighten the basic assumptions, but to facilitate intimate interaction between group members, thus minimizing and eventually eliminating the destructive forces that prevent the emergence of the overt tasks of the work group.

RESISTANCE TO INTIMACY IN GROUPS

However, the group leader will soon discover that facilitating intimacy in group is no easy task. While group members desire intimacy, they fear it at the same time. Each group member will reveal his or her own particular strategies for systematically sabotaging intimacy. This is particularly true for recovering alcoholics and addicts. The group leader's task is to identify how each member of his or her group will take elaborate precautions to prevent true intimacy. The group members' resistance is most strongly tied into their fear of intimacy. If alcoholics or addicts can find ways of preventing its occurrence, they will feel vindicated: "See, I was right; you can't really trust people."

If group leaders can discipline themselves to watch closely for the different ways that the group members resist intimacy, they will help members identify their own particular idiosyncratic styles. For instance, a group member may have the knack for saying the wrong thing at the wrong time in the wrong way to the wrong person. Sometimes, a group member will do all four at the same time.

Group therapy is the treatment of choice for resolving problems with intimacy. Resistance to intimacy is there because all addicts and alcoholics fear that if they risk being open to another, they will be rejected. Fears behind their resistance to intimacy must be resolved if individuals are to be able to get close to others on a mature level. Childhood fears of intimacy must be dispelled and replaced with mature intimate feelings.

> Steve, a thirty-nine-year-old sales manager, had entered group therapy at the request of his family therapist. He and his wife had been married for over fifteen years and had sought couples therapy because their sex life was unsatisfactory. After more than six months of couples therapy, it became obvious that their difficulty with their sexual relationship was a result of their difficulty with emotional closeness. They had been separated for nearly a year prior to entering couples therapy, and their relationship had been marked by vacillating periods of closeness and emotional distancing. Steve complained that his wife kept him at a distance and was withholding and uninterested in him sexually. She countered that every time she got close to him, he would do something to push her away and she was no longer willing to trust him because of his inconsistency. Because they had become locked into a power struggle around this issue, it was judged to be best for them to deal with their fears of intimacy individually. After a month of group therapy, Steve's pattern of vacillating between closeness and distancing became apparent to the group. While such an observation by his wife led to denial and anger, he found himself more open to the consensual observation of the other group members. Steve also talked freely about his occasional sexual affairs and consistent marijuana smoking. Since his wife grew up in a

home with an alcoholic father and was a recovering alcoholic herself with more than eight years of sobriety through AA, she reacted strongly to the inconsistent behavior Steve demonstrated when he was stoned. He objected to her accusations, saying that she had been brainwashed by AA. However, as the rest of the group, many of them recovering alcoholics, began to voice similar concerns, Steve began to admit that his marijuana use had indeed concerned him for some time, but that he was reluctant to admit it to his wife because this would be admitting she was right. As Steve's contradictory messages were challenged by the other group members, he started to question his own motives about his marijuana smoking and affairs. Every time he would get angry about his wife's coldness, he would get stoned in an effort to supress his anger because he "did not want to make matters worse." As she continued to pull away from him further as a result of his marijuana use, he felt justified in his getting his sexual needs met elsewhere. After a sexual liaison with another woman, his guilt would compel him to undo his anger and he would once again make an effort to get close to her. She would start to respond to his efforts, but was wary of his motives. As she withheld, the pattern would be repeated as it had been for the last ten years.

As the group began to point out Steve's uncomfortableness with closeness and his mixed messages, he came to identify his fears of intimacy. Finally, one evening in group, Steve admitted he was afraid to get close to his wife or commit himself to the marriage. "I have one foot in and one foot out." "I'm scared that if I go ahead and do make a consistent effort with her, she might still reject me. I don't want to take that risk." Steve was not willing to face the possibility that he might be rejected if he got close. Like the pairing assumption state in Bion's schema, Steve did not want to risk true intimacy because it would require he give up the hope of intimacy. His idealized fantasy must forever remain unborn. This was exactly his issue with his mother. She was cold, distant, and unwilling to accept Steve as he really was. True intimacy had always been absent from their relationship and Steve did not want to risk being rejected by another woman whom he cared for deeply. Steve's fear of intimacy was played out with his wife. If he risked being himself with her, he expected to be rejected. Since his own mother would only accept him if he met her wishes and expectations, he rebelled at complying with her wishes. Yet he feared openly expressing his anger toward his mother because this would only lead to her pushing him away further. As he does with his wife, Steve kept one foot in the relationship (i.e., wanting closeness) and one foot out of the relationship (fears rejection if he were to be truly intimate with her, because she would only accept him if he met her expectations).

Resistance to intimacy in group will always emerge if the group members are given enough time together. The group leader must allow members' resistance to manifest before their fears of intimacy can be observed and resolved. Observation of resistance in group will give the group leader much information about each member's fears of intimacy. As Freud once stated, "What people avoid telling you is more important than the content of their message of what they say they fear." Oscar Wilde expressed similar sentiments when he said, "People's masks tell you more than their faces."

Louis Ormont (1988) lists four major intimacy fears in groups:

1. Fear of Impulsivity
2. Fear of Merger
3. Fear of Abandonment
4. Fear of Vulnerability

Fear of Impulsivity

Group members, especially alcoholics and addicts, possess tremendous fears of their impulsivity. If they feel and show it, they fear it will get out of hand. Such fears are not limited to their anger or hostility, but also manifest in their caring for others, which frequently gets confused with sexuality. One male group member in particular would stiffen noticeably whenever he spoke to other men in the group. He feared that if he showed warm feelings to other men, he would be viewed as a homosexual. Many men and women struggle with issues of intimacy because they do not know how to be close without turning it into a sexual encounter. They fear if they get close to another, it will mean that they will have to act on their sexual feelings.

Fear of Merger

Many individuals, especially those who have grown up in a home with a controlling and intrusive parent, will possess strong fears of merger. They fear they will be taken over by the other person if they get close. They must remain separate or else they will lose themselves in the other. In the earlier reported case vignette, Steve's wife experienced such fears. She grew up in a home with a mother who tried very hard to control her because the mother was unable in any way to control her alcoholic husband. Steve's wife saw his efforts to get close as an attempt to control her since her mother used intimacy and closeness as a means of control.

Fear of Abandonment

Group members usually possess tremendous fears of abandonment. This is especially true for those who have been abandoned previously by another whom they deeply loved. Since group members want closeness and love, it would seem that the answer to their dilemma would be simple. Love and intimacy provide a rich source of gratification for both their instinctual and reality needs. The only problem with intimacy and closeness as a solution to their isolation is that it puts them at the mercy of their love object. Love, closeness, and intimacy leave individuals extremely vulnerable to the loss or a rejection by the love object. As Freud said, "We are never so defenseless against suffering as when we love, never so helplessly unhappy as when we have lost our love object or its love" (cited in Fancher, 1973, p. 229). People who have already experienced rejection are usually very reluctant to once again choose closeness and intimacy as a path to happiness. This point is clearly demonstrated in the following vignette:

> Mary was a thirty-six-year-old secretary who entered group because of her depression and lack of friends. She could never please her mother and father, as they were extremely critical of her appearance, intelligence, and even her gender. Her older brother, who was much preferred because he was a male, was an extremely successful student, athlete, and businessman. Mary would be extremely sensitive to any remarks that the group members made that could be interpreted, even in the slightest fashion, to be critical of her. She would also constantly put herself down, saying that no one in the group really liked her and she understood why. Anytime the group leader directed any of his attention toward another group member, she would attack that group member and accuse the group leader of not showing the same degree of concern for her problems. Her behavior drove the group to distraction. Their protests of her accusations were futile and led many of the members to avoid her because of their frustration with her behavior. Her fear of rejection compelled her to test everyone she came in contact with. Finally, one evening during group, she stated her fear directly to the group leader. "I know I'm worthless and I'd rather have you reject me now before I

start to care for you too much." Once the motive behind her behavior became obvious to the group and its members, the group leader would constantly interpret her actions to her and the other group members. Eventually, the group took over this confrontive process and did not "play out" their part in Mary's self-fulfilled prophecy. As they refused to succumb to her constant testing, they also began to show their concern for her. A repetitive pattern in Mary's life was consequently altered.

Fear of Vulnerability

Fear of vulnerability is the most common fear of intimacy. Group members fear that if they become truly intimate with another, they will be exposed as unworthy, undeserving, or lacking. They fear that the other group members will discover that they are really inept. Avoidance of vulnerability will take many forms. Some group members will avoid intimacy by fact-seeking ("What do you exactly mean by warmth?") or fault-finding ("Thank you for your concern, but do you have to keep repeating it?"). Others will set unrealistic conditions for intimacy ("Could you say that more softly?") or take another's intimate statement away ("That reminds me of my friend at work and how he has the same difficulty."). Sometimes the group member will turn off another intimacy by anger ("You are here now, but where were you last week?").

The group leader's task is to help his or her group members work through each of their fears of intimacy. At first, the members of the group will be puzzled by the leader's efforts because it will be contrary to all that they have learned about physical survival. Their early experiences have taught them it is not safe to be intimate, close, and open with another. Do not expect them to discard their old, maladaptive ways of coping. They must come to learn that their fears as children were unrealistic, but their early ways of relating need not continue to color their experiences as adults. As Shakespeare wrote, "What we cannot throw away, we must embrace." Group members must be encouraged to face their fears. They must experience them and know them completely. They must learn that their fears are a signal based on their childhood expectations. Keep pointing out what they are doing and constantly call it to the other group members' attention. Show them and the other group members how their behavior is an attempt on their part to ward off the fear of intimacy.

Group members possess their own early form of intimacy fears. In the initial stages of group, they will continue to harbor childhood fears and fantasies about intimacy. As they begin to talk about their fears in group, their position against intimacy will begin to soften. They will learn that their fears are grounded in their early bonding difficulties with their parents. These fears will get played out in group and they will come to learn about more mature forms of intimacy. They will eventually come to realize that their childhood expectations about intimacy are unfounded. One common fear is that their needs are bottomless. They feel ashamed of their needs, and their neediness usually frightens them because their needs were never appropriately met as a child. They were taught that it was dangerous to expect anything from others. They no longer have to deny their needs because of fears that admitting them will leave them vulnerable. This is why they do not let others know their needs. They fear that if others know, they will be seen as needy and will be rejected. Other members will learn their fear of intimacy is related to their fear of indebtedness. If they take from others, they fear that they will be indebted and must give back to the others. If they give to other members, they fear it will be expected of them in the future and that giving comes at a personal price.

As these issues and fears are resolved in group, mature desires for intimacy will be experienced by each of the group members. Intimacy and closeness will carry a vital sense of experience for them, an experience that is not just a happening, but one that sustains. It will become embedded in their character and incorporated into their being. The group will come to share a common intimacy where the expression and experience of the full range of emotions will be permitted. The whole group is always alive during an intimate moment.

RESISTANCE TO IMMEDIACY

Resistance can take many forms and can be triggered by numerous circumstances, topics, conditions, and situations. As demonstrated by his focus on resistance to intimacy in groups, Louis Ormont (1993) is very much aware that most resistances occur in the immediacy of the here and now. As he correctly points out, not only is transference (which was dealt with at length in Chapter 13), an interpersonal event, but "all resistances in group are also transference resistances (ego transference, id transference, and so on)" (p. 400). Ormont suggests that all resistance to communication has to do with transference and that the group with its circle array of different members provides numerous transference objects. Resistance to communication because of the transference to the group leader, its individual members, and the group as a whole usually leads to a group that is stale and directionless. Ormont believes that "The art of group therapy lies very much in keeping groups alive and in the moment" (Personal communication, 1985). Effectively dealing with resistances therefore requires the group leader to actively identify these resistances as they occur within the immediacy of the group and help the group members to deal with them. From Ormont's perspective, there are three common forms of resistance that will manifest in group and they all have to do with the avoidance of the here and now:

1. Group members' tendency to talk in the past tense instead of the present.
2. Group members' inclination to dwell on the future.
3. Group members' preference to occupy the group with issues related to their outside lives.

Ormont believes that group therapy succeeds or fails to the degree that the group leaders keep group members actively engaged in meaningful communication in the immediacy of the here and now. The extent to which the group leader is aware and able to identify the source of the resistances determines whether these resistances will be resolved or worked through. In many cases, the promotion of self-awareness, identification, and the resolution of resistances are the goals of treatment. To make the unconscious conscious was one of Freud's early aims for psychoanalysis. He often defined the goal of treatment as "Where Id is, Ego shall be." There are few patient populations that this is more true for than it is for alcoholics and addicts. Addiction is often called a disease of denial. No resistance is more primitive and destructive than denial. Addicted individuals' denial is just not limited to their denial that they are dependent on alcohol or drugs, it is also a denial that they need others and are limited, emotionally vulnerable human beings. Working through the resistance that they are alcoholics or addicts is just the first step toward working through the resistance that they are frail, needy human beings who have intense feelings that often guide or push them in directions they do not understand or are unaware that they need. Spinoza captured this sentiment many years ago when he wrote, "To the degree we are out of touch with our emotions and to the extent these emotions drive and influence our actions, we are essentially in human bondage to these emotions" (cited in Durant, 1926, p. 201). Staying in the immediacy of the here and now will help evoke the feelings that lie dormant and repressed from individuals' conscious awareness, allowing the feelings to be brought up to consciousness and eventually mastered.

RESISTANCE TO FEELINGS IN GROUP

Group therapy must be a place where all feelings, anger as well as happiness, can be expressed. The full range of feelings must be presentable in group. However, there will be both individual and group resistance to the expression and recognition of feelings. Group leaders must deal with the group resistance first before they tackle the individual resistances in group. Resistance is diminished whenever the feelings stirred up in group are appropriately dealt with. However, when feelings are too powerful, unconscious, or disavowed, the group and its members can become stuck in Bion's basic assumptions. Every resistance in group can be traced to a feeling that was triggered by other members in the group. Group leaders must be able to trace the resistance to a place and time when the group stopped being effective. While the group and its members will often be aware of their resistance, their awareness is usually superficial and poorly integrated with the rest of their experience. It is the leader's task to bring to their awareness the unconscious feelings that led to their resistance. Fancher (1973) addresses this issue succinctly when he writes about Freud's early discoveries concerning resistance:

> Freud was forced to the conclusion that the most important part of the resistance was not the most obvious part. The conscious distress and disgust experienced by a patient was only the most superficial manifestation of his resistance. His deepest resistance was embodied in his transference neurosis, which was a replica of his real neurosis, and of which he was completely unconscious. This suggested to Freud that at the most significant level an individual is unaware of his own resistance and of the real nature of his conflicts. That is, he is as unconscious of the process of repression itself as he is of the content of his repressions. (pp. 200-201)

Dealing with resistance and the obstacles to feelings is one primary task of the group leader. The leader must get the group and its members to be aware of the ways in which they are resisting and blocking emotions. Since the group members do this to avoid pain and the unpleasantness of emotions, they must come to realize that there is no danger in feeling. They must come to recognize that their faulty maneuvers at protecting themselves are no longer necessary.

It is the alleviation of the disturbance of a person's emotional life that constitutes the primary function of psychotherapy. There are limits to what psychotherapy can or cannot do. The primary effectiveness of therapy is achieved within the realm of the many ways in which an individual's subjective emotional experiences interfere with his or her ability to function interpersonally and intellectually. In order to accomplish this task in group, the group leader must have access to group members' feelings. This requires that there be an activation of their feelings in group. Group members must come to experience the wide range of their emotions in group since feelings cannot be changed or learned about just by talking about them. They must be experienced and observed in group. There is always an element of risk involved in the activation of feelings. However, the group leader and the person experiencing the emotions never know exactly where the feelings will go. Since feelings are often contagious, there is no way to predict the emotional responses of the other group members to their interactions in group. This reflects the advantage as well as the disadvantage of emotional expression in group. It is this risk and the fear of the unpredictability of emotions that leads members to resist the expression of feelings.

Feelings do not usually occur in a vacuum. An activation from another is required to energize feelings. The group leader needs to know how to facilitate the experience of emotions without interfering with the group members' experience. If the group and its members are working, it is best for the group leader to be quiet. When the person or the group is stuck, this is when the group leader must activate responses from other group members. It is often the interaction between the group members that evokes affect.

The belief that a person must be engaged on a real emotional level in order to uncover repressed feelings is a relatively new belief reflecting a shift from the intrapsychic model to one based on interaction and object relations. Freud's old, analytic belief was that it was only necessary to focus on feelings and the reasons (defenses) why individuals blocked their feelings. Strict adherence to his model does not focus enough emphasis on feelings that are evoked in response to exchanges that occur within the interpersonal context. Feelings have an adaptive significance and always serve a problem-solving function. It is within the interpersonal exchanges in the group that the group leader will learn how each group member has adapted to the feelings that are evoked by intimacy or anger.

Mental health is determined by the interplay between the individual and his or her feelings. The ability to experience one's feelings without resisting or running from them determines to a large degree whether a person is healthy or ill. (See Figure 14.2.)

Illness is usually the result of individuals' blockage of their feelings. It is the unhealthy individuals who remain unconnected with their emotions and out of touch with their feelings. Contrary to the popular belief held by most group members, healthy individuals are the ones who can experience

FIGURE 14.2

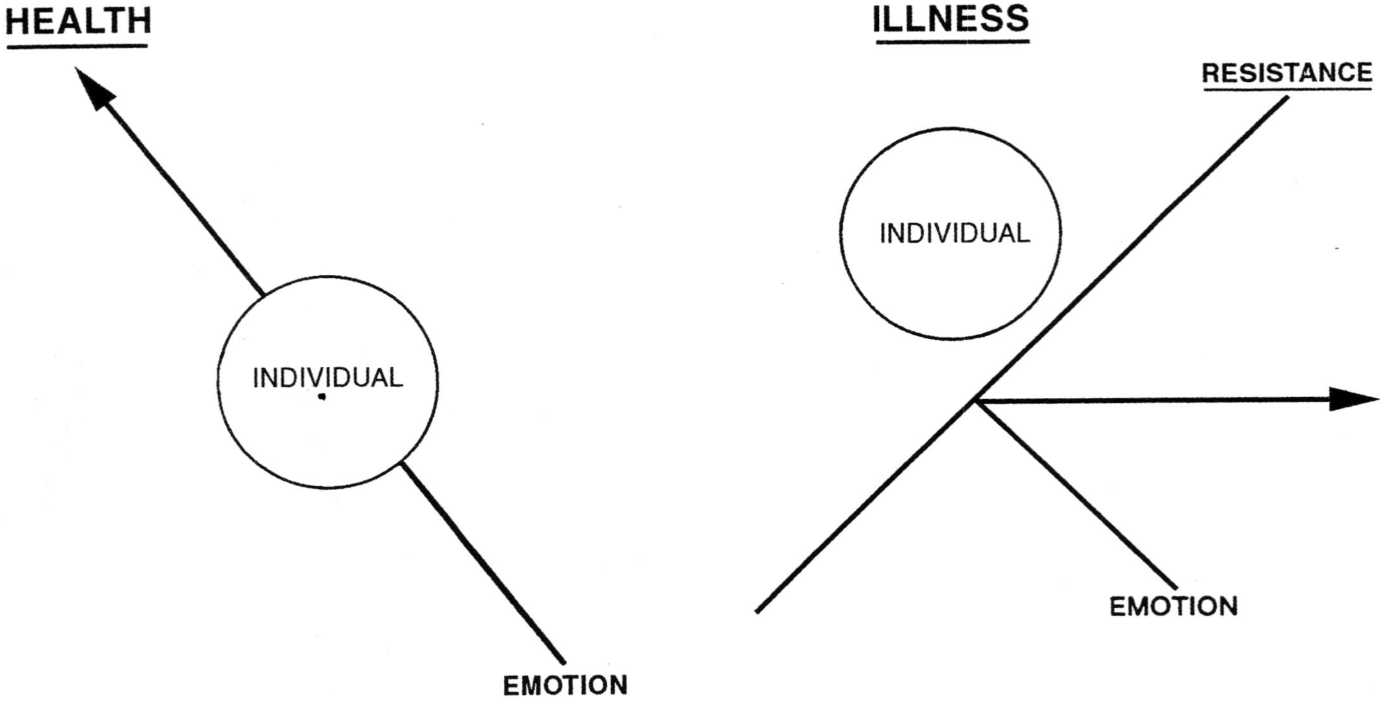

HEALTH
INDIVIDUAL
EMOTION
ILLNESS
RESISTANCE
INDIVIDUAL
EMOTION

their negative feelings, such as sadness, anger, envy, and anxiety. Many alcoholics and addicts erroneously attempt to reach an ideal state where they believe they will never have to experience negative emotions again. Alcohol and drugs temporarily confirm their illusion. However, the negative feelings that they fear and resist constantly push for expression. Resistance of negative feelings cannot be accomplished as selectively as the alcoholic and addict would like to believe. As negative feelings are denied and repressed, so are positive feelings. Group leaders must set the group in motion toward the expression of all repressed feelings. They must establish a climate in group of working toward health and away from illness.

It is when the group members direct their efforts toward the blocking and resistance of their feelings that problems arise. Healthy group members can explore their feelings and the reasons behind them. When anger is too frightening or pain too overwhelming, individual defenses become too rigid. Group members need the encouragement and the safety of the group before they will risk getting their impounded feelings out. Only after the feelings have been expressed can individuals come to a proper understanding of what has happened to them. Cognitive distortions will be eliminated and there will be a greater chance for reflection on the experience so that the present does not remain tied to or determined by the past. This requires feelings to come through to completion. If individuals are angry, it must be expressed. Once an emotion has been given its full expression, it will often be a freeing experience for the individuals. Ward (1984) expresses the importance of this principle when he speaks of the necessity of completing an experience before it can be understood. "After buying the sports car you always wanted, upon reflection, you will understand why it was so important for you to have it in the first place." Understanding the sequence of events that led to the expression of the anger or the purchase of the sports car will bring the experience to a close. An emotional expression not understood only leads to increased resistance of that emotion in the future.

The group leader will discover that some group members organize themselves to protect themselves against feelings. Spontaneity is resisted and rigidity is embraced. They become all form and no spirit. Conventionality rules their lives and this keeps them away from the spontaneous expression of anger and intimacy. Group members who are at ease in their interpersonal exchanges and comfortable with their emotional expressions are in good mental health.

Emotions can also interfere with individuals' intellectual functioning. Not only do they lose spontaneity in their intimate interactions, but they become rigid in their thinking and problem-solving. Actively explaining a problem to another involves putting their difficulty in some order and thus removes it far enough away from their emotional or mental set to free them from their stuck position. If individuals are frozen with anxiety and resistant to explore alternatives, they sometimes literally cannot think. They need the ability to shift mental sets. Individuals trapped into one mental set or emotional response can literally remain stuck. Ward (1984) gives an excellent example of such a condition:

> Company engineers had tried unsuccessfully for years to find the proper kind of solvent to dissolve the ink on newspapers so that the newspapers could be recycled for use at a savings of millions of dollars. Finally, distraught at their repeated failure, they sought the advice of an outside consultant. He rejected their initial requests to lead one of their research teams with the statement, "No, you have already thought about all the possible solvents. I doubt if I would be able to find a new one. Instead, let's look for an ink which will dissolve in one of the solvents you already have."

Rigid mental sets, as this illustration suggests, can freeze an individual's thinking process. Psychotherapy should be directed toward unfreezing and reframing a person's experience. Often just talking about a feeling will allow individuals to reorganize their conceptual understanding of the experience. Emotions can be like maps that freeze people in the center of their universe. As they get "the big picture," they will come to realize that their perception of the problem has exaggerated its magnitude. They will literally not be able to see the forest for the trees. Things that are closer to a person often look bigger than things that are far away. If individuals can put things in their proper historical and temporal arrangement, it will help reduce them to their proper size.

In interpersonal interactions, such as those that occur in group, members will evoke emotions in each other. The stronger the feelings produced, the more primitive the understanding of these emotions will be. If a person is very angry or hurt by another, it will seem as if the other did what he or she did only to anger or hurt the person. In childhood, everything is emotional. Through children's developmental process, they learn to better understand their emotions. Understanding helps reduce the intensity of the emotions and helps facilitate their proper expression. In group therapy, group members must learn the proper sequence of experiencing emotions and the understanding of their emotions. If they do not, they will either remain victims of their emotions or they will be emotionless. Understanding of feelings leads to less resistance to feelings and gives individuals the capacity to more fully express their feelings. This will allow them to modulate the appropriate expression of emotions rather than remain controlled by or out of touch with their feelings.

SPECIAL CONSIDERATIONS OF RESISTANCE TO ADDICTION

In the same way that chemical dependency impacts every aspect of a person's life, it will have a profound effect on treatment and group therapy. The group leader will often be presented with a set of treatment issues that are unique to this population. Resistance will take many different forms with the addict and alcoholic in group. Not only will group leaders have to deal with individual resistances and the typical resistances that occur with any therapy group, they also will have to find a way to effectively deal with the characterological defenses and acting out that is typically associated with this population. In an attempt to clarify the common resistance that addicts and alcoholics bring to group therapy, Marsha Vannicelli (1992) suggests that it is helpful to look at ways of "removing the roadblocks" by differentiating the resistances into three different categories:

1. Removing roadblocks or resistances in group.
2. Removing roadblocks or resistances with individuals in group.
3. Removing roadblocks or countertransference resistances in the group leader.

GROUP RESISTANCES

It is necessary to be able to distinguish group resistances from individual resistances. Sometimes it is difficult to discriminate between the two because they often interact with each other. As Vannicelli points out, what may appear at times to be an individual resistance may actually represent the group allowing or electing an individual member to "contain" some piece of resistance for the entire group. For instance, a group member may contain the feeling of fear of attack and judgment for the entire group. This may be voiced as the individual group member speaking to the issue of safety and trust in the group. If one of the group members voices this fear of attack and lack of a sense of safety or trust in the group, and if the group allows this one member to contain all of the group feelings on an individual level, the remaining group members can either spend their energies trying to convince the person it is safe or as is usually the case, they can attack the individual for distrusting them and "their group." What may appear as resistance on the individual's part may in this case actually represent resistance on the group's part to fail to deal realistically with an important stage of group development. Rather than deal with the ambiguity and uncertainty of life and all relationships, the group can retreat into a state of false cohesiveness where compliance is demanded and differences are not allowed. The group will, in effect, resist this healthy stage of development and instead will attack the deviant member for "not getting with the program."

Vannicelli, acknowledging the overlap among the three categories of resistances, suggests that it is helpful to look at group-as-a-whole resistance as falling into three categories:

1. *Distraction activities.* The group actively engages in one topic or issue as a way of avoiding a more important one, by focusing on outside-of-group crises, by joking around, or by engaging in patterned interactions.
2. *Avoidance defenses.* The group ignores painful material by acting as if it does not know what is going on, by behaving empathically, by clamming up (use of silence), by ignoring important self-disclosures, and by using other forms of flight.
3. *Displacement.* The group talks in a displaced way about the therapy group–for example, when the group talks about how much they hate their weekly meetings at work or particular A.A./Al-Anon meetings. (1992, p. 118)

INDIVIDUAL RESISTANCES

Even the most motivated and highly enthusiastic group member will manifest resistance. Resistance cannot be prevented and for the sake of recovery and progress in treatment, it should never be avoided. Dealing with resistance and in some cases, the resolution of it, is the source of the most vital and meaningful work that can happen in treatment. Unconscious wishes, fears, fantasies, ambivalence, and ingrained, habitual, characterological patterns all contribute to patients often behaving, acting, and even thinking in ways that are destructive and self-defeating. These actions and attitudes usually take place outside of their awareness and therefore are resistant to illumination and extinction. Only by bringing them sharply into a person's undeniable awareness can the individual have any chance to alter these habitual traits. Resistance must first be manifested and experienced if treatment is to progress.

One of the most potent and effective ways to permit resistance to manifest itself and be experienced is to provide the individual with something to push up against or resist. This is the purpose of the group contract. It is a set of groundrules, expectations, and working agreement that you expect the patient to violate. "The therapeutic contract sets a clear framework of expectations against which the deviations can be productively examined" (Vannicelli, 1992, p. 139). Ormont, as is usually the case, says the same thing more colorfully: "We give them these rules because we know they are going to break them. Then we ask them why and get them to look at and examine their reasons."

Every treatment program and therapy encounter has a set of expectations, assumptions, and working ground rules. The more explicit and clear this working contract is in the group, the better the treatment and the easier the tasks will be for the group leader. Because the contract defines the limits of the group leader's expectations and the individual's responsibilities, most of the important work in group will be directed toward managing the boundaries or the therapeutic frame of the group. Valuable information will be communicated by the group member who: (1) comes late; (2) doesn't come or call; (3) doesn't pay his or her bill; (4) avoids telling the meaningful stories of his or her life; (5) doesn't take an equal share of the talking time; (6) acts out sexually; (7) acts out with chemicals; (8) makes excessive outside contact with group members in the service of keeping secrets or forming subgroups; and (9) tries to form a special alliance with the group leader.

RESISTANCE IN THE GROUP LEADER

Resistance can also take many forms with the group leader. Many resistances on the part of group leaders have to do with their countertransference, which was dealt with more extensively in Chapter 13. However, it is important to comment here on the group leader who fails to hold up his or her end of the group contract. This requires that the group leader enforce the contract and actively inquire about absences, tardiness, acting out, fee payments, talking too much or too little, and the countless other boundary issues that need to be maintained in group.

As important as these issues are, they do not compare to the group leader who fails to address the most important issue that addicts and alcoholics must address in treatment–specifically, abstinence and their failure to stay chemically free. Failure to maintain that abstinence is the most crucial and primary requirement of treatment if a person is an addict or an alcoholic represents the most disturbing resistance a therapist can have when working with this population. It must be emphasized that not all heavy drinkers or heavy substance abusers are suffering from addictions, at least in the way that AA, NA, or CA define addiction. If the person meets the criteria for an addict or alcoholic as AA and other twelve-step programs describe addiction, he or she must remain abstinent. A therapist who concurs with the addict or alcoholic who believes that abstinence is an option and not a necessity, is engaging in the most troublesome and dangerous resistance that can present itself with this population.

THE GROUP LEADER'S EFFECT ON GROUP RESISTANCE

The importance of leadership style and the personality of the leader is often ignored in assessing resistance in group. As D. G. Brown (1985) stated, the basic assumption states that Bion wrote about "may owe their existence in a large part to the conditions imposed on the group by Bion, himself" (p. 192). Kernberg (1984) expressed similar sentiments when he asserted that both Bion's and Freud's explanations of group dynamics were observations determined to a large degree by their own influences upon the dynamics of the group. Kernberg goes on to state that there is a common and erroneously held belief that the leader has no quality that affects a group, an organization, or an institution. This is a result, Kernberg contends, of an organization's need to negate the personality of its leader. The point that Kernbergh wishes to make is that the leader cannot help but affect the group. More important, there are aspects of the leader that contribute and add to the resistance of the group.

While there are a number of treatment-destructive resistances that emerge in group, the attitude and the countertransference of the leader play a critical part in this resistance pattern. Many group members have been allowed to act out their tendencies in this direction because the group leader has either ignored their behavior or has only made half-hearted attempts at its resolution. Because the individual group member's resistance may evoke unacceptable feelings in the group leader, the group leader may try to circumvent his or her own anger, indifference, or anxiety instead of using it to confront the group member. Consequently, the group member's resistance never gets a chance to be completely aired and explored in group. The feeling behind the resistance remains shrouded in vagueness and denial and subsequently gets acted out by the group member. What is of critical importance is that once the resistance is sensed, it must be explored. Not to respond may contribute to the group member's destructive pattern and his or her eventual fleeing from treatment. Everything should take a back seat to resistance once it is observed. It must become the first order of business. There is never any therapeutic justification for postponing the confrontation of a treatment-destructive resistance. The group leader's primary objective must be to preserve the group and its existence for each of the group members.

While the group leader's countertransference issues may contribute to his or her reluctance to deal with individual resistances in group, there are specific characteristics of the leader that are certain to increase resistance in group:

1. Lack of empathy on the leader's part.
2. Failure to respond appropriately to group members at the right time.
3. Premature and incorrect interpretations to members of the group.
4. Hostile confrontation at an inappropriate time in group.

On the other hand, there are important qualities that group leaders must possess if they are going to minimize resistance in group. Group leaders must be:

1. Intelligent,
2. Honest and noncorruptible,
3. A little narcissistic,
4. A little paranoid.

If group leaders are not a little narcissistic, they will not possess the charisma and energy needed to keep a group viable and alive. If they are not a little paranoid, they will be easily fooled or misled by their group members. However, group leaders must have the ability to tone down their personality so as not to dominate the group and its members. They must be able, though, to use their personality and its effect on the group members to resolve resistances in group.

Resistance is never resolved if it is viewed as pathology. Focusing on it as pathology moves resistance from the realm of communication and puts it on the patient. Only when group leaders are able to ask themselves, "What is this patient communicating to me with his resistance?" will they be able to translate this back to the patient. This is what constitutes the essence of resolving resistance in treatment. Group leaders must first understand what the group member is conveying by his or her resistance and then they must explain it in a way that the group member will understand. Many group leaders have been taught that silence is neutral. Frequently, silence as neutrality is the therapist's intent. However, patients do not usually perceive silence as an act of neutrality. They perceive it as indifference or rejection. Just because group leaders care, they cannot expect their group members to know they care or that they are benevolent and listening unless they convey this information back to group members in a way they can understand.

The aim of psychotherapy is to experience what the patient experiences and convey this understanding back to them. If individuals are not understood, they will withdraw even farther. Group members must be given the power to agree, disagree, or change what the leader thinks he or she hears. If group members do not feel they have the right to correct the leader's comments, they will resist sharing more information. The curative process emerges out of the communication between the group members and their leader. Three things must occur if resistance is to be minimized and resolved:

1. Group members must feel safe enough to allow repressed material into their awareness.
2. The expressed feelings associated with this material must be accepted by the group leader and its members.
3. This material must be integrated into each group member's personality.

All individuals have a desire to experience a continuity in their lives. A sense of safety is crucial for the sharing of repressed or disavowed aspects of the self with others in a group setting. If this can be accomplished in group, the members will give way to their powerful needs to be understood and accepted as real by others. Empathic understanding and acceptance helps restore meaning and continuity to their lives. Empathic connections with others in group increase deeper introspection. Feeling understood by another as an adult is experienced by them in the same way that a child experiences being held. It firms up the person's sense of self. It is the consolidation of the self that leads to the capacity to change and diminishes the need to be resistant. There will no longer be a need for old defensive operations as the person feels more understood. If group leaders can avoid the pitfalls of focusing on resistance as defensive pathology, and instead focus on the reasons why the resistances have emerged, they will enhance the effectiveness of their group and the health of its members.

Chapter 15

The Curative Process in Group Therapy

Heinz Kohut (1984), in a book published after his death, asked the important question, How does analysis cure? While Kohut responded to this question from a self-psychology perspective, his answer needs to be extended because his formula does not take into consideration the special curative forces that exist in group therapy. Psychological cure is both a process and an event that is influenced by many different factors. Group therapy differs from individual therapy in that the circumstances influencing its occurrence are unique to group. However, as an event or goal, cure remains very similar for both individual and group therapy. Cure, from Kohut's perspective, is accomplished when a person can develop healthy object relationships. By this, he means that a psychologically healthy individual is one who possesses the capacity to engage in healthy interpersonal relationships with other healthy individuals. Interpersonal distortions, manipulations, pathological dependency, and unrealistic expectancies are all minimized. Most important, individuals who have obtained a healthy respect for themselves will be drawn to and choose others who are as healthy as they are. Kohut is operating on the principle that sick people attract sick people and healthy people are drawn to healthy people. Kohut is therefore suggesting that a person who is "cured" in therapy is one who develops the ability to pick and choose better friends, lovers, and partners. Kohut challenges the erroneous belief that healthy or "cured" people no longer need others and that they can operate completely independently of others' opinions, actions, or confirmations. Mental health, for Kohut, is not so much determined by complete autonomy from others as it is determined by individuals' ability to trade archaic and childish ways of getting their needs met for more mature ways of obtaining gratification in their adult relationships. As Kohut writes,

> Self-psychology holds that self-object relationships form the essence of psychological life from birth to death, that a move from depen-

> dence (symbiosis) to independence (autonomy) in the psychological sphere is no more possible, let alone desirable, than a corresponding move from a life dependent on oxygen to a life independent of it in the biological sphere. The developments that characterized normal psychological life must, in our view, be seen in the changing nature of the relationship between the self and its self-objects, but not in the self's relinquishment of self-objects. In particular, developmental advances cannot be understood in terms of the replacement of the self-objects by love-objects or as steps in the move from narcissism to object love. (1984, p. 47)

If one agrees with Kohut's description about the nature of cure and the definition of mental health, how is this to be obtained in group therapy? Kohut defines this process in individual therapy as being accomplished by the laying down of psychological structure. Kohut asks the question, "How does this accretion of psychological structure take place?" (1984, p. 98). He then answers his own question from a self-psychology perspective. Psychological structure is laid down (1) via optimal frustration and (2) in consequence of optimal frustration, via transmuting internalization (see Chapter 6). Cure is obtained when individuals, through a good-enough relationship with an appropriate mirroring and caring other, learn how to honor, accept, and take care of themselves while not allowing themselves to be treated with disrespect, harm, or injustice.

Group therapy parallels Kohut's description of cure in that it helps lay down psychic structure. The question that remains to be answered is how group therapy helps the individual obtain a firm sense of self through optimal frustration via transmuting internalization. Kohut is suggesting a firm sense of self is established as the group members work through their individual differences in group and learn more adaptive ways of resolving interpersonal and intrapersonal conflicts. The group enhances this process because it supplies each member with a source of support, identification, and acceptance while at the same time giving each individual a set of healthy values that can be internalized and incorporated. Eventually, each member's substitution of the group's healthy norms for the individual's destructive norms is reinforced by the group until these values become part of the individual's psychic structure.

Properly understanding how cure is obtained in a therapy group involves the investigation of two related, but distinctly different aspects of the curative forces operating in group. First, there are the identified curative factors that enhance a person's move from pathological behavior to psychological health. There is also a curative process in group that moves the individual through progressive and separate stages of increasing health, cure, and recovery. Yalom (1985) has done extensive research in identifying the curative factors in group and Rutan and Stone (1984) have done a comprehensive analysis of the curative process that exists in group. Each of their respective positions will be described in relation to Kohut's formula for the attainment of a healthy, cohesive self.

YALOM'S CURATIVE FACTORS

Cure for Yalom is an enormously complex process that "occurs through an intricate interplay of various guided human experiences" (1995, p. 1) that he refers to as curative factors. This complex process of cure is intricately tied up with what Yalom comes to identify as therapeutic change. Cure cannot be achieved unless a group member changes. To accomplish therapeutic change, the group leader must develop strategies and tactics that will enhance the curative process.

The effectiveness of a therapy group has been evaluated extensively by Yalom (1995). He has gained valuable information by asking group members and group leaders to identify qualities that they found helpful in a therapy group. While Yalom acknowledges that the process of cure in a therapy group is an intricate one and that different people in group respond differently to the many varying influences of group, he feels that even at the risk of oversimplifying these complicated processes, much can be gained by attempting to identify and categorize these varying curative factors. Numerous studies (Yalom, 1985) have been conducted over the years in an attempt to identify the order of importance of these curative forces. In most of the studies, group members have been asked to rank statements describing twelve potential helpful attributes of their group experience from most to least helpful. The twelve curative factors are summarized in Table 15.1.

To help understand the implications that these curative factors have on an alcoholic's and addict's recovery, each will be explored in relation to the special circumstances that are created when the addicted patient is treated in a therapy group.

CURATIVE FACTORS IN GROUP

Cohesiveness

Group cohesiveness is more likely to be an important factor with alcoholics than with non-alcoholics because of the dependency conflicts typi-

TABLE 15.1. Curative Factors Operating in Psychotherapy Group

1. *Altruism.* The feeling that a member is helping others and is important in their lives. Patients forget themselves momentarily, at least, and focus on helping others. People need to feel they are needed.
2. *Catharsis.* Expressing negative and positive feelings toward other members and the group leader. Acceptance for openness and personal change as a result of trying out new behavior begins to emerge. Feelings are no longer held inside. The process of learning how to express one's feelings emerges.
3. *Existential Factors.* Individuals learn there are limits in the world and that they alone are responsible for their life.
4. *Group Cohesiveness.* Emotional sharing and acceptance. A feeling of belonging and approval, with a feeling of warmth and closeness. There is mutual support and then heightened self-esteem. A sense of "we-ness" is established. This is a precondition for effective therapy.
5. *Guidance.* The imparting of information (i.e., "Why don't you try this?"; advice giving). Early stage group.
6. *Identification.* Individuals learn vicariously by listening and watching others in group.
7. *Instillation of Hope.* Seeing others getting better, knowing that the group has helped others gives members faith in the treatment mode. The expectation of effectiveness is established.
8. *Interpersonal Input.* Seeing how one relates to others and how others relate to oneself and then working on achieving more satisfying interpersonal relationships.
9. *Interpersonal Output.* Patients express feelings openly, and the group is supportive. The group allows patients to examine an incident with the consensual validation from others.
10. *Insight.* Patients gain a more objective perspective regarding interpersonal behavior. Patients gain some understanding into *what* they are doing to and with other people. There is an understanding as to why.
11. *Recapitulation of the Primary Family.* The group resembles the family in many aspects. Unresolved family issues are recapitulated and corrected.
12. *Universality.* Feeling that one is not that different from others. "We're all in the same boat." As common denominators emerge, *support* occurs.

cally associated with alcoholism. As Brown and Yalom (1977) suggest, cohesiveness is not in itself a curative factor but is instead a necessary precondition for effective therapy. Brown and Yalom have shown that, early in the life of the group, the issue of drinking serves as a unifying theme and members are often held together by this common bond until other sources of cohesion develop. It is essential that the therapist take advantage of this bond. Later, as Yalom showed, it is possible to differentiate each patient by examining with the group the different defensive functions each person's drinking has played in his or her life. The support and reinforcement of the group can serve as a powerful incentive for the primary goal of sobriety. Interpersonal and intrapersonal changes can be facilitated after a supportive and caring atmosphere has been established.

Universality

Considering the evidence for a post-alcoholic personality, the concept of universality is even more curative for alcoholics than for non-alcoholics. Brown and Yalom (1977) found that alcoholics generally had difficulty in distinguishing between thought and action; many would respond to fantasies with the same guilt and fear that would accompany actual behavior. While this eliminates fantasy work as a therapeutic option in group, it does indicate the importance that universality can play in quieting the alcoholics' thoughts that they are unique in their wretchedness. This sense of uniqueness is heightened for alcoholics by their social isolation and the guilt feelings associated with their drinking behavior. The phenomenon that Yalom describes as a process of "being welcomed back" to the human race results from sharing similar concerns and experiences and is an important curative factor in the early stages of alcoholics' recovery. Often, for the first time in their life, alcoholics will realize that they are not alone with their own personal and unique hell. The understanding that there are others who share their plight can serve as a powerful incentive to recovery, forgiveness, and acceptance of self.

Instillation of Hope

Group members often remark at the end of therapy how important it was for them to have observed the improvement of others (Yalom, 1985). A group therapist should by no means be above exploiting this factor by periodically calling attention to the improvement that members have shown. As a matter of fact, one of the great strengths of Alcoholics Anonymous is that each recovering alcoholic is a living inspiration to others. It is more than a mere coincidence that AA meetings involve members telling of their downfall and salvation.

Equally important is the fact that, at the beginning of therapy, alcoholics are usually in a crisis. They have attempted to control their drinking numerous times in the past and have failed. This, plus the dependency and passivity characteristics typical of alcoholic patients, requires that therapists be directive and convey the message that they know they can be of help. In fact, it may often be beneficial to state openly that, if the patient chooses to follow the recommendations of both AA and the therapist, chances are excellent that the client will remain sober and be abstinent at the end of treatment two years later. This is especially important considering that 90 percent of relapses occur during the first year of sobriety (Chalmers and Wallace, 1978).

Imparting of Information

The imparting of information is generally not highly valued as a curative mode in most therapy groups (Yalom, 1985). However, this situation is probably reversed in alcoholism treatment. If not highly valued, it is at least very important that the array of information about alcoholism be conveyed to recovering alcoholics. The disease concept, tolerance, physiological complications, and the addiction process are all simple but crucial matters of which all alcoholics should be aware. Alcoholics who come to construe their alcoholism as a physiological disorder complicated by psychological, sociological, and cultural factors show the best chances of recovery (Wallace, 1978b).

In the early stages of sobriety, because guilt is counterproductive to both treatment and the acceptance of the disease concept of alcoholism, patients should not be encouraged to delve deeply (beyond superficial drinking experiences) into prior life problems. Therapy time should be spent, instead, on the imparting of information on what alcoholism is and how to avoid drinking. This fulfills alcoholics' need for structure and direction while at the same time helping them to interpret their alcoholic behavior within the confines of what Wallace and Yalom respectively call the "exotic belief" and "vital lies." Fehr (1976) agrees that, in the early stages of treatment, when the therapist works individually with each patient, interaction between members of the group should be limited. This beginning part of therapy is described as the diagnostic-teaching phase wherein the patient explores those problems contributing to and associated with excessive alcohol consumption. In this process, alcoholics can learn how to become agents for themselves and other group members. Thus, in the early stages of treatment, the group therapy time is utilized more efficiently in individual diagnostic work with each patient.

Existential Factors

Yalom (1975) emphasizes a crucial principle for interpersonal change: "This principle–that change is preceded by a state of dissonance or incongruity–has considerable clinical and social psychological research backing" (p. 263). This is especially true for alcoholics, who, through their excessive drinking, have created a deep rift between their sober values and their alcoholic behavior. Unlike the typical neurotic patient, alcoholics have experienced "a stay in their own personal underworld, an experience which AA members refer to as hitting bottom. Some alcoholics emerge from this experience with an increased degree of integration. Many do not, however" (Brown and Yalom, 1977, p. 447).

Hitting bottom has a dual meaning for therapy; it is at once an impediment and a potentially invaluable reference point. An urgent experience (or in Jaspers' phrase, a "boundary situation") can, if properly integrated, lead to growth (Jaspers, 1975). "As patients face their limits, their symbolic deaths, they are often able to make some massive shifts in their life perspective. They may rearrange their priority of needs and trivialize the trivia in life" (Brown and Yalom, 1977, p. 448).

It is Yalom's experience that neurotics in therapy frequently avoid religious and existential factors in group, even though they are of great concern to them. Yalom feels that therapy groups with neurotics often tend to water down the tragedy of life, but that members who plunge deeply into themselves, who confront their fate most openly and resolutely, pass into a mode of existence that is richer than prior to their illness. Never is this more applicable than with alcoholic patients, who recognize and share a common theme that is widely addressed by the AA philosophy (Alcoholics Anonymous, 1955). The development of authenticity of character after being pushed to the edge of the psychic abyss is a theme that is also expressed by the most popular existential writers (Buber, 1960; Camus, 1960; Heidegger, 1963; Sartre, 1956). Yalom agrees with Camus when he expresses the idea that no human beings consider their life with absolute seriousness until they come fully to terms with their power to end it.

Such themes as suicide, hitting bottom, and the tragedy of life are far more meaningful in alcoholic groups than they normally are in non-alcoholic groups. The therapist, if he or she is to help patients integrate their experience in a healthy fashion, must not be frightened away by the patients' dread, but must gently and repeatedly lead the alcoholics back to their experience. "Any horror revisited long enough becomes detoxicated" (Brown and Yalom, 1977, p. 477).

Altruism

Although the alcoholic's behavior while drinking may suggest otherwise, alcoholics do not like interpersonal conflict, nor do they handle it well. They will support each other emotionally in group, and if they sense that another is experiencing too much discomfort, they will rescue that person, often interfering with important and necessary therapeutic catharsis. The therapist will soon discover that alcoholics do best in relationships characterized by complementary rather than competitive interactions. Brown and Yalom describe the alcoholics in their study as unusually conscientious and, rather than happy-go-lucky, "they were exceedingly prone to assume blame and guilt for dysphoric events in the group or distress suffered by others" (p. 450). These patients were inordinately cautious and generally experienced a deep sense of responsibility for others. Above all they avoided any behavior that might cause pain to another. This deep feeling of caring and support, evident in alcoholic groups, can be a powerful therapeutic asset. Yalom explained that this hypervigilance resulted in a constant surveying for signs of disturbance; group members would frequently submerge their own needs in an effort to be helpful to others. It was evident to Yalom that this was part of a deeper and shared character structure common to all the subjects in his study.

Identification, Interpersonal Input and Output

Through interaction with the therapist and the group, the alcoholic will often learn for the first time how to relate with others in a meaningful and sober manner. Usually all socializing in the past was either influenced by or a product of alcoholic consumption. For some individuals lacking intimate relationships, the group can represent the first opportunity for accurate interpersonal feedback. The alcoholic's general feeling of separateness and isolation must give way to the feeling of being a part of, and in some kind of harmony with, what is going on around him or her. In many cases, the group can fulfill the need quite adequately.

Catharsis

As Yalom illustrates, the intensity of the emotional expression is highly relativistic. Consequently, the expression of emotion must be appreciated from the perspective of the individual. For an alcoholic or addict, seemingly muted expression of emotion may represent an event of considerable intensity. Contrary to what many people think, alcoholics and addicts do not handle the expression of emotion well. They are usually incapable of modulating the expression of their own feelings. Part of this problem is related to the fact that alcoholics and addicts have usually had poor and inadequate models for the appropriate demonstration of affect. Alcoholics and addicts are usually adept at the suppression of uncomfortable feelings and frequently keep the recognition of the true affective state far from their conscious awareness. An often unrecognized fear is that once they start to express emotion, they will either be overwhelmed or explosive. However, if alcoholics or addicts do not get in touch with their feelings and if they fail to learn to master these impulses, treatment is likely to be impaired. Consequently, group therapists must constantly monitor their group and guide them between what Wallace cautions as too little emotional expression and too much emotional expression. The basic task of group therapists, therefore, involves the choosing of a safe course between two equally hazardous alternatives. It is important to lessen denial and encourage increased self-awareness and the affective arousal associated with self-disclosure while simultaneously keeping anxiety at a minimal level (Wallace, 1978b). This means that group therapists must be content with the gradual deepening of self-disclosure rather than demanding dramatic breakthroughs.

Unlike neurotics, whose defenses are usually inadequate, alcoholics and addicts are adept at keeping troublesome feelings out of their awareness. However, if a group therapist pushes an alcoholic or addict to feel and express his or her emotions too quickly, the consequence is usually an overwhelming flooding of emotions. During the early stages of recovery, such an occurrence must be avoided. It is this author's experience that many of the early and premature cathartic experiences in group often have long-term detrimental results. While it is often self-satisfying for the therapist to get past the defenses of alcoholics and addicts so that they get in touch with feelings that have been long buried, the usual result is individuals avoiding treatment. Therefore, the work of a group therapist with this population is what many psychodynamics theorists refer to as the building of ego strength.

As Erv and Miriam Polster (1973) write, an individual's defenses are there for a reason and the defenses must not be stripped away too quickly. Wallace agrees and points out that "denial is there for a purpose, it is the glue that holds an already shattered self-esteem system together. And it is a tactic through which otherwise overwhelming anxiety can be contained"

(Wallace, 1977, p. 15). On the other hand, as Yalom writes, there is little chance that permanent change will occur unless there is an affective arousal state accompanying the self-understanding. Self-understanding by itself only feeds the alcoholic's and addict's defensive system and makes treatment more difficult. The consequence of insight without catharsis is an alcoholic or addict who can tell you all the reasons why he or she drinks and does drugs while at the same time continuing to drink and do drugs. Certainly, alcoholics and addicts need little help in that area of their recovery.

Family Reenactment

As Yalom illustrates, and research addressing the importance of different cultural factors substantiates, the recapitulation of the primary family experience is usually not ranked as helpful by group members. However, as Yalom points out, only successful encounter groups' members cited this factor as important. Yalom thus implies that the issue of family reenactment is important even though group members may not identify it as such. I believe this is also true with addictive patients in group. One of the best predictors of alcoholism is the kind of home alcoholics come from. A broken home is the background for 40 percent of alcoholics, and 40 percent (some overlapping) report problem drinking in at least one parent (Ray, 1972). Group therapy therefore allows group members to understand their own attitudes and defenses about drinking by observing those same attitudes and defenses in others who are struggling with similar problems.

However, as Yalom suggests, even though the specter of early family experiences often haunts the members of the group, it is generally unproductive to focus explicitly on this subject. Rather, the shift in perspective about the past and the understanding of the influence of the early family experience will occur because of the vitality of the work that the alcoholic or addict does in the present. Change is less likely to occur through a direct inquiry into the experiences with the family in the past. Talking about the parents in the past can also become a defense against exploring the feelings and issues that the members have toward each other and their current struggles to remain abstinent from alcohol and drugs. Addicts and alcoholics are usually adept at "playing the psychotherapy game" and discover early that this is a topic that professionals usually love to "jump on because it is such a hot item." Consequently, focusing directly on the parental influences and experiences often leads to a discussion that only feeds the alcoholic's and addict's defensive system and impedes productive group work in the present.

Self-Understanding

Yalom criticizes the naive and popular conceptualization that views psychotherapy as a "detective search. . . . a digging or a stripping away" of defenses until individuals discover and identify the true negative aspects of themselves. Self-understanding, as it was ranked in importance by group members in Yalom's original study, referred instead to self-understanding as "discovery and accepting previously unknown or unacceptable parts of myself" (Yalom, 1975, p. 92). Therefore, self-understanding as it is intended here, refers to group members discovering previously unknown and unidentified positive aspect of themselves. Group therapy with alcoholics and addicts must be run on this principle. Because addicted individuals generally possess such strong feelings of shame, embarrassment, and self-loathing, it is extremely curative when they learn that they can be viewed by others in a positive manner. As Kurtz (1982) writes, the alcoholic suffers from deep feelings of shame. In fact, Kurtz views Alcoholics Anonymous as a program for the treatment of shame. While most contemporary forms of Western-based psychotherapy are directed toward the treatment of guilt, Alcoholics Anonymous directs its healing toward a more primitive emotional arrestment. Guilt, according to Kurtz, implies, "I feel bad for something I have done." Shame, a more profound feeling all alcoholics and addicts struggle with, implies, "I feel bad because of what I am." Addiction from this viewpoint implies that group therapy must enhance the self-understanding and the acceptance that one is worthwhile despite one's strong feelings of self-loathing. As Kurtz suggests, the healing of shame requires more than talking about shame. It requires that alcoholics and addicts identify feelings of self-loathing in others and eventually accept the others who are feeling what the alcoholic and addict feels. This principle–before individuals can be healed, they have to know they can heal another–is what Searles (1973) identifies as the "therapeutic symbiosis." While Searles was referring to the therapist in his description, this principle also applies to group members. It is this opportunity to learn that one has the ability to act as a healer to help another that supports the use of group psychotherapy. In fact, this is the very same principle that AA applies within the twelfth step of its twelve-step program for recovery. Alcoholics and addicts maintain their own sobriety by helping another alcoholic or addict become sober.

CURATIVE FACTORS IN AA

It is important to remember that Yalom's curative factors operate not only in therapy groups, but in AA as well. While the conditions for change and the therapeutic mechanisms of change may differ in each group, the process of cure is similar, even though each may place more emphasis or value on different curative factors. Emrick, Lassen, and Edwards (1977) investigated this possibility and searched through the literature on AA for direct or indirect reference to Yalom's twelve curative factors. Their research showed that ten of Yalom's twelve curative factors were operating in AA groups. Table 15.2 lists their findings and the ranked order of importance of each curative factor.

As Emrick, Lassen, and Edwards (1977) concluded, "If the factors more frequently mentioned play more central roles in AA, then the composition for and mechanisms of change operating in AA is reflected in the ranking of the factors" (p. 130). Comparing these rankings with those of Yalom (1985), Emrick and colleagues hypothesized that AA groups were different in the centrality and importance of these curative factors. Apparently, AA groups place more emphasis on guidance, identification, and instillation of hope, while professional group therapy relies more on interpersonal learning, catharsis, insight, and existential awareness. In order to determine the degree of similarity between the two, Emrick, Lassen, and Edwards (1977) felt it would be valuable to explore this comparison by randomly assigning alcoholics to psychotherapy groups and AA groups and later administering Yalom's instrument for measuring members' perceptions of the curative factors. Further, it may be important to explore the possible matching and differentiation of treatment effects based on the personality characteristics that Emrick et al. (1977) have identified as being differentially suited either to AA or to professional care. They maintain that

> clients appropriate for AA seem to be those who are responsive to peers, drawn towards a spiritually oriented approach, comfortable talking about their alcoholism in front of large groups and enjoy socializing with reformed alcoholics. Uniquely suited for professional care seem to be those alcoholics who . . . are responsive to professionals, are strongly invested in introspection, view alcoholism as a psychological problem, wish to talk at most to a few people . . . . (p. 138)

CURATIVE FACTORS OPERATING IN DIFFERENT TYPES OF THERAPY GROUPS

Kanas and Barr (1982) sought to answer the question of how an outpatient therapy group for alcoholics might differ from therapy groups with

TABLE 15.2. Frequency of Publications (N=26) Referring to Curative Factors Operative in AA Groups

Curative Factor	Number of Publications
Altruism	21
Group cohesiveness	20
Identification	14
Instillation of hope	12
Guidance	12
Universality	10
Catharsis	8
"Insight"	6
Interpersonal learning, "output"	2
Family reenactment	1
Interpersonal learning, "input"	0
Existential awareness	0

Source: Emerick, Lassen, and Edwards (1977)

alcoholic inpatients. They also compared the rankings of these curative factors with non-alcoholic outpatients and inpatients. Table 15.3 lists the results of their study.

Tables 15.2 and 15.3 reveal the importance of cohesion in a therapy group. Although none of the individual studies specifically ranked cohesiveness as the number one curative factor, a composite rank of the individual curative factors reveals the universal importance of cohesion in groups. As Yalom repeatedly states, "Group cohesiveness is the *sine qua non* of effective long-term group therapy, and the effective group therapist must direct his or her efforts towards maximal development of these therapeutic resources" (1985, p. 111). In describing the curative factors that exist in groups, Yalom draws the distinction between those curative factors that are mechanisms of change and those curative factors that are conditions for change. The importance of the attainment of cohesion in group cannot be overstated. Repeated studies and Yalom's own clinical opinion continually point to the necessity of first establishing an atmosphere of safety and trust before the group's curative forces can be activated. While cohesiveness itself may not be more important than any of the other curative factors, it is an essential condition that allows the other mechanisms of change and cure to be set in motion.

MECHANISMS OF CHANGE AND CURE IN GROUP THERAPY

Yalom's interactional group therapy model provides group leaders with a unique opportunity to assess their group members' capacity to engage in healthy or destructive interpersonal relationships. In light of Kohut's description of cure given earlier in this chapter, it is vitally important that the interpersonal and intrapersonal distortions possessed by group members be modified if they are to attain psychological health. This is important for two reasons. First, as Carl Rogers, Heinz Kohut, and other object-relations theorists have emphasized, having the potential to engage in healthy, authentic human relationships is in itself a powerful, ongoing curative process. Second, people generally treat and relate to others as they treat and relate to themselves. For instance, critical, punishing people are usually critical and punishing of themselves. Forgiving, caring, and honest people are more likely to treat themselves in a similar manner. External exchanges with others are usually clear representations of a person's internal reality. There are a variety of windows into the world of the unconscious. Transference, free associations, slips of the tongue, body language, character

TABLE 15.3. Group Therapy Curative Factors in Different Populations

Study	Yalom (1975)	Maxmen (1973)	Feeney and Dranger (1976)	Kanas and Barr (1981)	
Population	20 psychiatric outpatients	100 psychiatric inpatients	20 alcoholic inpatients	8 alcoholic outpatients	
# Hourly sessions	64 (approx.)	9	35 (approx.)	36.8	
Mean duration	16 months	18 days	49 days	25.9 weeks	
Ranking method	Q-sort	Questionnaire	Q-sort	Questionnaire	
Ranking order					Composite Ranks
Interpersonal input	1	5	3	7	3.7 (2)
Catharsis	2	8	1	6	5.7 (6)
Group cohesiveness	3	2	4	3	3.0 (1)
Insight	4	9	2	8	5.7 (6)
Interpersonal output	5	7	7	4	5.0 (5)
Existential factors	6	6	6	9	4.2 (4)
Universality	7	4	8	5	4.0 (3)
Instillation of hope	8	1	5	1	5.7 (6)
Altruism	9	3	9	2	6.7 (7)
Family reenactment	10	11	10	11	10.4 (10)
Guidance	11	10	11	10	11.0 (11)
Identification	12	12	12	12	12.0 (12)

Source: Kanas and Barr (1982)

styles, dreams, compulsions, and resistances are other ways of getting through to a person's internal world. Watching a person's object-relations and interpersonal exchanges with other members in the group is just another excellent avenue for understanding the individual's internal unconscious process.

Group leaders working in the Sullivanian, Rogerian, or object-relations tradition stress here and now relationships and the corrective emotional experience over classical insight as major curative forces. As Rutan and Stone write, "In group therapy the presence of a network of human relationships, rather than just the single relationship to the analyst, increases the opportunities for multiple experiences that can produce change" (1984, p. 53).

Rutan and Stone also state that in order to achieve the structural changes needed in rebuilding a person's fragmented or flawed ego, a safe, trusting, and cohesive atmosphere must first be established in group. They also feel that an unintrusive group leader is required if the group members are going to let down their defenses long enough to allow their parataxic distortions and fragmented selves emerge so that they can ultimately be examined and altered.

Rutan and Stone outline the three mechanisms of change that are required if people are to be cured in group. These mechanisms are:

1. Imitation
2. Identification
3. Internalization

Imitation

As members of a group watch others benefit from the open sharing and expression of emotions, they will be encouraged to do the same because of their desire to gain symptom relief and their need to belong and be accepted by others in the group. Rutan and Stone write:

> In therapy groups individuals have the opportunity to observe many interactions, styles of relating, and problem-solving techniques. Much of the early learning in groups is imitative. Patients who have difficulty tolerating and sharing strong emotions can first observe as other members interact intensely. As they learn that members are not harmed, but rather are typically drawn closer by such exchanges, such patients see some hope for change and, as a consequence, can begin to share feelings by imitating those who are more successful in that task. Though primarily used early in group mem-

> bership, imitation remains one of the ways in which members gain new behavioral options throughout their treatment. The successes following imitative behavior make the group more attractive, enhance a wish to belong, and increase cohesiveness. This furthers identifications among the members. The use of imitation is both a result of feeling that others have been successful and a means of discovering alternative ways of thinking, expressing, or behaving. It is by no means limited to group therapy; but group therapy, by virtue of the multiple interactions and relationships, expands the opportunities for change through imitative learning. (1984, p. 54)

Identification

Identification has long been a favorite theoretical mechanism to explain how children develop broad attributes and generalized behavior patterns similar to those of their parents. Classically, identification is the unconscious process through which individuals come to emulate or model another whom they admire, respect, or wish to be like. As the members in the therapy group and the group itself become cohesive and attractive, this furthers identifications among the members. Rutan and Stone described the importance of this process in stimulating the curative forces in group:

> Identifications arise not only from the content of the memories, associations, and feelings, but with the process of telling about them as well. Consciously these identifications may be expressed as feelings of attraction, belonging, and attachment to the members and the group. These are the building blocks from which group cohesiveness develops. Similarly, universalization, the development of the sense that one is not alone in his or her feelings, furthers group attraction and identifications among members. A circular process begins that enhances these powerful influences members have upon one another. In turn the resultant identifications alter fundamental ways in which the members perceive and respond. The incremental building of identifications forms the base for lasting change. (1984, p. 56)

Internalization

The third and final stage of change and cure culminates in the group members internalizing the values, norms, and behavior of other members in the group. This signals a true independent move to psychological health and cure. Group members no longer have to rely on more primitive external sources of identification or imitation to produce change in themselves. Through the resolution of conflicts and continual examination of emotional interactions in group, psychic structure has been slowly and methodically laid. Rutan and Stone summarized the importance of this change:

> Internalization produces greater flexibility in handling both internal and interactive states and is the result of working through conflicts or building new psychic structure to handle previously disruptive anxiety. The therapist can facilitate healthy internalization by detailed examination and reexamination of emotionally laden interactions. Through identification, clarification, and interpretation, individuals integrate knowledge gained in the here-and-now transactions with their sources and prior assumptions. This results in an increased integration of affects and object relationships as well as diminished inner conflict. The outcome can be observed in the therapy setting where a patient might indicate a new way of behaving to recurrent stimuli. (1984, p. 57)

The mechanisms of change that Rutan and Stone described as occurring in group are also active in AA. As alcoholics proceed through the initial stages of their recovery, they begin with the first stage in which they imitate the behavior of other alcoholics by stating "I can't drink." Attending numerous AA meetings, newly recovering alcoholics realize that if they are to stay sober, they must imitate the behavior of their fellow AA members. This is the initial stage where a great deal of external control is necessary (i.e., hospitalization, detoxification, Antabuse, etc.). At this stage, alcoholics need protection against their own impulses to drink. The second phase is what Wallace (1978b) calls the "I won't drink" stage and alcoholics now identify with their fellow AA members. Their desire to remain abstinent is not determined by external pressures, but more by their own desire to remain sober and active in AA. The third and final stage is the stage of internalization, which Wallace calls the "I don't have to drink" stage. Conflict resolution is obtained. Alcoholics have successfully worked the twelve steps of the AA program and have obtained a high degree of serenity in their recovery. While the danger of a relapse is never completely eradicated in any alcoholic, the alcoholics' recovery is much more stabilized than at any other stage of their recovery. (See Table 15.4.)

THE CURATIVE PROCESS

Rutan and Stone believe that the mechanisms of change inherent in imitation, identification, and internalization are enhanced by a curative

TABLE 15.4. Stages of Treatment

STAGES	PATIENT STATUS	TREATMENT
Stage I	"I can't drink." (need for external control) Imitation	Detoxification Antabuse AA (first four steps) Directive Psychotherapy Hospitalization Education
Stage II	"I won't drink." Identification	Supportive Psychotherapy AA (All twelve steps)
Stage III	"I don't have to drink." Internalization	AA=Sponsorship and twelfth-step work Insight-Oriented Psychotherapy

Adapted from Zimberg (1978).

process that requires confrontation, clarification, interpretation, and working through. Each of these factors is stage-specific to the curative process.

Confrontation

In treating addicted patients in a group setting, confrontation is essential at the beginning of treatment. The focus should not be on the alcoholics' or addicts' unconscious assumptions; rather, the group leader must constantly point out to them the external aspects of their behavior. The purpose of treatment during the initial stages of recovery is to do for the alcoholics or addicts what they are unable to do for themselves. Because their denial is so strong and their pathological defenses so rigid, they require a strong, caring relationship with a group leader who will serve as a container for their anger and anxiety while pointing out, in a nonpunitive manner, the destructive patterns of their behavior.

Learning to successfully confront requires (1) timing, (2) the capacity to form an alliance, and (3) empathy. If these skills are not adequately developed, group members will respond defensively, withdraw emotionally, attack the group and its members because of their own fears, or drop out of treatment.

Confrontations can take many forms, however. Rutan and Stone point out the many ways confrontation can be manifested in group. Confrontations in group can be contagious and can affect each group member differently.

> Most confrontations take place among members or between therapists and members. However, one form of confrontation in groups is distinct. Looking into the hall of mirrors, patients might observe others involving themselves in unproductive and pathological behavior and begin to be curious about the extent to which they too engage in identical or similar behaviors. This is a form of self-confrontation. In a therapy group no confrontation is given in isolation. Every member of the group hears and is affected, even though the confrontation may have been directed primarily at another member. Thus interventions must take into account more than an appreciation of the openness of a particular individual to hear them: they must include an awareness that the other members will have their own responses (1984, p. 61).

Clarification

Clarifications in group follow from interactions and confrontations. They serve the purpose of placing the individual interactions and exchanges in sharp focus. Clarifications help group members see repeated patterns in their behavior. As the group progresses in its development, the varied patterns of each individual member will begin to emerge. This is a middle phase process of group therapy in which each group member's behavioral constellation is brought to his or her as well as the rest of the group members' attention. A cold, distant group member might be told, "This is a common complaint of your wife and is the reason you find yourself without friends. It might be helpful for you to explore in group what it is that leads you to affect others in the way you do."

Interpretations

Interpretations differ from clarifications in that they are aimed at the unconscious in an attempt to get the group members' repressed unconscious material to their awareness by helping them gain an understanding of their hidden motives and conflicts. A later stage process of group therapy, successful interpretations require an emotional and cognitive component to their delivery. However, the timing of an interpretation is crucial. If given in the midst of an emotional storm or if too intellectually derived, they will fail to have an impact on a group member's understanding and behavior.

Working Through

Confrontation, clarification, and interpretation help group members become aware of their patterns of behavior and unconscious conflicts, but they alone are insufficient to bring about deep and lasting change. In working through, the emphasis is on increasing members' capacity to examine themselves and understand their areas of conflict and vulnerability. As they develop the capacity to interpret their own behavior, they will also develop a more varied and flexible defensive system that will protect them more adequately from undue anxieties while allowing more authentic intimacy with others.

Working through consumes the major portion of time in an ongoing therapy group. As each group member comes to understand and identify disturbing, self-defeating behavior, the associated thoughts and feelings are worked on and resolved. However, the consolidation of these thoughts, feelings, and behaviors will continue to emerge in a slightly disguised form repeatedly throughout the person's treatment in group. An example will help clarify this point.

> Martha, a thirty-two-year-old freelance photographer sought psychotherapy because of her severe depression and suicidal ideation. Two weeks into individual therapy, it was discovered that her depression was closely related to her excessive alcohol consumption. When encouraged to stop drinking and enter AA, Martha quickly complied. In fact, as therapy progressed, Martha readily complied to all the therapist's numerous requests. She had developed an acute idealizing transference in which she perceived her therapist to be "just perfect." Since the symptoms that had originally brought her to psychotherapy had quickly subsided, her therapist did not want to challenge her description of him as perfect too quickly for fear it would either prompt her to relapse or trigger a recurrence of her depression. As Martha's psychotherapy progressed, it became more apparent that she had at times come dangerously close to withdrawing into her own fantasy world where everything was perfect. She related that as a child, she had been sent by her school to see a psychiatrist because of her autistic-like self-absorption. Her early family life was marred by a distant father and a hostile, intrusive mother who demanded that Martha be perfect in her behavior, ap-

pearance, and schoolwork. At the age of thirteen, Martha discovered, through a reading of her sister's diary and some documents she found hidden in a closet, that she had been adopted. When she confronted her mother with her concerns, her mother exploded and denied all the evidence to the contrary. This only drove Martha to pursue her perfect fantasy world with more determination, since her reality-based world was too chaotic, threatening, and erratic.

After six months of individual therapy, Martha continued to insist that she had made the perfect choice in her therapist and believed that through his guidance in therapy everything would be perfect. All she had to do in order to be perfect was to perfectly perform all his requests since she sincerely believed he was perfect. After three more months of behaving perfectly, Martha began to realize that things were not turning out perfectly. She still felt angry, sad, and upset at varying times. Finally, she confronted her therapist, stating angrily that she was doing all he wanted, but that she still was not perfectly happy. Assured by him that he had not given her any formulation or suggestions, Martha confessed that she had inferred these formulas from their conversations. He then pointed out to her how she was attempting to create in the therapy situation the same circumstances that had existed in her early home life with her parents. Specifically, she believed if she did all things perfectly, the end result would turn out perfectly.

Encouraged by this insight, Martha proceeded to progress in therapy and began to make plans for termination. However, as she came closer to the termination date, her despair once again returned. Eventually, Martha came to understand that her despair was triggered by her realization that as she came closer to ending therapy, she had to face the fact that she was not yet perfect. She had held onto the fantasy that somehow, she would be perfect when therapy ended. Encouraged further by this insight, Martha decided to continue therapy to ensure that she was not fooling herself once again.

However, her need for perfection surfaced again in another form. After two difficult sessions in which she left the therapist's office feeling worse than when she had entered, Martha was struck by another important realization. Her therapist had twice made comments that had hurt her. She could not understand why he had done that. Since she still continued to perceive him as perfect, he must have hurt her on purpose. When she learned that her therapist had not hurt her intentionally, but apparently had made a mistake in his understanding of her feelings, she was forced once again to deal with the despair that this realization produced.

Transferred to a therapy group after another few months of individual therapy, her perfection fantasy resurfaced again. She had secretly bargained with herself that this time things would indeed really be perfect. Again, this was worked through only to have it resurface in another form. Two years after entering therapy, Martha's constant retreat into her perfect fantasy was rekindled by a new relationship with a man. The same theme emerged. She held onto the belief that this man and this relationship would now be perfect. After each progressive stage was worked through in therapy, Martha's reliance on her perfect fantasy diminished in its intensity and length of duration.

Taken in the proper sequence, confrontation, clarification, and interpretation can help the group members work through their various conflicts, resistances, and self-defeating, repetitive patterns. To enhance this process in its correct sequence, the group leader must:

1. *Confront the defense first.* For example, a withdrawn group member might be confronted with the following observation: "You deny your need for people. But, it is obvious to all of us in group that you are easily upset when people don't respond favorably to you. It is also obvious that you take great joy in the attention that others give you."
2. *Clarify the defense.* "There, you are doing it again. Every time someone reaches out to you, you do something to push them away."
3. *Interpretation.* "You keep denying your need for others because you are so frightened that they will get close to you and then reject you just as your mother did repeatedly when you were growing up."
4. *Working through.* The pattern will emerge again and again in varying forms. The group leader's task is to keep pointing out its occurrence in a nonjudgmental manner and help the group member come to a personal resolution about his or her fears, fantasies, and catastrophic expectations.

WORKING THROUGH WITH THE ADDICTED PATIENT

In working through with the typical addicted patient, group leaders must accomplish a sequence of tasks if they are to keep their group members sober. First, they must get the members to stop using chemicals. Through coercion, confrontation, encouragement, or appeal, this must be the first goal of treatment.

Second, group leaders must guide each member through a corrective emotional experience. The purpose of group treatment at this point is not insight–to make the unconscious conscious–but rather to promote the reliving of old experiences in group so that they can be reexperienced by a sober and more mature psyche. Alcoholics and addicts must come to discharge their old, pent-up emotions in a safe and constructive way so that they can work through the depression and hurt that is always buried underneath the anger. They must then come to identify and break the cycle of "The world and everyone in it is terrible. I am also terrible." Destructive relationships must be altered or severed, and healthy relationships with healthy people must be substituted. Self-esteem, which is always negatively affected by this cycle, is eventually restored. The grandiose, false self-organization that has been erected as a defensive facade must be given over to the true self so that authentic relationships can be established. As the sense of self is firmly established, members will then develop the capacity to make more autonomous decisions and healthy choices. Destructive dependencies will be altered and individuals will be free to engage in true intimate relationships without losing themselves in archaic needs and expectancies.

STAGES OF CURE IN A THERAPY GROUP

Cure in group therapy requires that the group leader carefully monitor the stage-specific behavior of the group. Do not expect the group to say goodbye before they say hello. Do not expect the group to share true intimacy before trust has been established. Group leaders who are finely tuned to the stage-consistent behavior of the group ares more likely to have a successful group experience with their group members. An understanding of group development and the curative process will help group leaders guide their group successfully through the difficult and different developmental stages that are sure to confront the group.

In the pages that follow, the six different phases of group development will be presented and discussed. The first two phases of group must be resolved before the group will be ready to move on to the more intimate phases of interpersonal interaction. (See Table 15.5.)

1. Dependence

Safety and trust are crucial during this phase. Like the chatter that occurs at a cocktail party, the group members' exchanges will be directed more by their desire to be accepted. What they have to say at this phase is not as meaningful as their interest in presenting themselves as a valuable and important asset to the group. Like the conversation at a cocktail party, after people have worked through their initial anxiety, they will then say, "Oh! What did you say your name was?" Now, they are ready to engage each other on a more meaningful level.

The group members rely on the group leader extensively during this phase. As they enter the group, they have a vague expectation that the group will somehow magically help them. But they also fear they will be traumatized and defeated by the group as they were by their parents. Their

TABLE 15.5. Phases of Group Development

1. *DEPENDENCE*
   - A. Each member enters group with the curative fantasy
   - B. Flight from intimacy and the here and now is prominent
   - C. Parallel talk is pronounced
   - D. Pseudo-cohesion develops
2. *COUNTERDEPENDENCE*
   - A. Rebellion dominates
   - B. Scapegoating
   - C. Intimacy is avoided by fighting
3. *RESOLUTION OF POWER/AUTHORITY ISSUES*
   - A. Pairing and fusion are pronounced
   - B. Disappointment and disillusionment
   - C. The group and the leader are found to be lacking
4. *STAGE OF REAL COHESION*
   - A. Deeper intimacy develops after anger and disappointment are resolved
5. *INTERDEPENDENCE*
   - A. Consensual validation of ambiguity
   - B. Group maturity and true intimacy
6. *TERMINATION*
   - A. Separation/individuation

curative fantasy will be pronounced as they try to get from the group leader what they had wanted from their parents in the past. Many members hope they will be accepted, affirmed, and not be rejected by the group. This is often all they want. Just to be told by the group that they are okay will often confirm their sense of self and for many will be initially therapeutic.

Group will be used frequently by the members to strengthen certain deficient parts of themselves. Kohut, in particular, placed extensive emphasis on individuals' intuitive drive to repair fragmented egos and defective selves. Their intuitive fantasy is that their sense of self will be mended and strengthened through their interaction and acceptance by the group.

2. Counterdependence

Although the group may shift its focus to more emotionally arousing issues, their fears of intimacy are still dominant. The group members will test the leader and the group to ensure that they are safe from humiliation and threat. Their basic question remains: "Will I and whatever I say be accepted here?" They must come to realize that the boundaries of the group are clearly set and safely managed.

3. Resolution of Power/Authority Issues

After anger is finally expressed and worked through in group, a stage of pseudo-cohesion develops. Hope is prominent in group and Bion's basic assumption of pairing is central to this phase of the group's development (see Chapter 14).

4. Stage of Real Cohesion

This is a phase that the group strives to attain but unfortunately is only temporary. However, while it lasts, it is warm, genuine, and authentic. But just when the group begins to feel as if it will be more cohesive, it falls apart. This is to be expected. If the group leader needs to have and believe in a continual, safe, trusting group, he or she will be disappointed. This is much like the mother who during the child's separation/individuation stage of development requires the child to stay in her lap and behave. The group leader must not interfere with this developmental stage, but must be able to contain the group's aggression and anger without allowing it to turn into harmful scapegoating.

5. Interdependence

This is the phase that Alonso (1985) refers to as the borderline existence of the group. Splitting and projective identification occurs repeatedly among the group members. The group and the leader are found lacking. People threaten to leave. Competition and fighting among group members emerge. The group members change and their working through the group conflicts occurs in a helix during this phase. The same issues emerge and re-emerge. As each issue is worked through in group, the members progress to a deeper stage each time until their conflicts are resolved.

The group enters the final stage of maturity. Each member has the opportunity to learn that he or she is independent and separate from the group.

The principle of "I must learn that I can live without you before I can be intimate with you" is experienced on more deepening levels. Separation is the key. This is a process of reparation and forgiveness. Members realize that "no one, not you or myself is perfect." However, the group and its members eventually acknowledge that although they are not perfect they are good enough.

6. Termination

Termination is the last phase of treatment and is an event, if handled properly, that can have important therapeutic implications for the entire group, not just the individuals who are leaving. Conversely, if handled poorly, it can provoke an entire host of dire consequences for those leaving, as well as for those group members who are staying. A poorly managed termination in group can have a long-standing ripple effect on the entire group that will reverberate throughout the life of the group, long after the departing group member has gone. Because termination is such an important event and the discussion of its proper management is often ignored, it is crucial that the group leader effectively manage its occurrence. Termination takes on even more significance for the group and its members because, other than those rare occasions when an entire group terminates together, it is unusual for individuals to have the opportunity to say goodbye to someone who is leaving them on good terms. Termination in group is a public event and it is rare in our society for people to have the chance to deal with departures in a healthy and honest fashion. Termination in group allows this to be experienced, not just for the departing member, but even more important, it permits the remaining group members to have an opportunity to share in an experience that may be new and powerfully corrective for a number of different reasons.

Termination, especially in individual therapy, is usually thought of in context of a patient's readiness to leave therapy. While this is also an important component in group therapy, the termination process (contemplation, discussion, announcement, and departure) itself has much more significance for the group because, unlike individual therapy where the therapist is left, a termination in group means that it is the patient, or more correctly, many patients that are being left. This provides an entirely different array and wider range of emotional stimuli than one individual leaving one therapist can ever provide. Despite the relevant differences between the event and process, it is still important to list some of the ideal goals that need to be obtained before individuals are considered ready for termination. Some of the most commonly cited goals of treatment are:

1. Resistance and transference are understood and worked through. This means individuals are less likely to be reactive to authorty and intimacy. However, it is understood that transference is never completely resolved. We are transferential animals. Individuals not only understand the sources of their resistance (against change, insight, reality, etc.), but are also willing to let go of these resistances.
2. Defenses are loosened and individuals can be more flexible in their responses to others. There is less reliance on primitive defenses (i.e., denial) and more of an ability to utilize other higher level defenses (i.e., sublimation). Changes in overall patterns or styles include less stereotyped and automatic defensive responses, more flexible and adaptive use of defenses, and less reliance on limited defensive mechanisms.
3. Drives are sublimated and frustration tolerance is established. Omnipotence is attenuated and the capacity for recognizing limitations is achieved (in the case of an alcoholic, this means "I cannot drink"). Reality testing and acceptance is achieved with the related attributes of love of truth, courage to be sincere, and willingness to check one's perceptions with those of others.
4. Observing ego is established with the associated capacity for insight, self-honesty, and reflection. Individuals are driven less by impulses and have the capacity to delay acting out of their feelings alone. Instead, the capacity to use feelings as signals is established.
5. Identity is established with a firmer sense of self as responsible agent. Autonomy is achieved without sacrificing the capacity to

need, be dependent upon, or temporarily merge self with another. Purpose, meaning, pride, and strength (i.e., self-esteem) in one's beliefs, values, and convictions are achieved and more firmly held.

6. Psychic structure is laid and integration of self is achieved. Previous levels of developmental arrestment are resolved, resulting in a greater capacity for trust, separation, individualization, healthy guilt/shame, assertiveness, and sexuality. The ability to manage happiness without excessive guilt or resorting to pleasure-seeking is achieved. The capacity for enjoyment, gratification, joy, relaxation, pleasure, and play is increased.
7. Object relations are improved and a capacity for intimate relations with others is obtained. The reduction of narcissism and self-centeredness and the ability to empathically relate to others is achieved. Individuals become less preoccupied with unusual and unrealistic private wishes and fantasies.
8. Symptomatology is reduced with greater emotional and physical health. The capacity for pleasure and acceptance and the tolerance for ambivalence is increased. There is an increase in the fullness of experience with the increased capacity of access to all affective states (i.e., anger, joy, sadness, grief, happiness, etc.).

ADDICTION AND GOALS OF TERMINATION

While all of the above-mentioned goals are applicable to addiction, there are some other essential elements that apply specifically to addiction. Acceptance that one is an alcoholic or addict and cannot use substances or chemicals is fully integrated. This means that individuals have truly taken the first step of the twelve-step program and that they acknowledge their addiction as a disease that is chronic and cannot be cured, but only arrested. On a more symbolic level, they come to recognize and admit they are not God (Kurtz, 1982). With this recognition come important existential implications about one's acceptance of the human condition, which for Kurtz and other existential writers, lies at the heart of all addictions.

A. *Limits.* The first limit alcoholics or addicts must recognize is that they cannot use chemicals. They must accept that they do not possess the capacity for unlimited happiness, control of others, or control of their own emotions, and must integrate the painful truth that life has its limits. They must accept that it is their nature as human beings to grow old and die. They must also accept that everything they love and cherish will change, grow old, die, or go away. Finally, they must realize that they cannot escape the consequences of their actions. As Sartre says, we are the sum of our actions.

B. *Needing Others.* Alcoholics and addicts must admit they cannot do it (life, sobriety, etc.) alone. They need others and by allowing themselves to need and be needed, they become fully human.

C. *Imperfectness.* Alcoholics and addicts develop the capacity to admit their faults, shortcomings, and imperfections. They relinquish the narcissistic defenses of specialness and grandiosity that is a false self erected to protect them from shame. This means their shame is worked through on a healthy level. Not only arc they accepting of their failures, but they are accepting of others whot are as flawed as they are.

D. *Authenticity.* They become real, complete human beings who develop more of a capacity for true, honest mutuality in their relationships with others and self. They live more in the moment (one day at a time) and learn that their actions are more important than their words or promises (Walk your talk).

The Termination Process

Despite all attempts to get the alcoholic and addict ready for termination, not everyone will leave group having fully obtained everything that is hoped for or required. Vannicelli (1992) suggests that group leaders accept the reality that a great many patients will leave group before they are ready or when they are on the very brink of working through an important but difficult issue. As group leaders, we cannot or should not try to force individuals to stay even if we believe or know it would be better for them if they did not leave group at this time. However, getting them to talk about their feelings, thoughts, and reasons for considering leaving the group can be extremely beneficial for a number of reasons. Foremost among these reasons is that feelings talked about are less likely to be acted upon. Vannicelli has categorized group terminators into three classifications. Not only is it helpful for the group leader to have these categories, but Vannicelli suggests that the potential terminators be asked to classify themselves into one of the three categories, thus providing a forum for their discussion in the group. These three categories are:

1. *Completers.* Completers have essentially finished the work that they came in for and are sufficiently educated regarding the benefits of group work that they understand, also, the impact of doing the last

phase of work, saying good-bye. They also understand that saying good-bye is a process—something that we all need to learn how to do better—and that the therapy group offers a unique opportunity to learn how to do this. These patients are able to review their goals and gains in therapy, as well as reflect upon their losses, as they think about giving up the group and how it will feel, ultimately, to be gone.

2. *Plateauers.* These patients have done some of the work that they came in for, but have a sense that they are not really finished. Rather, for the time being, they are "stuck." Plateauers have no clear sense of what more can be accomplished at the present time. (Often these patients return to treatment at a later point.) These patients are able to do some of the work of saying good-bye although usually in a more abbreviated way than completers. The good-byes serve as the last focused project that the patient can gain from working on.
3. *Flee-ers.* (This group may also be referred to as "Flyers.") These patients experience a pressing need to "get out." In fact, the pressure to leave is often the telling signal of the fleer. Such patients cannot take the time to terminate, but rather, feel tremendous pressure to leave in haste. Generally patients in this category are avoiding something in the group, or in themselves, that they feel uncomfortable about and from which they wish to flee as rapidly as possible. (1992, p. 178)

Termination in Groups

A successful termination in group is a unique experience because it is one of the few instances in many individuals' lives where they get to witness and be part of something that is ending positively and completely. Most relationships end without ever being finalized in a healthy way. Even in extreme cases where a relationship is brought to an end by death or divorce, there are complex emotional issues that prevent true closure. With death, because of denial or the suddenness of it, people often do not have the opportunity to work through it successfully. In divorce, it is usually an angry and bitter and disappointing separation that is often never completely resolved. People usually experience leaving in two common ways. Either they sneak away, gradually leave the relationship and fade apart slowly, or they storm out in an angry, abrupt manner. It is for many individuals a rare event to allow someone to depart in a caring and permissive manner. Individual therapy is usually a gradual fading away, a reduction of sessions until the person stops, usually with an understanding that they can return anytime they choose. Once a person leaves group, they can never come back to the same group.

Terminations are always difficult. They can be even more difficult or more damaging in new groups if the termination is premature or the result of unresolved conflicts and disagreements. Such a departure can have a contagious effect on the group if not adequately processed and dealt with. It may produce guilt ("Maybe it was my fault, could I have done more?") or envy ("I wish it was me leaving instead of having to deal with these difficult issues"), as well as abandonment and anger.

Termination is difficult even when everyone is in agreement that treatment is complete and the person is ready to graduate. Someone leaving, of course, never depends on a group vote; it is the individual's decision alone to make, even though it is crucial that the other group members be included in the discussion of the decision-making process. Hopefully, individuals will have been talking about their considerations about leaving long before they make the final announcement. It is recommended that they give the group a four-week notice, so that everyone is given the opportunity to deal with the feelings that their departure may trigger. Some of the reasons why terminations, even good ones, are difficult are:

1. Saying good-bye produces deep and sometimes painful affect. Some individuals, especially alcoholics and addicts, have extreme difficulty tolerating any affect. Sadness, grief, and tears are emotional expressions to be avoided at all costs because they have not yet learned the advantages of emotions freely expressed.
2. Termination evokes many old and unresolved losses, deaths, endings, and incomplete good-byes.
3. Individuals can often feel tremendous guilt about leaving, feeling as if they are letting the others down and abandoning them. The important developmental process of individualization/separation has been arrested for many individuals. They have a history of never being permitted to leave or individuate in a healthy and encouraging manner. Their history is usually marked by rebellion, abrupt departures, and angry separations.
4. Many individuals will have difficulty leaving because it provokes exceedingly high fears of disappointing or hurting others. Patients who have a history of taking on too much responsibility, blame, and shame will find it extremely difficult to leave, or do anything that is beneficial for themselves if it in any way proves even remotely difficult or painful for others.
5. Saying good-bye and leaving can be exorbitantly difficult for many individuals because they possess strong fears that no one will notice or care that they are gone. The group leader will have to help them face these fears lest they give in to them and allow themselves to

sneak out or fade away rather than face the catastrophic expectation that they matter so little to everyone. Often, there is a great surprise at learning that their presence and their leaving has such a strong impact on others.

CONCLUSION

It is fitting to end this book with a chapter that ends with the topic of termination in group. I hope I have been able to leave the reader with the same message and feeling that I would like the group leader to leave his or her group members with when they terminate and depart from the therapy group. Specifically, I hope the reader and group members leave with a better understanding of addiction, less confusion about group therapy, some direction and specific guidelines for their recovery, and, most important, some hope for their future. Despite all our efforts to give, guide, and support, each of us is ultimately alone when it comes to our life, recovery, and growth. This is the inevitable plight of the human condition. As the existentialists repeatedly say, we are ultimately alone and solely responsible for our fates. Nevertheless, while we are individually alone and responsible, this does not mean that we cannot be helped, supported, and encouraged by others in our life and in our community.

As group leaders, while we have our group members in our therapy groups, we can hopefully give them something that they will be able to carry with them after group ends. Specifically, we can give them what everyone wants–an experience and a sense of community where they feel they are accepted and belong. Feeling alienated, empty, and misunderstood is a struggle that all chemically dependent people experience. The therapy group gives them a sense of belonging and being understood at a very basic level. This is why the theme of cohesion, trust, and safety has been such a prominent one throughout this book. While everyone wants to be accepted, loved, and recognized, they want it unconditionally. The primary conflict for us all, the addicted as well as the non-addicted, is to belong and be connected to something larger than ourselves without losing ourselves. Alcoholics and addicts perhaps feel this a little more intensely and this may be the reason their demand for autonomy and independence takes on such rebellious, self-centered, and demanding properties. They fear that belonging to someone or something will cost them their individuality. This is a constant theme for all of us. Can I be close and truly intimate without losing myself, without my separateness coming at the expense of my independence? Can I tolerate my separateness without compromising my autonomy in order to get my need for human closeness met?

Group therapy, directed along the lines prescribed in this book, can meet the needs of both poles of this human dilemma. It first allows chemically dependent individuals to get close and be intimate with others who are accepting of them without it costing their identity and autonomy. It then encourages their individuality while giving them the tools to get close to others without compromising their separateness. Ultimately, it allows alcoholics and addicts to deal with the emotions triggered by all intimate encounters without relying on alcohol and drugs to sedate, buffer, or alter their feelings.

In many ways, group therapy, much like Alcoholics Anonymous, can be viewed as a holding environment–a cohesive, safe community where people can get at the depth of understanding the relationship between their private and public selves. At the same time, they can be encouraged and allowed to evolve in separate ways at their own pace. As suggested by Wallace earlier in this book, recovery is a time-dependent process. During the early stages of recovery, alcoholics and addicts need to be welcomed to join a safe, trusting, and healing culture. Later, as they gradually evolve through different stages, they will be encouraged to separate while learning how to be close without losing their identity or isolating themselves from others. As AA so correctly points out, AA members are recovering alcoholics. They are never recovered. Growth and evolution continues throughout life. Group therapy, as a part of alcoholics' or addicts' recovery, helps propel this process. It is a process that does not end once they leave group therapy or attain sobriety, for the issues of belonging and being alone remain constant themes in their lives. Group therapy helps recovering individuals learn ways to successfully adapt to this very central human process.

References

Ackerman, R. J. (1979). *Children of alcoholics: A guidebook for educators, therapists, and parents*. Holmes Beach, FL: Learning Publication, Inc.

Adler, G. (1994). Transference, countertransference and abuse in psychotherapy. *Harvard Review of Psychiatry, 2*, 151-159.

Agazarian, Y. M. (1992). Contemporary theories of group psychotherapy: A systems approach to the group-as-a-whole. *International Journal of Group Psychotherapy, 42*, 177-203.

Agazarian, Y. M. & Alonso, A. (1993). *Discussions around shame in a shamed group*. Philadelphia: Blue Sky Video.

Agazarian, Y. M. & Peters, R. (1981). *The visible and invisible group*. London: Routledge & Kegan Paul.

Albrecht, G. L. (1969). *The assessment of Fulton County adolescents' behavior, knowledge and attitudes in relation to the legal system: A preliminary report.* Fulton County Juvenile Court. Atlanta, GA.

Alcoholics Anonymous. (1939). *Alcoholics Anonymous.* New York: AA World Services.

Alcoholics Anonymous. (1955). *Alcoholics Anonymous: The story of how many thousands of men and women have recovered from alcoholism.* New York: AA World Services.

Alcoholics Anonymous. (1960). *Is A.A. for you?* AA Grapevine. New York: AA World Services.

Alcoholics Anonymous. (1990). *Alcoholics Anonymous 1989 membership survey.* New York: AA World Services.

Alcoholics Anonymous. (1992). *Alcoholics Anonymous 1992 membership survey.* New York: AA World Services.

Alexander, F. (1950). *Psychosomatic medicine.* New York: W. W. Norton.

Alibrandi, L. A. (1978). The folk psychotherapy of Alcoholics Anonymous. In S. Zimberg, J. Wallace, & S. B. Blume (Eds.), *Practical approaches to alcoholism psychotherapy* (163-180). New York: Plenum Press.

Allen, M. (1990). Group psychotherapy–past, present and future. *Psychiatric Annals, 20* (7), 358-361.

Alonso, A. (1985, Nov.). Lecture given at Harvard Medical School seminar on group psychotherapy. Boston, MA.

Alonso, A. & Rutan, J. S. (1988). The experience of shame and the restoration of self-respect in group psychotherapy. *International Journal of Group Psychotherapy, 38*, 3-14.

Alonso, A. & Rutan, J. S. (1993). Character change in group therapy. *International Journal of Group Psychotherapy, 43*, 439-452.

American Psychiatric Association (1994). *Diagnostic & statistical manual of mental disorders* (4th ed.). Washington, DC: APA.

Angyal, A. (1965). *Neurosis & treatment: A holistic theory.* New York: John Wiley & Sons.

Apfeldorf, M. (1978). Alcoholism scales of the MMPI: Contributions and future directions. *International Journal of Addictions, 13*, 17-53.

Bacal, H. A. (1985). Object-relations in the group from the perspective of self-psychology. *International Journal of Group Psychotherapy, 35*, 483-501.

Bacal, H. A. (1992). Contributions from self-psychology. In R. H. Klien, H. S. Bernard, & D. L. Singer (Eds.), *Handbook of group psychotherapy* (55-86). Madison, CT: International University Press.

Back, K. W. (1972). Beyond words: The story of sensitivity training and the encounter movement. *Psychology Today,* May.

Bailey, M. B. & Leach, B. (1965). *Alcoholics Anonymous, pathway to recovery: A study of 1,058 members of the AA fellowship in New York City.* New York: National Council on Alcoholism.

Bailey, M. B. (1965). Al-Anon family groups as an aid to wives of alcoholics. *Social Work N.Y., 10*, 68-74.

Bakan, A. (1972). *On method.* San Francisco: Jossey-Bass.

Bakeland, F. L., Lundwall, L., & Kissin, B. (1975). Methods for the treatment of chronic alcoholism: A critical appraisal. In R. J. Gibbins, Y. Israel, H. Kalant, R. E. Popham, W. Schmidt, & R. G. Smart (Eds.), *Research advances in alcohol and drug problems* (Vol. 2). New York: John Wiley & Sons.

Barnes, G. E. (1979). The alcoholic personality. *Quarterly Journal of Studies on Alcohol, 40*, 571-634.

Barnett, L. (1948). *The universe and Dr. Einstein.* New York: Bantam Books.

Barrett, C. L. (1985). Who are the alcoholics? Where are the devils? *Bulletin of the Society of Psychologists in Addictive Behaviors, 4*(1), 17-28.

Basch, M. F. (1980). *Doing psychotherapy.* New York: Basic Books.

Bateson, G. (1971). Thc cybernetics of self: A theory of alcoholism. *Psychiatry, 34*, 1-18.

Becker, E. (1973). *The denial of death.* New York: Free Press.

Berger, F. (1983). Alcoholism rehabilitation: A supportive approach. *Hospital and Community Psychiatry, 34*(11), 1040-1043.

Bergin, A. E. (1971). The evaluation of therapeutic outcomes. In A. E. Bergin & S. L. Garfield (Eds.), *Handbook of psychotherapy and behavior change: An empirical analysis* (36-51). New York: John Wiley & Sons.

Bergin, A. E. (1981). Psychotherapy & religious values. *Journal of Consulting and Clinical Psychology, 48*(1), 95-105.

Bergin, A. E. & Lambert, M. J. (1978). The evaluation of therapeutic outcomes. In S. L. Garfield & A. E. Bergin (Eds.), *Handbook of psychotherapy and behavior change* (2nd ed., 139-190). New York: John Wiley & Sons.

Berne E. (1961). *Transactional analysis in psychotherapy.* New York: Grove Press.

Beutler, L. E. (1979a). Individual, group and family therapy modes: Patient therapy value compatibility and treatment effectiveness. *Journal of Counseling and Psychotherapy, 32*, 43-59.

Beutler, L. E. (1980). Personal communication. University of Arizona Health Science Center. Tucson, AZ.

Bibb, R. E. (1970). The outpatient treatment of the alcoholic. *Ohio State Medical Journal, 66*, 686-689.

Bion, W. R. (1961). *Experiences in groups*. New York: Basic Books.

Bixenstine, E. (1956). Thc value-fact antithesis in behavioral science. *Journal of Humanistic Psychology, 16*, 35-57.

Blanck, G. & Blanck, R. (1974). *Ego Psychology: Theory and practice.* New York: Columbia University Press.

Blane, H. T. (1968). *The personality of the alcoholic: Guises of dependency.* New York: Harper & Row.

Blatt, S. J. (1974). Levels of object representation in analytic and introjective depression. *Psychoanalytic Study of the Child, 29*, 107-157.

Bollerud, K. (1995, March). A model for treating sexually abused substance abusers. Paper presented at workshop, The Addictions. Harvard Medical Shool, Boston, MA.

Borowitz, G. H. (1964). Some ego aspects of alcoholism. *British Journal of Medical Psychology, 37* (3), 257-263.

Bourne, E. & Fox, R. (1973). *Alcoholism: Progress in research & treatment.* New York: Academic Press.

Bowlby, J. (1958). The nature of the child's tie to the mother. *International Journal of Psychoanalysis, 39*, 350-373.

Bowlby, J. (1980). *Attachment and loss: Vol. III, Loss.* New York: Basic Books.

Bradshaw, J. (1993). *Healing the shame that binds you*. Deerfield Beach, FL: Health Communications.

Brandsma, J. & Pattison, E. M. (1985). The outcome of group psychotherapy in alcoholics: An empirical review. *American Journal of Drug & Alcohol Abuse*, *11*(1), 151-160.

Brix, D. J. (1983). Use of a group-centered psychotherapy group with the inpatient treatment of alcoholism. *Bulletin of the Society of Psychologists in Addictive Behaviors*, *2*(14), 253-258.

Bronowski, J. (1973). *The ascent of man*. Boston/Toronto: Little, Brown & Co.

Brown, D. G. (1985). Bion and Foukles: Basic assumptions and beyond. In M. Pines. (Ed.), *Bion and group psychotherapy* (192-219). London: Tavistock/Routledge.

Brown, N. O. (1959). *Life against death*. Middletown, MA: Wesleyan University Press.

Brown, S. (1985). *Treating the alcoholic: A developmental model of recovery*. New York: John Wiley & Sons.

Brown, S. (1988). *Treating adult children of alcoholics: A developmental perspective*. New York: John Wiley & Sons.

Brown, S. & Beletsis, S. (1986). The development of family transference in group for adult children of alcoholics. *International Journal of Group Psychotherapy*, *36*, 97-114.

Brown, S. & Yalom, I. (1977). Interactional group psychotherapy with alcoholic patients. *Journal of Studies on Alcohol*, *38*, 426-456.

Buber, M. (1955a). *Hasidism and modern man*. (M. Friedman, Trans.). New York: Horizon Press.

Buber, M. (1955b). *The life of dialogue*. (M. Friedman, Trans.). London: Routledge.

Buber, M. (1960). *I and thou*. (W. Kaufmann, Trans.). New York: Scribner & Sons.

Buber, M. (1963). *Pointing the way*. (M. Friedman, Trans.). New York: Harper Torchbooks.

Buber, M. (1964). In M. Friedman (Ed.), *The worlds of existentialism* (385-395). New York: Random House.

Buhler, C. & Lefever, D. W. (1956). A Rorschach study on the psychological characteristics of alcoholics. *Quarterly Journal of Studies on Alcohol*, *17*, 163-281.

Butters, N. & Cermak, L. S. (1980). *Alcoholic Korsakoff syndrome: An information-processing approach to amnesia*. New York: Academic Press.

Button, A. D. (1956). A study of alcoholics with the MMPI. *Quarterly Journal of Studies on Alcohol, 11*, 163-281.

Cahn, S. (1970). *The treatment of alcoholics: An evaluative study.* New York: Oxford University Press.

Camus, A. (1960). *The myth of Sisyphus, and other essays.* New York: Vintage.

Canter, F. M. (1969). Motivation for self-confrontation in alcohol patients. *Psychotherapy: Theory, Research & Practice, 6*(1), 21-23.

Carkhuff, R. (1969). *Helping & human relations, Vol. 2, Practice & research.* New York: Holt, Rinehart & Winston.

Cassell, E. J. (1985). The healer's art. Cambridge, MA: MIT Press.

Cermak, L. S. & Peck, E. (1982). Continuum versus premature aging theories of chronic alcoholism. *Alcoholism: Clinical and Experimental Research, 6*(1), 89-95.

Cermak, T. L (1984). Children of alcoholics and the case for a new diagnostic category of codependence. *Alcohol, Health and Research World, 8*(4) 38-42.

Cermak, T. L. & Brown, S. (1982). Interactional group therapy with adult children of alcoholics. *International Journal of Group Psychotherapy, 32*, 375-389.

Chafetz, M. E. (1968). Research in the alcoholic clinic. *American Journal of Psychiatry, 124*, 1674-1679.

Chaftez, M. E., Blane, H. T., & Hill, M. J. (1970). *Frontiers of alcoholism.* New York: Science Hours.

Chalmers, D. & Wallace, J. (1978). Evaluation of patient progress. In S. Zimberg, J. Wallace, & S. Blume (Eds.), *Practical approaches to alcoholism psychotherapy* (255-277). New York: Plenum.

Clavell, J. (1986). *Shogun.* New York: Dell.

Collins, G. B. (1995). Why treatment for alcohol dependence is changing. In N. S. Miller (Ed.), *Treatment of the addictions: Applications of outcome research for clinical management* (23-40). New York: The Haworth Press.

Cummings, N. (1979). Turning bread into stones. *American Psychologist, 34*(12), 1119-1129.

Dahany, S. A. (1977). The effects of assertive training with inpatient alcoholics on measures of assertive behavior, self-esteem, field-dependence. PhD Diss., University of Arizona.

Devito, R. A. (1969). New dimensions in treatment of alcoholism. *Illinois Medical Journal, 124*, 389-392.

DiClemente, C. C., Carbonari, J. P., & Velasquez, M. M. (1992). Alcoholism treatment mismatching from a process of change perspective. *Drug and Alcohol Abuse Reviews*, *3*, 115-142.

Dies, R. R. (1977). Group therapist transparency: A critique of theory and research. *International Journal of Group Psychotherapy*, *27*, 177-200.

Dies, R. R. (1992a). The future of group therapy. *Psychotherapy*, *29*(1), (Spring), 58-64.

Dies, R. R. (1992b). Models of group psychotherapy: Sifting Through Confusion. *International Journal of Group Psychotherapy*, *42*, 1-18.

Dies, K. R. & Dies, R. R. (1993). Directive facilitation: A model for short-term group treatments (Part 2). *The Independent Practioner*, *13*, 177-183.

Disterfano, N., Pryer, L. W., & Garrison, J. L. (1972). Internal-external control among alcoholics. *Journal of Clinical Psychology*, *28*, 36-37.

Dodes, L. K. (1988). The psychology of combining dynamics psychotherapy and Alcoholics Anonymous. *Bulletin of the Menninger Clinic*, *52*, 283-293.

Dolliver, R. (1981). Some limitations in Perls' gestalt therapy. *Psychotherapy: Theory, Research and Practice*, *18*(1), 38-45.

Donovan, D. M. & O'Leary, M. R. (1975). Comparison of perceived and experienced control among alcoholics and nonalcoholics. *Journal of Abnormal Psychology*, *84*,112-126.

Dostoyevsky, F. (1957). *The brothers Karamazov*. New York: Basic Books.

Dublin, J. (1976). Gestalt therapy. Existential-gestalt therapy and/versus "Perlism." In E. W. L. Smith (Ed.), *The growing edge of Gestalt therapy* (57-69). Secaucus, NJ: Citadel Press.

Dubourg, G. O. (1969). After care for alcoholics: A follow-up study. *British Journal of Addiction*, *64*, 155-163.

Durant, W. (1926). *Story of philosophy*. New York: Simon & Schuster.

Durkin, H. E. (1964). *The group in depth*. New York: Interactional Universities Press.

Early, P. H. (1994). Is everything I do an addiction? *Ridgeview Insight*, 3-7, Atlanta, GA.

Eliot, T. S. (1943). *Little Gidding. In four quartets*. New York: Harcourt Brace Jovanovich.

Emrick, C. D. (1974). A review of psychological oriented treatment of alcoholism, I: The use and interrelationships of outcome criteria and drinking behavior following treatment. *Quarterly Journal of Studies on Alcohol*, *36*, 523-549.

Emrick, C. D. (1979). Perspectives in clinical research: Relative effectiveness of alcohol abuse treatment. *Family and Community Health*, *2*(2), 71-88.

Emrick, C. D. (1989). Alcoholics Anonymous: Membership characteristics and effectiveness as treatment. In M. Galanter (Ed.), *Recent developments in alcoholism* (37-53). New York: Grune & Stratton.

Emrick, C., Lassen, C. L., & Edwards, M. T. (1977). Nonprofessional peers as therapeutic agents. In A. S. Gurman and A. M. Razin (Eds.), *Effective psychotherapy: A handbook of research* (120-161). New York: Pergamon.

English, J. (1975). Personality differences in alcohol treatment. *Quarterly Journal of Studies on Alcohol*, *36*, 52-61.

Ettin, M. F. (1988). By the crowd they have been broken, by the crowd they shall be healed: The advent of group psychology. *International Journal of Group Psychotherapy*, *38*(2), 139-168.

Eysenck, H. J. (1952). The effects of psychotherapy: An evaluation. *Journal of Consulting Psychology*, *16*, 319-324.

Ezriel, H. (1973). Psychoanalytic group psychotherapy. In L. R. Wolberg & E. K. Schwartz (Eds.), *Group Therapy* (183-210). New York: Stratton Intercontinental Medical Books.

Faber, L. (1966). *The ways of will*. New York: Basic Books.

Fairbairn, W. R. D. (1952). *Psychoanalytic studies of the personality*. London: Tavistock Publications.

Fancher, R. E. (1973). *Psychoanalytic psychology. The development of Freud's thought*. New York: W. W. Norton.

Fehr, D. (1976). Psychotherapy: Integration of individual and group methods. In R. E. Tarter & A. A. Sugarman (Eds.), *Alcoholism: Interdisciplinary approaches to an enduring problem* (637-654). Reading MA: Addison-Wesley.

Festinger, L. (1954). A theory of social comparison processes. *Human Relations*, *7*, 117-140.

Fischer, R. (1976). On creative psychotic & ecstatic states. In L. Allen & D. Jaffe (Eds.), *Consciousness as role & knowledge. Readings in abnormal psychology. Contemporary perspectives*. New York: Harper & Row.

Flores, P. (1985). Alcoholism treatment & the relationship of Native-American's cultural values to recovery. *International Journal of the Addictions*, *20*, 1707-1726.

Flores, P. (1988a). Alcoholics Anonymous: A phenomenological and existential perspective. *Alcoholism Treatment Quarterly*, *5*, 73-94.

Flores, P. (1988b). *Group psychotherapy with addicted populations.* New York: The Haworth Press.

Flores, P. (1993). Group psychotherapy with alcoholics, substance abusers and adult children of alcoholics. In H. I. Kaplan & B. J. Sadock (Eds.), *Comprehensive group psychotherapy* (3rd ed., 429-442). Baltimore, MD: Williams & Wilkins.

Flores, P. & Mahon, L. (1993). The treatment of addiction in group psychotherapy. *International Journal of Group Psychotherapy, 43*(2), 143-156.

Fox, R. (1967). Disulfiram as an adjunct in the treatment of alcoholism. In R. Fox (Ed.), *Alcoholism: Behavioral research, therapeutic approaches* (242-255). New York: Springer.

Fox, R. (1973). Treatment of the problem drinker by the private practitioner. In P. G. Bourne & R. Fox (Eds.), *Alcoholism: Progress in research and treatment* (227-241). New York: Academic Press.

Frank, J. (1961). *Persuasion and healing.* Baltimore, MD: Johns Hopkins Press.

Frank, J. (1972). Remarks. In M. E. Chafetz (Ed.), *Proceedings of the 2nd annual alcoholism conference of NIAAA* (242-244). Washington, DC: U. S. Government Printing Office.

Frank, J. (1978). *Psychotherapy and the human predicament.* New York: Schocken Books.

Frankel, C. (1971). *The case for modern man.* Boston: Beacon Press.

Frankl, V. (1969). *The will to meaning.* Cleveland, OH: New American Library.

Freimuth, M. (1994). Psychotherapy and twelve-step programs: A commentary on Humphreys. *Psychotherapy, 31*, 551-552.

Freud. S. (1910). The future prospects of psycho-analytic therapy. *The standard edition of the complete psychological works of S. Freud, Vol. 11* (139-152). London: Hogarth Press.

Freud, S. (1921). *Group psychology and the analysis of the ego. Complete psychological works of Sigmund Freud.* London: Hogarth Press.

Fromm, E. (1941). *Escape from freedom.* New York: Farrar and Rinehart.

Gallant, D. M. (1983). Prediction of cortical atrophy in young alcoholics. *Alcoholism: Clinical & Experimental Research, 7*(4), 448.

Gartner, A. & Riessman, F. (1984). *The self-help revolution.* New York: Human Sciences Press.

Gauron, E. F. & Rawlings, E. I. (1975). Procedure for orienting new members to group psychotherapy. *Small Group Behavior, 6*, 293-307.

Gelormino, G. (1995). Harm reduction: A response to the article by Alan Marlatt. *The Addictions Newletter, 2*, 9-10.

Gerard, D. C. (1962). *Troubled employees program*. Center City, MN: Hazelden.

Gitlow, S .E. (1973). Alcoholism: A disease. In P. G. Bourne & R. Fox (Eds), *Alcoholism: Progress, research and treatment* (1-9). New York: Academic Press.

Glatzter, H. T. (1969). Working through in analytic group psychotherapy. *International Journal of Group Psychotherapy*, *19*, 292-306.

Goodwin, D. (1979). Alcoholism and heredity: A review and hypothesis. *Archives of General Psychiatry*, *36*, 57-61.

Goss, A. & Morosko, T. E. (1970). Relation between a dimension of internal-external control and the MMPI with alcoholic population. *Journal of Consulting and Clinical Psychology*, *8*, 189-192.

Goulding, M. (1980, July). Personal communication. Western Institute for Group and Family Therapy. Watsonville, CA.

Goulding, R. L. & Goulding, M. M. (1979). *Changing lives through redecision therapy*. New York: Brunner/Mazel.

Gozali, J. & Sloan, J. (1971). Control orientation as a personality dimension among alcoholics. *Quarterly Journal of Studies on Alcohol*, *32*, 159-161.

Grant, I., Reed, R., & Adams, K. (1980). Alcohol & drug-related brain disorder: Implications for neuropsychological research. *Journal of Clinical Neuropsychology*, *2*(4), 321-331.

Grotjahn, M. (1983). The qualities of the group psychotherapist. In H. I. Kaplan & B. J. Sadock (Eds.), *Comprehensive group psychotherapy* (294-301). Baltimore, MD: Williams & Wilkins.

Guntrip, H. (1971). *Psychoanalytic theory, therapy and the self*. New York: Basic Books.

Haley, J. (1976). *Problem-solving therapy*. San Francisco: Jossey-Bass.

Har Paz, N. (1994). Failure in group psychotherapy: The therapist variable. *International Journal of Group Psychotherapy*, *44*, 3-20.

Hartocollis, P. (1964). Some phenomenological aspects of the alcoholic condition. *Psychiatry*, *27*, 345-348.

Hartocollis, P. & Hartocollis, C. (1980). Alcoholism, borderline & narcissistic disorders: A psychoanalytic overview. In W. Fann, I. Karacan, A. Porkory, & R. S. Williams (Eds.), *Phenomenology & treatment of alcoholism* (93-110). New York: Medical & Scientific Books.

Hartocollis, P. & Shaefer, D. (1963). Group psychotherapy with alcoholics: A critical review. *Psychiatric Digest*, *29*, 15-22.

Hartup, W. W. (1970). Peer interaction & social organization. In P. H. Mussen (Ed.), *Carmichael's manual of child psychology, Vol. 2* (3rd Ed.). New York: John Wiley & Sons.

Heidegger, M. (1963). *Being and time.* (J. MacQuarrie, & E. Robinson, Trans.) New York: Harper & Row. (original 1927).

Heitler, J. (1976). Preparatory techniques in initiating expressive psychotherapy with lower class, unsophistocated patients. *Psychology Bulletin, 3*, 339-352.

HEW. (1974). *Alcoholism treatment & rehabilitation.* National Institute on Alcohol Abuse & Alcoholism. Washington, DC: Department of HEW Publications.

Heyman, S. E. (1995, March). *What can neuroscience teach us about addiction*? Paper presented at workshop, The Addictions, Harvard Medical School, Boston, MA.

Hibbard, S. (1987). The diagnosis and treatment of adult children of alcoholics as a specialized therapeutic population. *Psychotherapy, 24*, 779-788.

Hoffman, H., Loper, R. G., & Kammeier, M. L. (1974). Identifying future alcoholics with MMPI alcoholism scales. *Quarterly Journal of Studies on Alcohol, 35*, 490-498.

Holder, H., Longabaugh, R., Miller, W. R., & Rubonis, A. V. (1993). The cost-effectiveness of treatment for alcoholism: A first approximation. *Journal of Studies on Alcohol, 52*, 517-203.

Horner, A. (1976). Oscillating patterns of object relations and borderline patient. *International Review of Psycho-Analysis*, 479-482.

Horner, A. (1979). *Object relations and the developing ego in therapy.* New York: Jason Aronson.

Horvath, A. T. (1993). Enhancing motivation for treatment of addictive behavior: Guidelines for the therapist. *Psychotherapy, 30*(3), 473-480.

Humphreys, K. (1993). Psychotherapy and the twelve-step approach for substance abusers: The limits of integration. *Psychotherapy, 30*, 207-213.

Hutchinson, J. A. (1969). *Paths of faith.* New York: McGraw-Hill.

Imhof, J., Hirsch, R., & Terenzi, R. E. (1984). Countertransferential and attitudinal considerations in the treatment of drug abuse and addiction. *Journal of Substance Abuse Treatment, 1*, 21-30.

Inkeles, A. (1968). *Socialization & society.* Boston: Little, Brown & Co.

Jacobson, G. R. & Ritter, D. P. (1977). Purpose in life and personal values among adult alcoholics. *Journal of Clinical Psychology, 33*, 314.

James, W. (1902). *The varieties of religious experience.* New York: Longmans.

James, W. (1907). *Pragmatism.* New York: Longmans.

Jarmas, A. L. & Kazak, A. E. (1990). Young adult children of alcoholic fathers: Depressive experiences, coping styles and family systems. *Journal of Consulting and Chemical Psychotherapy, 60*(2), 244-251.

Jaspers. K. (1975). On my philosophy. In W. Kaufman (Ed.), *Exisential-ism from Dostoevsky to Sartre*. New York: New American Library (original 1941).

Jellinek, E. M. (1960). *The disease concept of alcoholism*. New Haven, CT: College & University Press.

Johnson, V. E. (1973). *I'll quit tomorrow*. New York: Harper & Row.

Jones, R. K. (1970). Sectarian characteristics of Alcoholics Anonymous. *Sociology*, *4*, 181-195.

Kahn, E. (1985). Heinz Kohut & Carl Rogers: A timely comparison. *American Psychologist*, *40*(8), 893-904.

Kanas, N. (1982). Alcoholism and group psychotherapy. In E. M. Pattison & S. E. Kaufman (Eds.), *Encyclopedic handbook of alcoholism* (1011-1021). New York: Gardner Press.

Kanas, N. & Barr, M. A. (1982). Outpatient alcoholics view group therapy. *Group, the Journal of the Eastern Group Psychotherapy Society*, *6*, 17-20.

Kassell, J. D. & Wagner, E. F. (1993). Processes of change in Alcoholics Anonymous: A review of possible mechanisms. *Psychotherapy*, *30*, 222-234.

Kaufman, E. & Reoux, J. (1988). Guidelines for the successful psychotherapy of substance abusers. *American Journal of Drug and Alcohol Abuse*, *14*(2), 199-209.

Kaufmann. W. (1956). *Existentialism from Dostoevsky to Sartre*. New York: Meridian Books.

Kellogg, S. (1993). Identity and recovery. *Psychotherapy*, *30*, 235-250.

Kelly, G. (1955). *The psychotherapy of personal constructs: Clinical diagnosis and psychotherapy, Vol. 2*. New York: W. W. Norton.

Kemker, S. S., Kibel, H. D., & Mahler, J. C. (1993). On becoming oriented to inpatient treatment: Inducing new patients and professionals to recovery movement. *International Journal of Group Psychotherapy*, *43*, 285-302.

Kernberg, O. F. (1970). *New developments in psychoanalytic object-relations theory*. Topeka, KS: Menninger Foundation.

Kernberg, O. F. (1975). *Borderline conditions and pathological narcissism*. New York: Jason Aronson.

Kernberg, O. F. (1983). The borderline patient. *Psychiatry* (Audio Digest), *11*, No. 16.

Kernberg, O. F. (1984). The couch at sea: Psychoanalytic studies of group and organizational leadership. *International Journal of Group Psychotherapy*, *34*(1), 5-23.

Khantzian, E. J. (1982). Psychopathology, psychodynamics & alcoholism. In E. M. Pattison & S. E. Kaufman (Eds.), *Encyclopedic handbook of alcoholism* (581-597). New York: Gardner Press.

Khantzian, E. J. (1985). On the psychological predisposition for opiate & stimulant dependence. *Psychiatry Letter, 3*(1), 1-3.

Khantzian, E. J. (1994). Alcoholics Anonymous–Cult or corrective? Paper presented at Fourth Annual Distinguished Lecture. Manhasset, NY: Cornell University.

Khantzian, E. J. & Treece, C. J. (1977). Psychodynamics of drug dependence: An overview. In J. D. Blaine & D. A. Julius (Eds.), *Psychodynamics of drug dependence.* NIDA Research Monograph No. 12. DHEW Publication No. ADM 77-470. Washington, DC: Superintendent of Documents, U. S. Government Printing Office.

Khantzian, E. J., Halliday, K. S., & McAuliffe, W. E. (1990). *Addiction and the vulnerable self.* New York: Guilford Press.

Klein, R. H., Orleans, J. F., & Soule, C. R. (1991). The Axis II group: Treating severely characterologically disturbed patients. *International Journal of Group Psychotherapy, 41*, 97-116.

Kline, E. B. (1983, Jan.). Personal communication. University of Cincinnati, Cincinnati, OH.

Kohut, H. (1977a). Preface. In J. D. Blaine & D. A. Julius (Eds.), *Psychodynamics of drug dependence.* NIDA Research Monograph No. 12. DHEW Publication No. ADM 77-470. Washington, DC: Superintendent of Documents, U.S. Goverment Printing Office.

Kohut, H. (1977b). *The restoration of the self.* New York: International Universities Press.

Kohut, H. (1984). *How does analysis cure?* Chicago: University of Chicago Press.

Kohut, H. & Wolfe, E. S. (1978). The disorders of the self and their treatment: An outline. *International Journal of Psychoanalysis, 60*, 413-425.

Kopp, S. B. (1971). *Guru: Metaphors from a psychotherapist.* Palo Alto, CA: Science & Behavior Books.

Kosinski, J. (1977). Horatio Algers of the nightmare. *Psychology Today*, December, 59-64.

Kosseff, J. W. (1975). The leader using object-relations theory. In Z. A. Liff (Ed.), *The leader in group* (212-242). New York: Jason Aronson.

Kritsberg, W. (1985). *The adult children of alcoholics syndrome: From discovery to recovery.* Pompano Beach, FL: Health Communications, Inc.

Krystal, H. (1982). Character disorders: Characterological specificity and the alcoholic. In M. E. Pattison & E. Kaufman (Eds.), *Encyclopedic handbook of alcoholism* (607-618). New York: Gardner Press.

Krystal, H. & Raskin, H. A. (1993). *Drug dependence. The disturbances in personality functions that create the need for drugs*. Northvale, NJ: Jason Aronson.

Kuhn, T. S. (1962). *The structure of scientific revolutions*. Chicago: University of Chicago Press.

Kurtz, E. (1979). *Not-God: A history of Alcoholics Anonymous*. Center City, MN: Hazelden.

Kurtz, E. (1981). *Shame and guilt: Characteristics of the dependency cycle*. Center City, MN: Hazelden.

Kurtz, E. (1982). Why AA works. The intellectual significance of Alcoholics Anonymous, *Quarterly Journal of Studies on Alcohol*, *43*(1), 38-80.

Kurtz, E. (1983, Feb.). *Shame and alcoholism*. Paper presented at the Conference for National Association of Alcohol and Drug Abuse Counselors. Atlanta, GA.

Laing, R. D. (1969). *The self and others*. London: Tavistock Publications.

Laing, R. D. (1972). *The divided self: An existential study in sanity and madness*. Baltimore, MD: Penguin.

Langs, R. (1976). *The bipersonal field*. New York: Jason Aronson.

Lemere, F. (1958). Alcoholism & the worker. *Quarterly Journal of Studies on Alcohol*, *19*, 419-428.

Leszcz, M. (1989). Group psychotherapy of the characterologically difficult patient. *International Journal of Group Psychotherapy*, *39*, 311-336.

Leszcz, M. (1992). The interpersonal approach to group psychotherapy. *International Journal of Group Psychotherapy*, *42*, 37-62.

Leuba, J. H. (1896). A study in the psychology of religious phenomena. *American Journal of Psychology*, *7*, 309-385.

Levy, S. (1984). *Principles of interpretation*. New York: Jason Aronson.

Lew, D. (1973). *Realities of alcoholism in industry*. Rockville, MD: NIAAA Publications.

Lichtenstein, H. (1961). Identity & sexuality: A study of their interrelationship in man. *Journal of American Psychoanalytic Association*, *9*, 179-260.

Lieberman, M. A. & Borman, L. D. (1979). *Self-help groups for coping and crisis: Origins, members, processes & impact*. San Francisco: Jossey-Bass.

Lieberman, M., Yalom, I. D., & Miles, M. (1973). *Encounter groups: First facts*. New York: Basic Books.

Lomranz, J., Lakin, M., & Schiffman, H. (1972). Variants of sensitivity training and encounter: Diversity of fragmentation? *Journal of Applied Behavior Science, 8*, 399-420.

Lowen, A. (1969). Bio-energetic group therapy. In H. Rouiten (Ed.), *Group therapy today* (279-290). New York: Atherton.

MacLeod, J. A. (1968). Management of the initial phase of psychotherapy: Optimal frustration as a guide to technique in psychotherapy. *Comprehensive Psychiatry, 9*(4), 400-406.

Madsen, W. (1974). *The American alcoholic*. Springfield, IL: Charles C Thomas.

Mahler, M. S. (1968). *On human symbiosis and the vicissitude of individuation*. New York: International University Press.

Mahler, M. S. (1979). *The selected papers of Margaret Mahler, Volumes I and II*. New York: Jason Aronson.

Mahler, M. S., Pine, F., & Bergman, H. (1975). *The psychological birth of the human infant*. New York: Basic Books.

Malcolm, J. (1984). *In the Freud archives*. New York: Alfred Knopf.

Mann, M. (1973). *The disease concept of alcoholism*. San Francisco: Faces West Productions.

Marlatt, G. A. (1983). The controlled drinking controversy: A commentary. *American Psychologist, 38*, 1097-1111.

Masterson, J. F. (1981). *The narcissistic & borderline disorders*. New York: Brunner/Mazel.

Matakas, F., Koester, H., & Leidner, B. (1978). Which treatment for which alcoholic? A review. (Selected translation of international alcoholism research). *Psychiatrische Praxis, 5*, 143-153.

Matano, R. A. & Yalom, I. (1991). Approaches to chemical dependency: Chemical dependency & interactive group therapy–a synthesis. *International Journal of Group Psychotherapy, 41*(3), 269-294.

May, R. (1983). *The discovery of being*. New York: W. W. Norton.

McCrady, B. S. (1985). Comments on the controlled drinking controversy. *American Psychologist, 40*(3), 370-371.

McDougall, J. (1989). *Theaters of the body*. New York: W. W. Norton.

McNeel, J. (1977). The seven components of redecision therapy. In G. Barnes (Ed.), *Transactional analysis after Eric Berne*. New York: Harpers College Press.

Miller, N. S. (1995). *Treatment of the addictions: Applications of outcome research for clinical management*. New York: The Haworth Press.

Miller, N. S. & Hoffman, N. G. (1995). Addiction treatment outcomes. In N. S. Miller (Ed.), *Treatment of the addictions: Applications of outcome research for clinical management.* (41-56). New York: The Haworth Press.

Miller, W. R. & Hester, R. K. (1986). Matching problem drinkers with optimal treatments. In W. M. Miller & N. Heather (Eds.), *Treating addictive behaviors: Process of change* (175-203). New York: Plenum Press.

Minkoff, K. (1995, March). *Assessment and treatment of dual diagnosis: Serious mental illness and substance abuse disorder.* Paper presented at workshop, The Addictions. Harvard Medical School, Boston, MA.

Minovitz, M. (1973). *Using industrial alcoholism programs as a model for health & welfare agencies*. Rockville, MD: NIAAA Publications.

Modell, W. (1955). *The relief of symptoms*. Philadelphia: Saunders.

Monte, C. F. (1980). *Beneath the mask: An introduction to theories of personality* (2nd ed.). New York: Holt, Rinehart & Winston.

Moore, R. A. (1973). *Psychotherapeutics of alcoholism*. Proceedings of the 2nd Annual Alcoholism Conference of NIAAA. Pub #73-9083.

Moore, R. A. & Buchanan, T. K. (1966). State hospitals and alcoholism: A nation-wide survey of treatment techniques and results. *Quarterly Journal of Studies on Alcohol, 27*, 459-468.

Moreno, J. L. (1971). Psychodrama. In H. Kaplan & B. Sadock (Eds.), *Comprehensive group psychotherapy.* Baltimore, MD: Williams and Wilkins.

Morrison, A. P. (1989). *Shame: The underside of narcissism*. Hillsdale, NJ: Analytic Press.

Mueller, S. R., Suffer, B. H., & Prengaman, T. P. (1982). A short-term intensive treatment program fo the alcoholic. *The International Journal of Addictions, 17*(6), 931-943.

Muggeridge, M. (1980). *Do we need religion or religious institutes?* Sussex, England: Firing Line.

Murray, T. (1973). *The fight to save alcoholic executives*. Rockville, MD: NIAAA Publications.

Muus, R. E. (1968). *Theories of adolescence* (2nd ed.). New York: Random House.

National Institute on Alcohol Abuse and Alcoholism. (1995). *Distinctive features of the alcohol treatment system.* NIAAA Research Publication, Washington, DC, June.

National DWI Conference. (1976). *Alcohol and the impaired driver.* Chicago: National Safety Council.

Neibergh, N. (1993, Feb.). Presentation on group psychotherapy at American Group Psychotherapy Conference, San Diego, CA.

Nemiah, J. (1961). *Foundations of psychopathology.* New York: Oxford University Press.

Nietzsche, F. (1968). *Basic writings of Nietzsche* (W. Kaufman, Trans.). New York: Modern Library.

Ogden, T. H. (1982). *Projective Identification and psychotherapeutic technique.* New York: Jason Aronson.

Ogden, T. H. (1983a). The concept of internal object relations. *International Journal of Psychoanalysis, 64,* 227-241.

Ogden, T. H. (1983b). *The primitive edge of experience.* Northvale, NJ: Jason Aronson.

Ormont, L. (1985, Nov.). *Intimacy and group psychotherapy.* Paper presented at Harvard Medical School Seminar on group psychotherapy. Boston, MA.

Ormont, L. (1988). The leader's role in resolving resistances to intimacy in the group setting. *International Journal of Group Psychotherapy, 38,* 29-46.

Ormont, L. (1990). The craft of bridging. *International Journal of Group Psychotherapy, 40,* 3-18.

Ormont, L. (1992). *The group therapy experience.* New York: St. Martin's Press.

Ormont. L. (1993). Resolving resistances to immediacy in the group setting. *International Journal of Group Psychotherapy, 43,* 399-418.

Ornstien, P. (1981). The bipolar self in the psychoanalytic treatment process: Clinical & theoretical considerations. *Journal of American Psychoanalytic Association, 29,* 353-375.

Osborne, J. W. & Baldwin, J. R. (1982). From one state of illusion to another? *Psychotherapy: Theory, Research, and Practice, 19,* 266-275.

Oziel, L. J., Obitz, F. W., & Kerpon, M. (1972). General & specific perceived locus of control in alcoholics. *Psychological Reports, 30,* 957-958.

Parsons, O. A. & Farr, S. P. (1981). The neuropsychology of alcohol & drug use. In S. B. Felskov & T. J. Boll (Eds.), *Handbook of clinical neuropsychology* (320-365). New York: John Wiley & Sons.

Patterson, G. R. & Anderson, D. (1964). Peers as social reinforcers. *Child Development, 35,* 951-960.

Pattison, E. M. (1966). A critique of alcoholism treatment concepts: With special reference to abstinence. *Quarterly Journal of Studies on Alcohol, 27,* 49-71.

Pattison, E. M. (1979). The selection of treatment modalities for the alcoholic patient. In J. H. Mandelson & N. K. Mello (Eds.), *The diagnosis and treatment of alcoholism* (229-255). New York: McGraw-Hill.

Pendery, M. L., Maltzman, I. M., & West, L. J. (1982). Controlled drinking by alcoholics? New findings and a reevaluation of a major affirmative study. *Science, 217*, 169-174.

Perls, F. S. (1969). *Gestalt thearpy verbatim*. Lafayette, CA: Real People Press.

Perls, F. S., Hefferline, R., & Goodman, P. (1951). *Gestalt therapy: Excitment and growth in the human personality*. New York: Julian Press.

Perls, L. (1976). Comments on the new directions. In E. W. L. Smith (Ed.), *The growing edge of Gestalt therapy*. Secaucus, NJ: Citadel Press, 36-51.

Pesso, A. (1991). Ego function and Pesso System/Psychomotor Therapy. In A. Pesso & J. Crandall (Eds.), *Moving Psychotherapy* (41-50). Franklin, NH: Brookline Books.

Piaget, J. (1954). *The construction of reality in the child*. New York: Basic Books.

Pines, M. (1992). *Contrasting views of representative group events*. Garden Grove, CA: Info Medix Audio Tape.

Polster, E. (1975). Techniques and experience in Gestalt therapy. In F. D. Stephenson (Ed.), *Gestalt therapy primer* (75-91). Springfield, IL: Charles C Thomas.

Polster, E. (1981, July). Resistance & Gestalt therapy. Lecture given at the Gestalt Institute of San Diego. LaJolla, CA.

Polster, E. & Polster, M. (1973). *Gestalt therapy integrated*. New York: Brunner/Mazel.

Polster, E. & Polster, M. (1974). Notes on the training of Gestalt therapy. *Voices: The Art and Science of Psychotherapy, 10*(3), 38-44.

Polster, E. & Polster, M. (1976). Therapy without resistance: Gestalt therapy. In A. Burton (Ed.), *What makes behavior change possible?* (259-277). New York: Brunner/Mazel.

Prochaska, J. O. & DiClemente, C. C. (1992). Stages of change in the modification of problem behaviors. In M. Hersen, R. M. Eisler, & P. M. Miller (Eds.), *Progress in behavior modification, Vol. 28* (184-214). Sycamore, IL: Sycamore Press.

Prochaska, J. O., DiClemente, C. C., & Norcross, J. C. (1992). In search of how people change: Applications to addictive behaviors. *American Psychologist, 47*(9) , 1102-1114.

Rachman, A. W. & Heller, M. E. (1974). Anti-therapeutic factors in therapeutic communities for drug rehabilitation. *Journal of Drug Issues, 4*, 393-403.

Raubolt, R. (1974). Games addicts play: Implications for group treatment. *Corrective and Social Psychiatry, 20*, 7.

Rawson, R. A., Obert, J. L., McCann, M. J., & Marinelli-Casey, P. (1993). Relapse prevention models for substance abuse treatment. *Psychotherapy, 30*, 284-298.

Ray, O. (1972). *Drugs, society & human behavior.* St. Louis, MO: C.V. Mosby Co.

Rice, A. K. (1965). *Learning for leadership*. London: Tavistock Publications.

Rice, C. A. & Rutan, J. S. (1981). Boundary maintenance in inpatient therapy groups. *International Journal of Group Psychotherapy, 31*, 297-309.

Rice, C. (1988). Paper presented at Conference on Group Psychotherapy. Atlanta, GA, October 28-29.

Rinpoche, S. (1992). *The Tibetan Way of Living and Dying*. San Francisco: Harper.

Rogers, C. (1942). *Counseling & psychotherapy.* Boston: Houghton Mifflin.

Rokeach, M. (1973). *The nature of human values*. New York: New York Press.

Roman, P. M. (1989). *Inpatient alcohol and drug treatment: A national study of treatment centers*. Executive report. Institute for Behavioral Research, University of Georgia. (1-22).

Rossi, J. J. (1972). Motivational issues in capturing alcoholism patients into a rehabilitation program. In *Selected papers from the twenty-third annual meeting of alcohol & drug problems association* (51-56). Atlanta, GA.

Rotter, J. B. (1966). Generalized expectancies for internal vs. external control. *Psychological Monographs, 80*, 1-28.

Rutan, J. S. (1983, Feb.). Transference & group psychotherapy. Paper presented at 40th Annual American Group Psychotherapy Association Conference, Toronto, Canada.

Rutan, J. S. & Stone, W. (1984). *Psychodynamic group psychotherapy.* Lexington, MA: The Collamore Press.

Rutan, J. S. & Stone, W. (1993). *Psychodynamic group psychotherapy* (2nd. Ed.). New York: The Guilford Press.

Ryan, C. & Butters, N. (1980). Further evidence for a continuum of impairment encompassing male alcoholic Korsakoff patients and chronic alcoholic men. *Alcoholism, 4*, 190-198.

Sartre, J. P. (1956). *Being and nothingness*. New York: Philosophical Library.

Schaffer, H. J. (1995, March). A clinical update on the addictions. Paper presented at workshop, The Addictions. Harvard Medical School, Boston, MA.

Scheidlinger, S. (1983, Feb.). Current theories in group psychotherapy. Paper presented at 40th Annual American Group Psychotherapy Association Conference, Toronto, Canada.

Schiff, A. & Schiff, J. L. (1971). Passivity. *Transactional Analysis Journal, 1*, 71-77.

Schmidt, W. (1968). *Social class and the treatment of alcoholism*. Monograph 7. Toronto: University of Toronto Press.

Schuckit, M. A. (1973). Alcoholism & sociopathy. Diagnostic confusion. *Quarterly Journal of Studies on Alcohol, 37*, 157-164.

Schultz, W. (1969). *Joy*. New York: Grove Press.

Scott, E. M. (1961). The technique of psychotherapy with alcoholics. *Quarterly Journal of Studies on Alcohol, 22*, 69-80.

Scott, M. (1970). In D. Calahan (Ed.), *Problem drinkers*. San Francisco: Jossey-Bass.

Searles, H. (1973). Concerning therapeutic symbiosis. *Annals of Psychoanalysis, 1*, 247-262.

Sexias, F. (1976). *Tie in with local council on alcoholism. DWI rehabilitation programs*. Falls Church, VA: AA Publications, World Services.

Shestov, L. (1932). *On Job's balance*. (Coventry & Macartney, Trans.). London: Dent & Sons.

Shore, J. J. (1981). Use of paradox in the treatment of alcoholism. *Health and Social Work, 38*, 11-20.

Simkin, J. (1976). *Gestalt therapy mini-lectures*. Millbrae, CA: Celestial Arts.

Simmel, G. (1950). *Sociology of George Simmel* (K. Wolff, Trans.). New York: Free Press.

Singer, D. L., Astrachan, B. M., Gould, L. J., & Klein, E. B. (1975). Boundary management in psychological work with groups. *Journal of Applied Behavioral Science, 11*(2), 137-176.

Smart, R. T., Schmidt, W., & Moss, M. K. (1969). Social class as a determinant of the types and duration of therapy received by alcoholics. *International Journal of Addictions, 4*, 543-556.

Sobell, M. B. & Sobell, L. C. (1973a). Individualized behavior therapy for alcoholics. *Behavior Therapy, 4*, 49-72.

Sobell, M. B. & Sobell, L. C. (1973b). Alcoholics treated by individualized behavior therapy: One-year treatment outcome, *Behavior Research and Therapy, 11*, 599-618.

Sobell, L. C. (1995). Natural recovery from alcohol problems. Paper presented at workshop, The Addictions, Harvard Medical School, Boston, MA.

Sollod, R. H. (1993). Reply to Humphreys: On the compatibility of twelve step programs and psychotherapy. *Psychotherapy, 31*, 549-550.

Stace, W. (1966). What is mysticism? In P. Struhl & K. Struhl (Eds.), *Philosophy now!* (235-251). New York: Random House.

Stachnik, T. J. (1980). Priorities for psychology in medical education and health care delivery. *American Psychologist, 35*(1), 8-15.

Starbuck, E. D. (1899). *The psychology of religion*. New York: Scribner & Sons.

Stein, A. & Friedman, W. H. (1971). Group therapy with alcoholics. In H. I. Kaplan & B. J. Sadock (Eds.), *Comprehensive group psychotherapy.* Baltimore, MD: Williams & Wilkens.

Steiner, C. M. (1969). The alcoholic game. *Quarterly Journal of Studies on Alcohol, 30*, 920-938.

Steiner, C. M. (1971). *Games alcoholics play.* New York: Grove Press.

Sterne, M. & Pittman, D. (1965). The concept of motivation: A source of institutional & professional blockage in the treatment of alcoholics. *Quarterly Journal of Studies on Alcohol, 26*, 41-57.

Stewart, D. A. (1985). Control or freedom? *American Psychologist, 40*(3), 373-374.

Stinson, D., Smith, W., Arnidjaya, I., & Kaplan, J. (1979). System of care and treatment outcomes for alcoholic patients. *Archives of General Psychiatry, 36*, 535-539.

Stone, L. (1961). *The psychoanalytic situation*. New York: International University Press.

Strupp. H. H. (1972). Freudian analysis today. *Psychology Today*, July, 33-40.

Strupp, H. H. (1978). A reformation of the dynamics of the therapist's contribution. In A. German & A. Rozier (Eds.), *The therapist's contribution to effective psychotherapy: An empirical assessment* (62-91). Elmsford, NY: Pergamon Press.

Strupp, H. H. & Hadley, S. W. (1979). Specific versus nonspecific factors in psychotherapy: A controlled study of outcome. *Archives of General Psychiatry, 36*, 1125-1136.

Sullivan, H. S. (1953). *The interpersonal theory of psychiatry.* New York: W. W. Norton.

Surkis, A. (1989). The group therapist's quandary: To lead or to treat? Workshop presented at Tenth International Congress of Group Therapy, Amsterdam.

Szasz, T. S. (1966). Alcoholism: A socio-ethnical perspective. *Western Medicine, 7*, 15-21.

Tarter, R. E. & Sugerman, A. A. (1976). *Alcoholism: Interdisciplinary approaches to an enduring problem*. Reading, MA: Addison-Wesley.

Thune, C. E. (1977). Alcoholism and the archetypal past: A phenomenological perspective on Alcoholics Anonymous. *Quarterly Journal of Studies on Alcohol, 38*, 75-88.

Tiebout, H. M. (1953). Surrender vs. compliance in therapy with special reference to alcoholism. *Quarterly Journal of Studies on Alcohol, 14*, 58-68.

Tiebout, H. M. (1954). The ego factors in surrender in alcoholism. *Quarterly Journal of Studies on Alcohol, 15*, 610-621.

Tiebout, H. M. (1961). Alcoholics Anonymous: An experiment of nature. *Quarterly Journal of Studies on Alcohol, 22*, 52-68.

Tournier, R. E. (1979). Alcoholics Anonymous as treatment and as ideology. *Quarterly Journal of Studies on Alcohol, 40*, 230-239.

Truax, C. B. & Wargo, A. G. (1969). Effects of vicarious therapy pretraining and alternative sessions on outcome in group psychotherapy with outpatients. *Journal of Consulting and Clinical Psychology, 33*, 440-447.

Twelve steps and twelve traditions (1952). New York: AA World Services, Inc.

Twerski, A. J. (1983). Early intervention in alcoholism: Confrontational techniques. *Hospital & Community Psychiatry, 34*(11), 1027-1030.

Vaillant, G. (1983). The natural history of male alcoholism. Is alcoholism the cart or horse to sociopathy? *British Journal of Addictions, 78*, 317-320.

Vaillant, G. (1995, Feb). The natural history of alcoholism: A fifty-year follow up. Paper presented at workshop, The Addictions. Harvard Medical School, Boston, MA.

Vaillant, G. & Milofsky, E. (1982). The etiology of alcoholism: A prospective viewpoint. *American Psychologist, 37*(5), 494-503.

Vannicelli, M. (1982). Group psychotherapy with alcoholics: Special techniques. *Journal of Studies on Alcohol, 41*(1), 17-37.

Vannicelli, M. (1988). Group therapy aftercare for alcoholic patients. *International Journal of Group Psychotherapy, 35*(3), 337-353.

Vannicelli, M. (1991). Dilemmas and countertransferences considerations in group psychotherapy with adult children of alcoholics. *International Journal of Group Psychotherapy, 41*, 295-312.

Vannicelli, M. (1992). *Removing the road blocks: Group psychotherapy with substance abusers & family members*. New York: The Guilford Press.

Verinis, J. S. (1995). Treatment of the socially disadvantaged alcoholic. In N. S. Miller (Ed.), *Treatment of addictions: Applications of outcome studies for clinical management* (93-112). New York: The Haworth Press.

Wald, P. (1974). *Right of alcoholic & addicted prisoners to refuse treatment: Some preliminary perimeters*. Presented at Washington area council on alcohol & drug abuse symposium. Washington, DC.

Wallace, J. (1975). *Tactical and strategic use of the preferred defense structure of the recovering alcoholic*. New York: National Council on Alcoholism.

Wallace, J. (1977a). Alcoholism from the inside out: A phenomenological analysis. In N. J. Estes & M. E. Heinemann (Eds.), *Alcoholism, development, consequences, and interventions* (51-69). St. Louis, MO: C.V. Mosby Co.

Wallace, J. (1977b). Between Scylla and Charybdis: Issues in alcoholism therapy. *Alcohol, Health & Research World* (Summer), 15-22.

Wallace, J. (1978a). Behavioral modification methods as adjuncts to psychotherapy. In S. Zimberg, J. Wallace, S. B. Blume (Eds.), *Practical approaches to alcoholism psychotherapy* (99-117). New York: Plenum Press.

Wallace, J. (1978b). Working with the preferred defense structure of the recovering alcoholic. In S. Zimberg, J. Wallace, & S. Blume (Eds.), *Practical approaches to alcoholism psychotherapy* (19-29). New York: Plenum Press.

Wallace, J. (1984a). Comments on the controlled drinking controversy. *American Psychologist, 40*(3), 372-373.

Wallace, J. (1984b). Myths and misconceptions about Alcoholics Anonymous! About AA. New York: AA World Services.

Wallace, J., Forbes, R., & Chalmers, D. K. (1979). Alcoholism treatment revisited. *World Health Project, 2*(1), 1-28.

Ward, R. (1984, May). Lecture given at Atlanta Psychoanalytic Interest Group, Atlanta, GA.

Washton, A. M. (1992). Structured outpatient group therapy with alcohol & substance abusers. In J. Lowinson, P. Ruiz, & R. Millman (Eds.), *Substance abuse: A comprehensive textbook*. Baltimore, MD: Williams & Wilkens.

Watzlawick, P. (1978). *The language of change*. New York: Basic Books.

Wedel, H. L. (1965). Involving alcoholics in treatment. *Quarterly Journal of Studies on Alcohol, 26*, 468-479.

Weinberg, J. (1976). *Why do alcoholics deny their problem?* Center City, MN: Hazelden.

Weiner, M. F. (1983). The assessment & resolution of impasse in group psychotherapy. *International Journal of Group Psychotherapy, 33*, 313-331.

Wells, C. (1982). Chronic brain disease: An update on alcoholism, Parkinson's disease, and dementia. *Hospital and Community Psychiatry, 33*(2), 111-126.

Whitaker, C. A. & Malone, T. P. (1953). *The roots of psychotherapy.* New York: Blakiston.

White, M. (1972). *Documents in the history of American philosophy.* New York: Oxford University Press.

Whitehead, A. N. (1925). *Science and the modern world.* New York: The Free Press.

Whitehead, A. N. (1933). *Adventures of ideas.* New York: The Free Press.

Whitfield, C. L. (1987). *Healing the child within: Discovery and recovery for adult children of dysfunctional families.* Deerfield Beach, FL: Health Communications, Inc.

Wilkenson, D. A. & Carlen, P. L. (1981). Chronic organic brain syndromes associated with alcoholism: Neuropsychological & other aspects. In Y. Israel, F. Glace, H. Kalanet, R. E. Popham, W. Schmidt, & R. G. Smart (Eds.), *Research advances in alcohol and drug problems, Vol. 6.* New York: Plenum Press.

Winnicott, D. W. (1965). *The maturation process in the facilitating environment.* New York: International University Press.

Witkin, H. A. & Oltman, P. K. (1967). Cognitive styles. *International Journal of Neurology, 6*, 119-137.

Witkin, H. A., Karp, S. A., & Goodenough, D. R. (1959). Dependence in alcoholics. *Quarterly Journal of Studies on Alcohol, 20*, 493-504.

Wogan, M., Getter, H., Anidur, M. J., Nichols, M. F., & Okman, G. (1977). Influencing interaction and outcome in group psychotherapy. *Small Group Behavior, 8*, 26-46.

Wolfe, A. & Schwartz, E. K. (1962). *Psychoanalysis in groups.* New York: Grune & Stratton.

Wood, B. L. (1987). *Children of alcoholism: The struggle for self & intimacy in adult life.* New York: New York University Press.

Wurmser, L. (1978). *The hidden dimension: Psychodynamics in compulsive drug use.* New York: Jason Aronson.

Yalom, I. D. (1974). Group therapy and alcoholism. *Annals of the New York Academy of Sciences, 233*, 85-103.

Yalom, I. D. (1975). *The theory and practice of group psychotherapy* (2nd Ed.). New York: Basic Books.

Yalom, I. D. (1980). *Existential psychotherapy.* New York: Basic Books.

Yalom, I. D. (1983). *Inpatient group psychotherapy.* New York: Basic Books.

Yalom, I. D. (1985). *The theory and practice of group psychotherapy* (3rd Ed.). New York: Basic Books.

Yalom, I. D. (1995). *The theory and practice of group psychotherapy* (4th Ed.). New York: Basic Books.

Yalom, I. D. & Rand, K. H. (1966). Compatibility and cohesiveness in therapy groups. *Archives of General Psychiatry, 15*, 267-276.

Yalom, I. D., Houts, P. S., Newell, A. B., & Rand, K. H. (1967). Preparation of patients for group therapy. *Archives of General Psychiatry, 17*, 416-428.

Yalom, I. D., Block, S., Bond, G., Zimmerman, E., & Qualls, B. (1978). Alcoholics in interactional group therapy: An outcome study. *Archives of General Psychiatry, 35*, 419-425.

Zax, M. (1961). Demographic characteristics of alcoholic outpatients and the tendency to remain in treatment. *Quarterly Journal of Studies on Alcohol, 22*, 98-105.

Zimberg, S. (1978). Principles of alcoholism psychotherapy. In S. Zimberg, J. Wallace, & S. Blume (Eds.). *Practical approaches to alcoholism psychotherapy* (3-18). New York: Plenum Press.

Zimberg, S. (1980). *The clinical management of alcoholism.* New York: Brunner/Mazel.

Zinker, J. (1977). *Creative process in Gestalt therapy.* New York: Brunner/Mazel.

Index